Complications of
Urologic Surgery and Practice

Complications of Urologic Surgery and Practice

Diagnosis, Prevention, and Management

Edited by

Kevin R. Loughlin

Harvard Medical School
Brigham and Women's Hospital
Boston, Massachusetts, USA

informa

healthcare

New York   London

Informa Healthcare USA, Inc.
52 Vanderbilt Avenue
New York, NY 10017

International Standard Book Number-10: 0-8493-4028-4 (Hardcover)
International Standard Book Number-13: 978-0-8493-4028-4 (Hardcover)

Library of Congress Cataloging-in-Publication Data

Complications of urologic surgery and practice : diagnosis, prevention, and management/edited
   by Kevin R. Loughlin.
     p. ; cm.
   Includes bibliographical references and index.
   ISBN-13: 978-0-8493-4028-4 (Hardcover : alk. paper)
   ISBN-10: 0-8493-4028-4 (Hardcover : alk. paper)
   1. Genitourinary organs—Surgery—Complications.
   I. Loughlin, Kevin R.
   [DNLM: 1. Urologic Surgical Procedures—adverse effects. 2. Intraoperative
     Complications—prevention & control. 3. Postoperative
     Complications—prevention & control. WJ 168 C7369 2007]

RD571.C654 2007
617.4′601--dc22   2006103362

Visit the Informa Web site at
www.informa.com

and the Informa Healthcare Web site at
www.informahealthcare.com

You will make all kinds of mistakes, but as long as you are generous and true,
and also fierce, you cannot hurt the world or even seriously distress her.
She was made to be wooed and won by youth.

—Winston Churchill

To my teachers, the urologists of the last generation.
To my colleagues, the urologists of this generation.
To my residents, the urologists of the next generation.

—Kevin R. Loughlin

Preface

A surgical career is interspersed with incredible highs and incredible lows. The exhilaration one feels when a procedure goes well can be followed the next day by a devastating complication. Yet, we learn much more from our failures, the complications, than we do from our successes, the triumphs. In fact, surgery is one of the few professions where usually, on a weekly basis, we discuss and analyze our complications and try to learn from them. Urologic surgical practice has seen enormous changes in the past decade. The practicing urologist is now faced with a wide array of procedures that were not even performed a few short years ago. Therefore, it is more important now than ever before to have a one-volume source that reviews the diagnosis, management, and prevention of urologic complications.

This book is divided into five sections: perioperative complications, complications of open surgical procedures, pediatric surgical complications, complications of minimally invasive procedures, and miscellaneous complications. These divisions are intended to facilitate the use of the book by urologists who emphasize different aspects of urology in their practice. The book places special emphasis on some of the newer minimally invasive and laparoscopic procedures that are becoming a large part of urologic practice.

I have invited the contributors of this book to provide their insight into the prevention and management of complications that can occur during urologic surgery and practice. I want to thank each of the authors for sharing their expertise and experience with the reader. All aspects of surgery are changing rapidly in today's world, but perhaps nowhere more than in urology. Urologists have already witnessed the impact of technology and the aging of the population on their practice. Urologic care will continue to evolve rapidly in the future and it is my hope that the readers of this book will use it as a trusted companion throughout their urologic careers.

Kevin R. Loughlin

Contents

Contributors

Gregory S. Adey   Division of Urologic Surgery, Mercy Hospital, Portland, Maine, U.S.A.

Linda S. Aglio   Department of Anesthesiology, Perioperative and Pain Medicine, Brigham and Women's Hospital, Boston, Massachusetts, U.S.A.

Paul D. Allen   Department of Anesthesiology, Perioperative and Pain Medicine, Brigham and Women's Hospital, Boston, Massachusetts, U.S.A.

Gerald L. Andriole, Jr.   Division of Urologic Surgery, Washington University School of Medicine, St. Louis, Missouri, U.S.A.

Alberto A. Antunes   Division of Urology, University of Sao Paulo Medical School, Sao Paulo, Brazil

Demetrius Bagley   Department of Urology, Thomas Jefferson University, Philadelphia, Pennsylvania, U.S.A.

Elisabeth M. Battinelli   Division of Hematology and Oncology, Department of Medicine, Beth Israel Deaconess Medical Center, Harvard Medical School, Boston, Massachusetts, U.S.A.

Clair Beard   Department of Radiation Oncology, Dana-Farber/Brigham and Women's Cancer Center, Boston, Massachusetts, U.S.A.

Stephen D. W. Beck   Department of Urology, Indiana University School of Medicine, Indianapolis, Indiana, U.S.A.

Arie S. Belldegrun   Division of Urologic Oncology, Department of Urology, David Geffen School of Medicine at UCLA, Los Angeles, California, U.S.A.

Akshay Bhandari   Vattikuti Urology Institute, Henry Ford Health System, Detroit, Michigan, U.S.A.

Richard Bihrle   Department of Urology, Indiana University School of Medicine, Indianapolis, Indiana, U.S.A.

David Bloom   Department of Urology, University of Michigan, Ann Arbor, Michigan, U.S.A.

Joseph G. Borer   Department of Urology, Children's Hospital and Harvard Medical School, Boston, Massachusetts, U.S.A.

Travis L. Bullock   Division of Urologic Surgery, Washington University School of Medicine, St. Louis, Missouri, U.S.A.

Maurizio Buscarini   Department of Urology, University of Southern California, Norris Comprehensive Cancer Center, Los Angeles, California, U.S.A.

Jeffrey A. Cadeddu   Department of Urology, University of Texas Southwestern Medical Center, Dallas, Texas, U.S.A.

Anthony A. Caldamone   Division of Pediatric Urology, Hasbro Children's Hospital, Brown Medical School, Providence, Rhode Island, U.S.A.

Craig V. Comiter   Department of Surgery, Section of Urology, University of Arizona Health Sciences Center, Tucson, Arizona, U.S.A.

Stephen S. Connolly   Department of Urology, Mater Misericordiae Hospital, University College, Dublin, Ireland

Douglas M. Dahl   Harvard Medical School and Department of Urology, Massachusetts General Hospital, Boston, Massachusetts, U.S.A.

Marc A. Dall'Era   Department of Urology, University of Washington School of Medicine and The VA Puget Sound Health Care System, Seattle, Washington, U.S.A.

Sean P. Elliott   Department of Urologic Surgery, University of Minnesota, Minneapolis, Minnesota, U.S.A.

Ehab A. Eltahawy   Ain Shams University, Cairo, Egypt

Robert C. Eyre   Division of Urologic Surgery, Beth Israel Deaconess Medical Center, Boston, Massachusetts, U.S.A.

James Chen-tson Fang   Division of Cardiovascular Medicine, University Hospitals of Cleveland, Case Western Reserve University, Cleveland, Ohio, U.S.A.

John M. Fitzpatrick   Academic Department of Surgery, Mater Misericordiae Hospital and University College, Dublin, Ireland

Robert C. Flanigan   Department of Urology, Loyola University Medical Center, Maywood, Illinois, U.S.A.

Richard S. Foster   Department of Urology, Indiana University School of Medicine, Indianapolis, Indiana, U.S.A.

Patricio C. Gargollo   Harvard Medical School and Department of Urology, Massachusetts General Hospital, Boston, Massachusetts, U.S.A.

Marc B. Garnick   Division of Hematology and Oncology, Department of Medicine, Beth Israel Deaconess Medical Center, Harvard Medical School, Boston, Massachusetts, U.S.A.

Jonathan D. Gates   Division of Vascular and Endovascular Surgery, Harvard Medical School and Division of Trauma, Burns, and Surgical Critical Care, Trauma Center, Brigham and Women's Hospital, Boston, Massachusetts, U.S.A.

Brian T. Helfand   Department of Urology, Feinberg School of Medicine, Northwestern University, Chicago, Illinois, U.S.A.

Jeffrey M. Holzbeierlein   Department of Urology, University of Kansas Medical Center, Kansas City, Kansas, U.S.A.

Gerald H. Jordan   Urology of Virginia and Department of Urology, Eastern Virginia Medical School, Norfolk, Virginia, U.S.A.

Louis Kavoussi   Smith Institute for Urology, North Shore-Long Island Jewish Health System, New Hyde Park, New York, U.S.A.

John N. Krieger   Department of Urology, University of Washington School of Medicine and The VA Puget Sound Health Care System, Seattle, Washington, U.S.A.

Sanjaya Kumar   Division of Transplant Surgery, Brigham and Women's Hospital, Boston, Massachusetts, U.S.A.

Jeffrey C. La Rochelle   Department of Urology, Rush University Medical Center, Chicago, Illinois, U.S.A.

Larissa J. Lee   Department of Radiation Oncology, Massachusetts General Hospital and Harvard Medical School, Boston, Massachusetts, U.S.A.

Laurence A. Levine   Department of Urology, Rush University Medical Center, Chicago, Illinois, U.S.A.

James E. Lingeman   Clarian Health, Indiana University School of Medicine and International Kidney Stone Institute, Indianapolis, Indiana, U.S.A.

Kevin R. Loughlin   Harvard Medical School and Division of Urology, Brigham and Women's Hospital, Boston, Massachusetts, U.S.A.

Michael J. Malone   Division of Transplant Surgery, Brigham and Women's Hospital, Boston, Massachusetts, U.S.A.

José L. Maymí   Department of Urology, University of Iowa, Iowa City, Iowa, U.S.A.

Jack W. McAninch   Department of Urology, University of California at San Francisco, San Francisco General Hospital, San Francisco, California, U.S.A.

W. Scott McDougal   Harvard Medical School and Department of Urology, Massachusetts General Hospital, Boston, Massachusetts, U.S.A.

Brian K. McNeil   Department of Urology, Loyola University Medical Center, Maywood, Illinois, U.S.A.

Kevin T. McVary   Department of Urology, Feinberg School of Medicine, Northwestern University, Chicago, Illinois, U.S.A.

Mani Menon   Vattikuti Urology Institute, Henry Ford Health System, Detroit, Michigan, U.S.A.

Amy Leigh Miller   Division of Cardiovascular Medicine, Brigham and Women's Hospital, Boston, Massachusetts, U.S.A.

Nicole L. Miller   Department of Endourology and Minimally Invasive Surgery, Clarian Health, Indiana University School of Medicine and International Kidney Stone Institute, Indianapolis, Indiana, U.S.A.

Kris M. Mogensen   Metabolic Support Service, Department of Surgery, Brigham and Women's Hospital, Boston, Massachusetts, U.S.A.

Stephen Y. Nakada   Division of Urology, School of Medicine and Public Health, University of Wisconsin, Madison, Wisconsin, U.S.A.

Michael A. O'Donnell   Department of Urology, University of Iowa, Iowa City, Iowa, U.S.A.

John Park   Department of Urology, University of Michigan, Ann Arbor, Michigan, U.S.A.

Sangtae Park   Department of Urology, University of Washington Medical Center, Seattle, Washington, U.S.A.

Erik Pasin   Department of Urology, University of Southern California, Norris Comprehensive Cancer Center, Los Angeles, California, U.S.A.

Sutchin R. Patel   Division of Pediatric Urology, Hasbro Children's Hospital, Brown Medical School, Providence, Rhode Island, U.S.A.

Alan B. Retik   Department of Urology, Children's Hospital and Harvard Medical School, Boston, Massachusetts, U.S.A.

Malcolm K. Robinson   Metabolic Support Service, Department of Surgery, Brigham and Women's Hospital, and Harvard Medical School, Boston, Massachusetts, U.S.A.

Brian M. Shuch   Department of Urology, David Geffen School of Medicine at UCLA, Los Angeles, California, U.S.A.

Miguel Srougi   Division of Urology, University of Sao Paulo Medical School, Sao Paulo, Brazil

John P. Stein   Department of Urology, University of Southern California, Norris Comprehensive Cancer Center, Los Angeles, California, U.S.A.

James A. Street   Department of Anesthesia, Emerson Hospital, Concord, Massachusetts, U.S.A.

Aaron Sulman   Medical College of Wisconsin, Milwaukee, Wisconsin, U.S.A.

J. Brantley Thrasher   Department of Urology, University of Kansas Medical Center, Kansas City, Kansas, U.S.A.

Stefan G. Tullius   Division of Transplant Surgery, Brigham and Women's Hospital, Boston, Massachusetts, U.S.A.

Ramon Virasoro   Department of Urology, Eastern Virginia Medical School, Norfolk, Virginia, U.S.A.

Thomas J. Walsh   Department of Urology, University of Washington School of Medicine and The VA Puget Sound Health Care System, Seattle, Washington, U.S.A.

Julian Wan   Department of Urology, University of Michigan, Ann Arbor, Michigan, U.S.A.

C. Charles Wen   Division of Urology, School of Medicine and Public Health, University of Wisconsin, Madison, Wisconsin, U.S.A.

Elizabeth R. Williams   Division of Urologic Surgery, Washington University School of Medicine, St. Louis, Missouri, U.S.A.

Brent Yanke   Department of Urology, Thomas Jefferson University, Philadelphia, Pennsylvania, U.S.A.

Anthony L. Zietman   Department of Radiation Oncology, Massachusetts General Hospital and Harvard Medical School, Boston, Massachusetts, U.S.A.

1 | Infectious Complications of Urologic Surgery

Marc A. Dall'Era, Thomas J. Walsh, and John N. Krieger
Department of Urology, University of Washington School of Medicine and The VA Puget Sound Health Care System, Seattle, Washington, U.S.A.

INTRODUCTION

This chapter reviews infectious complications of urologic surgery from our perspective as practicing urologists. We focus on the urinary tract and surgical site infections (SSIs) that are of most interest to other urologists. Because of limited space, we omitted important postoperative problems that are less relevant to urological practice, such as respiratory infections and antibiotic-associated bowel problems. We highlight studies of special interest and outline our own clinical approach to management of urologic patients with postoperative infectious complications.

URINARY TRACT INFECTIONS COMPLICATING UROLOGIC PROCEDURES

The risk of urinary tract infection (UTI) following endoscopic urologic procedures is a complex and highly controversial topic. Much of the controversy reflects the difficulties of defining and classifying UTI, and in distinguishing among the varied urologic procedures. This section begins by defining and categorizing UTI and urologic endoscopic procedures to provide an overview of the pertinent literature and to offer a systematic approach for diagnosing and managing postoperative UTIs.

Postprocedural UTIs—A Clinical Approach

Classically, UTI is defined as the inflammatory response of the urothelium to bacterial invasion. UTI is associated with bacteriuria and with pyuria. While this definition seems straightforward, further categorization of UTI is necessary to facilitate clinical decisions.

From a clinical perspective, we prefer a simple classification of UTI into three categories: asymptomatic bacteriuria, uncomplicated UTI, and complicated UTI including urinary sepsis syndrome. This classification helps determine the appropriate clinical approach.

Asymptomatic Bacteriuria

Asymptomatic bacteriuria is defined as the presence of bacteria in the urine in a patient who has no symptoms or signs. This definition presumes that such bacteria are not contaminants from the skin, vagina, or prepuce. Further, the definition also presumes that the specimen has been "handled properly," meaning that it has been transported promptly to the laboratory for processing. Asymptomatic bacteriuria represents one of the most commonly measured and reported urologic infections.

The literature contains considerable debate about the concentration of bacteria in urine that is considered "significant." The traditional threshold was >100,000 colony-forming units (CFU) per mL of a single species. This definition was based on older population surveys where patients were required to have repeated samples showing $>10^5$ CFU/mL (1). More recent literature suggests that $>10^2$ CFU/mL represents significant bacteriuria in a patient with urinary tract symptoms, but the precise definition of significant bacteriuria in an asymptomatic patient remains a subject of debate (2).

Complicated vs. Uncomplicated Urinary Tract Infection

The practice of classifying UTIs based upon the organ of origin (pyelonephritis, cystitis, etc.) is common in clinical practice. However, such classification makes little contribution to clinical management. The reason is that localization studies have shown that it is exceedingly difficult to distinguish bladder infection from renal infection in many populations based upon clinical signs and symptoms (3). Further, at least in outpatient women, such distinction may be arbitrary because patients with upper and lower UTIs do equally well on similar antibiotic regimens if the infections are uncomplicated.

We prefer to classify patients with clinical signs or symptoms of UTI into two groups: uncomplicated UTIs and complicated UTIs. Uncomplicated UTIs occur in patients with structurally normal urinary tracts with intact voiding function. The uncomplicated category includes most isolated or recurrent bacterial cystitis as well as acute uncomplicated pyelonephritis in women.

Complicated UTIs are infections that occur in patients with structural or functional impairment of the urinary tract. Examples of such impairments include urinary tract obstruction from stone, edema, or foreign body, or the inability to void as is the case with bladder outlet obstruction or neurologic impairment. The reason we prefer this clinical approach to UTI reflects the efficacy of antimicrobial therapies. Specifically, complicated infections often do not respond to medical therapy alone and may require relief of structural or functional obstruction, drainage of an abscess, or other urologic measures (4).

Urosepsis

Urosepsis is a syndrome resulting from a complicated UTI in a patient with one or more of the following signs: tachypnea, tachycardia, hyperthermia or hypothermia, or evidence of inadequate end-organ perfusion. Inadequate tissue perfusion is often accompanied by elevated plasma lactate, oliguria, or hypoxemia. Septic shock refers to sepsis syndrome that is accompanied by hypotension. Septic shock is a rare event after urologic procedures. Fortunately, septic shock following urologic procedures (often termed "urosepsis") has a more favorable prognosis than septic shock from diseases of other organ systems because many urologic disorders are correctable. After correction of underlying urologic factors, the pathophysiology of urosepsis is often reversible.

Urinary Tract Infection Risk Associated with Urologic Procedures

Procedures performed by urologists vary widely and are associated with markedly different risks for infection. Therefore, we will consider the risks with common urologic procedures separately.

Urethral Catheterization

Urinary catheters represent an essential part of medical care that is widely employed to relieve structural or functional obstructions of the urinary tract. However, when used inappropriately or left in place too long, urethral catheters represent a significant risk factor for development of UTI and other complications. Catheter-associated UTIs account for roughly 40% of all nosocomial infections that increase the duration of hospitalization, as well as morbidity and costs. Further, the use of antimicrobial therapy in the setting of indwelling urethral catheters often leads to selection of antibiotic-resistant microorganisms and nosocomial outbreaks of infection caused by multi-drug-resistant strains (5).

Cystoscopy

Traditionally, cystoscopy is considered a "clean" procedure that does not merit routine prophylactic antimicrobial therapy. Most reports indicate that symptomatic infections occur following fewer than 5% of procedures, provided the urine is sterile preoperatively (6). However, asymptomatic bacteriuria has been reported after as many as 35% of cystoscopy procedures in some series, with most series in the 10% range (7,8).

In a randomized controlled trial of 162 patients undergoing office cystoscopy, Rane et al. compared preoperative, intramuscular gentamicin to no antimicrobial therapy. Only 4.9% of the gentamicin group developed post-procedural bacteriuria compared to a 21.3% bacteriuria rate among untreated controls (P = 0.004) (8). Although there was no adverse reaction to gentamicin, this study did not evaluate the presence of symptoms, and results were based on a single urine specimen from each patient.

Kortmann et al. addressed the question of symptomatic UTI in a study of 104 patients having office cystoscopy without prophylaxis. The outcomes included both urine culture and a follow-up symptom questionnaire. They found a 3% symptomatic UTI rate and a 9% asymptomatic bacteriuria rate (9). In contrast, Manson found an asymptomatic bacteriuria rate of only 2.2% among 138 patients who had cystoscopy without antimicrobials (10). Such low symptomatic UTI rates following cystoscopy led Kraklau et al. to conclude that "low-risk" patients undergoing cystoscopy do not require prophylactic antimicrobials (7).

In our opinion, these and other studies suggest that patients with a history of UTI, voiding dysfunction, presence of a foreign body, or immunosuppression should be considered at "high risk" for symptomatic UTI. Such high-risk patients merit either a single dose or short course of antimicrobial prophylaxis.

Ureteroscopy

Ureteroscopy often represents the first-line approach for treating renal and ureteral calculi, as well as diagnosis and treatment of upper tract urothelial tumors. Thus, ureteroscopy has become one of the most common "same day" urologic procedures. In contrast to cystoscopy and other transurethral procedures, there are remarkably few data on the infectious complications of ureteroscopy. Following ureteroscopy, reported UTI rates range from 3.9% to 25%, and use of routine, perioperative, prophylactic antimicrobials is virtually ubiquitous.

In one case series of 378 patients undergoing ureteroscopy, Puppo et al. reported postoperative fever after 3.9% of procedures for ureterolithiasis (11). Because the focus of this report was not on the infectious complications, routine postoperative urine cultures were not obtained. Further, this report did not describe the use of antimicrobials. In 1991, Rao et al. described a series of 117 patients undergoing endoscopic treatment of renal and ureteral stones (12). Bacteremia occurred in almost one-quarter of patients; however, this information is of limited use because they include many more invasive procedures such as percutaneous nephrolithotomy in this series. Although not the primary focus of their study, Hendrikx et al. collected infection data in a randomized trial comparing extracorporeal shock wave lithotripsy to ureteroscopy for treatment of mid-to-distal ureteral stones in 156 patients. Of patients undergoing ureteroscopy, 3.5% had signs of pyelonephritis with septicemia, including fever greater than 38.5°C and symptomatic UTI in 3.5% and 4.5%, respectively (13). Details of prophylactic antimicrobial regimens were not provided. In 2003, Knopf et al. randomized 113 patients undergoing ureteroscopy for stone removal without clinical evidence of UTI to a single oral dose of levofloxacin versus no prophylaxis (14). Although no patient in either group developed a symptomatic UTI, there was a significant reduction in postoperative bacteriuria from 12.5% to 1.8% in the antimicrobial therapy group.

Although limited, these data support the standard practice of prophylactic antimicrobial therapy for patients undergoing ureteroscopy and suggest that such treatment is associated with reduced rates of infectious complications.

Nephroscopy

Percutaneous access to the renal collecting system is necessary for treating large renal calculi, patients who fail shock-wave lithotripsy, and stones in anatomically abnormal kidneys. As with ureteroscopy, remarkably few data are available on the infectious risks of nephroscopy. Given the need to transverse the renal parenchyma, there is particular concern for causing bacteremia and sepsis syndrome.

In the series of 27 patients undergoing percutaneous nephrolithotomy, nearly 40% developed sepsis syndrome despite routine use of prophylactic antibiotics (12). The clinical importance of this was underscored by O'Keefe et al. in a series of 700 patients undergoing percutaneous procedures for upper tract stones. Sepsis syndrome occurred in 1.3%, with an associated mortality rate of 66% (15). Mariappan et al. described 54 patients who underwent percutaneous nephrolithotomy. Patients were monitored closely for sepsis syndrome defined using strict criteria. Despite routine perioperative therapy with intravenous gentamicin, 5.6% developed sepsis syndrome (16). The most accurate predictors of sepsis were culture-positive renal pelvis urine, and culture-positive stones.

These limited observations support routine antimicrobial prophylaxis for patients undergoing nephroscopy, especially for treatment of stones. Infectious complications occur commonly. It may be difficult to identify patients with risk factors such as positive renal pelvis urine or culture-positive stones preoperatively.

Transurethral Prostatic Resection

Benign prostatic hypertrophy is one of the most common urologic problems among older men. With the development of selective alpha-antagonists and 5-alpha reductase inhibitors in the 1980s and 1990s, the need for surgical intervention has decreased drastically. Many "minimally invasive" techniques have been engineered to facilitate removal or destruction of obstructing prostatic adenomas. However, transurethral prostatic resection (TURP) remains the "gold standard" therapy for medically-refractory prostatic obstruction.

Historically, TURP was considered an Altermeier class II ("clean contaminated") procedure that did not merit routine perioperative antimicrobial therapy (17). However, postoperative bacteriuria rates up to 60% have been reported (18,19). The precise pathophysiology of infection following TURP is unknown, but most likely results from urethral abrasion and disruption of the prostatic bed (18). Potential sources of bacteria leading to infection include the prostatic adenoma, urethral flora, bladder colonization, or perioperative contamination (20).

The clinical significance of asymptomatic bacteriuria following TURP is debatable. Reported rates of urosepsis from post-TURP bacteriuria range from 1% to 4%, with an associated mortality rate of 13%. Mortality rates for post-TURP sepsis increase to more that 20% in men over 65 years old. Additionally, postoperative hospital stays may be prolonged by 0.6 to 5 days as a result of bacteriuria (21), based on studies from the older literature when hospital stays were much longer than in current practice.

In 2002, Berry and Barratt reported a meta-analysis of 32 randomized controlled trials evaluating antimicrobial prophylaxis for TURP in patients with sterile preoperative urine (18). These studies included a total of 4260 patients, with 1914 randomized to receive no antimicrobials, and 2346 randomized to receive various perioperative regimens. The primary endpoints were development of bacteriuria, symptomatic infection, or sepsis syndrome. Antimicrobial prophylaxis was associated with reduced rates of bacteriuria (9.1% vs. 26%, P < 0.01), and postoperative sepsis syndrome (0.7% vs. 4.4%, P < 0.01), corresponding to relative risk reductions of 65% and 77%, respectively. The effectiveness of various regimens was also analyzed, with aminoglycosides, co-trimoxazole, and cephalosporins all decreasing relative risks by 55% to 67%. Although evaluated in fewer studies, fluoroquinolone administration was associated with a relative risk reduction of 92%. Duration of prophylactic antimicrobial therapy appeared important, with short-course (<72 hours) therapy proving more effective than a single preoperative dose. There was little improvement for therapy extended beyond 72 hours. The 2346 patients who received prophylactic antimicrobials had 19 treatment-related adverse events (0.8%), with only two (0.09%) considered moderate or severe.

More recently, Qiang et al. confirmed the findings of Berry and Barratt in their systematic review of 28 randomized clinical trials of antimicrobial prophylaxis for TURP (20). They also noted a lower rate of postoperative fever in patients receiving prophylaxis (13.5% vs. 2.6%).To identify risk factors for postoperative bacteriuria, Colau et al. collected prospective data on 101 patients undergoing TURP. These patients had negative preoperative urine cultures and had received a single preoperative dose of a cephalosporin (19). Although one quarter of patients developed bacteriuria, all were treated readily, and no patient developed sepsis. Multivariate analysis found that risks for bacteriuria included long operative times, disconnection of the closed urethral catheter drainage, and increased duration of postoperative catheterization.

Taken together, these studies support the following conclusions on antimicrobial prophylaxis for patients undergoing TURP: (*i*) Assure that the patient has a negative urine culture preoperatively, if possible; (*ii*) a single dose of perioperative antimicrobial therapy may decrease rates of postoperative bacteriuria and, perhaps postoperative symptomatic UTI rates; and (*iii*) maintaining closed urinary drainage and minimizing the duration of postoperative catheterization substantially reduce postoperative infection rates.

Transurethral Resection of Bladder Tumor

Compared to TURP, very few data have been published on the infectious complications of transurethral resection of bladder tumor (TURBT). In 1990, Badenoch et al. prospectively reviewed the complications related to TURBT in 51 patients. Infected tumors were identified in 18% of males and 75% of females. Tumor infection correlated with preoperative urine culture results (22).

Based on analogies with the data for TURP, the following recommendations appear prudent: (*i*) avoid TURBT in patients with bacteriuria, if possible; (*ii*) although few data suggest that routine antimicrobial prophylaxis results in improved results, such therapy should be recommended for high-risk patients; (*iii*) maintain sterile closed urinary drainage; and (*iv*) minimize the duration of postoperative catheterization.

Prostate Needle Biopsy

During the past 15 years, technological advances in screening and diagnosis of clinically localized prostate cancer have revolutionized the practice of urology. Hodge et al. first introduced the concept of sextant biopsies for detecting prostate cancer, representing a marked improvement from the earlier practice of directed biopsies of palpable lesions or abnormalities visualized by transrectal ultrasound (23).

Although it is common practice to administer prophylactic antimicrobials before and after prostate biopsy, data supporting such therapy are conflicting. Aron et al. randomized 231 men to receive placebo for three days, single-dose oral antimicrobial therapy, or oral prophylaxis for three days. Significantly more patients in the placebo arm developed infectious complications and no additional benefit was noted by increasing the duration of prophylaxis from single dose to three days (24). Other studies reported similar results and support the routine use of single-dose therapy but no studies have examined the duration of therapy (25–27).

If a patient has a history of valvular heart disease, the American Heart Association recommends 2 g of parenteral ampicillin plus 80 mg of gentamicin at least 30 minutes before the procedure to prevent bacterial endocarditis (28).

Following total joint replacements, an expert panel from the American Urologic Association and the American Academy of Orthopedic Surgeons recommended that patients at highest risk for joint infection included: those within two years of joint implant surgery, immunocompromised patients, previous joint infections, or medical conditions such as diabetes or malignancy. This panel recommended either a single oral quinolone dose taken one to two hours before biopsy or 2 g of parenteral ampicillin (or 1 g intravenous vancomycin for patients allergic to penicillin) plus 80 mg of gentamicin at least 30 minutes before the procedure (29).

Historically, an enema was part of the routine pre-biopsy preparation. This practice has been examined by multiple investigators. A recent study by Carey and Korman included 410 patients who received three days of oral ciprofloxacin. Two hundred twenty-five patients received enemas prior to biopsy and 185 did not receive any bowel preparation. In this cohort, a pre-biopsy enema provided no clinically significant advantage (30). Lindert et al. randomized 50 patients to receive either a pre-biopsy enema or no enema, with both arms receiving post-biopsy oral antibiotics. Patients were evaluated with post-biopsy urine and blood cultures prior to antibiotic administration. While there was no difference in post-biopsy bacteriuria rates, patients who had received enemas were much less likely to develop bacteremia (16%) than those who had not received enemas (87%, P = 0.003) (31).

In summary, prophylactic antimicrobial therapy (e.g., an oral quinolone) is recommended prior to prostate biopsy. In contrast, there is no consensus on the value of pre-biopsy enemas to decrease infectious complications.

Presentation and Clinical Approach

The clinical presentation of UTI varies widely depending on the anatomic origin, the severity of infection, the patient's immune response, sensory, and communication capabilities. In addition, irritative urinary symptoms and hematuria are present routinely following urologic procedures, further complicating the diagnosis of UTI.

In cases where postoperative infection is suspected, a thorough history, focusing on the cardinal symptoms of UTI is necessary. Systemic symptoms and signs may aid in determining whether the patient has developed bacteremia, or is progressing to sepsis syndrome. Some patients may not experience any symptoms. For other patients, it may prove difficult to determine whether symptoms result from the procedure itself or whether symptoms result from UTI.

The physical examination should concentrate on the genitourinary tract. A more general examination is also indicated because UTI can ascend from the lower to the upper urinary tract and local infections can cause systemic symptoms and signs. Vital signs and urine production must be monitored closely for evidence of bacteremia or impending sepsis, characteristically heralded by fever, tachycardia, or low urinary output. When these findings are accompanied by hypotension, septic shock is present.

Urine cultures are key to making a diagnosis. In contrast, urinalysis has limited value. Following urologic instrumentation, urinalysis routinely shows erythrocytes, pyuria, and proteinuria, presence of bacteria in a fresh, unspun urine sample may prove helpful for diagnosis of UTI in a symptomatic patient following urologic procedures.

Whenever possible, a mid-stream, clean-catch urine sample should be collected. Depending upon the specific procedure, symptoms and signs, additional studies may be warranted. For example, in the setting of suspected pyelonephritis after ureteroscopy or nephroscopy, radiographic studies should be performed to determine whether the collecting system is obstructed or whether there are signs of an abscess. The optimal imaging study depends on the clinical setting and may include an antegrade nephrostogram, renal-bladder ultrasonography, computed tomography, or abdominal plain film to assess the position of a previously placed stent or tube.

In the setting of fever and presumed bacteremia, we also obtain a complete blood count and serum chemistries, as well as two peripheral blood cultures.

We have several general recommendations: (*i*) it is important to assure the patency of urethral catheters, nephrostomy, stents, or other urologic tubing; (*ii*) in all cases of presumed post-procedure UTI, quantitative urine cultures should be speciated, and antimicrobial sensitivities obtained. Ideally, these urine specimens should be obtained prior to initiating therapy; (*iii*) if started prior to availability of culture results, therapy should be modified based on sensitivity data and the patient's clinical response; and (*iv*) appropriate imaging may indicate other factors that require attention. Patients with complicated UTIs often require correction of underlying anatomic factors, such as relief of obstruction or drainage of an abscess.

SURGICAL SITE INFECTIONS

In the late 1800s, Sir Joseph Lister was disturbed to find that most of his amputation patients died shortly after surgery from wound sepsis (32). Because Sir Joseph Lister hypothesized that microbes from the air caused these deaths, he began to practice "antiseptic surgery." After learning that carbolic acid was being used successfully to treat raw sewage, Lister began using carbolic acid-soaked dressings and began soaking the surgical instruments and surgeons' hands in carbolic acid to prevent infections in the operating room. Lister also began spraying carbolic acid around the operating room and into his patients' wounds. These practices resulted in a dramatic decrease in postoperative wound infection rates.

Although we have progressed to the era of aseptic surgery, SSIs still cause considerable morbidity and mortality for urologic patients. SSIs represent the second most common nosocomial infections (after pneumonia) with about 500,000 documented in fections per year (33). SSIs complicate 1% to 2% of clean, extra abdominal procedures and up to 12% of abdominal procedures (33). SSIs significantly increase patient morbidity and mortality, and greatly increase hospital stays and healthcare costs (34).

Definition and Classification of Surgical Site Infections

The Centers for Disease Control and Prevention (CDC) has published guidelines for the diagnosis of SSIs (34a). The recommended definition of an SSI is an infection occurring between 0 and 30 days after a surgical procedure or up to one year later if prosthetic materials were implanted. Overt signs and symptoms of infection, such as erythema, pain, or localized swelling, are sufficient to diagnose superficial wound infections. In addition, diagnosis can be based on a positive, aseptically obtained bacterial wound culture. SSIs are further categorized as incisional (superficial and deep) and organ or surgical space-related, such as abdominal or retroperitoneal.

Risk Factors for Surgical Site Infection

Traditionally, SSI risk was estimated solely based on the wound category (35). Rates ranged from 1% to 4% for clean wounds to 12% to 40% for dirty wounds (Table 1) (35). It is now evident that a combination of patient factors, surgical factors, and microbiological factors must be assessed to accurately estimate SSI risk (36).

Patient Factors

Recent data suggest that intraoperative factors, including maintenance of normothermia, tight control of perioperative blood glucose, and a high inhaled oxygen tension (80%), are associated with reduced SSI risk (37–39). Other important patient-related factors include the presence of comorbid conditions, medications, or drug usage (Table 2) (40). Several classes of medications are associated with increased SSI risk. Steroids and chemotherapy, for example, can significantly increase SSI risk by inhibiting the immune response (40,41). There is some suggestion that coumadin or heparin prophylaxis for venous thrombosis may also be associated with increased rates of prosthetic infections after joint replacement (42). This increase might simply reflect an increased risk for seroma or hematoma development. It is reasonable to expect that similar risk factors also increase prosthetic infection rates after urologic surgery.

Surgical Factors

Local surgical factors that influence SSI risk include methods of preoperative hair removal, wound drainage, seroma/hematoma prevention, and the presence of foreign bodies (40,43,44). Studies have clearly shown that clipping hair immediately before surgery is associated with fewer SSIs than shaving, which is no longer recommended (43). Prevention of seromas or hematomas by appropriate drains is also important for reducing SSI risk (40). In general, studies suggest that closed suction drains are associated with lower SSI rates than more passive drainage systems (44). Appropriate wound irrigation is important to decrease bacterial counts after surgical procedures, especially procedures involving the gastrointestinal or genitourinary tracts.

Microbiological Factors

Micro-organism–related factors include the overall degree of wound contamination, or bacterial load, at the surgical site as well as virulence-associated traits of the particular organisms involved. Bacteria have developed a variety of methods to survive and flourish in specific environments. For example, in the healthcare environment one common survival mechanism is the evolution and transmission of antibiotic resistance. Detailed discussion of this topic is beyond the scope of this chapter. With the widespread use of antimicrobials and increased numbers of compromised patients, multiple drug-resistant organisms, such as methicillin-resistant *Staphylococcus aureus* and vancomycin-resistant Enterococcus are encountered with increasing frequency (45).

Coagulase-negative *Staphylococcus* species and Enterococcus remain the most common organisms identified in SSI followed specifically by *Staphylococcus aureus* and *Candida*

TABLE 1 Surgical Wound Category Definitions and SSI Risk

Wound class	Description	Risk of SSI (%)
Clean	GI/GU/respiratory tract not entered	1–4
Clean-contaminated	GI/GU/respiratory tract entered without contamination	3–8
Contaminated	Open accidental wounds, gross GI contamination, inflammation	8–15
Dirty	Old traumatic wounds, perforated viscous, existing infection	12–40

Abbreviations: GI, gastrointestinal; GU, genitourinary; SSI, surgical site infection.
Source: From Ref. 35.

TABLE 2   Risk Factors for Surgical Site Infection

Patient related	Procedure related	Bacteria related
Hypothermia	Seroma/hematoma	Wound contamination
Hyperglycemia	Hair removal method	Bacterial load
Advanced age (>70 yr)	Closed suction drains	Antibiotic resistance
Diabetes mellitus	Foreign bodies	
Malnutrition	Wound irrigation	
Immunosuppression		
Obesity		
Chronic alcohol use		
Malignancy		

Note: Documented univariate risk factors for surgical site infection risk. Estimating individual patient risk is based on the interaction between several risk factors.
Source: From Refs. 37–41, 43–45.

albicans (46). These organisms represent ubiquitous components of the normal human flora. *Pseudomonas aeruginosa*, enterics such as *Escherischia coli* and *Bacteroides fragilis* are also encountered commonly. Depending on wound type, many other bacteria may be encountered. While bacterial resistance to multiple antibiotics is on the rise, it is exceedingly important to consider local antimicrobial sensitivity patterns and trends in individual practice settings to select optimal therapy.

Need for a Comprehensive Approach

The SSI risk assessment must consider multiple factors simultaneously. For example, one large multivariate analysis identified the following independent risk factors for SSIs: wound type, length of procedure, American Society of Anesthesiology (ASA) score, hypothermia, hypoxia, presence of remote site infection, and preoperative shaving (47). Accurately estimating SSI risk proved complex involving multiple variables, supporting the need for a more useful, practical and objective measure to estimate an individual patient's SSI risk.

The national nosocomial infection surveillance system (NNIS) score was devised to more accurately classify individual patients' risk based on the concept that SSI risk reflects the interaction among multiple factors (35). The NNIS score concentrates on three primary risk factors: wound category, ASA score, and length of procedure (>75th percentile is considered high risk). Contaminated or dirty wounds are scored as one point, ASA score of III, IV, or V is scored as one point, and >75th percentile for procedure length is scored as one point. The total NNIS score predicts an individual's SSI risk (Table 3).

Diagnosis of Surgical Site Infection

The classical physical signs of infection include redness, swelling, and pain over the incision, with purulent drainage or foul odor. Deeper infections may present initially with more systemic

TABLE 3   NNIS Score and SSI Risk

NNIS Score	Risk of SSI (%)
0	1.5
1	2.9
2	6.8
3	13.0

Note: Because it is difficult to estimate an individual patient's risk of SSI based on traditional risk factors outlined in Table 2, the NNIS score was developed to consider the interaction between multiple risk factors and provide individualized SSI risk assessments. Estimates are based on over 84,000 procedures with 2376 documented SSIs. To calculate NNIS score, contaminated and dirty wounds are given 1 point, an ASA score of III or greater is given 1 point, and length of procedure >75th percentile is given 1 point.
Abbreviations: NNIS, National Nosocomial Infection Surveillance System; SSI, surgical site infection.
Source: From Ref. 35.

symptoms, such as fever, chills, and rigors. One must maintain a high index of suspicion for infection when a patient is not recovering as expected after a surgical procedure. Laboratory findings including leukocytosis, hyperglycemia, acidosis, C-reactive protein elevation, and procalcitonin elevation support the diagnosis of infection (48,49).

If imaging is needed to document and localize an SSI (which is not necessary in a patient with a superficial infection), the most useful studies are ultrasound, computerized tomography, and magnetic resonance imaging (50–52). All three imaging methods have equal sensitivity for detecting large, drainable abdominal and subcutaneous fluid collections (52). However, ultrasound imaging is very operator-dependent and may be less accessible than computerized tomography in some practice settings.

We prefer computerized tomography and magnetic resonance imaging. These methods have proved more sensitive for detecting small, deeper abscesses and provide far better anatomic detail for safe, percutaneous drain placement near vital structures (51,52). Because magnetic resonance imaging is significantly more expensive than other imaging methods, we reserve this approach for patients with contraindications to iodinated intravenous contrast.

Management of Surgical Site Infection

Superficial infections and cellulitis are treated with antimicrobial therapy and local wound care alone. Superficial abscesses should be drained by opening the surgical wound. Deeper fluid or abscess collections usually require drainage for diagnosis and management. In this situation, our preference is radiologically-guided percutaneous drainage, reserving traditional open surgical procedures for cases where percutaneous drainage is contraindicated or has failed. Up to 85% of intra-abdominal abscesses can be managed by percutaneous drainage and appropriate antimicrobial therapy (53). Purulent material should be carefully evaluated with Gram stain, culture, and antibiotic sensitivity testing.

Empirical antimicrobial selection should be based on Gram stain results and the suspected pathogens based upon the wound type, and local sensitivity patterns. Such therapy may be modified, if needed, depending on subsequent culture and sensitivity results. Most patients respond rapidly to appropriate therapy.

The clinical pearl is that subsequent clinical deterioration or nonprogression requires further evaluation. Such evaluation includes careful physical examination plus other measures such as repeated imaging, culturing, or a change in antimicrobial coverage. An undrained abscess and fungal or mycobacterial infections must also be considered when patients do not respond to therapy as expected.

Prevention of Surgical Site Infection

The NNIS guidelines recommend preoperative prophylactic antimicrobial therapy for procedures with an estimated SSI risk >1% based upon the NNIS score (54). Therefore, prophylactic antimicrobial therapy should be strongly considered for: (*i*) any clean-contaminated procedure, (*ii*) any clean procedure in a patient with an NNIS score >1, (*iii*) an immunocompromised patient, (*iv*) when any prosthetic material is inserted, or (*v*) when the operative area contains high bacterial counts, such as the axilla or scrotum.

Timing of antimicrobial prophylaxis administration is critical. A large study by Stone et al. found that the lowest SSI risk occurred when therapy was initiated within one hour of surgery (55). Patients who received therapy after the incision had nearly the same risk as patients who did not receive prophylaxis. More recent data corroborate the conclusion that timely preoperative antimicrobial administration can reduce SSI rates (56). These and other observations demonstrate the importance of obtaining therapeutic serum antimicrobial levels before the surgical incision and exposure to bacteria. Current guidelines suggest that prophylactic antimicrobials should be redosed appropriately for lengthy procedures and should stop within 24 hours of surgery (54).

Recent data support prophylactic antimicrobial therapy for trans-scrotal surgery based on high bacterial counts on the scrotum and perineum. In a retrospective review of 131 outpatient scrotal procedures, Kiddoo et al. found a 9.3% overall SSI rate among patients who did not receive prophylactic therapy (57). In contrast, Swartz et al. found a 4% SSI rate in over 100 trans-scrotal procedures with a mean follow-up of 36 months (Swartz M, Urology, University of Washington). Although the precise benefit of prophylactic antimicrobials cannot be ascertained by comparing such retrospective studies, these data do suggest that scrotal wounds merit consideration as clean-contaminated wounds that may warrant prophylaxis.

Prophylactic antimicrobial agents should be selected based on the most likely organisms encountered. Beta-lactam antibiotics, such as the cephalosporins, are the most common agents used for prophylaxis. Recommendations include cefazolin for clean abdominal procedures or cefotetan for clean-contaminated abdominal procedures involving the gastrointestinal tract (54). Clindamycin or vancomycin regimens are recommended alternatives for patients with documented beta-lactam allergies (54). Other possible regimens include combinations of either metronidazole or clindamycin with gentamicin or a floroquinolone. Currently, there is no evidence supporting the use of prophylactic vancomycin rather than other agents, even in hospitals with perceived high rates of bacterial resistance. Recommendations for specific urologic procedures are described next

Special consideration must be given to preventing bacteremia in surgical patients with prosthetic joints who are at risk for joint infections or patients with certain cardiac anomalies who are at risk for life-threatening endocarditis. The American Urological Association (AUA) and the American Heart Association (AHA) have published specific guidelines for antibiotic prophylaxis in these patient populations (as outlined previously) (29,58).

Transient bacteremia can occur after a variety of urologic procedures, especially if patients are instrumented during active UTI. Identification and treatment of active infections is strongly recommended prior to any elective procedure. Bacteremia is commonly associated with urologic procedures, with rates of 31% for patients undergoing TURP, 24% among patients undergoing urethral dilations, 44% in patients having prostate needle biopsy, and 7% in patients having office urodynamics (31,59,60).

The AHA recommends endocarditis prophylaxis for patients undergoing prostatic surgery, urethral dilations, cystoscopy, or ureteroscopy (58). Prophylaxis is not necessary for urethral catheterization or circumcision in the absence of clinical infections (58). Perioperative ampicillin or vancomycin with gentamicin is recommended for high-risk patients while moderate-risk patients can be treated with single-agent ampicillin or vancomycin (58). High-risk patients are defined by having prosthetic heart valves, previous histories of endocarditis, or complex congenital anomalies. Currently, the AUA recommends assessing patients' overall risk for artificial joint infection based on a combination of patient-related and procedure-related factors (as outlined previously) (29).

Examples of Our Approach to Urologic Surgical Site Infection Problems
Infected Artificial Urinary Sphincter
The first consideration is prevention of infection, if possible. Perioperative antimicrobial administration is imperative. We favor broad-spectrum coverage with particular attention to assure coverage for *Staphylococcus epidermidis* employing either a cephalosporin or beta-lactam agent. As with surgery not involving insertion of prosthetics, therapy must be administered within one hour of surgery and prolonged administration postoperatively is not supported by the literature. Control of intraoperative risk factors to limit SSI risk is also important (as outlined previously).

Infections complicate 4% to 21% of artificial urinary sphincter (AUS) insertions and large series document no difference in infection rates between men and women (61–64). Such infections represent some of the most difficult and frustrating complications in urology. *S. aureus* and coagulase-negative Staphylococcus species cause the vast majority of AUS infections (64,65). Multiple patient risk factors for infection have been identified including previous sphincter insertion, previous radiotherapy, and previous procedures for bladder neck insertions (64). Recent series indicate that with modern focused radiotherapy, the risk for AUS infection is comparable to rates in the general population (64,66). Improper urethral catheterization or endoscopy in patients with artificial sphincters also represent important risk factors for infection.

There is considerable debate on the merits of simultaneous bladder augmentation and AUS insertion for patients with neurogenic bladders. After such combined procedures sphincter infection rates range from 5% to 50%, depending on the bowel segment used (67–69). Miller et al. described an overall infection rate of 6.9% in 29 patients undergoing simultaneous procedures (67). Nineteen (66%) of the twenty-nine patients underwent gastrocystoplasty with no infections. In contrast, 2 (20%) of 10 patients had sphincter infections following ileal or colonic augmentations (67). Other studies support these findings, suggesting that the relatively sterile stomach environment allows simultaneous procedures to be performed (68,70).

Most patients with infected sphincters present with persistent pain over the prosthetic parts (65). Other symptoms, including dysuria, hematuria, or pump fixation against the scrotal wall, may represent the first indication of an infection. More obvious signs of infection include purulent drainage from the scrotum or exposed prosthetic parts. Other patients with infected sphincters may have few systemic symptoms, with only a mild leukocytosis or low-grade fever. Therefore, the clinician must have a high index of suspicion of infection when any patient with an AUS presents with vague symptoms of systemic infection or inflammation with no clear source.

Initial management depends on the clinical presentation and extent of infection. Stable patients with suspected artificial sphincter infections may undergo a trial of oral or parenteral antimicrobial therapy. However, resolution of true prosthetic infections is rare with medical management alone.

Persistent or progressive symptoms require surgical exploration and removal of the infected prosthesis. Regardless of the clinical presentation, more than half of patients have infections involving all three device components, supporting complete removal (61,62). Standard management includes removal of all parts with washout and debridement of any devitalized tissue. Selected patients may undergo AUS reinsertion several months later after the infection has completely resolved and all wounds have healed.

Some investigators have described success with salvage protocols for removal and immediate replacement of an infected device similar to that outlined below for infected penile prostheses (65). Bryan et al. described eight patients with infected artificial sphincters who underwent a salvage protocol with removal of the entire device, extensive washout of the wound with multiple solutions, and immediate replacement (65). Most patients in this series had post-radical prostatectomy incontinence and all patients were given an oral fluoroquinolone for one month after reinsertion. Seven (88%) of eight patients did well with a mean follow-up of 33 months.

These observations suggest that a salvage protocol for AUS infections might be feasible for highly selected patients. The advantages offered by immediate reinsertion following removal of an infected sphincter are not as pronounced as those for an infected penile prosthesis. Although patients enjoy immediate return of continence with simultaneous placement of a new sphincter, reinsertion once the infection has clearly resolved is often not much more difficult than primary insertions. Overall outcomes with regard to comfort and continence appear similar with primary and secondary insertions (71). Further data on optimal patient selection and long-term follow-up are needed to determine whether the risk of infection with reinsertion warrants general adoption of such salvage protocols for infected AUS.

Infected Penile Prosthesis

Consistent with our approach to management of infected urinary sphincters, we believe that the urologist's first goal should be to prevent infection of penile prostheses. In 1978, Small reported a markedly decreased infection rate in men undergoing placement of penile prostheses with prophylactic antimicrobial therapy (72). The infection rate decreased from 5 (25%) of 20 patients without antimicrobial prophylaxis to 1 (<1%) of 140 patients following institution of routine prophylaxis.

The absence of urinary tract, systemic, or cutaneous infection must be assured and the patient should be carefully shaved just before surgery. To better define the relative merits of different regimens, Schwartz et al. found no difference between oral and IV prophylactic antimicrobial therapy for penile prosthesis insertion in 20 men (73). The study documented a clear cost reduction because the oral therapy group did not require hospital admission.

Current AUA guidelines recommend broad-spectrum gram-positive and gram-negative prophylactic antimicrobial coverage, commonly employing the combination of an aminoglycoside plus a cephalosporin or vancomycin administered one hour prior to insertion (74). Broad-spectrum coverage should be continued for 24 to 48 hours postoperatively, which often requires an over-night hospital stay.

To further reduce the risk of infection, the industry has produced antibiotic and hydro-philic coatings for penile prostheses (75). Hopefully, clear data will document long-term clinical advantages of these modifications. Revision surgery for noninfectious problems with penile prostheses is associated with a significantly higher risk for infection. However, extensive wash-out procedures similar to the salvage protocol can reduce reinfection rates from 12% to 3% (76). Henry et al. reported infections in 4 (3%) of 140 penile prostheses removed for mechanical failure following extensive wound irrigation and immediate replacement compared with infections in 5 (12%) of 43 patients who were not irrigated prior to reinsertion (76).

Such data are consistent with the finding of sub-clinical bacterial colonization within protective biofilms and support extensive washout during revision surgery even for clinically noninfected prostheses (77). Several organisms are able to produce biofilms that protect the bacteria from host defenses and antibiotics (77,78). Bacteria in biofilms exist in colonies where individual organisms often have a low metabolic rate that further increases antimicrobial resist-ance. Such biofilms facilitate bacterial persistence on the prosthesis sub-clinically for extended periods and bacteriologic studies of clinically uninfected prostheses removed for mechanical failure report a 70% colonization rate, most commonly with *S. epidermidis* (79).

Postoperative infections complicate 1% to 8% of primary penile prosthesis insertions and up to 18% of reinsertions performed for mechanical failure (80–85). Most infections result from device contamination during implantation (79). Much less commonly, late hematogenous seeding may result in an infected penile prosthesis (86). *S. epidermidis* is the most common isolate from prosthetic infections (79,81,84). However, infections with Pseudomonas species, *E. coli*, Proteus species, and Enterobacter species have been described (79,87).

Most patients with infected prostheses present with fever, erythema, swelling, and pain over the affected parts (87). Traditionally, staged procedures were used to manage penile pros-theses infections. These procedures include complete device removal, wound debridement, and antimicrobial administration (88). Patients are typically candidates for reinsertion several months later once the infection has resolved completely. Unfortunately, reinsertion several months after removal of an infected device is often technically challenging. Corporal scar for-mation often results in penile shortening and higher complication rates than with primary insertions (89). At this point, these patients typically have few options for management of their erectile dysfunction which may substantially reduce their quality of life.

The ability to perform simultaneous removal of an infected prosthesis with immediate insertion of a new device holds substantial appeal. Penile length is maintained while difficult dissections due to significant scar formation are avoided. Early attempts at salvage procedures with penile prostheses were largely unsuccessful and the risks of reinfection at the time were unknown (89). However, direct exchange salvage protocols for infected hip arthroses have existed since the 1970s (90,91). In many ways, prosthetic joint infections parallel infections seen with urologic prosthetics. *S. epidermidis* is the most commonly isolated organisms with infected hip prosthetics and traditional management involving complete removal, washout, and delayed replacement of the joint (92). By the late 1970s orthopedic surgeons performed successful salvage procedures by removing the infected joint followed by extensive wound washout prior to insertion of a new prosthetic (90). Although reinfection rates are higher than with staged pro-cedures, selected patients benefit from immediate joint replacement (85). With up to 10 years of follow-up, reinfection rates after direct exchange arthroplasty are now on the acceptable order of 1% to 2%, especially with the introduction and widespread use of antibiotic-impregnated cements (92). On multivariate analysis, Berbari et al. found the lowest infection rates in patients undergoing direct removal and replacement of infected joints compared with patients undergo-ing debridement with joint retention or joint removal with delayed reinsertion (93).

In 1991, Mulcahy et al. published a salvage protocol for managing infected penile prostheses and other groups have adopted a similar strategy (94,95). The protocol includes sequential use of seven solutions for extensive irrigation of the involved tissue, followed by immediate insertion of a new device (Table 4). With a mean follow-up of 35 months, they had an 82% successful salvage rate for 65 men undergoing the salvage protocol. Risk factors for failure included early infection after initial placement of the prosthetic, extensive cellulitis upon presentation, and the isolation of

TABLE 4 Irrigation Solutions Used Sequentially Prior to Immediate Reinsertion
Following Removal of Infected Penile Prostheses

Irrigation solutions
1. Antibiotic irrigation (bacitracin 50,000 U/L and kanamycin 500 mg/L)
2. Half-strength hydrogen peroxide
3. Half-strength povidone iodine
4. Pressure irrigation with 1 g vancomycin and 80 mg gentamicin/L of solution
5. Half-strength povidone iodine
6. Half-strength hydrogen peroxide
7. Antibiotic irrigation

Note: Solutions are used in sequence after removal of infected prostheses as described by Mulcahy et al.
Source: From Ref. 94.

particularly virulent organisms such as methacillin-resistant *S. aureus* or vancomycin-resistant *Enterococcus* (81). Absolute contraindications to performing this salvage protocol include severe necrotizing infections, sepsis, or patient immunosuppression.

REFERENCES

1. Kunin CM. Guidelines for urinary tract infections. Rationale for a separate strata for patients with "low-count" bacteriuria. Infection 1994; 22(suppl. 1):S38–S40, discussion S1.
2. Stamm WE. Urinary tract infections. Infect Dis Clin North Am 2003; 17:xiii–xiv.
3. Kunin CM. Definition of acute pyelonephritis vs the urosepsis syndrome. Arch Intern Med 2003; 163:2393, author reply, 4.
4. Krieger JN. Urinary tract infections: what's new? J Urol 2002; 168:2351–2358.
5. Kunin CM. Nosocomial urinary tract infections and the indwelling catheter: what is new and what is true? Chest 2001; 120:10–12.
6. Grabe M. Perioperative antibiotic prophylaxis in urology. Curr Opin Urol 2001; 11:81–85.
7. Kraklau DM, Wolf JS, Jr. Review of antibiotic prophylaxis recommendations for office-based urologic procedures. Tech Urol 1999; 5:123–128.
8. Rane A, Cahill D, Saleemi A, Montgomery B, Palfrey E. The issue of prophylactic antibiotics prior to flexible cystoscopy. Eur Urol 2001; 39:212–214.
9. Kortmann BB, Sonke GS, D'Ancona FC, Floratos DL, Debruyne FM, De La Rosette JJ. The tolerability of urodynamic studies and flexible cysto-urethroscopy used in the assessment of men with lower urinary tract symptoms. BJU Int 1999; 84:449–453.
10. Manson AL. Is antibiotic administration indicated after outpatient cystoscopy. J Urol 1988; 140: 316–317.
11. Puppo P, Ricciotti G, Bozzo W, Introini C. Primary endoscopic treatment of ureteric calculi. A review of 378 cases. Eur Urol 1999; 36:48–52.
12. Rao PN, Dube DA, Weightman NC, Oppenheim BA, Morris J. Prediction of septicemia following endourological manipulation for stones in the upper urinary tract. J Urol 1991; 146:955–960.
13. Hendrikx AJ, Strijbos WE, de Knijff DW, Kums JJ, Doesburg WH, Lemmens WA. Treatment for extended-mid and distal ureteral stones: SWL or ureteroscopy? Results of a multicenter study. J Endourol 1999; 13:727–733.
14. Knopf HJ, Graff HJ, Schulze H. Perioperative antibiotic prophylaxis in ureteroscopic stone removal. Eur Urol 2003; 44:115–118.
15. O'Keeffe NK, Mortimer AJ, Sambrook PA, Rao PN. Severe sepsis following percutaneous or endoscopic procedures for urinary tract stones. Br J Urol 1993; 72:277–283.
16. Mariappan P, Smith G, Bariol SV, Moussa SA, Tolley DA. Stone and pelvic urine culture and sensitivity are better than bladder urine as predictors of urosepsis following percutaneous nephrolithotomy: a prospective clinical study. J Urol 2005; 173:1610–1614.
17. Childs SJ. Appropriate surgical prophylaxis in transurethral genitourinary surgery and potential reduction in nosocomial infections. Urology 1986; 27:15–20.
18. Berry A, Barratt A. Prophylatic antibiotic use in transurethral prostatic resection: a meta-analysis. J Urol 2002; 167(2 Pt 1):571–577.
19. Colau A, Lucet JC, Rufat P, Botto H, Benoit G, Jardin A. Incidence and risk factors of bacteriuria after transurethral resection of the prostate. Eur Urol 2001; 39:272–276.
20. Qiang W, Jianchen W, MacDonald R, Monga M, Wilt TJ. Antibiotic prophylaxis for transurethral prostatic resection in men with preoperative urine containing less than 100,000 bacteria per ml: a systematic review. J Urol 2005; 173:1175–1181.
21. Raz R, Almog D, Elhanan G, Shental J. The use of ceftriaxone in the prevention of urinary tract infection in patients undergoing transurethral resection of the prostate (TUR-P). Infection 1994; 22:347–349.

22. Badenoch DF, Murdoch DA, Tiptaft RC. Microbiological study of bladder tumors, their histology and infective complications. Urology 1990; 35:5–8.

23. Hodge KK, McNeal JE, Terris MK, Stamey TA. Random systematic versus directed ultrasound guided transrectal core biopsies of the prostate. J Urol 1989; 142:71–74, discussion 4–5.

24. Aron M, Rajeev TP, Gupta NP. Antibiotic prophylaxis for transrectal needle biopsy of the prostate: a randomized controlled study. BJU Int 2000; 85:682–685.

25. Griffith BC, Morey AF, Ali-Khan MM, Canby-Hagino E, Foley JP, Rozanski TA. Single dose levofloxacin prophylaxis for prostate biopsy in patients at low risk. J Urol 2002; 168:1021–1023.

26. Kapoor DA, Klimberg IW, Malek GH, et al. Single-dose oral ciprofloxacin versus placebo for prophylaxis during transrectal prostate biopsy. Urology 1998; 52:552–558.

27. Enlund AL, Varenhorst E. Morbidity of ultrasound-guided transrectal core biopsy of the prostate without prophylactic antibiotic therapy. A prospective study in 415 cases. Br J Urol 1997; 79:777–780.

28. Dajani AS, Taubert KA, Wilson W, et al. Prevention of bacterial endocarditis. Recommendations by the American Heart Association. JAMA 1997; 277:1794–1801.

29. Antibiotic prophylaxis for urological patients with total joint replacements. J Urol 2003; 169:1796–1797.

30. Carey JM, Korman HJ. Transrectal ultrasound guided biopsy of the prostate. Do enemas decrease clinically significant complications? J Urol 2001; 166:82–85.

31. Lindert KA, Kabalin JN, Terris MK. Bacteremia and bacteriuria after transrectal ultrasound guided prostate biopsy. J Urol 2000; 164:76–80.

32. Townsend CM. Sabiston Textbook of Surgery. 17th ed. St. Louis, Mosby: Saunders, 2004.

33. National Nosocomial Infections Surveillance (NNIS) System Report. Data summary from January 1992 through June 2004, issued October 2004. Am J Infect Control 2004; 32:470–485.

34. Kirkland KB, Briggs JP, Trivette SL, Wilkinson WE, Sexton DJ. The impact of surgical-site infections in the 1990s: attributable mortality, excess length of hospitalization, and extra costs. Infect Control Hosp Epidemiol 1999; 20:725–730.

35. www.cdc.gov/NCIDOD/dhqp/gl-surgicalsite.html

36. Culver DH, Horan TC, Gaynes RP, et al. Surgical wound infection rates by wound class, operative procedure, and patient risk index. National Nosocomial Infections Surveillance System. Am J Med 1991; 91:152S–157S.

37. Gaynes RP, Culver DH, Horan TC, Edwards JR, Richards C, Tolson JS. Surgical site infection (SSI) rates in the United States, 1992–1998: the National Nosocomial Infections Surveillance System basic SSI risk index. Clin Infect Dis 2001; 33(suppl 2):S69–S77.

38. Kurz A, Sessler DI, Lenhardt R. Perioperative normothermia to reduce the incidence of surgical-wound infection and shorten hospitalization. Study of Wound Infection and Temperature Group. N Engl J Med 1996; 334:1209–1215.

39. Belda FJ, Aguilera L, Garcia de la Asuncion J, et al. Supplemental perioperative oxygen and the risk of surgical wound infection: a randomized controlled trial. JAMA 2005; 294:2035–2042.

40. Grey NJ, Perdrizet GA. Reduction of nosocomial infections in the surgical intensive-care unit by strict glycemic control. Endocr Pract 2004; 10(suppl 2):46–52.

41. Heinzelmann M, Scott M, Lam T. Factors predisposing to bacterial invasion and infection. Am J Surg 2002; 183:179–190.

42. Fuenfer MM, Olson GE, Polk HC, Jr. Effect of various corticosteroids upon the phagocytic bactericidal activity of neutrophils. Surgery 1975; 78:27–33.

43. Asensio A, Ramos A, Munez E, Vilanova JL, Torrijos P, Garcia FJ. Preoperative low molecular weight heparin as venous thromboembolism prophylaxis in patients at risk for prosthetic infection after knee arthroplasty. Infect Control Hosp Epidemiol 2005; 26:903–909.

44. Alexander JW, Fischer JE, Boyajian M, Palmquist J, Morris MJ. The influence of hair-removal methods on wound infections. Arch Surg 1983; 118:347–352.

45. Raves JJ, Slifkin M, Diamond DL. A bacteriologic study comparing closed suction and simple conduit drainage. Am J Surg 1984; 148:618–620.

46. Furuno JP, Perencevich EN, Johnson JA, et al. Methicillin-resistant Staphylococcus aureus and vancomycin-resistant Enterococci co-colonization. Emerg Infect Dis 2005; 11:1539–1544.

47. Weiss CA III, Statz CL, Dahms RA, Remucal MJ, Dunn DL, Beilman GJ. Six years of surgical wound infection surveillance at a tertiary care center: review of the microbiologic and epidemiological aspects of 20,007 wounds. Arch Surg 1999; 134:1041–1048.

48. Christou NV, Nohr CW, Meakins JL. Assessing operative site infection in surgical patients. Arch Surg 1987; 122:165–169.

49. Falcoz PE, Laluc F, Toubin MM, et al. Usefulness of procalcitonin in the early detection of infection after thoracic surgery. Eur J Cardiothorac Surg 2005; 27:1074–1078.

50. Tegnell A, Aren C, Ohman L. Wound infections after cardiac surgery—a wound scoring system may improve early detection. Scand Cardiovasc J 2002; 36:60–64.

51. Noone TC, Semelka RC, Worawattanakul S, Marcos HB. Intraperitoneal abscesses: diagnostic accuracy of and appearances at MR imaging. Radiology 1998; 208:525–528.

52. Bydder GM, Kreel L. Computed tomography in the diagnosis of abdominal abscess. J Comput Tomogr 1980; 4:132–145.

53. Noone TC, Semelka RC, Chaney DM, Reinhold C. Abdominal imaging studies: comparison of diagnostic accuracies resulting from ultrasound, computed tomography, and magnetic resonance imaging in the same individual. Magn Reson Imaging 2004; 22:19–24.

54. Khurrum Baig M, Hua Zhao R, Batista O, et al. Percutaneous postoperative intra-abdominal abscess drainage after elective colorectal surgery. Tech Coloproctol 2002; 6:159–164.

55. Bratzler DW, Houck PM. Antimicrobial prophylaxis for surgery: an advisory statement from the National Surgical Infection Prevention Project. Am J Surg 2005; 189:395–404.

56. Stone HH, Haney BB, Kolb LD, Geheber CE, Hooper CA. Prophylactic and preventive antibiotic therapy: timing, duration and economics. Ann Surg 1979; 189:691–699.

57. Classen DC, Evans RS, Pestotnik SL, Horn SD, Menlove RL, Burke JP. The timing of prophylactic administration of antibiotics and the risk of surgical-wound infection. N Engl J Med 1992; 326:281–286.

58. Kiddoo DA, Wollin TA, Mador DR. A population based assessment of complications following outpatient hydrocelectomy and spermatocelectomy. J Urol 2004; 171(2 Pt 1):746–748.

59. Dajani AS, Taubert KA, Wilson W, et al. Prevention of bacterial endocarditis: recommendations by the American Heart Association. Clin Infect Dis 1997; 25:1448–1458.

60. Onur R, Ozden M, Orhan I, Kalkan A, Semercioz A. Incidence of bacteraemia after urodynamic study. J Hosp Infect 2004; 57:241–244.

61. Sullivan NM, Sutter VL, Mims MM, Marsh VH, Finegold SM. Clinical aspects of bacteremia after manipulation of the genitourinary tract. J Infect Dis 1973; 127:49–55.

62. Venn SN, Greenwell TJ, Mundy AR. The long-term outcome of artificial urinary sphincters. J Urol 2000; 164(3 Pt 1):702–706, discussion 6–7.

63. Hajivassiliou CA. A review of the complications and results of implantation of the AMS artificial urinary sphincter. Eur Urol 1999; 35:36–44.

64. Petero VG, Jr, Diokno AC. Comparison of the long-term outcomes between incontinent men and women treated with artificial urinary sphincter. J Urol 2006; 175:605–609.

65. Martins FE, Boyd SD. Postoperative risk factors associated with artificial urinary sphincter infection-erosion. Br J Urol 1995; 75:354–358.

66. Bryan DE, Mulcahy JJ, Simmons GR. Salvage procedure for infected noneroded artificial urinary sphincters. J Urol 2002; 168:2464–2466.

67. Gomha MA, Boone TB. Artificial urinary sphincter for post-prostatectomy incontinence in men who had prior radiotherapy: a risk and outcome analysis. J Urol 2002; 167(2 Pt 1):591–596.

68. Miller EA, Mayo M, Kwan D, Mitchell M. Simultaneous augmentation cystoplasty and artificial urinary sphincter placement: infection rates and voiding mechanisms. J Urol 1998; 160(3 Pt 1):750–752, discussion 2–3.

69. Holmes NM, Kogan BA, Baskin LS. Placement of artificial urinary sphincter in children and simultaneous gastrocystoplasty. J Urol 2001; 165(6 Pt 2):2366–2368.

70. Catto JW, Natarajan V, Tophill PR. Simultaneous augmentation cystoplasty is associated with earlier rather than increased artificial urinary sphincter infection. J Urol 2005; 173:1237–1241.

71. Ganesan GS, Nguyen DH, Adams MC, et al. Lower urinary tract reconstruction using stomach and the artificial sphincter. J Urol 1993; 149:1107–1109.

72. Raj GV, Peterson AC, Toh KL, Webster GD. Outcomes following revisions and secondary implantation of the artificial urinary sphincter. J Urol 2005; 173:1242–1245.

73. Small MP. Small-carrion penile prosthesis: a report on 160 cases and review of the literature. J Urol 1978; 119:365–368.

74. Schwartz BF, Swanzy S, Thrasher JB. A randomized prospective comparison of antibiotic tissue levels in the corpora cavernosa of patients undergoing penile prosthesis implantation using gentamicin plus cefazolin versus an oral fluoroquinolone for prophylaxis. J Urol 1996; 156:991–994.

75. Montague DK, Jarow JP, Broderick GA, et al. Chapter 1: The management of erectile dysfunction: an AUA update. J Urol 2005; 174:230–239.

76. Carson CC III. Efficacy of antibiotic impregnation of inflatable penile prostheses in decreasing infection in original implants. J Urol 2004; 171:1611–1614.

77. Henry GD, Wilson SK, Delk JR II, et al. Revision washout decreases penile prosthesis infection in revision surgery: a multicenter study. J Urol 2005; 173:89–92.

78. Nickel JC, Heaton J, Morales A, Costerton JW. Bacterial biofilm in persistent penile prosthesis-associated infection. J Urol 1986; 135:586–588.

79. Silverstein A, Donatucci CF. Bacterial biofilms and implantable prosthetic devices. Int J Impot Res 2003; 15(suppl 5):S150–S154.

80. Henry GD, Wilson SK, Delk JR II, et al. Penile prosthesis cultures during revision surgery: a multicenter study. J Urol 2004; 172:153–156.

81. Darouiche RO. Treatment of infections associated with surgical implants. N Engl J Med 2004; 350:1422–1429.

82. Mulcahy JJ. Long-term experience with salvage of infected penile implants. J Urol 2000; 163:481–482.

83. Merrill DC. Clinical experience with the Mentor inflatable penile prosthesis in 301 patients. J Urol 1988; 140:1424–1427.

84. Kabalin JN, Kessler R. Infectious complications of penile prosthesis surgery. J Urol 1988; 139: 953–955.

85. Montague DK. Periprosthetic infections. J Urol 1987; 138:68–69.

86. Minervini A, Ralph DJ, Pryor JP. Outcome of penile prosthesis implantation for treating erectile dysfunction: experience with 504 procedures. BJU Int 2006; 97:129–133.

87. Carson CC, Robertson CN. Late hematogenous infection of penile prostheses. J Urol 1988; 139: 50–52.

88. Jarow JP. Risk factors for penile prosthetic infection. J Urol 1996; 156(2 Pt 1):402–404.

89. Kaufman JJ, Lindner A, Raz S. Complications of penile prosthesis surgery for impotence. J Urol 1982; 128:1192–1194.

90. Wilson SK, Delk JR II. Inflatable penile implant infection: predisposing factors and treatment suggestions. J Urol 1995; 153(3 Pt 1):659–661.

91. Buchholz HW, Elson RA, Engelbrecht E, Lodenkamper H, Rottger J, Siegel A. Management of deep infection of total hip replacement. J Bone Joint Surg Br 1981; 63-B:342–353.

92. Miley GB, Scheller AD Jr, Turner RH. Medical and surgical treatment of the septic hip with one-stage revision arthroplasty. Clin Orthop Relat Res 1982; 170:76–82.

93. Ure KJ, Amstutz HC, Nasser S, Schmalzried TP. Direct-exchange arthroplasty for the treatment of infection after total hip replacement. An average ten-year follow-up. J Bone Joint Surg Am 1998; 80:961–968.

94. Berbari EF, Osmon DR, Duffy MC, et al. Outcome of prosthetic joint infection in patients with rheumatoid arthritis: the impact of medical and surgical therapy in 200 episodes. Clin Infect Dis 2006; 42:216–223.

95. Mulcahy JJ, Brant MD, Ludlow JK. Management of infected penile implants. Tech Urol 1995; 1: 115–119.

96. Kaufman JM, Kaufman JL, Borges FD. Immediate salvage procedure for infected penile prosthesis. J Urol 1998; 159:816–818.

2 | Cardiovascular Issues in Urologic Surgery

Amy Leigh Miller
Division of Cardiovascular Medicine, Brigham and Women's Hospital, Boston, Massachusetts, U.S.A.

James Chen-tson Fang
Division of Cardiovascular Medicine, University Hospitals of Cleveland, Case Western Reserve University, Cleveland, Ohio, U.S.A.

INTRODUCTION

Cardiovascular disease has been the leading cause of death in the United States for the past 50 years (1) and is the predominant concern in the preoperative assessment of the adult patient undergoing noncardiac surgery. Rates of perioperative cardiovascular complications range from 0.4% to 11%; an incidence of 2% was observed in an unselected population over age 50 (2). The number of perioperative cardiac events ranges from 500,000 to 900,000 per year (3). With urological surgery, cardiac mortality is on the order of 0.3%, accounting for just under one-fourth of all-cause mortality (4). However, the risk of cardiovascular complications is not fixed, and can be reduced by perioperative and intraoperative interventions (5), such as careful preoperative assessment and planning. In this review, we discuss the principles of preoperative cardiovascular assessment and care with special emphasis on the patient undergoing urologic procedures and surgery.

PATHOPHYSIOLOGIC CONSIDERATIONS

In general, perioperative cardiovascular complications refer to myocardial infarction (MI) or cardiac death, with the latter being attributable to complex arrhythmias, valvular heart disease, and cardiomyopathies. Although heart failure, arrhythmias, angina, and hypotension are important occurrences in the perioperative patient, they are only variably considered in most studies that have addressed cardiovascular risk.

A wide range of anatomic and physiologic conditions may result in a "vulnerable patient," even in the absence of a "vulnerable plaque" (6,7). The pathophysiology of perioperative MI likely involves excessive myocardial oxygen demand that is compromised by fixed obstructive coronary artery disease (8). However, occlusive rupture of a vulnerable plaque in an atherosclerotic coronary circulation may also be responsible, as is the case in nonoperative settings (9,10). Angiographic data in the perioperative period are limited but support both mechanisms of MI. A predominance of "demand" infarction due to inadequate collateralization to support myocardial perfusion during the stress of the perioperative period (3) has been noted; others have found infarcts that were not associated with high-grade stenoses, implying that plaque rupture within a nonobstructive stenosis was responsible (11). Both mechanisms are plausible since surgery involves not only hemodynamic changes that could produce demand-related ischemia, but is also associated with inflammatory responses that lead to a prothrombotic state and plaque rupture (3). In fact, the critical time for perioperative cardiovascular complications occurs in the hours to days after surgery when heart rate, blood pressure, and inflammation may be particularly elevated due to wound healing and inadequate postoperative pain control.

PREOPERATIVE CARDIAC RISK ASSESSMENT

Although preoperative cardiac risk assessment is often referred to as "cardiac clearance," "clearance" per se cannot be provided. In fact, cardiovascular risk in the perioperative period cannot be entirely eliminated; it can only be defined and modified. Furthermore, the preoperative evaluation provides a unique opportunity to review and treat the overall cardiovascular health of the patient independent of the need to get the patient through surgery. Generally, such an evaluation focuses on characterizing the relative risk of a perioperative cardiovascular complication from patient-related as well as procedure-related factors and, in certain cases, with further testing. In addition, strategies to lower that risk may be recommended during the periprocedural period. Importantly, while risk assessment is often triggered by the "need" to perform a procedure, the subsequent cardiovascular evaluation should not be any more exhaustive than a standard assessment based upon risk factors, functional capacity, and symptoms in a patient not scheduled for surgery. Such an approach is supported by consensus statements by a number of societies (12,13).

Two axes of assessment are required to properly assess preoperative cardiovascular risk: procedural risk and patient-related clinical factors (including functional capacity).

Procedural Characteristics

There are two predominant issues related to the procedure itself to be considered in the preoperative patient: (*i*) the urgency of the procedure and (*ii*) the hemodynamic burden imposed by the procedure. The accurate assessment of surgical urgency is paramount. Truly emergent procedures do not involve exhaustive preoperative cardiovascular studies because the very urgency of the procedure does not allow the time required to perform such tests. Furthermore, implicit in a decision to perform an emergent procedure is an acknowledgment that the emergent clinical issue is of such immediate threat to life or would result in such great morbidity that any level of cardiovascular risk is acceptable. Therefore, it is imperative that the surgeon and cardiovascular consultant together review the urgency of the proposed surgical intervention. In contrast, with urgent and elective procedures there is adequate preoperative time to perform indicated cardiovascular testing and/or risk-modifying interventions.

The hemodynamic burden imposed by a given procedure has been characterized in both human subjects and animal models. In general, fluid shifts and blood loss are the predominant hemodynamic stressors, resulting in tachycardia and hypotension. These stresses are present both intra- and postoperatively; in fact, postoperative ischemic electrocardiogram (EKG) changes are more predictive of a cardiovascular event than are intraoperative changes (14).

Tachycardia is the body's intrinsic response to decreases in intravascular volume, providing a defense against the decrease in cardiac output that would result otherwise. It is also part of the sympathetic response, occurring along with psychological stress and pain/discomfort, both of which can be dominating factors in the perioperative period. Interestingly, the timing of myocardial enzyme elevations postoperatively suggests that the onset of myocardial ischemia occurs at the end of a surgical procedure, presumably as a consequence of lightened sedation resulting in tachycardia and increased sympathetic drive (8). In dogs, tachycardia has been shown to produce subendocardial ischemia (15). Even in the presence of a coronary stenosis that is not hemodynamically significant at rest, subendocardial necrosis can occur (16).

Hypotension in the perioperative setting can be related to anesthetic agents, preoperative medications, and/or volume loss. Regardless of the mechanism, if coronary perfusion pressure is sufficiently decreased, myocardial ischemia can result, even in the absence of significant coronary stenoses. This ischemia will be more pronounced if coronary artery disease is present concomitantly. Retrospective analysis suggests that intraoperative hypotension is associated with an increased rate of perioperative cardiovascular events (17).

Surgical procedures are consequently divided into risk categories based upon their hemodynamic stress; these risk categories are well aligned with cardiovascular event rates observed in the coronary artery surgery study (CASS) registry (18), which are the bases of the current guidelines (19). High-risk procedures (cardiovascular event risk >5%) involve large fluid shifts and/or blood loss and include vascular (aortic and peripheral) surgeries and emergent procedures (particularly in elderly patients) (19). In contrast, low-risk procedures (cardiovascular event risk <1%) are associated with minimal blood loss, and include minor operations (dermatologic procedures, cataract surgery) and endoscopic procedures. Finally, intermediate-risk procedures (cardiovascular event risk 1–5%) include nonvascular intraperitoneal and intrathoracic procedures as well as orthopedic and head/neck surgery (including carotid endarterectomy). In general, urological procedures, including prostatic operations, fall into the intermediate-risk category. However, some common urological procedures like cystoscopy are generally associated with low cardiovascular risk.

Patient Characteristics

A variety of indices have been developed for perioperative cardiac risk prediction that use traditional patient-related risk factors (e.g., history of MI, diabetes, heart failure) (3). A widely used risk index, the revised cardiac risk index (RCRI) (3), was developed in a random population of patients undergoing elective noncardiac surgery (2). Its broad use stems from its simplicity in that risk is calculated by adding together both specific procedural and patient-related factors (Table 1). Alternatively, the current American College of Cardiology/American Heart Association (ACC/AHA) guidelines define three classes (Table 2) of risk factors (19), where the cardiovascular risk to patients is determined by the greatest risk class in which they have a clinical predictor. Importantly, the ability to assess functional capacity is assumed in this system.

The ACC/AHA guidelines include a detailed algorithm encompassing the management of patients for all levels of procedural risk (19). For the urologist, the focus of the ACC/AHA algorithm is the intermediate-risk-procedure algorithm. Patients whose functional capacity does not exceed four metabolic equivalents (METS) [gardening, raking leaves, or mowing a lawn with a power mower (20)] should undergo preoperative noninvasive cardiac testing to assess for ischemia, unless they have had recent testing (stress test/catheterization within the past two years without progression of symptoms) or revascularization (within the past five years without progression of symptoms) (19). In patients who are unable to provide a clear/reliable description of their functional status, the observed ability to walk up two flights of stairs is quantitatively equal to at least four METS. All other cases can proceed directly to intermediate/low-risk surgical intervention without preoperative cardiac testing (19). Therefore, the cardiovascular specialist's consultation will focus on the accurate quantification of a patient's functional status, review of prior cardiovascular testing and interventions, and most importantly, the ascertainment of new or progressive cardiovascular symptoms of angina, dyspnea, or syncope.

Preoperative Stress Testing/Ischemia Assessment

Who, then, should undergo further cardiovascular testing? In general, such testing should be reserved for those who either fall into an intermediate-risk category because of clinical criteria (see previously) or have an unclear functional capacity from a detailed history. In these situations, further testing can further refine risk (19). In contrast, for patients who have had coronary revascularization within the past five years (or stress testing/catheterization within the past two years) and stable symptoms in that time period, no further testing or evaluation is indicated in the preoperative setting (19). Similarly, risk cannot be further refined when patients are

TABLE 1 Revised Cardiac Risk Index

RCRI = no. of the following risk factors present:
      High-risk surgery
      Ischemic heart disease
      History of cerebrovascular disease
      History of congestive heart failure
      Presence of insulin-requiring diabetes
      Preoperative serum creatinine exceeding 2.0 mg/dL

RCRI class	RCRI score	Cardiovascular event rate[a]
Class I	0	0.5 (0.2, 1.1)
Class II	1	1.3 (0.7, 2.1)
Class III	2	3.6 (2.1, 5.6)
Class IV	>2	9.1 (5.5, 13.8)

[a]Cardiovascular event rates from the derivation patient cohort.
Abbreviation: RCRI, revised cardiac risk index.
Source: From Ref. 2.

TABLE 2   Classes of Clinical Predictors of Cardiovascular Risk

Major clinical predictors
 Unstable coronary syndrome[a]
 Decompensated congestive heart failure
 Significant arrhythmia[b]
 Severe/critical valvular disease

Intermediate clinical predictors
 Stable mild angina
 Prior (distant) MI (by history or EKG)
 History of heart failure/compensated congestive heart failure
 Diabetes mellitus
 Renal insufficiency

Minor clinical predictors
 Advanced age
 Significant EKG abnormality[c]
 Non-sinus atrial mechanism (e.g., atrial fibrillation)
 Low functional capacity
 Uncontrolled systemic hypertension
 History of stroke

[a]Unstable angina, severe chronic angina, acute (0–7 days) MI or recent (8–30 days from onset) MI.
[b]High-grade atrioventricular block, symptomatic ventricular arrhythmia, supraventricular arrhythmia with uncontrolled ventricular rate.
[c]Left bundle branch block, left ventricular hypertrophy, significant ST-T wave abnormalities, etc.
Abbreviations: EKG, electrocardiogram; MI, myocardial infarction.
Source: From Refs. 19, 34.

either at low or high risk as accessed by clinical criteria; consequently, in these cases, further testing is not required.

A variety of tests are available to assess myocardial ischemia, including ambulatory ischemic electrocardiography, exercise tolerance testing (ETT), myocardial perfusion scintigraphy, radionuclide ventriculography, dobutamine stress echocardiography, and dipyridamole stress echocardiography. When compared in a meta-analysis, no significant differences in sensitivity or specificity were found between these various tests (21). While significant differences have not been demonstrated, these various tests have their own individual strengths and weaknesses, and test selection should be tailored to the patient to provide the most specific information (e.g., valvular heart disease, systolic dysfunction, functional capacity, exertional symptoms). In fact, most clinicians favor studies that incorporate some assessment of functional capacity over pharmacologic stressors because of the prognostic power of objectively measured functional capacity. Finally, local expertise regarding specific testing modalities will also necessarily affect test selection. Although newer tests are also now available, that is, cardiac stress magnetic resonance imaging (MRI) and coronary computerized tomography (CT) angiography, their role in preoperative risk assessment has yet to be delineated. Ultimately, if testing is not going to change the therapeutic strategy for a given patient, testing is not recommended. In fact, the presence of ischemia by any test is not, in and of itself, sufficient rationale to revascularize to modify risk (see subsequently).

MODIFYING PERIOPERATIVE CARDIOVASCULAR RISK

Once the cardiovascular risk has been defined as outlined previously, the issue of decreasing the defined cardiovascular risk must be addressed. There are three classes of interventions that are employed perioperatively to reduce the risk of cardiac complications: hemodynamic/telemetric monitoring, medical therapy (for ischemia, heart failure, and arrhythmias), and preoperative revascularization of the coronary circulation (5).

Perioperative Monitoring

"Monitoring" refers to invasive monitoring [central venous lines, pulmonary artery catheters (PAC), arterial lines, etc.], cardiac telemetry, and/or an intensive care setting with associated sub-specialized staff. There are only limited studies that form the basis of current evidence-based guidelines for the role of any of these interventions. The role of cardiac telemetry has not been studied in the setting of perioperative cardiovascular complications, but is assumed to have reasonable cost-effective utility. For patients with known heart disease or at high risk for cardiovascular events, cardiac telemetry allows close surveillance of arrhythmias and ischemic events. Similarly, involvement of an intensivist and admission to an intensive care unit may be advisable for patients who require extensive nursing support, invasive monitoring, and/or frequent titration of hemodynamically active medications, with the understanding that the evidence supporting such a strategy remains relatively limited (22).

While telemetric monitoring and involvement of an intensivist are accepted components of aggressive perioperative management in high-risk situations (despite a lack of definitive evidence that they lower risk), the role of the PAC is even less clear. In fact, observational studies in the past decade (23,24) have suggested that PAC use *increases* morbidity and mortality. Prospective studies of PAC use in the perioperative setting have been complicated by considerable variability in the manner in which PACs were used to direct care in these trials (25), and even when specific hemodynamic goals are selected (goal-directed therapy), there is no real consensus of what these goals should be (26). Despite these limitations, even the largest and most contemporary randomized controlled study suggests that PACs are not very beneficial when routinely employed. In this trial, Sandham and others randomized high-risk [American Society of Anesthesiologists (ASA) class III/IV] patients undergoing intermediate- to high-risk (orthopedic, abdominal, thoracic, and vascular) procedures to goal-directed therapy with a PAC treatment versus standard medical care (including a central venous line, if desired). They found no statistically significant difference in mortality (27) but a significant increase in the frequency of pulmonary embolism (PE) in the PAC treatment group. While even this study remains a subject of much debate (28), routine PAC use cannot be justified. Finally, although there may be patient subsets that might benefit from such monitoring, this issue remains largely unsettled.

Perioperative Medical Therapy

The cornerstone of the medical management of the perioperative patient is beta-blockade, which has been known for a decade to decrease cardiovascular morbidity and mortality (29). Beta-blockers, through their antiadrenergic effects, reduce myocardial oxygen consumption by decreasing heart rate, wall stress, and contractility, as well as decreasing arrhythmias. Early trials (29,30) showed significant benefits of atenolol or bisoprolol, but showed variations in the timing of beta-blocker initiation and duration of therapy. More recently, a retrospective cohort study (31) raised concerns regarding beta-blocker use in low-risk patients. In that study, end-points were actually increased in low-risk patients on beta-blockade, relative to those not receiving beta-blockers. Given the retrospective nature of the study and limited information available regarding the impetus for beta-blockade in patients at low risk, the implications of the study are unclear (32).

In general, it does appear that the benefit of beta-blockade is relatively proportional to the preoperative risk of a cardiac event (33). At present, beta-blockers are indicated in high-risk patients. These agents should be continued in low- or intermediate-risk patients who have been on them prior to surgery, in order to avoid the deleterious effects of beta-blocker withdrawal in the perioperative period (32). In the recently published ACC/AHA guidelines, the writing committee found insufficient data to recommend for or against beta-blockade in low-risk patients underlying nonvascular surgery (34). For intermediate-risk patients undergoing intermediate- to high-risk procedures, perioperative beta-blockade receives a Class IIb recommendation (34). For high-risk patients, beta-blockade has a Class IIa recommendation (34). These are slightly broader recommendations than the guidelines published by the European Society of Cardiology (35). The optimal time to initiate beta-blocker therapy has not been determined, but earlier initiation relative to surgery is advisable in order to allow time for the drug to exert its effects prior to surgery.

The role for the routine use of other classes of pharmacological agents is less clear. Alpha-agonists (clonidine, mivazeral), nitroglycerin, and diltiazem have all been studied in the perioperative setting (5). While the majority of studies show no significant benefit from these drugs (5), there is some evidence that alpha-agonists may be beneficial (33,36,37), particularly as adjuncts to beta-blockade to improve blood pressure control (19). It is clear, however, that these agents are less effective than beta-blockade (33). Recently, interest has been focused on 3-hydroxy-3-methyl-glutaryl coenzyme A (HMG CoA) reductase inhibitors, or statins, as a potential treatment to reduce perioperative cardiac events. While statins were originally invoked to lower cholesterol levels, they are now widely recognized to have pleiotropic therapeutic effects on the cardiovascular system (38). Observational studies suggest that statins are beneficial perioperatively (39,40). Theoretical concerns regarding increased myopathy in the perioperative setting have largely been discounted (41), and a large randomized controlled trial is now underway assessing the efficacy of statin, beta-blockade, or statin plus beta-blocker in noncardiac surgery patients (42).

Antiplatelet therapy in the perioperative setting has also been considered. Traditionally, antiplatelet agents have been discontinued days in advance of surgical procedures, due to concern for increased bleeding associated with the procedure. Several observational studies have demonstrated decreased morbidity and mortality with cardiac surgery in patients receiving perioperative aspirin relative to those not on aspirin (43–45), but to date, there are no randomized controlled studies or even observational studies of aspirin in noncardiac surgery patients.

One special circumstance deserves mention. Patients who have had a coronary stent placed should, in particular, not have their antiplatelet therapy discontinued without specific consultation with an interventional cardiologist (see below).

Preoperative Revascularization

There is no evidence that routine percutaneous or surgical revascularization improves perioperative outcomes in stable patients with coronary artery disease undergoing noncardiac surgery. In the landmark CARP trial, 510 patients from 18 VA hospitals who were to undergo either abdominal aortic aneurysm (AAA) repair or lower extremity revascularization were randomized to either coronary revascularization [59% percutaneous coronary intervention (PCI), 41% coronary artery bypass graft surgery (CABG)] or medical therapy (46). There were no differences in perioperative outcomes (including perioperative MI and the three-year mortality rate) in this high-risk population undergoing high-risk surgery. Therefore, the indication to revascularize should be driven by other known mortality benefits (e.g., three vessel coronary artery disease with depressed ventricular function) or to improve symptoms (e.g., unstable angina) that can be sought at the time of cardiovascular preoperative assessment. The indications for coronary bypass surgery in the preoperative setting should therefore be no different from those in the nonsurgical setting (19). In summary, the need to undergo surgery is not an indication for coronary revascularization since there is no evidence that such a routine practice decreases cardiovascular risk.

Recent PCI may also complicate rather than improve perioperative outcomes with noncardiac surgery. For example, patients who have recently undergone percutaneous coronary stenting are at particular risk for catastrophic in-stent thrombosis if antiplatelet agents are discontinued prematurely to facilitate surgery. An observational study identified 40 patients who had bare metal coronary stents (BMS) placed less than six weeks prior to noncardiac (moderate to high-risk) general surgery. Seven patients suffered MI, with six MI-related fatalities (47). Risk of a cardiovascular complication was substantially higher in the patients who underwent stenting less than two weeks prior to their operative procedure, prompting the authors to recommend that elective/urgent surgery be delayed for a minimum of 14 days after coronary stenting, or that angioplasty without stenting be considered if surgery could not be safely delayed (47). A subsequent retrospective analysis from the Mayo clinic surgical database of 207 patients undergoing noncardiac surgery less than 60 days postcoronary stenting found a lower rate of events (eight major adverse cardiac events total), but confirmed that the risk of events was significantly increased in the early poststenting period, with maximal risk in the first six weeks poststenting (48).

The six-week high-risk period identified with BMS is believed to correspond to the time required for endothelialization of the stent (48). With BMS, dual antiplatelet therapy is recommended for a minimum of four weeks post-PCI. Because the time to adequate endothelialization is significantly prolonged with drug-eluting stents (DES) (and necessitates prolonged dual antiplatelet therapy), the vulnerable period is likely greater than six weeks post-DES stenting. Consequently, in patients who receive a DES, surgeons are faced with the choice of early surgery with an increased risk of bleeding on dual antiplatelet therapy, or a waiting period of three to six months before considering surgery. While the two currently available DES, the CYPHER and TAXUS stents, were released with recommendations for 3 and 6 months, minimum, of antiplatelet therapy respectively, subsequent data analysis had revealed a small but significant number of stent thromboses occurring beyond these time points. Based on recently convened consensus panel formed by the Food and Drug Administration (FDA), the current recommendation for patients with a DES is a minimum of 1 year of dual antiplatelet therapy following stent placement. Furthermore, given the possibility of late in-stent thrombosis with DES, continuation of aspiring therapy during the preoperative period is advisable if at all possible (49), regardless of the time since stent placement. In circumstances in which the surgical urgency precludes a three to six months delay, bare metal stenting or balloon angioplasty without stenting are alternative revascularization strategies, but are associated with lower long-term coronary patency rates. To date, there are no published studies comparing different management strategies in this difficult setting (50).

SPECIAL CASES
Valvular Heart Disease

In general, stenotic valvular lesions like mitral and aortic stenosis (AS) are a greater hemodynamic stressor for the patient undergoing noncardiac surgery than are regurgitant lesions, such as mitral regurgitation. Therefore, current recommendations advise that symptomatic stenotic valvular lesions be corrected (surgically or percutaneously) prior to an elective or urgent surgical procedure, if possible (19). Although patients with significant AS may easily become hemodynamically unstable, a retrospective analysis of a Mayo clinic experience suggests that it is possible to safely manage patients with severe AS through noncardiac procedures if prophylactic valve replacement is prohibited for some reason (51). The Mayo group advocates close attention to the "classic tenets" of AS management (51):

1. Avoid decreases in preload
2. Prevent tachycardia
3. Avoid decreases in contractility
4. Avoid decreases in systemic vascular resistance

While noncardiac surgery in patients with severe AS is possible when absolutely necessary, it is not without risk. In the Mayo clinic series, three patients with previously unknown AS required emergent balloon valvuloplasty postoperatively, due to florid pulmonary edema (51). Of note, patients in this series did not routinely undergo preoperative aortic valvuloplasty.

Regurgitant lesions in association with preserved systolic function are generally well tolerated and can be managed with close monitoring and medical therapy. When valve repair or replacement is clinically indicated independent of the preoperative situation, valve intervention can be safely delayed until after noncardiac surgery (19).

Cardiomyopathy

Patients with a history of heart failure or cardiomyopathy require a careful assessment of their hemodynamic profile and volume status. In patients with decompensated heart failure, elective or urgent surgical procedures should be delayed until their heart failure is well-compensated. Medical management should be optimized according to accepted treatment guidelines (52). In patients for whom heart failure/cardiomyopathy is a new diagnosis, investigation of the etiology of cardiomyopathy should be pursued preoperatively, as the management of cardiomyopathy will depend in part upon the specific physiology involved (19,52). Left ventricular function should be characterized preoperatively, in order to guide perioperative fluid management (19). Once the cause/type of cardiomyopathy has been identified and the volume status optimized, surgery can proceed with close attention to alterations in volume status and/or systemic perfusion. There is no evidence that the routine use of PAC is required in this setting, although patients with advanced heart failure may benefit.

Hypertrophic cardiomyopathy presents a particularly vexing hemodynamic milieu within which to perform surgery (19). As with stenotic valvular lesions, patients with hypertrophic cardiomyopathy are preload-dependent and can experience significant decreases in cardiac output with hypovolemia and/or vasoplegia (19). Interestingly, the risk of cardiovascular morbidity in the perioperative setting is not predicted by the typical echocardiographic measures of hypertrophic severity, but rather, appears to depend primarily on the procedure (duration/hemodynamic burden) (53).

Arrhythmia/Conduction System Disease and Devices

There are currently no specific recommendations for perioperative management of patients with a known history of arrhythmia (19). Rate/rhythm control agents should be continued throughout the perioperative period, unless there is a strong contraindication to doing so. In the latter case, a cardiologist should be consulted to assist in perioperative management.

In patients with permanent pacemakers (PPMs) or internal cardioverter/defibrillators (ICDs), preoperative workup should include identification of the device manufacturer, the indication for the device, and the current programming status (54). This information should be clearly documented in the preoperative history and physical, to facilitate device interrogation and reprogramming if required on an urgent basis in the perioperative period. With approximately 200 different models of PPM generators available with complex programming capacities (55), it is essential that device information is readily available.

If electrocautery will be used in the procedure, inappropriate device behavior may be triggered by resulting electromagnetic interference (EMI) (56); such inappropriate behavior may include inappropriate inhibition (device interprets EMI as a native cardiac impulse), mode switch to asynchronous pacing, or inappropriate defibrillation therapy (device interprets EMI as ventricular fibrillation) (19,54,56–58). While magnets have historically been used in the operating room to prevent untoward interference, the response to magnet application varies across devices (54,56–58), making this a potentially dangerous practice if the response of the device in question is different than expected. If electrocautery is planned in the scheduled operative procedure, the device should be interrogated both prior to the procedure (at which time reprogramming may be required to reduce the risk of deleterious responses to interference) and after the procedure (to insure that the device is functioning properly, and reverse any procedure-specific manipulations that have been made) (58,59). Specific programming changes include disabling rate-adaptive features, as well as changes in maximum sensitivity and noise reversion mode, if possible (57,58). In general, defibrillator-specific therapy [antitachycardia pacing (ATP) or defibrillation] should be disabled for the duration of operative procedures involving electrocautery (19,57,58). For patients with specific ICDs who are pacemaker-dependent, external pacing or temporary pacing wire placement may be required to prevent EMI-induced inhibition of pacing, due to the absence of asynchronous pacing modes in these models (57,58).

While not an operative procedure, shock-wave lithotripsy also has the potential to affect PPMs and ICDs. Prior to the lithotripsy procedure, rate-responsive/adaptive characteristics of the device should be disabled, and postprocedure device interrogation should be performed to insure appropriate function (59).

Postoperative arrhythmias can be triggered by a variety of abnormalities, including hypoxia, hypercarbia, cathecholamine surge (stress response), increased vagal tone, electrolyte imbalance, or ischemia (60). Management of postoperative arrhythmia is identical to arrhythmia management in other settings: restoring hemodynamic stability by pharmacological or electrical means, using pharmacotherapy to control rate and/or rhythm, and identifying and treating underlying precipitants if possible.

ANESTHESIA—CARDIOVASCULAR ISSUES
Neurocardiogenic Changes Intraoperatively

General anesthesia can be complicated by strong vagal responses, such as severe bradycardia (to the point of asystole) (61). Other hypotensive effects may be neurally-triggered in response to specific precipitants (pain/emotion, carotid sinus stimulation, micturition, anesthesia, hypovolemia) and are characterized by both peripheral vasodilation and bradycardia (61). In the setting of anesthesia, vasovagal reactions typically occur at induction and are associated with pain and/or emotional distress (61). The possible reduction in venous return that can occur with laparoscopy (62) may predispose patients to vasovagal reactions as well.

Regional anesthesia can similarly cause decreased venous return, and is associated with frequent bradycardia and hypotension (on the order of 5%, with approximately 0.3% incidence of life-threatening hemodynamic embarrassment) (61). Incidence of hypotension with regional anesthesia increases with age (63), making the elderly population common in urological procedures more likely to suffer hemodynamic compromise. The primary mechanism of regional anesthesia-induced hypotension appears to be decreased venous return, with decreased vascular resistance playing a more minor role (63).

In the mid-1990s, prostate anesthetic block was proposed as an alternative to spinal or general anesthesia for transurethral prostate procedures, in an attempt to minimize anesthesia-induced hemodynamic changes (64). This approach appears to significantly reduce (from approximately 55% to 0%, in a study of approximately 90 patients) the incidence of anesthesia-induced hypotension (65).

Clinicians should distinguish between vagal and vasovagal reactions in order to provide prompt and appropriate treatment. Whereas vagal reactions generally resolve spontaneously upon cessation of the stimulus precipitating the reaction, the peripheral vasodilation that occurs in a vasovagal reaction may not be as easily reversed (61). Immediate response should focus on augmenting venous return via mechanical (Trendelenberg positioning, elevation of lower extremities) and/or intravenous (fluid resuscitation) means, as well as administration of sympathomimetic agents (e.g., ephedrine) to improve peripheral vascular tone (61). In addition, neurocardiogenic changes can be minimized by institution of preventive measures, including limiting the maximum level of sensory blockade and optimizing volume status preoperatively, as the observed changes will be exaggerated in the setting of hypovolemia (63,66). Preoperative hydration should be guided by volume status rather than empiric, as empiric volume loading has not been shown to be beneficial (63,66).

While anesthesia is the primary cause of neurocardiogenic changes intraoperatively, it is important to remember that the psychological/emotional implications of genitourinary procedures may also facilitate vasovagal reactions, independent of anesthesia/medication administration. Such reactions are more common in patients with a history of syncope, which should be explored in the preoperative history and physical (61).

Other Effects of Mechanism of Anesthesia

In addition to the vasodilatory effects of anesthetic medications, additional hemodynamic changes are observed with general anesthesia, due to the institution of positive pressure ventilation. In this setting, central venous pressure (CVP) will be increased and venous return decreased due to the positive pressure provided by the ventilator. This can in turn affect Starling forces, and in fact, has been shown to reduce the rate of irrigational fluid absorption during transurethral resection of the prostate (TURP), relative to regional anesthesia (67).

PROCEDURE-SPECIFIC CARDIOVASCULAR ISSUES
Laparoscopy—Specific Cardiovascular Issues

Laparoscopic procedures are associated with a number of physiological changes including (62):

1. Increased mean arterial pressure (MAP)
2. Increased heart rate
3. Increased arterial CO_2 concentration ($PaCO_2$)
4. Alterations in CVP—increased at low intra-abdominal pressures in response to hypercarbia, but decreased at high intra-abdominal pressures due to decreased venous return

During laparoscopic surgery, CO_2 is used to produce pneumoperitoneum in order to minimize the risk of gas embolism. The target intra-abdominal pressure (~15 mmHg) is associated with small perturbations in hemodynamics (62). The cardiovascular safety of laparoscopy in high-risk patients is not well defined; for example, only two small studies (less than 25 patients combined) have reported outcomes in high-risk patients undergoing laparoscopic cholecystectomy (62). The surgical stress response appears reduced in patients undergoing laparoscopic procedures relative to open laparotomy. In a study comparing laparoscopic cholecystectomy to open cholecystectomy, Karayiannakis et al. found significantly decreased elevations in the levels of plasma cortisol, catecholamines, glucose, C-reactive protein (CRP), and IL-6 in patients undergoing laparoscopic procedures (68). This diminution of the surgically induced activation of sympathetic and hypothalamic/pituitary/adrenal axes may reduce the risk of MI.

Laparoscopic Nephrectomy

Pneumoperitoneum is associated with a decrease in renal perfusion. In renal transplant, this creates concerns not only for the recipient, given the possibility of ischemic damage to the donor organ, but also to the donor, whose remaining kidney may be damaged by laparoscopic harvest of the donor organ. Research in animal models suggests that volume expansion may minimize the hemodynamic effects of pneumoperitoneum, but such maneuvers are not fully protective against renal impairment (69). Retrospective comparison of laparoscopic and open nephrectomy suggests that renal impairment associated with laparoscopy is not permanent, with comparable creatinine levels after the first week in transplant recipients, and after the first year in transplant donors (70). While these long-term results are reassuring, further work is indicated to identify maneuvers that will reduce the short-term impact of laparoscopy on renal function.

Transurethral Resection of the Prostate

An Australian review of in-hospital deaths following urological surgery found that almost half of the observed deaths occurred after TURP, and were in general due to acute MI (71). This likely reflects an association between benign prostatic hyperplasia (BPH) and cardiovascular risk factors/disease, as cardiovascular mortality rates are similar in patients who undergo transurethral microwave thermotherapy (72). While observational studies have found that TURP is associated with higher cardiovascular event rates than open prostatectomy (73), this likely reflects a selection bias, with open procedures being preferred performed in healthier patients with fewer comorbidities (74).

As noted earlier, the amount of irrigant absorbed intraoperatively during a TURP depends in part upon the mode of anesthesia (67). In the extreme case, excessive/rapid absorption of irrigant can cause the so-called "TURP syndrome," characterized by hyperglycemia, hyperammonemia, and serum hypotonicity, with associated dilutional hyponatremia. These metabolic perturbations cause both central nervous system and cardiovascular changes, including hypertension, bradycardia, and in the extreme case, cardiovascular collapse (75). Historically, the only means to reduce the risk of TURP syndrome was to reduce surgical resection time and irrigating hydrostatic pressure (75). More recently, however, the development of bipolar TURP systems has enabled the use of normal saline as an irrigant in place of nonconductive irrigants (e.g., glycine), making TURP syndrome a historical footnote in facilities that employ the newer technology (76).

Lithotripsy

As noted earlier, lithotripsy can produce EMI that disrupts the function of PPMs and ICDs (59). Consequently, patients with these devices should be evaluated by an electrophysiologist prior to and immediately after any lithotripsy procedure.

CONCLUSIONS

Urologic procedures are generally associated with a low to intermediate levels of risk for cardiovascular complications. Preoperative assessment in the majority of cases can be achieved through a careful history and physical examination without specific cardiovascular testing prior to surgery. Preoperative revascularization is rarely indicated, except in unusual circumstances.

A cardiologist should be consulted if antiplatelet therapy is to be discontinued to facilitate surgery in a patient who has received a coronary stent. In patients at intermediate to high risk, beta-blockade should be provided throughout the perioperative period. Further investigation is needed to clarify the role of statins and aspirin in these patients. Careful attention to intra-abdominal pressures during laparoscopic procedures is essential, as these pressures largely determine the hemodynamic effects of the procedure.

REFERENCES

1. Cooper R, Cutler J, Desvigne-Nickens P, et al. Trends and disparities in coronary heart disease, stroke, and other cardiovascular diseases in the United States. Circulation 2000; 102(25):3137–3147.
2. Lee TH, Marcantonio ER, Mangione CM, et al. Derivation and prospective validation of a simple index for prediction of cardiac risk of major noncardiac surgery. Circulation 1999; 100(10):1043–1049.
3. Devereaux PJ, Goldman L, Cook DJ, Gilbert K, Leslie K, Guyatt GH. Perioperative cardiac events in patients undergoing noncardiac surgery: a review of the magnitude of the problem, the pathophysiology of the events and methods to estimate and communicate risk. CMAJ Can Medl Assoc J 2005; 173(6):627–634.
4. Boersma E, Kertai MD, Schouten O, et al. Perioperative cardiovascular mortality in noncardiac surgery: validation of the Lee cardiac risk index. Am J Med 2005; 118(10):1134–1141.
5. Fleisher LA, Eagle KA. Clinical practice. Lowering cardiac risk in noncardiac surgery. N Eng J Med 2001; 345(23):1677–1682.
6. Naghavi M, Libby P, Falk E, et al. From vulnerable plaque to vulnerable patient: a call for new definitions and risk assessment strategies: Part II. Circulation 2003; 108(15):1772–1778.
7. Naghavi M, Libby P, Falk E, et al. From vulnerable plaque to vulnerable patient: a call for new definitions and risk assessment strategies: Part I. Circulation 2003; 108(14):1664–1672.
8. Landesberg G. The pathophysiology of perioperative myocardial infarction: facts and perspectives. J Cardiothor Vasc Anesth 2003; 17(1):90–100.
9. Libby P. Current concepts of the pathogenesis of the acute coronary syndromes. Circulation 2001; 104(3):365–372.
10. Libby P, Theroux P. Pathophysiology of coronary artery disease. Circulation 2005; 111(25):3481–3488.
11. Ellis SG, Hertzer NR, Young JR, Brener S. Angiographic correlates of cardiac death and myocardial infarction complicating major nonthoracic vascular surgery. Am J Cardiol 1996; 77:1126–1128.
12. Guidelines for assessing and managing the perioperative risk from coronary artery disease associated with major noncardiac surgery. American College of Physicians. Ann Int Med 1997; 127(4): 309–312.
13. Eagle KA, Berger PB, Calkins H, et al. ACC/AHA guideline update for perioperative cardiovascular evaluation for noncardiac surgery-executive summary: a report of the American College of Cardiology/American Heart Association Task Force on Practice Guidelines (Committee to Update the 1996 Guidelines on Perioperative Cardiovascular Evaluation for Noncardiac Surgery). J Am Coll Cardiol 2002; 39(3):542–553.
14. Landesberg G, Luria MH, Cotev S, et al. Importance of long-duration postoperative ST-segment depression in cardiac morbidity after vascular surgery. Lancet 1993; 341(8847):715–719.
15. Canty JMJ. Effect of tachycardia on regional function and transmural myocardial perfusion during graded coronary pressure reduction in conscious dogs. Circulation 1990; 81:1815–1825.
16. Landesberg G, Zhou W, Aversano T. Tachycardia-induced subendocardial necrosis in acutely instrumented dogs with fixed coronary stenosis. Anesth Analg 1999; 88:973–979.
17. Steen PA, Tinker JH, Tarhan S. Myocardial reinfarction after anesthesia and surgery. JAMA 1978; 239(24):2566–2570.
18. Eagle KA, Rihal CS, Mickel MC, Holmes DR, Foster ED, Gersh BJ. Cardiac risk of noncardiac surgery: influence of coronary disease and type of surgery in 3368 operations. CASS Investigators and University of Michigan Heart Care Program. Coronary Artery Surgery Study. Circulation 1997; 96(6):1882–1887.
19. Eagle KA, Berger PB, Calkins H, et al. ACC/AHA guideline update for perioperative cardiovascular evaluation for noncardiac surgery-executive summary a report of the American College of Cardiology/American Heart Association Task Force on Practice Guidelines (Committee to Update the 1996 Guidelines on Perioperative Cardiovascular Evaluation for Noncardiac Surgery). Circulation 2002; 105(10):1257–1267.
20. Fletcher GF, Balady GJ, Amsterdam EA, et al. Exercise standards for testing and training: a statement for healthcare professionals from the American Heart Association. Circulation 2001; 104:1694–1670.
21. Kertai MD, Boersma E, Bax JJ, et al. A meta-analysis comparing the prognostic accuracy of six diagnostic tests for predicting perioperative cardiac risk in patients undergoing major vascular surgery. Heart 2003; 89:1327–1334.
22. Manthous C. Leapfrog and Critical Care: Evidence- and Reality-Based Intensive Care for the 21st Century. Am J Med 2004; 116:188–193.

23. Connors AF, Jr., Speroff T, Dawson NV, et al. The effectiveness of right heart catheterization in the initial care of critically ill patients. SUPPORT Investigators. JAMA 1996; 276(11):889–897.

24. Polanczyk CA, Rohde LE, Goldman L, et al. Right heart catheterization and cardiac complications in patients undergoing noncardiac surgery: an observational study. JAMA 2001; 286(3):309–314.

25. Hall JB. Searching for evidence to support pulmonary artery catheter use in critically ill patients. JAMA 2005; 294(13):1693–1694.

26. Shah MR, Hasselbad V, Stevenson LW, et al. Impact of the pulmonary artery catheter in critically ill patients: meta-analysis of randomized clinical trials. JAMA 2005; 294(13):1664–1670.

27. Sandham JD, Hull RD, Brant RF, et al. A randomized, controlled trial of the use of pulmonary-artery catheters in high-risk surgical patients. N Eng J Med 2003; 348(1):5–14.

28. Parsons PE. Progress in research on pulmonary-artery catheters. N Eng J Med 2003; 348(1):66–68.

29. Mangano DT, Layug EL, Wallace A, Tateo I. Effect of atenolol on mortality and cardiovascular morbidity after noncardiac surgery. N Eng J Med 1996; 335(23):1713–1720.

30. Poldermans D, Boersma E, Bax JJ, et al. The effect of bisoprolol on perioperative mortality and myocardial infarction in high-risk patients underoing vascular surgery. N Eng J Med 1999; 341:1789–1794.

31. Lindenauer PK, Pekow P, Wang K, Mamidi DK, Gutierrez B, Benjamin EM. Perioperative beta-blocker therapy and mortality after major noncardiac surgery. N Eng J Med 2005; 353(4):349–361.

32. Poldermans D, Boersma E. Beta-blocker therapy in noncardiac surgery. N Eng J Med 2005; 353(4): 412–414.

33. Stevens RD, Burri H, Tramer MR. Pharmacologic myocardial protection in patients undergoing noncardiac surgery: a quantitative systematic review. Anesth Analg 2003; 97:623–633.

34. Fleischer LA, Beckman JA, Brown KA, et al. ACC/AHA 2006 Guideline update on perioperative cardiovascular evaluation for noncardiac surgery: focused update on perioperative beta-blocker therapy. J Am Coll Cardiol 2006; 47(11):2243–2255.

35. Lopez-Sendon J, Swedberg K, McMurray J, et al. Expert consensus document on beta-adrenergic receptor blockers. Eur Heart J 2004; 25(15):1341–1362.

36. Wallace AW, Galindez D, Salahieh A, et al. Effect of clonidine on cardiovascular morbidity and mortality after noncardiac surgery. Anesthesiology 2004; 101(2):284–293.

37. Devereaux PJ, Goldman L, Yusuf S, Gilbert K, Leslie K, Guyatt GH. Surveillance and prevention of major perioperative ischemic cardiac events in patients undergoing noncardiac surgery: a review. CMAJ Can Med Assoc J 2005; 173(7):779–788.

38. Liao JK. Clinical implications for statin pleiotropy. Curr Opin Lipidol 2005; 16(6):624–629.

39. Kertai MD, Boersma E, Westerhout CM, et al. A combination of statins and beta-blockers is independently associated with a reduction in the incidence of perioperative mortality and nonfatal myocardial infarction in patients undergoing abdominal aortic aneurysm surgery. Eur J Vasc Endovasc Surg 2004; 28(4):343–352.

40. Kertai MD, Boersma E, Westerhout CM, et al. Association between long-term statin use and mortality after successful abdominal aortic aneurysm surgery. Am J Med 2004; 116(2):96–103.

41. Schouten O, Kertai MD, Bax JJ, et al. Safety of perioperative statin use in high-risk patients undergoing major vascular surgery. Am J Cardiol 2005; 95(5):658–660.

42. Schouten O, Poldermans D, Visser L, et al. Fluvastatin and bisoprolol for the reduction of perioperative cardiac mortality and morbidity in high-risk patients undergoing non-cardiac surgery: rationale and design of the DECREASE-IV study. Am Heart J 2004; 148(6):1047–1052.

43. Mangano DT. Aspirin and mortality from coronary bypass surgery. N Eng J Med 2002; 347(17): 1309–1317.

44. Dacey LJ, Munoz JJ, Johnson ER, et al. Effect of preoperative aspirin use on mortality in coronary artery bypass grafting patients. Ann Thorac Surg 2000; 70:1986–1990.

45. Bybee KA, Powell BD, Valeta U, et al. Preoperative aspirin therapy is associated with improved postoperative outcomes in patients underoing coronary artery bypass grafting. Circulation 2005; 112:286–292.

46. McFalls EO, Ward HB, Moritz TE, et al. Coronary-artery revascularization before elective major vascular surgery. N Eng J Med 2004; 351(27):2795–2804.

47. Kaluza GL, Joseph J, Lee JR, Raizner ME, Raizner AE. Catastrophic outcomes of noncardiac surgery soon after coronary stenting. J Am Coll Cardiol 2000; 35(5):1288–1294.

48. Wilson SH, Fasseas P, Orford JL, et al. Clinical outcome of patients underoing non-cardiac surgery in the two months following coronary stenting. J Am Coll Cardiol 2003; 42(2):234–240.

49. Serruys PW, Kutryk MJB, Ong ATL. Drug Therapy: Coronary-Artery stents. N Eng J Med 2006; 354:483–495.

50. Weitz HH. How soon can a patient undergo noncardiac surgery after receiving a drug-eluting stent. Cleveland Clin J Med 2005; 72(9):818–820.

51. Torsher LC, Shub C, Rettke SR, Brown DL. Risk of patients with severe aortic stenosis undergoing noncardiac surgery. Am J Cardiol 1998; 81(4):448–452.

52. Hunt SA, Abraham WT, Chin MH, et al. ACC/AHA 2005 Guideline update for the diagnosis and management of chronic heart failure in the adult. J Am Coll Cardiol 2005; 46(6):1–82.

53. Haering JM, Comunale ME, Parker RA. Cardiac risk of noncardiac surgery in patients with asymmetric septal hypertrophy. Anesthesiology 1996; 85:254–259.
54. Salukhe TV, Dob D, Sutton R. Pacemakers and defribrillators: anaessthetic implications. Br J Anaesth 2004; 93(1):95–104.
55. Rozner M. Pacemaker misinformation in the perioperative period: programming around the problem. Anesth Analg 2004; 99:1582–1584.
56. Madigan JDBA, Choudhri AFBS, Chen JMD, Spotnitz HMMD, Oz MCMD, Edwards NMD. Surgical Management of the Patient with an Implanted Cardiac Device: Implications of Electromagnetic Interference. Ann Surg 1999; 230(5):639.
57. Pinski SL. Emergencies related to implantable cardioverter-defibrillators. Crit Care Med 2000; 28(10 suppl):N174–180.
58. Pinski SL, Trohman RG. Interference in implanted cardiac devices, part II. Pacing Clinl Electrophysiol 2002; 25(10):1496–1509.
59. Goldschlager N, Epstein A, Friedman P, Gang E, Krol R, Olshansky B. Environmental and drug effects on patients with pacemakers and implantable cardioverter/defibrillators: a practical guide to patient treatment. Arch Int Med 2001; 161(5):649–655.
60. Hollenberg SM, Dellinger RP. Noncardiac surgery: postoperative arrhythmias. Crit Care Med 2000; 28 (suppl):N145–N150.
61. Kinsella SM, Tuckey JP. Perioperative bradycardia and asystole: relationship to vasovagal syncope and the Bezold-Jarisch reflex. Br J Anaesth 2001; 86(6):859–68.
62. Taylor GD, Cadeddu JA. Applications of laparoscopic surgery in urology: impact on patient care. Med Clin N Am 2004; 88(2):519–538.
63. Stienstra R. Mechanisms behind and treatment of sudden, unexpected circulatory collapse during central neuraxis blockade. Acta Anaesthesiol Scand 2000; 44(8):965–971.
64. Tabet BG, Levine S. Nerve block in prostate surgery. J Urol 1996; 156(5):1659–1661.
65. Niccolai P, Carles M, Lagha K, Raucoules-Aime M. Prostate anaesthetic block with ropivacaine for urologic surgery. Eur J Anaesthesiol 2005; 22(11):864–869.
66. Buggy D, Higgins P, Moran C, O'Brien D, O'Donovan F, McCarroll M. Prevention of spinal anesthesia-induced hypotension in the elderly: comparison between preanesthetic administration of crystalloids, colloids, and no prehydration. Anesth Analg 1997; 84(1):106–110.
67. Gehring H, Nahm W, Baerwald J, et al. Irrigation fluid absorption during transurethral resection of the prostate: spinal vs. general anaesthesia. Acta Anaesthesiol Scand 1999; 43(4):458–463.
68. Karayiannakis AJ, Makri GG, Mantzioka A, Karousos D, Karatzas G. Systemic stress response after laparoscopic or open cholecystectomy: a randomized trial. Br J Surg 1997; 84(4):467–471.
69. London ET, Ho HS, Neuhaus AM, Wolfe BM, Rudich SM, Perez RV. Effect of intravascular volume expansion on renal function during prolonged CO2 pneumoperitoneum. Ann Surg 2000; 231(2):195–201.
70. Lind MY, Zur Borg IM, Hazebroek EJ, et al. The effect of laparoscopic and open donor nephrectomy on the long-term renal function in donor and recipient: a retrospective study. Transplantation 2005; 80(5):700–703.
71. Gyomber D, Lawrentschuk N, Ranson DL, Bolton DM. An analysis of deaths related to urological surgery, reviewed by the State Coroner: a case for cardiac vigilence before transurethral prostatectomy. BJU Int 2006; 97(4):758–761.
72. Hahn RG, Farahmand BY, Hallin A, Hammar N, Persson PG. Incidence of acute myocardial infarction and cause-specific morality after transurethral treatments of prostatic hypertrophy. Urology 2000; 55(2):236–240.
73. Roos NP, Wennberg JE, Malenka DJ, et al. Mortality and reoperation after open and transurethral resection of the prostate for benign prostatic hypertrophy. N Eng J Med 1989; 320:1120–1124.
74. Seagrott V. Mortality after prostatectomy: selection and surgical approach. Lancet 1995; 346:1521–1524.
75. Jensen V. The TURP syndrome. Can J Anaesth 1991; 38(1):90–97.
76. Issa MM, Young MR, Bullock AR, Bouet R, Petros JA. Dilutional hyponatremia of the TURP syndrome: a historical event of the 21st century. Urology 2004; 64:298–301.

3 Metabolic Complications Following the Use of Intestine and Metabolic Abnormalities Occurring with Irrigants in Urologic Surgery

W. Scott McDougal
Harvard Medical School and Department of Urology, Massachusetts General Hospital, Boston, Massachusetts, U.S.A.

INTRODUCTION

The use of intestine in the urinary tract results in altered solute reabsorption, which has protean manifestations and has the potential to alter normal homeostatic mechanisms. In the presence of a normally functioning kidney with adequate renal reserve, most of these untoward effects are blunted so that they do not become clinically significant. On occasion, however, when intestinal segments are substantial or renal function is compromised, severe and oftentimes debilitating metabolic derangements occur. As a general rule, ileum and colon have similar abnormalities, whereas jejunum and stomach have distinct and separate metabolic consequences. What follows is a description of specific metabolic abnormalities and how each segment contributes to alterations in homeostasis (1,2,3). Finally, the metabolic complications of commonly used irrigants in urologic practice is considered.

ELECTROLYTE ABNORMALITIES

Each segment of the gastrointestinal tract when exposed to urine has specific absorption characteristics. If the segment chosen is the stomach, a hypokalemic metabolic alkalosis may occur. This abnormality is rarely significant except in circumstances where there is compromised renal function, severe sepsis intervenes, or if the patient is subject to dehydration and the bowel segment is distended. Since protons are secreted by the stomach with the net addition of bicarbonate to the systemic circulation, the kidney must be efficient in excreting the excess bicarbonate load. If it is not, then systemic metabolic alkalosis occurs. In selected circumstances, when the segment is distended and the patient is dehydrated, the alkalosis can become severe, which is referred to as the syndrome of severe metabolic alkalosis. Patients particularly prone to the syndrome are those who have a high resting level of serum gastrin. This is due to the fact that the relationship between serum bicarbonate and gastrin is sigmoidal. At high resting levels of serum gastrin, small incremental increases in its level due to distention of the gastric segment results in large changes in serum bicarbonate; whereas, at medium levels of serum gastrin, substantial changes in its concentration result in small changes in serum bicarbonate. Those most likely to develop the syndrome are those who have high normal resting levels of gastrin, thus placing them on the tail of the sigmoid curve. When they become dehydrated and allow their segment to become distended, a slight increase in gastrin results in a large increase in serum bicarbonate. Since dehydration compromises the ability of the kidney to excrete the excess bicarbonate, persistent alkalosis ensues. The patient may present with muscle weakness, lethargy, and seizures. If allowed to progress, the condition may lead to death. The treatment for this disorder is hydration, decompression of the gastric segment, and in severe cases the use of proton pump inhibitors such as omiprozol.

When jejunal segments are employed, the metabolic derangement, which may occur is a hyponatremic, hypochloremic, hypokalemic metabolic acidosis. These electrolyte abnormalities may be minimized by keeping the segment short. Dehydration and hypovolemia exacerbate the syndrome and in severe situations, lethargy, nausea, vomiting, dehydration, weakness, and fever may occur. Treatment includes hydration, sodium chloride repletion, and correction of the acidosis. When short segments of jejunum are used for urinary diversion, the syndrome rarely occurs.

With the use of ileum and colon, the metabolic abnormality, which occurs is a hyperchloremic metabolic acidosis. This results from the substitution of ammonium ion for sodium in the sodium/hydrogen antiport of the colon. To maintain electrical neutrality, chloride is absorbed in exchange for bicarbonate. Thus, ammonium chloride is reabsorbed with the excretion of carbonic acid. The carbonic acid disassociates into CO_2 and water with a net absorption of ammonium chloride. Patients who are particularly prone to hyperammonemia and hyperchloremic metabolic acidosis are those with compromised renal function and those with impaired hepatic function. When ileum is employed, total body potassium loss may also occur over the long term. This may occur with the colon as well, but potassium depletion is more likely to occur when long segments of the ileum are used. Treatment includes correction of the acidosis and repletion of potassium. Both may be accomplished with balanced citrate solutions or the administration of sodium bicarbonate along with potassium chloride, as needed.

CALCULUS FORMATION

Patients with urinary intestinal diversions are at a higher risk for development of urinary calculi. This may be due to several mechanisms, which include infection, dehydration, foreign bodies in the reconstructed segment, abnormal mucus production, and increased secretion of calcium and oxalate by the kidney. Treatment generally centers around citrate supplementation as well as hydration and eradication of infection, and stasis. If a foreign body, such as staples, is responsible, it should be removed.

NUTRITIONAL DISTURBANCES

It has been shown that children who undergo a urinary intestinal diversion, over the long term, may demonstrate growth and bone disturbances. When distal ileum or the antrum of the stomach is used, vitamin B_{12} deficiencies may occur. If the segment removed from the gastrointestinal tract results in bile salts irritating the colon, steatorrhea, and fat-soluble vitamin deficiencies (A, D, E, and K) may also occur. Finally, achievement of normal growth and development has been shown to be diminished in children with long-standing urinary intestinal diversions.

BONE DISTURBANCES

Patients who have persistent metabolic acidosis are prone to increased bone reabsorption resulting in osteomalasia. This has been well described in patients with severe and prolonged metabolic acidosis. Osteomalasia in adults and rickets in children have been observed in patients with ureterosigmoidostomies, ileal ureters, and augmentation cystoplasties. It has been shown that if patients are kept in balance with respect to acid–base status, these abnormalities of the bone are less likely to occur.

GLUCOSE METABOLISM, HEPATIC METABOLISM, AND ABNORMAL DRUG METABOLISM

Patients who have a significant impairment of liver function are prone to abnormalities in drug metabolism. Drugs may reach toxic proportions when they are incompletely metabolized, excreted unchanged in the urine, and reabsorbed by the intestinal segment. Hyperammonemia also may occur particularly in patients who have compromised hepatic function. Diabetics may on occasion have reabsorption of glucose excreted in the urine by the intestinal segment, thereby resulting in hyperglycemia. Adjusting insulin dosage is therapeutic. Of particular concern is the reabsorption of antimetabolites given for malignant conditions. Placing the segment on catheter drainage and establishing a diuresis blunts these effects.

ABSORPTION OF IRRIGANTS

A number of irrigants are used in the genitourinary system during urologic procedures. These include irrigants used to dissolve stones, that is, renacidin, Suby's Solution G, and irrigants used for endoscopic procedures, which include water, glycine, sodium chloride, sorbatol, and urea. Each one of these irrigants may have significant untoward effects particularly if excessive absorption occurs. With the use of renacidin or Suby's Solution G, magnesium intoxication may occur with increased salivation followed by hypotension, seizures, and coma. It is particularly dangerous to utilize these solutions in the presence of infection as sepsis may be a sequelae. The use of water, glycine, sorbatol, and urea as irrigants may result in volume overload and severe hyponetremia—termed the transurethral resection syndrome. Significant volume overload results in an increased pulse pressure, bradycardia and in the case of severe hyponetremia, visual disturbances followed by seizures, coma, and death. The correction of these abnormalities, if hyponetremia is a major component, includes diuresis with restoration of systemic sodium. In severe cases of hyponatremia in patients who are symptomatic, half of the sodium deficit is replaced with hypertonic saline. It should be noted that diuretics do not work in patients with severe hyponetremia. Therefore, repletion may be necessary before a loop diuretic is effective. The use of saline as an irrigant results in volume overload and volume expansion without hypernatremia. A diuretic and fluid restriction are therapeutic. On occasion ammonium intoxication may occur with the use of glycine.

In summary, there are a number of metabolic derangements, which may be a consequence of intestine interposed in the urinary tract and the use of irrigants in the genito urinary tract. Prevention of untoward long-term sequelae is best accomplished by recognition of the potential problems and correcting the metabolic abnormalities early, even though they may be of minor degree.

REFERENCES

1. Gerharz EW, McDougal WS. Urinary diversion. World J Urol 2004; 22:155–234.
2. Tanrikut C, McDougal WS. Metabolic implications and electrolyte disturbances. In: Webster GD, Goldwasser B, eds. Urinary Diversion: Scientific Foundation in Clinical Practice. 2nd ed. London: Oxford, Isis Medical Media, 2005, Chapter 3.
3. McDougal WS. Metabolic complications of urinary intestinal diversion. J Urol 1992; 147:1199–1208.

4 | Anesthesia for Urogenital Surgery

Linda S. Aglio
Department of Anesthesiology, Perioperative and Pain Medicine, Brigham and Women's Hospital, Boston, Massachusetts, U.S.A.

James A. Street
Department of Anesthesia, Emerson Hospital, Concord, Massachusetts, U.S.A.

Paul D. Allen
Department of Anesthesiology, Perioperative and Pain Medicine, Brigham and Women's Hospital, Boston, Massachusetts, U.S.A.

INTRODUCTION

Patients requiring anesthesia for genitourinary procedures are often of advanced age. With aging, physiological changes occur, as well as an increased incidence of cardiovascular and respiratory disease. Evaluation of medical conditions that might influence anesthetic management and monitoring depends upon a good history and physical examination as part of the preoperative assessment. Urologic procedures are performed on the kidney, adrenals, ureters, urinary bladder, prostate, urethra, penis, scrotum, testes, and spermatic cord. The sensory supply of these structures is mostly the thoracolumbar and sacral outflow, making many of these procedures well suited for regional anesthesia. This chapter reviews the more commonly performed genitourinary procedures and describes anesthetic implications and management.

TRANSURETHRAL PROCEDURES
Cystoscopy
Preoperative Considerations

The most commonly performed urologic procedure is cystoscopy. This procedure may be performed using a flexible or rigid cystoscope, either for diagnostic or therapeutic purposes. Hematuria, recurrent urinary infections, and obstruction are the most common indications. Bladder biopsies, removal of bladder and prostate tumors, renal stone extraction, retrograde pyelography, and placement of urinary catheters and stents are generally performed with rigid cystoscopy.

Anesthetic Management
The choice of anesthetic technique varies with the patient and the type of procedure. For most flexible cystoscopies, topical anesthesia with lidocaine is used successfully (1), particularly in women because of the short urethra. Diagnostic rigid cystoscopy of the urethra with topical anesthesia is also well tolerated by most women. In addition, intravenous sedation with a short-acting benzodiazepine, opioid, or propofol may be used. For diagnostic procedures, most male patients require regional or general anesthesia. Regional or general anesthesia is required for most operative cystoscopies.

Some patients may be anxious and prefer to be asleep. General anesthesia may be used for these patients, particularly if they are undergoing long procedures. If general anesthesia is selected, thiopental or propofol with oxygen in nitrous oxide and an inhalation agent may be used. The airway may be managed with conventional endotracheal intubation or a laryngeal mask airway. Controlled ventilation with an endotracheal tube is the best option in patients who are obese, since limited pulmonary reserve may lead to arterial oxygen desaturation when the obese patient is placed in the lithotomy or Trendelenburg position.

Regional anesthesia with a T6 sensory level will provide satisfactory anesthesia for most cystoscopy procedures, including ureteroscopy and stone extraction. Spinal anesthesia is most often used. Transient neurologic symptoms are a concern with lidocaine use, and hyperbaric 0.75% bupivacaine, in the usual dose range of 10 to 15 mg, has become the drug of choice. For short procedures, a 7.5-mg dose will be sufficient in most cases. Studies fail to demonstrate that immediate elevation of the legs after intrathecal hyperbaric anesthesia solution increases the level of anesthesia or the incidence of hypotension (2). In addition, Trendelenburg position does not always increase cephalad spread of hyperbaric local anesthesia during spinal anesthesia (3). However, the site of injection does seem to influence cephalad spread, with the sensory level appearing to be several dermatomes higher than the site of injection (4).

Regional anesthesia does not block the obturator reflex unless obturator nerve blocks are also performed. Muscle contractions are only reliably blocked by paralysis during general anesthesia. Electrocautery current through the lateral wall of the bladder can cause external rotation and adduction of the thigh, with the potential to cause the surgeon to perforate the bladder with the cystoscope.

Patients with spinal cord lesions often require repeated cystoscopies. If the lesion is above T_6-T_7, the patient is at elevated risk for autonomic hyper-reflexia. This disorder is characterized by a paroxysm of generalized sympathetic hyperactivity in response to stimulation below the level of the cord lesion. Such patients typically present with severe hypertension and bradycardia. Pallor, piloerection, somatic and visceral contraction, and increased spasticity occur below the lesion. Flushing of the face, congestion of the mucous membranes, sweating, and mydriasis occur above the lesion. Episodes can be self-limiting, but may result in hypertensive encephalopathy, stroke, arrhythmias, myocardial ischemia, and death if not treated.

Transurethral Resection of the Prostate
Preoperative Considerations

Benign prostatic hypertrophy (BPH) is a disease seen in the elderly male population, and may require surgical removal of the prostate gland. Surgical intervention becomes necessary when obstruction of urinary outflow through the prostatic urethra becomes symptomatic. Transurethral resection of the prostate (TURP) is preferred over suprapubic, retropubic, and perineal approaches, which allow better surgical exposure, but carry a higher morbidity. Because this approach necessitates the use of large volumes of nonelectrolyte irrigating fluid for endoscopic resection, TURP carries unique complications. Systemic absorption of irrigating fluid can produce circulatory overload, hyponatremia, hypoproteinemia, and the presence of irrigating fluid solutes in the circulation.

The prostate gland is located at the base of the bladder, surrounding the prostatic urethra. The gland is pear-shaped and has five lobes. Only the median and lateral lobes are enlarged and surgically excised in primary idiopathic prostatic hypertrophy. In the majority of males older than 50 years of age, the submucosal glands and the smooth muscle of the prostate undergo glandular and leiomyomatous hyperplasia, a process stimulated by testicular hormones. Consequently the normal prostatic tissue is pressed against the fibrous capsule of the gland, forming a "surgical capsule," consisting of compressed normal prostatic tissue and veins, infiltrated by nodular or new growth. Compressed prostatic veins are entered during TURP and irrigating fluid is absorbed into the intravascular compartment. Fibrosis of the hypertrophied gland can occur, reducing the vascularity of the gland. Less bleeding occurs and less fluid enters the circulation when a fibrotic gland is resected.

TURP is performed through a resectoscope. The hypertrophied tissue of the prostate gland is excised with an electrically energized wire loop. Bleeding is controlled with a coagulating current. The bladder is distended, and dissected prostatic tissue is washed away, with a continuous flow of irrigating fluid. The use of distilled water provides the best visibility. However, the absorption of large quantities of water can lead to water intoxication. This, in turn, results in red blood cell hemolysis, dilutional hyponatremia, and central nervous system symptoms which range from confusion to convulsions and coma. This phenomenon is termed TURP syndrome. Although approximately isotonic electrolyte solutions, such as normal saline or Ringer's lactate, do the least amount of harm when absorbed into the systemic circulation, they are highly ionized and therefore promote dispersion of current from the resectoscope.

The use of distilled water has, in general, been abandoned in favor of nonelectrolyte solutions. Solutions of sorbitol and mannitol (Cytal), or of glycine, which are hypo-osmolar to the blood, are used predominantly (5,6).

Intravascular absorption of irrigating fluid occurs via the large venous sinuses of the hypertrophied gland. The amount of fluid absorption is governed by several factors, including the hydrostatic pressure driving fluid into the prostatic veins and sinuses, the vascularity of the gland, and the duration of resection (7). Hydrostatic pressure of the irrigating solution is determined by the height of the reservoir above the operating table. In relation to resection time, it is estimated that 10 to 30 mL of fluid is absorbed per minute of resection time. In prolonged cases, as much as 6 to 8 L may be absorbed over a two-hour period (7,8). Therefore, limiting resection time one hour or less is desirable (9).

In addition to TURP syndrome, other significant complications of TURP include hypothermia, bacteremia, blood loss and perforation of the bladder, or urethra with extravasation of irrigation fluids.

Since these patients are more likely to have coexisting cardiopulmonary problems, they generally carry greater anesthetic risk, and it is essential to the anesthetic management that the patient's preoperative condition be optimized. Common findings in males older than 60 years of age include hypertension, angina, congestive heart failure, cardiac rhythm management devices, diabetes mellitus, neurologic dysfunction, and renal insufficiency. Patients should be in the best possible condition prior to surgery, since TURP is an elective procedure.

Transurethral Resection of the Prostate Syndrome

During the intraoperative or immediate postoperative period of a TURP, a patient may manifest an untoward reaction. This reaction is initially characterized by headache, restlessness, confusion, nausea and vomiting, skeletal muscle twitching, bradycardia, and hypertension. Symptoms may evolve to hypotension, dyspnea, cyanosis, cardiac dysrhythmias, seizures, unconsciousness, and occasionally death (6–10). Severe dilutional hyponatremia is a major component of TURP syndrome, but fluid overload, serum hypo-osmolarity, hyperglycinemia, and hemolysis may contribute to morbidity and mortality. Adverse hemodynamic and central venous system changes can occur because of fluid shifts and cardiovascular compromise (11–13).

The most commonly used irrigating solutions for TURP are glycine and Cytal. Cytal is a combination of 2.7% sorbitol and 0.54% mannitol. It is nonelectrolytic, iso-osmolar, and is cleared from the plasma rapidly. Glycine 1.5% in water is most commonly used because of low cost relative to Cytal, but is a slightly hypo-osmolar solution (230 mOsm/L). Thus, hemolysis and many of the sequelae associated with the use of distilled water have been reduced or eliminated with the use of these new irrigating solutions. The problem of overhydration, however, still remains. Furthermore, the absorption of glycine and its metabolic product, ammonia, may raise the possibility of potential chemical toxicity (14–17).

There is considerable variability in the amounts of irrigating solution absorbed during TURP. The area of raw surface exposed by surgical resection, the hydrostatic pressure exerted by the irrigating solution, the duration of the procedure, and the vascularity of the gland are all important considerations (15). Blood proteins, as well as electrolytes, are diluted by the nonelectrolytic solution entering the vascular compartment. Movement of fluid from the vascular compartment to the interstitial space is favored as a result of increased intravascular pressure and decreased protein oncotic pressure (18). Ordinarily, only 20% to 30% of a crystalloid solution remains in the intravascular space and the remainder enters the interstitial space. For every 100 mL of fluid entering the interstitial compartment, 10 to 15 mEq of sodium also moves with it (10). The movement of fluid into the interstitial space and the development of pulmonary edema are favored when venous pressure is increased. The amount and speed of absorption of irrigating fluid, the extent of surgical blood loss, and the preoperative cardiovascular status will determine whether patients will develop symptoms of circulatory overload. It is crucial, therefore, to monitor patients undergoing TURP very carefully. Clearly, an awake patient has the advantage of being able to verbalize potential cardiopulmonary and central nervous system problems during surgery. Therefore, spinal or epidural anesthesia is preferred. The sympathetic blockade, which regional anesthesia produces increases the venous capacitance. This tends to protect against intraoperative fluid overload during TURP. When the block dissipates, however, the venous capacitance can acutely decrease, thereby precipitating circulatory overload in the immediate postoperative period.

Hyponatremia, arising from water intoxication, can seriously impair the electrophysiology of neurons and myocardial cells. For effective depolarization and the production and propagation of action potentials, extracellular sodium concentrations must be in a physiologic range. Central nervous system symptoms will occur and cardiac dysrhythmias may develop if brain and myocardial cells, respectively, are incapable of producing effective impulses. The development of serious reactions seems to occur with a threshold serum sodium level of about 120 mEq/L or less. At this point, restlessness and confusion may occur. Widening of the QRS complex and ST elevation on the electrocardiogram can occur when the serum sodium level falls below 115 mEq/L. In severe hyponatremia, cardiac dysrhythmias, hypotension, and pulmonary edema may also occur secondary to cardiovascular dysfunction (19). Loss of consciousness and seizures may occur at serum sodium levels below 100 mEq/L (20). The TURP syndrome must be recognized early and therapy instituted immediately. For fluid overload and dilutional hyponatremia, hypertonic saline and diuretics are useful therapy. The patients' serum electrolytes and osmolarity must be carefully monitored.

Visual impairment and even transient blindness have been reported following TURP. The absorption of glycine, a nonessential amino acid, and its metabolic byproduct, ammonia, have been implicated as possible causes (14,15). Both glycine and ammonia can produce central nervous system impairment, which includes (16), mild depression, confusion, transient blindness, and even coma. Pharmacologic doses of glycine have been shown to inhibit visual evoked potentials, both in animals (17) and in TURP patients (20).

Glycine has a distribution in the central nervous system similar to gamma aminobutyric acid (GABA), an inhibitory transmitter in the spinal cord and in the brain (21,22). During an episode of blindness in one patient, plasma glycine levels were as high as 1029 mg/L (14) compared to normal plasma glycine levels of 13–17 mg/L. Twelve hours later the patient's vision had returned and the plasma glycine level had fallen to 143 mg/L (14). The oxidative biotransformation of glycine to ammonia may also result in central nervous system toxicity (15,16). Elevated blood ammonia concentration, more than 10 times the upper limit of normal, was associated with encephalopathy after TURP in three patients (15). The production of false neurotransmitters and a suppression of norepinephrine and dopamine release may result from high ammonia concentrations in the central nervous system after neutral amino acid metabolism, an etiology of encephalopathy, which has been hypothesized in a subset of patients who develop TURP syndrome (15). Thus, although fluid overload, hyposmolarity and hyponatremia are recognized factors in TURP syndrome, hyperglycinemia and elevated blood levels of ammonia may also play a role. The information to date remains inconclusive.

Blood Loss in Transurethral Resection of the Prostate

Visual estimation of blood loss in TURP is often grossly inadequate (23,24). Furthermore, the usual hemodynamic responses to blood loss may be obscured by the increase in intravascular volume accompanying absorption of irrigating solution. The intraoperative hematocrit will also be an unreliable guide to blood loss, since it is influenced by the amount of irrigating solution absorbed. Intraoperative blood transfusion generally is not necessary, but should be based on the preoperative hematocrit, duration of the resection, and the clinical assessment of the patient's condition. It has been estimated that two units of blood may be required for transfusion if the predicted weight of a gland is 30 to 80 g, while resection of glands larger than 80 g may require transfusion of four units. In addition, these patients have a high incidence of fibrinolysis (25), which may contribute to intraoperative and postoperative bleeding. It has been hypothesized that prostatic tissue releases urokinase, which stimulates the transformation of plasminogen to plasmin, which, in turn, causes lysis of fibrin (25).

The vascularity of the prostate gland, the surgeon's experience and technique, the weight of the prostate resected, and the length of the operation are all factors determining blood loss during TURP (26–30). For comparative purposes, blood loss may be expressed in mL/g of prostate resected per minute. Abrams and his group (26) reported a reduction in blood loss when regional anesthesia was employed (median of 0.25 mL/g/min) compared to general anesthesia (median of 0.38 mL/g/min). There was no correlation between blood pressure and blood loss during the operation. Those patients undergoing TURP for carcinoma of the prostate, in general, have less blood loss than patients with benign prostatic hyperplasia (BPH) (27). Levin and his group (25) demonstrated that blood loss during TURP was fairly constant at about 15 mL/g. The severity of bleeding increased with the duration of the operation. Therefore, if the surgeon feels that he cannot complete his resection within one hour, a two-stage resection or an open operation may be preferable.

Hypothermia During Transurethral Resection of the Prostate
Geriatric patients tolerate hypothermia poorly. There is an age-related decline in the function of the autonomic nervous system and in the ability to increase heat production, which results in thermoregulatory impairment (31,32). The constant irrigation of cold fluid through the bladder, in addition to its intravascular absorption, can rapidly lower core body temperature. Furthermore, these patients are in cold operating rooms, and receive intravenous fluids at ambient temperature. The anesthetic technique used, general or regional, does not appear to influence intraoperative hypothermia (32,33). However, the use of warm intravenous and irrigating fluids, warming mattresses, and even warmed anesthetic gases, will help minimize the problem of excessive heat loss. Shivering, a direct consequence of hypothermia, causes increased oxygen consumption. Therefore, supplemental oxygen should be used in every patient. Shivering also increases venous pressure and promotes hemorrhage. Maintaining body temperature is an important consideration in providing for optimal care of TURP patients.

Bacteremia
Bacteremia is a common occurrence following TURP. Prior to surgery, infection of the prostate should be controlled with appropriate antibiotic therapy. Bacteremia may be manifested as fever, rigors, or cardiovascular collapse after TURP. In addition to hemodynamic supportive measures, blood cultures should be obtained and broad-spectrum antibiotic therapy should be instituted based on the preoperative urine culture results.

Perforation of the Bladder
Perforation of the bladder may occur during TURP. The incidence of perforation is estimated at 1.1% (34). Perforations are most often made by the cutting loop or the knife electrode, although the tip of the resectoscope is sometimes responsible. Overdistension of the bladder with irrigating fluid can also result in a perforation. Most perforations are extraperitoneal. In the awake patient, pain may occur in the periumbilical, inguinal, or suprapubic region. If the irrigation fluid fails to return as it normally does, perforation of the prostatic capsule is suspected. Occasionally, damage to the wall of the bladder may cause an intraperitoneal perforation, or a large extraperitoneal perforation may extend into the peritoneum. In such cases, pain might be referred from the diaphragm to the precordial region or the shoulder, or may be more generalized to the upper abdomen. Additional warning signs or symptoms may include pallor, diaphoresis, abdominal rigidity, nausea, vomiting, hypotension, or hypertension. Hiccups and shortness of breath may result from subdiaphragmatic irritation. Intraperitoneal fluid will usually be extruded by the kidney although catheter drainage may be necessary. Significant extravasation may need to be drained suprapubically (35).

Anesthetic Management
Each patient scheduled for TURP should be assessed on an individual basis and patient preferences should be taken into consideration. A conscious patient undergoing regional anesthesia provides the advantage of early symptomatic warning of fluid overload, hyponatremia, or perforation. Regional anesthesia may benefit patients with coronary artery disease and prior myocardial infarction undergoing TURP. The awake patient can communicate symptoms of myocardial ischemia. Additionally, the reinfarction rate for spinal anesthesia has been reported to be less than 1% versus 2% to 8% for general anesthesia (34). However, many patients prefer to be asleep and general anesthesia is an acceptable alternative, particularly when difficulties in placement of a local anesthetic in the subarachnoid or epidural space are anticipated. Although general anesthesia may mask the early signs and symptoms of TURP syndrome, it may be more

desirable in patients who require pulmonary support. Loss of sympathetic tone associated with regional anesthesia may be problematic in some patients, and the treatment of hypotension with intravenous fluids may be poorly tolerated in those with limited cardiac reserve. These patients may require invasive monitoring. Central venous or pulmonary artery pressure monitoring may be helpful under such conditions.

Spinal anesthesia has been advocated as the anesthetic choice for TURP. As stated earlier, symptoms of fluid overload, hyponatremia, and urinary bladder perforation can be recognized promptly in the awake patient. Spinal anesthesia produces a predictable sensory block using small amounts of local anesthetic agents. A continuous epidural anesthetic may be employed, but does not offer much advantage over spinal anesthesia, since the duration of resection is usually not more than one hour. Additionally, the block is less predictable than that achieved with subarachnoid local anesthetics, and sacral segments may sometimes be missed with lumbar epidural blockade. A T_9-T_{10} sensory level is desirable in order to block the uncomfortable sensation associated with bladder over-filling. However, an S_3 level has been shown to be adequate in approximately 25% of patients. An anesthetic level higher than T_{10} is not recommended, since the pain on perforation of the capsule of the prostate would not be apparent. Spinal anesthesia with lidocaine was a popular choice before the phenomenon of transient neurologic irritation became widely appreciated. More recently, hyperbaric 0.75% bupivacaine has been commonly employed for TURP. A caudal anesthetic may be suitable if a patient has had previous spine surgery or has an osteoarthritic spine. Local anesthesia, with intravenous supplementation with sedatives, has been used in patients with small to moderate prostate glands (34). 0.25% bupivacaine, 1% lidocaine, or both were injected into the prostate transurethrally, and transperineal infiltration into the gland was with a lidocaine–bupivacaine mixture.

It has been advocated that blood loss during TURP can be minimized with the use of a regional technique (26). Other investigators found no difference in blood loss in comparing patients under spinal versus those under general anesthesia, either breathing spontaneously or during mechanical ventilation of the lung. A significant cause of blood loss may be a rise in venous pressure resulting from straining or coughing. This can occur as a result of a partially obstructed airway or from painful stimuli. Abolishing these factors could conceivably cause a decrease in hemorrhage.

Morbidity and Mortality

Although spinal anesthesia offers certain distinct advantages over general anesthesia for TURP surgery, many markers of patient outcomes have been similar for both groups. What constitutes the safest anesthetic for prostatectomies was debated as early as 1924, with advocates of regional anesthesia gaining ground thereafter (36).

Some studies have shown that this procedure appears to carry a significantly higher mortality than the average anesthetic mortality (37,38). Factors which contribute to the morbidity associated with this surgical procedure include the anatomy of the pathologic hypertrophic gland, the size of the gland, and the skill of the surgeon. Currently, the 30-day mortality rate associated with TURP is reported to be 0.2% to 0.8% (39). Mortality rates are reported to be similar in patients receiving regional anesthesia or general anesthesia (40). Increasing mortality was found in patients with resections exceeding 90 minutes, gland size greater than 45 g, acute urinary retention, and age older than 80 years (39).

Postoperatively, these patients may benefit from diuresis, to prevent clot formation, and to remove the excess water and glycine from the body. Postoperative fluid balance should be monitored. There is little discomfort from this operation and postoperative analgesia is usually not a problem.

The incidence of postoperative complications, namely myocardial infarction, pulmonary embolism, cerebrovascular accidents, transient ischemia attacks, renal failure, hepatic insufficiency, and the need for prolonged ventilation is similar when comparing patients receiving regional anesthesia with those receiving general anesthesia (39,41).

Regardless of whether general or regional anesthesia is selected, a careful evaluation of cardiopulmonary parameters is vital. A high degree of expertise and vigilance is required for these patients, both from an anesthetic and a surgical point of view.

LAPAROSCOPIC SURGERY IN UROLOGY

Pelvic lymph node dissection used to be the most commonly performed laparoscopic urologic procedure in adults. Recently, the use of laparoscopy has been extended to other urologic procedures. These include varicocelectomy, hernia repair, adrenalectomy, percutaneous stone retrieval from the renal pelvis or ureter, nephrectomy, and radical prostatectomy. The laparoscopic approach reduces perioperative mortality, and also allows better preservation of periprostatic vascular, muscular, and neurovascular structures (42).

There are two unique problems associated with the laparoscopic approach to these procedures. First, the urogenital system is mainly retroperitoneal. The retroperitoneal space and its communication with the thorax and subcutaneous tissues are exposed to insufflated carbon dioxide. Subcutaneous emphysema is frequent and may extend to the head and neck (43). In severe cases, the upper airway is at risk for pharyngeal swelling secondary to submucous carbon dioxide, an issue that should be kept in mind at the time of extubation. Second, these procedures are lengthy and absorption of carbon dioxide may result in acidemia and marked acidosis (44). The patient is also positioned in a steep Trendelenburg position. For these reasons, general anesthesia with controlled ventilation is the method of choice.

Intraoperative oliguria may occur despite adequate hydration and diuresis may occur in the immediate postoperative period. The mechanism is unknown, but may be due to perirenal pressure exerted by the insufflated gas in the retroperitoneal space. Most clinicians avoid nitrous oxide to prevent bowel distension and expansion of residual intra-abdominal gas.

RADICAL SURGERY IN UROLOGY

Radical surgery in urology is becoming common. Procedures include radical nephrectomy, radical retropubic prostatectomy, and radical cystectomy. These surgeries have some common features. There may be sudden and significant blood loss, with preservation of renal function becoming an important consideration.

The flank position is used for radical nephrectomy. Cardiac and respiratory changes associated with positioning may occur. Respiratory changes include decreases in thoracic compliance, tidal volume, vital capacity, and functional residual capacity. Hypoxemia may result from dependent atelectasis. Pneumothorax may occur secondary to surgical entry into the thorax, and chest tube placement is not uncommon. Blood pressure may decrease when the kidney bar is raised due to compression of the inferior vena cava. Venous return may decrease from tumor extension into the vena cava.

Peripheral nerve injuries can also occur. These include cervical plexus, brachial plexus, and common peroneal neuropathies.

SURGERY FOR RENAL CANCER
Preoperative Considerations

Radical nephrectomy is most commonly performed for adenocarcinoma of the kidney. This disease has a peak incidence in the fifth and sixth decades of life, with a male to female ratio of 2:1. Risk factors include smoking, obesity, and hypertension. Only 10% of patients present with the classic triad of hematuria, flank pain, and a palpable mass. This carcinoma is frequently associated with a paraneoplastic syndrome, including erythrocytosis, hypercalcemia, hypertension, and nonmetastatic hepatic dysfunction. Approximately 30% of patients present with metastatic disease, most commonly involving the lung, soft tissues, bone, liver, and central nervous system. Computed tomography (CT) and magnetic resonance imaging (MRI) scans are used for tumor staging. Surgery is usually only performed for nonmetastatic disease, although 5% to 10% of tumors extend into the renal vein and the inferior vena cava as thrombus.

These tumors are usually large and vascular, and so extensive blood loss can be anticipated. Preoperative arterial embolization may reduce blood loss.

Preoperative assessment should define the degree of renal impairment, which usually depends on the size of the tumor and the presence of hypertension and diabetes. The high incidence of coronary artery disease and chronic destructive lung disease in this population should also be taken into account in the preoperative assessment. Most patients are anemic, although some may present with erythrocytosis.

Anesthetic Management

An anterior subcostal, flank, midline, or thoracoabdominal incision may be used. The kidney rest is used with the flank position. The thoracoabdominal approach is used for large tumors, or those, which extend superiorly into the thoracic inferior vena cava.

General endotracheal anesthesia is used for this procedure. In most patients, direct arterial pressure monitoring is performed. Arterial hypotension may occur due to retraction of the inferior vena cava or blood loss. Central venous pressure monitoring is indicated in some patients. Patients with severe cardiac dysfunction may require a pulmonary artery catheter. Reflex renal vasoconstriction may occur in the unaffected kidney. Infusion of mannitol for preservation of renal function is advised before the dissection begins.

If the pleura is entered, either intentionally or incidentally, a pneuomothorax will occur. A postoperative chest X-ray is recommended and some patients may receive a chest tube.

Tumor extension into the inferior vena cava and right atrium occurs mostly with right-sided renal cell carcinoma. To operate on these patients safely, the extent of the lesion must be defined preoperatively. Cardiopulmonary bypass is required in some cases.

The thoracoabdominal approach is almost always used. The presence of a large thrombus greatly complicates the anesthetic management. Multiple large bore intravenous catheters and invasive pressure monitoring are necessary. Central venous pressure is usually high reflecting the degree of venous obstruction by the thrombus. A pulmonary artery catheter is contraindicated if the thrombus extends into the right atrium. A low-lying central venous pressure catheter would be equally detrimental. Transesophageal echocardiography may be used (45).

Blood loss may require extensive use of blood and blood products, including platelets, fresh frozen plasma and cryoprecipitate may be required. Complications associated with massive blood transfusion are to be expected.

MAJOR CANCER SURGERIES

Adenocarcinoma of the prostate is the most common malignancy in men. It is the second most common cause of death in men over the age of 55 years. Prostate cancer is a disease of the elderly male, with an estimated incidence of 75% in patients over 75 years of age (46), reaching a peak incidence at the age of 80 years.

Radical intrapelvic prostactomy is often performed in conjunction with a pelvic node dissection. It is indicated for localized prostate cancer, or as a salvage procedure after radiation (47). The entire prostate gland, the seminal vesicles, ejaculatory ducts, and part of the bladder neck are removed. The prostate is approached anteriorly, and the dissection then proceeds from the bladder downward (Walsh) to preserve sexual function. The remaining bladder neck is anastomosed directly to the urethra over an indwelling catheter. Indigo carmine is given intravenously to visualize the ureters. Although blood loss varies, this procedure carries the potential for major blood loss. Two large bore intravenous catheters are required. Some patients will need direct arterial blood pressure monitoring. Some individuals advocate central venous pressure monitoring (48). Although it is seldom used, Albin et al. (49) suggested the use of a precordial Doppler to monitor for venous air embolism.

Anatomic factors that may affect blood loss include pelvic anatomy, positioning, and the size of the prostate. Surgical factors may include technique, early ligation of the dorsal vein of the penis plexus, and temporary clamping of the hypogastric artery. Blood loss is similar in patients receiving general anesthesia versus regional anesthesia (50). Preoperative analogous blood donations may be considered, although its value as a cost effective strategy has been questioned (48,51,52).

Prostatectomy surgery can be performed under general, epidural, or spinal anesthesia. Postoperative morbidity appears to be similar in patients receiving epidural and general anesthesia (53). A T_6 sensory level is required for regional anesthesia. Regional anesthesia requires heavy sedation because the hyperextended supine position is not well tolerated. In addition, the administration of large amounts of fluid and the steep Trendelenburg position may result in airway edema, which may complicate the anesthetic management should endotracheal intubation become necessary. For these reasons, regional techniques are rarely used.

Shir et al. (54) reported that epidural anesthesia may have a pre-emptive analgesic effect, and may decrease postoperative pain requirements, although this could not be demonstrated in patients receiving combined epidural and general anesthesia. The use of epidural narcotics for postoperative analgesia does not appear to be superior to IV patient-controlled analgesia (PCA) (54–56). Liu et al. (56) found no difference in pain relief or recovery between patients receiving hydromorphine either epidurally or by IV PCA. The IV PCA group did require less hydromorphone. Ketorolac may be used as an adjuvant to epidural narcotics, where it improves analgesia and promotes earlier return of bowel function (57). The same effect may be expected with ketorolac and IV narcotics administered by PCA.

Dissection near the pelvic veins may increase the risk of a thromboembolic event. The use of epidural anesthesia may reduce the evidence of deep vein thrombosis (58). Many surgeons use warfarin prophylactically to reduce the incidence of deep vein thrombosis and pulmonary embolus. The beneficial antithrombotic effect of epidural anesthesia is most likely masked with warfarin therapy, which may also increase the risk of an epidural hematoma.

Other surgical complications include bleeding, injury to the obturator nerve, ureter, rectum, and urinary incontinence and impotence.

SURGERY FOR BLADDER CANCER AND URINARY DIVERSION

Bladder cancer is the second most common malignancy of the genitourinary tract, with transitional cell carcinoma being the most common variety. It occurs mostly in the elderly with a 3:1 male-to-female ratio.

Preoperative Considerations

Cigarette smoking is associated with bladder cancer. It contributes to coexisting coronary artery and chronic destructive pulmonary disease seen in these patients. Impaired renal function can also be a factor in this patient population, either from urinary tract obstruction, or from associated conditions, such as hypertension and diabetes.

Anesthetic Management

Radical cystectomy is a surgery associated with considerable blood loss (59). The procedure is performed through a large midline incision that extends from the pubis to the xiphoid. In men, all anterior pelvic organs are removed, including the bladder, prostate, seminal vesicles, and part of the urethra. In women, the resection includes the uterus, cervix, ovaries, anterior vaginal vault, and part of the urethra. A bilateral pelvic node dissection is also performed. Urinary diversion is performed after the pelvic node dissection is complete.

General endotracheal anesthesia with a muscle relaxant is most often used. Controlled hypotensive anesthesia may be considered, since it has been shown to reduce intraoperative blood loss and transfusion requirements (60). General anesthesia may be supplemented by epidural anesthesia, which can facilitate the hypotensive technique and reduce anesthesia requirements. In addition, an epidural catheter is an effective route for postoperative analgesia. It should be realized that regional anesthesia may cause increased peristalsis from unopposed parasympathetic activity.

Monitoring intravascular volume and blood loss is essential during these procedures. All patients require direct intra-arterial pressure monitoring. Multiple large-bore intravenous catheters are required. If a patient has limited cardiac reserve, or limited vascular access, a central venous pressure catheter is recommended. In cases where a patient has severely impaired ventricular function, a pulmonary artery catheter should be considered. Urinary output should be monitored and correlated with the progress of the surgery. The urinary path is interrupted early in most of these procedures, and a low threshold for placement of central venous pressure monitoring is appropriate.

Several urinary diverting procedures are currently used, but all require implanting the ureters into a segment of bowel. The bowel segment may be left in situ, or divided with its mesenteric blood supply and attached to a stoma or urethra. The isolated bowel can function as a conduit (ileal conduit) or be reconstructed to form a reservoir (Koch pouch). Conduits are formed from the ilieum, jejum, or the colon. Urinary diversions include ureterosigmoidostomy and small bowel (Koch, Camey), large bowel (Indiana), and gastric reservoirs.

The patient should be kept well hydrated to maintain a brisk urine output. As stated, central venous pressure monitoring may be used to guide intravenous fluid administration. When the ureters are divided, an abrupt decrease in urine output occurs, and the ability to follow volume status by urine output is lost. If regional anesthesia is used, the sympathetic block may leave parasympathetic activity unopposed. The resulting hyperactive bowel may result in a technically difficult reconstruction of the ileal reservoir. This problem can be alleviated with an anticholinergic agent, such as glycopyrrolate. Metabolic disturbances can arise from the urine being in contact with bowel mucosa. These include hyponotremia, hypochloremia, and hyperkalemic metabolic acidosis seen after jejunal conduits. In contrast, hyperchloremic metabolic acidosis can be seen with colonic and ileal conduits.

SURGERY FOR TESTICULAR CANCER
Preoperative Considerations

Germ cell tumors constitute 95% of all testicular tumors. They are either seminomas or nonseminomas. The initial management is radical (inguinal) orchiectomy. Subsequent management depends on the histology of the tumor.

Seminomas are radiosensitive, and respond well to radiation therapy. Except for choriocarcinoma, all testicular tumors spread lymphatically. Chemotherapy is used after radiation. Patients with large seminomas, or those associated with increased alpha-fetoprotein levels, are treated with chemotherapy. A combination of cisplatin, vincristine, and bleomycin is an example of one such regimen. Patients who have residual tumor after chemotherapy require a retroperitoneal lymph node dissection (RPLND).

Patients with nonseminomatous germ cells are usually managed with an RPLND, or a RPLND and chemotherapy if they have high-grade disease. These patients are usually young men aged 15 to 35 years. They are at risk from the morbidity associated with the use of chemotherapeutic agents, for example, pulmonary fibrosis after bleomycin, renal impairment after cisplatin, and neuropathy after vincristine.

Anesthesia Management

Radical orchiectomies may be performed under regional or general anesthesia, although most patients prefer general anesthesia. During this procedure, the anesthesia provider should be prepared to treat reflex bradycardia, which may occur as a result of traction on the spermatic cord.

The staging and management of nonseminomatous testicular cancers is performed with an RPLND. This requires a large thoracoabdominal incision extending from the posterior axillary line over the eighth to tenth ribs to a paramedian line halfway between the xiphoid and the umbilicus. Another approach may be a midline transabdominal incision. All the lymph node tissue from the renal vessels to the iliac bifurcation is removed. In the process, sympathetic fibers are disrupted, resulting in loss of ejaculation and infertility. To preserve fertility a modified technique may be used. The dissection below the inferior mesenteric artery is limited to the nodal tissue on the ipsilateral side of the tumor.

Patients receiving bleomycin preoperatively seem to be at increased risk of developing postoperative pulmonary insufficiency (61,62). High oxygen inspired concentration has been associated with the development of adult respiratory distress syndrome (ARDS). Anesthetic management in these patients involves the use of low inspired oxygen concentration, with less than 0.30% oxygen being considered optimal. An air–oxygen mixture is used, since absorption of nitrous oxide may be associated with bowel enlargement. Intravenous fluid administration should also be carefully monitored. Fluid replacement should be sufficient to maintain an adequate urinary output of at least 0.5 mL/kg/hr. Evaporative and redistributive fluid losses occur as a result of a large wound and extensive surgical resection.

Before dissection near the renal arteries mannitol (0.5 g/kg) is usually given. Mannitol is thought to increase renal blood flow and tubular flow, thereby diminishing the likelihood of ischemic renal injury from surgically induced spasm of the renal arteries.

The postoperative pain associated with RPLND can be severe. Patients are frequently unable to take a full tidal volume breath because of splinting. This can result in atelectasis and hypoxemia. Therefore, it is important to have a plan for effective postoperative analgesia. Epidural analgesia, interpleural analgesia, and intercostal blocks have been used. Currently epidural analgesia is the most popular.

It is important to realize that dissection of the left intercostal arteries where the artery of Adamkiewicz arises, can compromise the blood supply to the lower posterior segment of the spinal cord. Although rare, motor function could be compromised. In addition, in the modified RLND, unilateral sympathectomy may result in the upsilateral leg being warmer than the contralateral leg.

ROBOTIC SURGERY

Robotic surgery is the next step in the evolution of minimally invasive surgery. The robotic device allows precise control of surgical instruments. Benefits include less pain and trauma, shorter hospital stay, quicker recovery, and a better cosmetic result. Anesthesiologists must keep abreast of these changes and their impact on patient care and safety.

Guillonneau and Vallancien were the first to perform a laparoscopic radical prostatectomy (63). The feasibility of robotically assisted prostatectomy has been shown at several hospital centers (64,65).

General anesthesia is administered in the standard fashion, as for the conventional radical prostatectomy. Intravenous catheters and direct arterial catheters must be placed prior to the surgical positioning of the patient. All four extremities become inaccessible during the procedure itself. The patient is placed in a supine lithotomy position with a 30° Trendelenburg incline. The thighs are spread to allow the approach of the robotic system between them. If the patients are less than six feet tall they are placed in a frog-leg position.

Patients with a history of stroke or cerebral aneurysm may not be good candidates for prolonged Trendelenburg position. Silicone gel pads are placed at all pressure points. The patient is prepped and draped and a urinary catheter inserted. A pneumoperitoneum is created with an umbilical puncture needle. The maximum pressure is set to 15 mmHg. The trocar is inserted according to the five-trocar arrangement, with a sixth in the suprapubic area (66). A modified Montsaurtis technique is used (67).

REFERENCES

1. Harioka T, Murakawa M, Noda J, et al. Effect of continuously warmed irrigating solution during transurethral resection. Anaesth Intensive Care 1988; 16:324.
2. Schmidt KA, Snyder SA. Effect of horizontal lithotomy position on hyperbaric tetracaine spinal anesthesia. Anesth Analg 1988; 67:894.
3. Sinclair CJ, Scott DB, Edstrom BH. Effect of the Trendelenburg positionon spinal anesthesia with hyperbaric bupivacaine. Br J Anaesth 1982; 54:497.
4. Touminen M, Taivainen T, Rosenberg PH. Spread of spinal anaesthesia with plain 0.5% bupivacaine: influence of the certebral interspace used for injection. Br J Anaesth 1989; 62:358.
5. Desmond J. Serum osmolality and plasma electrolytes in patients who develop dilution hyponatremia during transurethral resection. Can J Surg 1970; 13:116.
6. Nesbit T, Carter OW, Tudor JM, et al. Complications of transurethral prostatectomy and their management. South Med 1966; 5:.
7. Hagstrom RS. Studies on fluid absorption during transurethral prostatic resection. J Urol 1955; 73:852.
8. Marz GF, Orkin LR. Complications associated with transurethral surgery. Anesthesiology 1962; 23:802.
9. Fillman EM, Hanson OL, Gilbert LO. Radioisotopic study of effects of irrigation fluid in transurethral prostatectomy. JAMA 1959; 171:1488.

10. Norris HT, Aasheim GM, Sherrard DJ, et al. Symptomatology, pathophysiology, and treatment of the transurethral resection of the prostate syndrome. Br J Urol 1973; 45:420.

11. Harrison RH, Boren JS, Robinson JR. Dilutional hyponatremia shock: another concept of the transurethral prostatic resection reaction. J Urol 1956; 75:95.

12. Wakim KG. The pathophysiologic basis for the clinical manifestations and complications of transurethral prostatic resection. J Urol 1961; 106:719.

13. Hurlbert BJ, Wingard DW. Water intoxication after fifteen minutes of transurethral resection of the prostate. Anesthesiology 1979; 50:355.

14. Mani M. Transurethral prostatic surgery revisited. Anesthesiol Rev 1976; 16:.

15. Aasheim GM. Hyponatremia during transurethral surgery. Can Anaesth Soc J 1973; 20:247.

16. Henderson DJ, Middleton RG. Coma from hyponatremia following transurethral resection of prostate. Urology 1980; 15:267.

17. Hoekstra PT, Kahnoski R, McCamish MA, et al. Transurethral prostatic resection syndrome—a new perspective: encephalopathy with associated hyperammonemia. J Urol 1983; 130:704.

18. Ovassapian A, Joshi CW, Brunner EA. Visual disturbance: an unusual symptom of transurethral prostatic resection reaction. Anesthesiology 1982; 57:332.

19. Roesch RP, Stoelting RK, Lingeman JE, et al. Ammonia toxicity resulting from glycine absorption during a transurethral resection of the prostate. Anesthesiology 1983; 58:577.

20. Wang JM, Wong KC, Creel DJ, et al. Effects of glycine on hemodynamic responses and visual evoked potentials in the dog. Anesth Analg 1985; 64:1071.

21. Apreson MH, Werman R. The distribution of glycine in cat spinal cord and roots. Life Sci 1965; 4:2075.

22. Snyder SH, Enna EJ. The role of central receptors in the pharmacologic actions of benzodiazepines. Adv Biochem Psychopharmacol 1975; 14:81.

23. Desmond J. A method of measuring blood loss during transurethral prostatic surgery. J Urol 1973; 109:453.

24. Jansen H, Berseus O, Johansson JE. A simple photometric method for determination of blood loss during transurethral surgery. Scand J Urol Nephrol 1978; 12:1.

25. Levin K, Nyren O, Pompeius R. Blood loss, tissue weight and operating time in transurethral prostatectomy. Scand J Urol Nephrol 1981; 15:197.

26. Abrams PH, Shah PJR, Bryning K, et al. Blood loss during transurethral resection of the prostate. Anaesthesia 1982; 37:71.

27. Perkins JB, Miller HC. Blood loss during transurethral prostatectomy. J Urol 1969; 101:93.

28. Madsen RE, Madsen PO. Influence of anaesthesia form on blood loss in transurethral prostatectomy. Anaesth Analg 1967; 46:330.

29. Collins KJ, Dore C, Exoton-Smith AN, et al. Accidental hypothermia and impaired temperature homeostasis in the elderly. Br Med J 1977; 1:353.

30. Stjerstrom H, Henneberg S, Eklund A, et al. Thermal balance during transurethral resection of the prostate: a comparison of general anesthesia and epidural analgesia. Acata Anaesthesiol Scand 1985; 29:743.

31. Jenkins J, Fox J, Sharwood-Smith G. Changes in body heat during transvesical prostatectomy. Anaesthesia 1983; 38:748.

32. Whitfield HN, Hendry WF. Endoscopic surgery. In: Whitfield H, Hendry W, eds. Textbook of Genitourinary Surgery. Vol. 2. Edinburgh: Churchill-Livingstone, 1985:1373–1374.

33. Kenton HR. Perforation in transurethral operations: techniane for immediate diagnosis and management of extravasations. JAMA 1950; 142:798.

34. Sinha B, Haikel G, Lange PH, et al. Transurethral resection of the prostate with local anesthesia in 100 patients. J Urol 1986; 135:719.

35. Holtgrewe HL, Valk WL. Factors influencing the mortality and morbidity of transurethral prostatectomy: a study of 2015 cases. J Urol 1962; 87:450.

36. Burrows R. Anesthesia for prostatectomies. Anesth Analg 1924; 228–229.

37. Melchoir J, Valk WL, Forest JD, et al. Transurethral prostatectomy: computerized analysis of 2223 consecutive cases. J Urol 1974; 112:634.

38. Desmond J. Complications of transurethral prostatic surgery. Can Anaesth Soc J 1970; 17:25.

39. Mebust WK, Holtgreive HL, Cockett ATK, et al. Transurethral prostatectomy—immediate and postoperative complications. A cooperative study of 13 participating institutions evaluating 3885 patients. J Urol 1989; 141:243.

40. Cullen DJ, Apolone G, Greenfield S, et al. ASA physical status and age predict morbidity after three surgical procedures Ann Surg 1994; 220:3 (abstract).

41. Hatch PD. Surgical and anaesthetic considerations in transurethral resection of the prostate. Anaesth Intensive Care 1987; 15:203.

42. Guillonneau B. Laparoscopic radical prostatectomy: assessment after 240 procedures. Urol Clin North Am 2001; 28:189–202.

43. Weingram J, Sosa RE, Stein B, Poppas D. Subcutaneous emphysema (SCE) during laparoscopic pelvic lymph node dissection (LPLND). Anesth Analg 1993; S460.

44. Roesch RP, Stoelting RK, Lingeman JE, et al. Ammonia toxicity resulting from glycine absorption during a transurethral resection of the prostate. Anesthesiology 1983; 58:577.

45. Swenson JD, Hullander RM, Nolan JF, et al. Renal cell carcinoma in the inferior vena cava demonstrated by transesophageal echocardiography. J Cardiothorac Vasc Anesth 1993; 7:335.
46. Linke CL, Merin RG. A regional anesthetic approach for renal transplantation. Anesth Analg 1976; 55:69.
47. Catalona WJ. Surgical management of prostatic cancer: contemporary results with anatomic radical prostatectomy. Cancer 1995; 75:1903.
48. Monk TG. Cancer of the prostate and radical prostatectomy. In: Malhorta V, ed. Anesthesia for Renal and Genitor-Urologic Surgery. New York: McGraw-Hill, 1996:481–482.
49. Albin MS, Ritter RR, Reinhart R, et al. Venous air embolism during radical retropubic prostatectomy. Anesth Analg 1992; 74:151.
50. Shir Y, Raja SN, Frank SM, et al. Intraoperative blood loss during radical retropubic prostatectomy: epidural versus general anesthesia. Urology 1995; 45:993.
51. Goodnough LT, Grishaber JE, Birkmeyer JD, et al. Efficacy and cost effectiveness of autologous blood predeposit in patients undergoing radical prostatectomy. Urology 1994; 44:226.
52. Yamada AH, Lieskovsky G, Skinner DG, et al. Impact of autologous blood transfusion on patients undergoing radical prostatectomy using hypotensive anesthesia. J Urol 1993; 149:73.
53. Shir Y, Frank SM, Brendler, et al. Postoperative morbidity is similar in patients anesthetized with epidural and general anesthesia for radical prostatectomy. Urology 1994; 44:232.
54. Shir Y, Raja SN, Frank SM. The effect of epidural versus general anesthesia on postoperative pain and analgesic requirements in patients undergoing radical prostatectomy. Anesthesiology 1994; 80:49.
55. Allaire PH, Messick JM, Oesterling JE, et al. A prospective randomized comparison of epidural infusion of fentanyl and intravenous administration of morphine by patient controlled analgesia after radical prostatectomy. Mayo Clin Proc 1992; 67:1031.
56. Liu S, Carpenter RL, Mulroy MF, et al. Intravenous versus epidural administration of hydromorphone: Effects on analgesia and recovery after radical retropubic prostatectomy. Anesthesiology 1995; 82:682.
57. Grass JA, Sakima NT, Valley M, et al. Assessment of ketorolac as an adjuvant to fentanyl patient-controlled epidural anesthesia after radical prostatectomy. Anesthesiology 1993; 78:642.
58. Hendolin H, Mattila MAK, Poikolainen E. The effect of lumbar epidural analgesia on the development of deep vein thrombosis of the legs after open prostatectomy. Acta Chir Scand 1981; 147:425.
59. Ryan DW. Anesthesia for cystectomy. Anaesthesia 1982; 37:557.
60. Ahlering TE, Henderson JB, Skinner DG. Controlled hypotensive anesthesia to reduce blood loss in radical cystectomy for bladder cancer. J Urol 1983; 129:953.
61. Mathes DD. Bleomycin and hyperoxia exposure in the operating room. Anesth Analg 1995; 81:624.
62. Waid-Jones MI, Coursin DB. Perioperative considerations for patients treated with bleomycin. Chest 1991; 99:993.
63. Guillonneau B, Vallancien G. Laparoscopic radical prostatectomy: the Montsouris experience. J Urol 2000; 163:418–422.
64. Binder J, Kramer W. Robotically-assisted laparoscopic radical prostatectomy. BJU Int 2001; 87:408–410.
65. Rassweiler J, Binder J, Frede T. Robotic and telesurgery: will they change our future? Curr Opin Urol 2001; 11:309–320.
66. Rassweiler J, Sentker L, Seemann O, et al. Heilbronn laparoscopic radical prostatectomy. Technique and results after 100 cases. Eur Urol 2001; 40:54–64.
67. Tewari A, Peabody J, Sarle R, et al. Technique of da Vinci robot-assisted anatomic radical prostatectomy. Urol 2002; 60:569–572.

5 Nutritional Considerations in Urologic Surgery

Kris M. Mogensen
Metabolic Support Service, Department of Surgery, Brigham and Women's Hospital, Boston, Massachusetts, U.S.A.

Malcolm K. Robinson
Metabolic Support Service, Department of Surgery, Brigham and Women's Hospital, and Harvard Medical School, Boston, Massachusetts, U.S.A.

INTRODUCTION

The response to surgery and critical illness is a complex process designed to provide energy and other essential compounds for reparative processes. This process also serves to protect the host from microbial invasion and optimize the function of vital organs. Compounds are released from the periphery and taken up by visceral organs for use in these functions, which often expedite recovery. The flow of substrates is initiated and maintained by a variety of mediators and neural signals. The catabolic process appears well orchestrated but errs on the side of abundant substrate delivery. Hence, the physiologic and metabolic alterations that characterize the surgical response may be deleterious when prolonged or severe. There is degradation of total body protein and an increase in systemic metabolism, which can result in death if nutritional and cardiopulmonary reserves are exhausted. While these metabolic changes are usually well tolerated on a short-term basis, prolonged catabolic illness may be harmful even if appropriately managed by the attending clinician. The primary goal of nutritional support is to enhance those salutary processes of the response to surgical stress while minimizing the adverse affects of this response (1). This chapter focuses on nutritional support of the urology patient and those with pathological conditions of the urinary system.

Malnutrition in the urology patient can have a significant impact on outcome and lead to increased length of hospital stay and subsequent costs. Early identification of malnutrition and implementation of an aggressive nutrition repletion plan may improve outcome. Although this chapter primarily focuses on preventing or treating underfeeding of calories and protein, it is important to note that malnutrition includes both "under-nutrition" and "over-nutrition." Both states of malnutrition can lead to poor outcome and increased risk of disease. For example, obesity carries with it increased risk of diabetes, hypertension, and hyperlipidemia and is associated with increased risk of kidney stones, prostate cancer, and renal cancer.

OUTCOMES ASSOCIATED WITH MALNUTRITION

Malnutrition has been associated with negative outcomes in surgical patients including infectious complications, poor wound healing, and wound dehiscence. For example, Kuzu et al. (2) assessed the nutritional status and postoperative complications of 460 surgical patients. Patients with malnutrition had a significantly higher incidence of infectious and noninfectious complications compared to the well-nourished. The malnourished patients also took significantly longer to return to normal activity.

Given the increased incidence of complications in malnourished patients, it is not surprising that they often have longer lengths of stay in the hospital. In a study (3) of both medical and surgical patients, those patients classified as having a "likelihood of malnutrition" had longer lengths of stay than those who were not likely to be malnourished. Kuzu et al. (2) also found that malnourished patients had longer lengths of stay compared to well-nourished patients (mean length of stay 20.78 days vs. 17.77 days; P = 0.001).

NUTRITION SCREENING AND ASSESSMENT

The first step in evaluating patients for nutrition intervention is nutrition screening and assessment. There are a variety of methods available to determine the presence of malnutrition or nutritional risk, ranging from very simple tools to more complex prognostic indicators. Assessment typically begins with a diet history. In the clinical setting, a basic nutritional interview may include a simple 24-hour diet recall or food frequency questionnaire. Questions should be asked about food allergies or intolerances, ability to chew/swallow food, and cultural or religious practices associated with food habits (4). The clinician can then evaluate the adequacy of oral intake as well as use the information about specific food limitations for development of the nutrition care plan.

Height- and weight-based screening methods can be simple for the practitioner to implement as well. However, the practitioner must be wary of self-reported height and weight, as they are often inaccurate, with men overestimating and women underestimating (5). Hence, measuring both height and weight is important for accurate assessment of nutritional status.

A consistently reliable indicator of malnutrition is the presence of unintentional weight loss. This was first demonstrated by Studley (6) in 1936 when he assessed 46 patients requiring surgery for peptic ulcer disease. Postoperative mortality was approximately 33% in those with >20% unintentional weight loss, compared to 3.5% in those patients with <20% weight loss. Seltzer et al. (7) found that loss of at least 10 pounds unintentionally increased postoperative mortality and Roy et al. (8) found that just a 6% weight loss increased the risk of postoperative complications. Frequently, 10% unintentional weight loss, or 90% or less of usual body weight, is considered clinically significant, especially if there are additional symptoms of functional impairment. It is important to note that although one may be overweight or obese, recent unintentional weight loss still increases surgical risk.

Circulating proteins can also be used as part of the nutrition-screening process. Serum albumin is a frequently used measure of chronic visceral protein status, with low serum albumin suggesting poor nutritional status. In the National Veterans Affairs Surgical Risk Study (9), preoperative serum albumin was the most important predictor of 30-day mortality for all surgeries as well as urology as a subspecialty. Unfortunately, there are many other factors besides nutritional status that affect serum albumin, including volume overload, liver disease, trauma, and inflammation. In addition, albumin also has a long half-life of approximately 21 days, and thus, it may not accurately reflect acute changes in nutritional status. Hence, while albumin may correlate well with chronic nutritional status, it is a poor indicator of nutritional status in acutely-ill patients or for assessing acute changes in nutritional status (10).

Prealbumin, or transthyretin, is another circulating protein that can be used in screening for nutritional risk, assessment of nutritional status, and monitoring response to nutritional therapy. Robinson et al. (11) demonstrated that prealbumin is an excellent screening tool, correlating well with a dietitian's assessment of nutritional status. However, as with albumin, prealbumin can also be depressed as a result of inflammatory states and can also be elevated in cases of renal failure and with steroid therapy, thus, these conditions must be taken into account when interpreting measured levels. Other circulating proteins can be used for nutritional assessment, including retinol-binding protein and transferrin, but these also have the limitations outlined with albumin and prealbumin (10).

Some practitioners prefer predictive formulas, which combine several pieces of data to determine nutritional status to make up for the unreliability of using one index of nutrition alone. A variety of prognostic indices are available. For example, the prognostic nutritional index (PNI) was developed by Buzby et al. (12) to determine the degree of malnutrition and related surgical risk. The PNI uses weighted values of serum albumin, triceps skinfold, transferrin, and presence of delayed hypersensitivity to determine a score that predicts risk of postoperative complications. A simpler index, the nutrition risk index (NRI), was developed for use in surgical patients to determine presence of mild, moderate, severe, or no malnutrition. Only serum albumin and percent usual body weight are used in the calculation (13).

GENERAL CONSIDERATIONS IN NUTRITIONAL THERAPY FOR THE UROLOGIC SURGERY PATIENT

Once a malnourished patient or a person at risk for malnourishment is identified, an individualized nutritional plan should be developed and implemented to decrease the risk of complications and improve outcomes. Two major categories of nutritional support can be considered: enteral and parenteral nutrition (PN). A decision algorithm for selecting enteral or PN is outlined in Figure 1.

Enteral Nutrition

Enteral nutrition (EN) is the feeding modality of choice. Outcomes associated with EN versus PN in patients with functioning intestinal tracts have been recently reviewed (14). Generally, EN, when feasible, is associated with decreased complications compared to PN. In addition, EN is typically less expensive than PN because the former is typically made in a large manufacturing facility, while PN needs to be prepared individually for each patient by a pharmacist.

Enteral nutrition includes both oral nutrition and nutrition fed via a tube accessing the intestinal tract. Ideally, the least invasive method of nutritional support should be used. Patients who are taking an inadequate oral diet may respond to use of liquid oral nutritional supplements provided either with or between meals. For example, Gariballa et al. (15) conducted a randomized, double-blind, placebo-controlled study assessing the effectiveness of provision of a concentrated liquid oral nutritional supplement to 445 hospitalized older adults (age >65, admitted to medical and surgical services) daily for six weeks. The supplemented group had a significantly lower re-admission rate compared to the placebo group (29% vs. 40%). Others have found similar positive results with oral supplements in surgical patients (16).

For patients with a functional gastrointestinal tract who are unable to take oral nutrition, for example, as a result of a swallowing disorder, altered mental status, or anorexia, enteral tube feeding is the next choice. There are four main types of enteral formulas designed to be

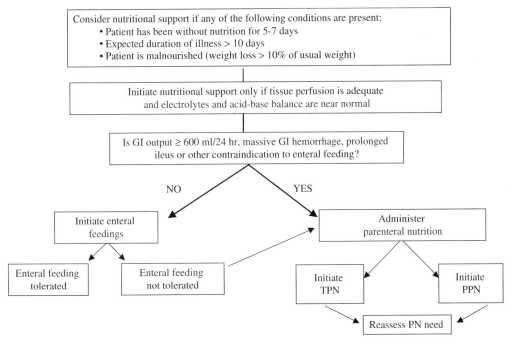

FIGURE 1 Algorithm for determining route of nutritional support. *Abbreviations*: GI, gastrointestinal; TPN, total parenteral nutrition; PPN, peripheral parenteral nutrition.

administered via feeding tubes: polymeric, elemental, disease-specific, and modular. Polymeric formulas are those comprised of intact protein, starch and glucose polymers, and polyunsaturated fats. These formulas are designed for patients with normal gastrointestinal function, who can digest and absorb nutrients easily. Elemental, also known as "defined diet," formulas are comprised of free amino acids or small peptides, small glucose polymers, and a blend of medium-chain triglycerides and long-chain fats. These formulas are designed for patients with maldigestive and/or malabsorptive disorders. Disease-specific formulas can fall into either the polymeric or elemental categories. These formulas have specific modifications making them appropriate for patients with conditions requiring adjustments in nutrient delivery. For example, products designed for patients with renal failure are restricted in sodium, potassium, and phosphorus and may contain limited protein. Finally, modular products are a single macronutrient (protein, carbohydrate, or fat) that can be used to modify a specific formula or can be added to a patient's food to increase protein or energy intake. All formulas, except for the modular products, are fortified with vitamins and minerals (17).

Formula choice depends on careful evaluation of a patient's energy, protein, and fluid requirements, and then consideration of any specific nutritional concerns (e.g., need to restrict or supplement specific nutrients). The location of the tube will help to guide the method of formula delivery.

There are three methods for infusing EN: continuous, pump-assisted feedings; intermittent feedings (either pump-assisted or gravity drip); and bolus feedings. Continuous feedings run constantly for a set period of time, anywhere between 10 and 24 hours. An enteral feeding pump is required to regulate the flow of formula into the intestine. This method is most appropriate for patients with jejunal feeding tubes as the small intestine does not have the reservoir capacity to tolerate large-volume infusions as with bolus feedings. Continuous feedings are also appropriate for patients who require consistent infusion of nutrients, for example, patients at risk of aspiration who may be at further risk with a large amount of formula in the stomach (18).

Intermittent feedings can be infused using a feeding pump or gravity-drip bags. This method is typically used for patients who want to infuse enteral formula three to four times per day to approximate a typical "eating" plan, but cannot tolerate a large amount of formula in the stomach at once. Bolus feedings are appropriate for ambulatory patients with normal gastric emptying and minimal risk of aspiration. The patient typically uses a large syringe as a funnel to pour formula (typically 1–2, 240-mL cans) into the gastric tube. As with intermittent feedings, the patient will infuse formula three to four times per day. As mentioned previously, bolus feeding into the jejunum should be avoided because of the lack of reservoir capacity and increased risk of complications such as bloating, abdominal distention, and diarrhea (18).

The type of enteral access selected depends on the estimated length of therapy. Nasoenteric feeding tubes can stay in place for up to six to eight weeks. This short-term access is best when it is anticipated that the patient will eventually regain the ability to eat by mouth. Feeding tubes intended for the long term, including gastrostomy tubes and jejunostomy tubes, are selected when it is anticipated that the patient will require enteral tube feeding support for more than six to eight weeks. Recent in-depth reviews of enteral access procedures and devices have been published (19–21).

Complications associated with EN can be divided into four broad categories: mechanical, infectious, gastrointestinal, and metabolic. Typical complications are listed in Table 1.

Mechanical complications are those associated with the tube itself and may include the formation of granulation tissue around the feeding tube with associated pain and cracked/leaking or clogged tubes (22,23).

Aspiration has been categorized as a mechanical complication associated with enteral feeding. This complication can be life-threatening and the best treatment is prevention. At-risk patients should be fed with strict aspiration precautions, including keeping the head portion of the bed elevated 30° to 45°. Continuous feedings may be beneficial compared to bolus feedings, particularly for patients with delayed gastric emptying. Monitoring gastric residual volume (GRV) may be useful for patients being fed into the stomach. A GRV > 150–200 mL may be suggestive of delayed gastric emptying, increasing the risk of aspiration. Feeding beyond the pylorus may be helpful for some patients, but this does not prevent the patient from aspirating his or her own

TABLE 1 Selected Complications Associated with Enteral Nutrition

Category	Complications	Prevention/treatment strategies
Mechanical	Aspiration	Keep head of bed elevated while formula is infusing
		Avoid bolus feeding in high-risk patients
		Consider post-pyloric feeding
	Clogged feeding tube	Flush with warm water
		Flush with a solution of pancreatic enzymes and sodium bicarbonate
		Use a commercial declogging device (avoid wires)
		Do not flush with cola or cranberry juice (these will further coagulate proteins, worsening the clog)
Infectious	Diarrhea	Check stool culture, treat with appropriate antibiotics
		Consider use of probiotics
		Use clean technique when handling enteral formulas
	Sinusitis (naso-enteric tubes only)	Change to an oro-gastric tube
		Consider change to long-term enteral feeding access
	Infection around insertion site	Meticulous tube care
Gastrointestinal	Abdominal discomfort/bloating	Assess for intestinal obstruction or ileus
		Assess for constipation
		Decrease rate of infusion
		Avoid infusion of cold enteral formula
		Change from bolus feeding to continuous infusion
	Constipation	Change to fiber-containing formula
		Assure adequate provision of fluid
		Disimpaction
		Initiate bowel regimen
	Diarrhea	Antibiotics if infectious source
		Change to fiber-containing formula
		Change to isotonic formula
		Add antidiarrheal medications to enteral formula
		Trial of elemental formula
	Nausea/vomiting	Assess for delayed gastric emptying
		Avoid narcotics
		Consider use of prokinetic agents
		Decrease rate of infusion
		Change to a low-fat formula
		Avoid infusion of cold formula
		Consider change to a postpyloric feeding tube
Metabolic	Dehydration	Change to dilute enteral formula
		Provide free water flushes
	Electrolyte and acid/base disturbances	Monitor electrolytes and acid/base status daily when initiating enteral nutrition; correct abnormalities promptly
		Monitor long-term enteral patients every 1–3 months depending on risk
	Hyperglycemia	Avoid overfeeding
		Consider fiber-containing formula
		Provide insulin as needed
	Vitamin, mineral, trace-element deficiencies	Assure that enteral formula meets 100% of requirements
		Provide multivitamin/mineral elixir if necessary
		Consider monitoring levels every 6–12 months

oro-pharyngeal secretions (23). The outdated practice of using blue food coloring to detect aspiration has been abandoned due to several reports of deaths associated with its use (24).

Infectious complications include infections around the tube insertion site, which may require antibiotic treatment. Diarrhea can also develop and may or may not be related to the tube feeding. If a patient is complaining of diarrhea, appropriate evaluation should take place before starting antidiarrheal medications to rule out an infectious etiology. For patients with a naso-gastric or naso-enteric tube, sinusitis is a possible complication. If patients develop this complication, options include changing to an oro-gastric or oro-enteric tube (if tolerated) or consideration of long-term enteral access (22,23).

Gastrointestinal complications include nausea, vomiting, bloating, and diarrhea. In a survey of home enteral patients (22), 29% experienced abdominal pain with feedings and 24% experienced diarrhea. It is important to address these issues as they can have a negative impact on the quality of life. Of note, 44% of the patients surveyed avoided activities because of the tube feedings. Suggestions for evaluating gastrointestinal issues associated with enteral feedings are presented in Table 1 (23).

Metabolic complications associated with EN include fluid and electrolyte imbalances, acid/base disturbances, hyperglycemia, and vitamin, mineral, and trace-element deficiencies. Appropriate monitoring should occur on a regular basis, with the monitoring schedule individualized for the patient (23).

Parenteral Nutrition

PN should be reserved for patients who cannot be fed enterally. Indications for PN include severe gastrointestinal bleeding, obstruction or pseudo-obstruction of the gastrointestinal tract, certain intestinal motility disorders, inflammatory bowel disease, short bowel syndrome, and severe pancreatitis. Relative contraindications to PN include use in patients with a functional gastrointestinal tract, with microbiologic evidence of bacteremia, or when the risk of nutritional support outweighs the benefits (25).

There are two types of PN: peripheral parenteral nutrition (PPN) and central parenteral nutrition (CPN), which is also referred to as total parenteral nutrition (TPN). PPN solution is infused through a peripheral vein and thus the osmolality of the solution must be <900 mOsm/L. The solution is dilute in calories as a result of this limitation, so patients may require up to 3 L of the PPN solution to begin to meet maintenance energy and protein requirements. In addition, PPN solutions are high in fat (as this helps to keep the osmolality low), which increases the risk of infectious complications because excessive intravenous fat is immunosuppressive (26). Since CPN solutions are infused directly into the central venous system, the solution may be more calorically dense, allowing one to meet stress or repletion requirements in less volume (27). There are many choices for central venous access devices. Central venous access devices for short- and long-term access have been recently reviewed (28,29).

PN prescriptions must be carefully reviewed by a pharmacist specializing in compounding these solutions to assure that there are no incompatibilities or imbalances in the electrolyte components that may cause complications such as calcium and phosphate precipitation or lipid emulsion separating from the rest of the solution "cracking" (30).

Since malnourished patients are at risk for postoperative complications, the United States Department of Veterans Affairs Medical Research Service designed a study (31) to assess the effect of perioperative PN on postoperative complications in malnourished patients undergoing major abdominal and thoracic surgeries. The 395 malnourished patients (99% male) were randomized to receive either 7 or 15 days of PN prior to surgery and three days after, or no PN (the control group). There were no significant differences in the incidence of major complications at 30 days and in 90-day mortality. However, there were more infectious complications in the PN group as a whole compared to the control group. When the groups were compared by nutritional status, patients categorized as borderline or moderately malnourished had significantly more infectious complications compared to the severely malnourished group. However, the severely malnourished group derived the most benefit from PN, having significantly fewer noninfectious complications compared to the control group, without an increase in infectious complications. This led to the conclusion that perioperative PN should be reserved for patients who are severely malnourished.

Heyland et al. (32) conducted a meta-analysis to assess the effectiveness of PN in surgical patients. Provision of PN did not make a difference in mortality rates in well-nourished or malnourished patients. However, there was a reduction in major complication rates in all patients and in malnourished patients receiving PN compared to patients receiving "conventional" therapy (oral diet plus intravenous dextrose). In general, one can conclude that PN is beneficial to those who are (*i*) moderately to severely malnourished or at risk for such and (*ii*) cannot be fed by the enteral route for a prolonged (e.g., more than 7–10 days) period.

TABLE 2 Selected Complications Associated with Parenteral Nutrition

Category	Complications	Prevention/treatment strategies
Mechanical	Catheter occlusion	Treat with a thrombolytic agent or other pharmacological agent
		Consider low-dose anticoagulation
		For long-term patients, appropriate education for routine flushing and catheter care
	Catheter malfunction	Replace the catheter
		Choose the appropriate catheter for the patient's needs
Infectious	Catheter-related blood stream infection	Use sterile technique with insertion and routine catheter care
		Use a dedicated port for PN infusion
		Consider use of antibiotic-impregnated catheters for high-risk patients
		For long-term patients, education on appropriate technique for catheter care
Gastrointestinal	Intestinal atrophy	Transition to enteral nutrition as soon as feasible
		For long-term patients, allow small amounts of enteral nutrients if possible
	Parenteral-associated liver disease	Avoid overfeeding
		Avoid excessive lipid delivery
		Assess for carnitine, choline, and vitamin E deficiency; correct deficiency state as needed
		Cycle PN
Metabolic	Dehydration/volume overload	Assess fluid requirements carefully, accounting for additional sources of fluid losses (e.g., fistula output, severe diarrhea) or need for volume restriction (e.g., renal failure)
		Monitor weight daily
		Dilute or concentrate PN solution as needed
		Give supplemental intravenous fluids or treat with diuretics as indicated
	Electrolyte disturbances	Monitor daily when initiating PN, correct abnormalities promptly as indicated
		Once stable, monitor weekly, correcting abnormalities as indicated
	Metabolic bone disease	Assure adequate calcium, phosphorus, and vitamin D delivery
		Yearly dual-energy absorptiometry scans
		Initiate appropriate therapy as indicated
	Vitamin/trace-element deficiency or excess	Monitor full vitamin/trace-element panel every 6 months
		Correct individual deficiencies or excesses as indicated
	Essential fatty acid deficiency	Monitor essential fatty acid panel every 6 months
		Asssure adequate lipid delivery

Abbreviation: PN, parenteral nutrition.

As with EN, complications associated with PN can be divided into four major categories: mechanical, infectious, gastrointestinal, and metabolic. Table 2 summarizes the common complications associated with PN.

Mechanical complications are related to the catheter. Typical mechanical complications include catheter occlusion related to either thrombotic or nonthrombotic causes. Thrombotic occlusions are typically treated with a thrombolytic agent. For nonthrombotic causes, such as occlusion from medication, other pharmacologic agents may be used. Catheter malfunctions, such as a broken catheter, are also categorized as mechanical complications and would require the catheter to be replaced (33).

The most important infectious complication associated with PN is catheter-related blood stream infection (CR-BSI). PN has been identified as an independent risk factor for CR-BSIs and may increase the catheter infection risk by 10 to 20-fold (34). A variety of techniques should be employed to decrease the risk of infectious complications, including using a dedicated port for PN on a multi-lumen catheter and using sterile technique for line insertion and catheter care. The Centers for Disease Control and Prevention have published detailed guidelines for the prevention of catheter-related infections (35).

Gastrointestinal complications associated with PN are typically related to non-use of the gastrointestinal tract. Liver function tests may become elevated within the first few weeks of PN therapy. This is often related to excessive energy delivery. If excessive energy delivery continues, steatosis may develop. The etiology of PN-associated liver disease is unclear, but potential risk factors have been identified including severe protein-deficient malnutrition, carnitine deficiency, choline deficiency, vitamin E deficiency, excessive energy delivery, and lipid overload syndrome (provision of >2.5–3 g lipid/kg) (36,37). It is important to monitor liver function tests regularly and intervene early.

Metabolic complications associated with PN include electrolyte imbalances, acid/base disturbances, volume imbalance, essential fatty acid deficiency, and vitamin, mineral, and trace-element deficiencies. Hospitalized patients should have electrolytes measured daily, and patients treated in their homes should have electrolyte monitored weekly initially, and once stable, monitoring can decrease to every other week to once per month. Essential fatty acids, vitamins, minerals, and trace elements should be measured every six months and appropriate adjustments made to correct low or high levels. Patients receiving long-term PN are also at risk for osteoporosis and osteopenia, and should undergo yearly monitoring to assess bone mineral density (36).

SPECIAL CONSIDERATIONS FOR THE UROLOGIC SURGERY PATIENT
Nutritional Management of Nephrolithiasis

Nutrition can play a significant role in the management of nephrolithiasis. Obesity and weight gain in adulthood increase the risk of kidney stones. In addition, obese patients tend to have higher urine osmolality, and concentrations of uric acid, sodium, oxalate, sulfate, and phosphate, and lower urine pH, all conditions that can precipitate stone formation. Other obesity-related conditions, including type II diabetes and hypertension, can also predispose these patients to kidney stones (38,39). Hence, treatment of kidney stones should include counseling about weight loss in overweight patients.

Patients with a history of fat malabsorption, including those with cystic fibrosis, chronic pancreatitis, Crohn's disease, and short bowel syndrome are at risk for nephrolithiasis. Saponification occurs when unabsorbed fat and bile acids react with calcium in the intestine. This decreases the amount of calcium available to bind with oxalate, leading to increased oxalate absorption and subsequent hyperoxaluria (40). The important factor in this group is to minimize the amount of fat available for saponification. This can be achieved through adequate management of the disorder, through a combination of a low-fat diet, pancreatic enzyme therapy, and alternate fat sources (such as medium-chain triglycerides).

The nutritional management typically depends on the type of stone formed, as well as the implementation of other broad dietary modifications as indicated, such as pursuing weight loss if obesity is a factor. Table 3 summarizes the modifiable dietary factors to consider (41–43).

Previously, patients with hypercalciuria in whom calcium oxalate stones were formed were advised to follow a low-calcium diet. However, results from the Health Professionals Follow-Up Study, the Nurses' Health Study II, and controlled dietary studies have all demonstrated that those with a normal calcium intake have a lower relative risk for the development of kidney stones than those with a low calcium intake (44–48). It is thought that low dietary calcium intake increases oxalate absorption, thereby contributing to increased development of oxalate stones. Ensuring adequate calcium intake may decrease risk, however, calcium intake in excess of 1200 mg/day does not have any additional benefit (49).

Protein and sodium intake can also increase urinary calcium losses. Excessive protein intake, greater than 0.8–1.0 g/kg body weight, has been implicated in the formation of calcium oxalate stones. A high-protein diet carries a large dietary acid load, which requires buffering from the bones. This increases calcium resorption from bone, increasing urinary calcium excretion (42,43). Thus, a protein intake of 0.8–1.0 g/kg is advisable. Those patients on high-protein, high-fat diets (e.g., the Atkins diet) should be advised against following this type of diet if they develop kidney stones. The recommended dietary allowance for adults as set by the Institute of Medicine's Food and Nutrition Board is 0.8 g/kg (50). Since sodium also contributes to urinary calcium losses, intake should be restricted to less than 3000 mg/day (42,43).

TABLE 3   Dietary Modifications for Management of Kidney Stones

Increase fluid consumption to 2.5–3 L/day
Limit protein intake to 0.8–1.0 g/kg
Restrict oxalate intake
High-oxalate foods
Beets
Chocolate
Coffee
Cola
Nuts
Rhubarb
Spinach
Strawberries
Tea
Wheat bran
Restrict sodium intake
Consume adequate calcium (1000–1200 mg/day)
Avoid excessive vitamin C supplementation
Consider vitamin B$_6$ supplementation
Weight loss for obese patients

Patients should be counseled to limit dietary oxalate in order to decrease the amount available for absorption and subsequent excretion in the urine (42,43,51). Many resources are available that have lists of oxalate content of foods, but those listed in Table 3 are considered to have high oxalate content and should be limited (51,52). Ideally, the patient should see a registered dietitian for individualized assessment of typical dietary intake and counseling on minimizing oxalate intake.

Vitamin supplementation can contribute to or protect from kidney stone formation. Excessive vitamin C intake can be a contributor to kidney stones because a small amount of vitamin C is metabolized to oxalate, thus, contributing to hyperoxaluria (47,53). Massey et al. (53) demonstrated that subjects taking 1000 mg vitamin C twice daily had increased urinary oxalate production. In the health professionals follow-up study, Taylor et al. (47) found that those men consuming more than 1000 mg vitamin C per day were at increased risk of developing kidney stones. Interestingly, this was not found in the Nurses' Health Study analysis (54). Supplementation with vitamin B6 may be beneficial as some patients experience decreased oxalate excretion with high doses of this vitamin (54).

Nutritional Considerations in the Urinary Diversion Patient

Patients undergoing urinary diversion are at risk for some nutritional and metabolic disturbances. The type of disturbance depends on the section of the gastrointestinal tract used for reconstruction, as the intestine retains its normal physiologic function (55).

The ileum and the colon are used most frequently in urinary diversion procedures. Both absorb chloride and ammonium from the urine, increasing the risk of the patient developing hyperchloremic metabolic acidosis. Hypokalemia may also be an issue, particularly in patients with colonic segments as the colon is not as efficient as the ileum in reabsorbing potassium. Patients with impaired renal function have difficulty compensating for the acidosis and are more likely to be symptomatic. Patients with continent diversions may also be more symptomatic as there is increased exposure of the mucosa of the intestinal segment to urine. Patients should be monitored carefully and acidosis and hypokalemia should be corrected (55). For patients who have had a section of ileum used, regular monitoring for vitamin B12 deficiency is necessary.

The jejunum has been associated with the greatest metabolic complications when used in urinary diversion procedures and, therefore, is typically the last choice for these procedures. The jejunum secretes sodium, chloride, and water, and reabsorbs potassium and hydrogen ions. The patient is at risk for dehydration, hyponatremia, and hypochloremic metabolic acidosis because of the properties of the jejunum and resultant hormonal responses from the kidney.

With severe metabolic disturbances, patients can present with jejunal conduit syndrome, described as lethargy, nausea, vomiting, dehydration, weakness, and fevers. Treatment for this includes correction of dehydration, repletion of salt losses, and correction of acidosis (55).

A long-term complication associated with urinary diversion procedures may be bone disease as a result of decreased calcium and vitamin D absorption (particularly after ileal resections) and alterations in vitamin D metabolism as a result of acidosis. Patients who fall into high-risk groups for bone disease (children, adolescents, and patients with renal impairment) require regular monitoring, which may include yearly dual-energy X-ray absorptiometry or other measurements to assess bone density (56).

Nutritional Considerations for Prostate Cancer

Many dietary factors are thought to play a role in the development of prostate cancer (57,58). Observational studies have shown a correlation between a high-fat diet and incidence of prostate cancer. Fatty fish may be protective with some, but not all, studies showing decreased incidence of prostate cancer and prostate cancer progression in men with high fish intake (59). This may be due to the high omega-3 fatty acid content of fish, the beneficial omega-3:omega-6 fatty acid ratio, or the high content of naturally occurring vitamin D in fish (58,59).

Obesity is associated with prostate cancer mortality (60,61). A recent study (62) of 526 men with prostate cancer assessed the effect of obesity as well as the effect of weight gain from age 25 to the time of diagnosis. Obese patients at the time of diagnosis had marginally significant ($P = 0.07$) higher rates of "biological failure" [defined as a rise in prostate specific antigen (PSA) ≥ 0.1 ng/mL] over time compared to nonobese men. Men with an annual weight gain of >1.5 kg/yr from age 25 to diagnosis were also at increased risk of biological failure after diagnosis (62). It is recommended that overweight men with prostate cancer be advised to lose weight, with professional help to do so.

Dietary changes after diagnosis may have a beneficial effect on disease progression. Lycopene is a carotenoid that has been shown to have prostate-specific antioxidant properties. It is most bioavailable in cooked tomato products (63,64). Data from the Health Professionals Follow-Up Study (59) demonstrated that men with prostate cancer who were in the highest quartile for tomato sauce intake had a 40% reduced risk of cancer progression compared to those in the lowest quartile. However, men in the highest quartile for fresh tomato consumption had a 58% increased risk of progression compared to the lowest quartile. The cause for this is unclear and warrants further research.

Ornish et al. (65) conducted a lifestyle intervention trial with 93 men with a serum PSA of 4–10 ng/mL and cancer Gleason scores <7 who chose not to undergo conventional treatment for prostate cancer. The men were randomized to follow an intensive lifestyle program (summarized in Table 4) that included dietary changes as well as exercise and stress management or standard lifestyle changes as recommended by their personal physician. At one year, the experimental group had a 4% decrease in PSA from baseline and the control group had a 6% increase in PSA. The experimental group also inhibited serum-stimulated LNCaP cell growth by 70% and the control group by only 9%. There was a trend for decreased C-reactive protein in the experimental group as well, suggesting decreased inflammation.

TABLE 4   Intensive Lifestyle Program for Prostate Cancer

Vegan diet supplemented with soy (1 daily serving of tofu plus 58 g of a fortified soy protein powdered beverage)
Total dietary fat restricted to <10% of total energy intake
3 g fish oil supplement/day
400 IU vitamin E/day
200 mcg selenium/day
2 g vitamin C/day
30 minutes aerobic activity 6 days/wk
60 minutes/day of stress management techniques (stretching, breathing, meditation, imagery, and progressive relaxation)

Many patients are seeking out complementary and alternative medicine (CAM) along with conventional treatment for prostate cancer. These therapies can include simply taking a multivitamin daily to more complex antioxidant and herbal supplements. Table 5 summarizes popular supplements used by prostate cancer patients (63,64,66–76). In a survey (77) of 2582 men with prostate cancer, one-third were using some type of CAM. The most common were oral supplements (26% of the men surveyed), including vitamins and minerals (26%), herbal supplements (16%), antioxidants (13%), and supplements specifically designed for prostate health (12%). These patients often do not inform health care providers of the use of complementary and alternative therapies. Because some of these therapies can have associated toxicities or interact with other therapies, it is important to ask the patient about the use of CAM.

As with other types of cancer, patients with advanced prostate cancer are at risk for developing malnutrition (78). Hence, all malnourished men with prostate cancer should receive appropriate nutritional intervention, preferably enteral nutrition.

Nutritional Considerations for Renal Cancer

As with prostate cancer, nutrition also plays a role in the development of renal cancer. For both men and women, obesity is a risk factor for the development of renal cell carcinoma (RCC). In The Netherlands Cohort Study on diet and cancer (79), a high body mass index (BMI) as well as weight gain from age 20 was associated with increased risk of development of this cancer. Interestingly, those with a BMI between 27 and 30 kg/m2 had the greatest risk of RCC. Data from the European Prospective Investigation into Cancer and Nutrition (80) do not fully support the Netherlands Cohort Study data (79), with the increased risk for men only seen in those with a BMI ≥ 30 kg/m^2 and for women, increased risk for RCC was seen starting with a BMI ≥ 25 kg/m^2. It has also been shown that a high total energy intake also increases the risk of RCC. This is likely reflective of the energy intake required to promote obesity (81).

Prior studies have demonstrated that fruits and vegetables may have a protective effect against RCC, but not all studies are conclusive. In a study (82) assessing the fruit and vegetable intake in Swedish women, those eating >75 servings of fruits and vegetables/month had a decreased risk of RCC, however, the results were not statistically significant. Other studies have also shown trends with specific fruits or vegetables, or no benefit at all (83–85). Daily multivitamin intake does not have a significant impact on incidence of RCC, however, vitamin E and calcium supplements have been found to be associated with decreased risk of RCC in both men and women, and in women only B complex vitamins, vitamin C, and zinc also seem to decrease the risk of RCC (83). Excessive protein intake has also been identified as a risk factor for the development of RCC (81). Given the other health benefits associated with high fruit and vegetable intake, it would be prudent to continue to encourage increased consumption of these foods.

Nutritional Considerations for Urinary Bladder Cancer

Obesity does not play a role in the development of urinary bladder cancer, but it can have an influence on postoperative outcomes. In a study of 498 patients (86) undergoing radical cystectomy primarily for bladder cancer (10 patients had benign disease), those categorized as morbidly obese (defined as BMI ≥ 35 kg/m^2) had a greater risk of postoperative complications compared to those patients categorized as being normal weight, overweight, or obese. The morbidly obese group had more complications as well as more patients with more than one postoperative complication. Specifically, the morbidly obese patients had greater incidences of cardiopulmonary issues, ileus, total wound disturbances, and urinary tract infections compared to all other weight groups. Knowledge of these potential complications for this weight group may help to develop appropriate intervention to help minimize these postoperative complications.

For prevention of urinary bladder cancer, high fruit and vegetable intake may be beneficial. In a case-control study (87) from Serbia, where urinary bladder cancer is one of the most prevalent types of cancer, a high intake of kale, carrots, cereals, tangerines, and cabbage was found to have a protective effect. Intake of liver, pork, canned meats, eggs, and pickled vegetables increased the risk of urinary bladder cancer (87). The risk associated with these foods could

TABLE 5   Selected Complementary and Alternative Medicine Used in Prostate Cancer

Supplement	Potential mode of action	Potential adverse reactions
Carotenoids (beta carotene, lycopene)	Antioxidant; may inhibit prostate cancer cell growth	None known
Vitamin A	May inhibit prostate cancer cell growth	Toxicity can occur with a single dose of >100×the RDA or chronic intake of >25,000 IU for 6 years or >100,000 IU for >6 months. Toxicity effects include osteoporosis, liver damage, desquamation of skin, anorexia
Vitamin C	Antioxidant	Diarrhea, nephrolithiasis, rebound scurvy if abruptly discontinued
Vitamin D	Inhibits proliferation and promotes differentiation of certain tumor cell types; inhibits overall invasion, cell adhesion, and migration in the DU 145 and PC-3 prostate cancer cell lines; inhibition of angiogenesis and enhanced apoptosis	Hypercalcemia, hyperphosphatemia, hypertension, anorexia, nausea, weakness, confusion, lethargy, polyuria, polydipsia, nephrocalcinosis, nephrolithiasis, soft tissue calcification
Vitamin E	Decreased proliferation and increased apoptotic activity; inhibition of cancer cell growth	Nausea, diarrhea, muscle weakness, fatigue; large doses may increase bleeding
Omega-3 fatty acids	Decreased risk of development of prostate cancer with high intake; have anti-inflammatory properties	Nausea, flatulence, diarrhea, "fishy" odor/taste, increased bleeding time
Phytoestrogens	May create a more favorable hormonal pattern; inhibits growth of prostate tissue	In an animal model, supplementation with soy showed enhancement in androgen-independent tumor growth
Selenium	Antioxidant; decreased risk of prostate cancer with high intake	Chronic dermatitis, hair and nail loss, fatigue, dizziness, headache, nausea, vomiting, pulmonary edema, circulatory collapse; may also impair activity of natural killer cells, production of thyroid hormones, growth hormone, and insulin-like growth factor-1
Saw palmetto	Used primarily for benign prostatic hyperplasia, but also used by prostate cancer patients. Inhibits binding of dihydrotestosterone to androgen receptors in prostate cells; inhibits 5-alpha-reductase, the enzyme responsible for converting testosterone to dihydrotestosterone	Headache, nausea, upset stomach
PC-SPES: a combination of *Chrysanthemum morifolium, Isatis indigotica, Glycyrrhiza glabra* (licorice), *Ganoderma lucium, Panax pseudoginseng, Rabdosia rubescens, Serona repens* (saw palmetto), *Scutellaria biacalensis*	Inhibits cell growth; induces cell-cycle arrest of certain cancer cell lines; induces apoptosis in a dose-dependent fashion	Contains diethylstilbestrol which may increase risk of thromboembolic events; may contain indomethacin and warfarin which may increase risk of hemorrhagic events. Has been recalled by the manufacturer as a result of these adverse events
Green tea	Induces apoptosis; dose-dependent inhibition of cell growth	Insomnia, fatigue; caution as some green teas have high vitamin K content
Garlic	Inhibits growth of androgen-dependent prostate cancer cells	May increase the risk of bleeding when used with anticoagulants; heartburn, flatulence, sweating, lightheadedness, allergic reactions
Shark cartilage	Angiogenesis	Hypercalcemia from high calcium content
Modified citrus pectin	Inhibits cancer cell adhesion, aggregation, and metastasis	Loose stools

Abbreviation: RDA, recommended dietary allowance.

be due to the fat content, especially since these foods are often fried, or to the preservatives in the canned meats and pickled vegetables. For the protective foods, the folate content could be the source of protection as fruits, vegetables and grains are high in this B vitamin. Schabath et al. (88) conducted a case-control study assessing the incidence of urinary bladder cancer based on folate intake. Those in the highest quartile of folate intake had a significantly lower risk of incidence of bladder cancer compared to those in the lowest quartile. Unfortunately, not all studies have shown decreased risk of urinary bladder cancer with high fruit and vegetable intake (89,90). However, the general population should still be encouraged to increase fruit and vegetable intake as there are many other health benefits associated with this practice.

SUMMARY AND CONCLUSIONS

Nutrition can play a key role in improving surgical outcomes and can have a specific role in urological surgery patients and patients with urinary tract pathology. Malnutrition needs to be identified early so that appropriate nutritional intervention (oral supplements, enteral tube feeding, or PN) can be initiated to improve outcomes in these patients. For specific urological concerns, specific nutritional guidelines can be very useful to decrease the incidence of recurrent nephrolithiasis, decrease complications associated with urinary diversion procedures, and decrease the incidence of prostate cancer, RCC, and urinary bladder cancer.

REFERENCES

1. Wilmore DW, Robinson MK. Metabolism and nutrition support. In: Fischer JE, ed. Surgical Basic Science. St. Louis, MO: Mosby, 1993:125–169.
2. Kuzu MA, Terzioglu H, Genc V, et al. Preoperative nutritional risk assessment in predicting postoperative outcome in patients undergoing major surgery. World J Surg 2006; 30:378–390.
3. Reilly JJ, Hull SF, Albert N, Waller A, Bringardener S. Economic impact of malnutrition: a model system for hospitalized patients. JPEN J Parenter Enteral Nutr 1988; 12:371–376.
4. Thompson FE, Subar AF. Dietary assessment and methodology. In: Coulston AM, Rock CL, Monsen ER, eds. Nutrition in the Prevention and Treatment of Disease. San Diego, CA: Academic Press, 2001:3–30.
5. Pirie P, Jacobs D, Jeffery R, Hannan P. Distortion in self-reported height and weight. J Am Diet Assoc 1981; 78:601–606.
6. Studley HO. Percentage of weight loss: a basic indicator of surgical risk in patients with chronic peptic ulcer. JAMA 1936; 106:458–460.
7. Seltzer MH, Slocum B, Cataldi-Betcher EL, Fileti C. Instant nutritional assessment: absolute weight loss and surgical mortality. JPEN J Parenter Enteral Nutr 1982; 6:218–221.
8. Roy LB, Edwards PA, Barr LH. The value of nutritional assessment in the surgical patient. JPEN J Parenter Enteral Nutr 1985; 9:239–241.
9. Khuri SF, Daley J, Henderson W, et al. Risk adjustment of the postoperative mortality rate for the comparative assessment of the quality of surgical care: results of the National Veterans Affairs Surgical Risk Study. J Am Coll Surg 1997; 185:325–338.
10. Fuhrman MP, Charney P, Mueller CM. Hepatic proteins and nutrition assessment. J Am Diet Assoc 2004; 104:1258–1264.
11. Robinson, MK, Trujillo EB, Mogensen KM, et al. Improving nutritional screening of hospitalized patients: the role of prealbumin. JPEN J Parenter Enteral Nutr 2003; 27:389–395.
12. Buzby GP, Mullen JL, Matthews DC, Hobbs CL, Rosato EF. Prognostic nutritional index in gastrointestinal surgery. Am J Surg 1980; 139:160–167.
13. Buzby GP, Williford WO, Peterson OL, et al. A randomized clinical trial of total parenteral nutrition in malnourished surgical patients: the rationale and impact of previous clinical trials and pilot study on protocol design. Am J Clin Nutr 1988; 47(suppl 2):366–381.
14. Zaloga GP. Parenteral nutrition in adult inpatients with functioning gastrointestinal tracts: assessment of outcomes. Lancet 2006; 367:1101–1111.
15. Gariballa S, Forster S, Walters S, Powers H. A randomized, double-blind, placebo-controlled trial of nutritional supplementation during acute illness. Am J Med 2006; 119:693–699.
16. Lawson RM, Doshi MK, Barton JR, Cobden I. The effect of unselected post-operative nutritional supplementation on nutritional status and clinical outcome of orthopaedic patients. Clin Nutr 2003; 22:39–46.
17. Ideno KT. Enteral nutrition. In: Gottschlich MM, Matarese LE, Shronts EP, eds. Nutrition Support Dietetics Core Curriculum. 2nd ed. Silver Spring, MD: American Society for Parenteral and Enteral Nutrition, 1993:71–104.

18. Charney P. Enteral nutrition: indications, options, and formulations. In: Gottschlich MM, Fuhrman MP, Hammond KA, Holcombe BJ, Seidner DL, eds. The Science and Practice of Nutrition Support. A Case-Based Core Curriculum. Silver Spring, MD: American Society for Parenteral and Enteral Nutrition, 2001:141–166.

19. Vanek VW. The ins and outs of enteral access. Part 1: Short-term enteral access. Nutr Clin Pract 2002; 17:275–283.

20. Vanek VW. The ins and outs of enteral access. Part 2: Long-term access—esophagostomy and gastrostomy. Nutr Clin Pract 2003; 18:50–74.

21. Vanek VW. The ins and outs of enteral access. Part 3: Long-term access—jejunostomy. Nutr Clin Pract 2003; 18:201–220.

22. Crosby J, Duerksen D. A retrospective survey of tube-related complications in patients receiving long-term home enteral nutrition. Digest Dis Sci 2005; 50:1712–1717.

23. Russell M, Cromer M, Grant J. Complications of enteral nutrition therapy. In: Gottschlich MM, Fuhrman MP, Hammond KA, Holcombe BJ, Seidner DL, eds. The Science and Practice of Nutrition Support. A Case-Based Core Curriculum. Silver Spring, MD: American Society for Parenteral and Enteral Nutrition, 2001:189–209.

24. Maloney JP, Halbower AC, Fouty BF, et al. Systemic absorption of food dye in patients with sepsis. N Engl J Med 2000; 343:1047–1048.

25. A.S.P.E.N. Board of Directors and the Clinical Guidelines Task Force. Guidelines for the use of parenteral and enteral nutrition in adult and pediatric patients. JPEN J Parenter Enteral Nutr 2002; 26(suppl 1):1SA–138SA.

26. Seidner DL, Mascioli EA, Istfan NW, et al. Effects of long-chain triglyceride emulsions on reticuloendothelial system function in humans. JPEN J Parenter Enteral Nutr 1989; 13:614–619.

27. Mirtallo JM. Introduction to parenteral nutrition. In: Gottschlich MM, Fuhrman MP, Hammond KA, Holcombe BJ, Seidner DL, eds. The Science and Practice of Nutrition Support. A Case-Based Core Curriculum. Silver Spring, MD: American Society for Parenteral and Enteral Nutrition, 2001: 211–223.

28. Vanek VW. The ins and outs of venous access. Part 1. Nutr Clin Pract 2002; 17:85–98.

29. Vanek VW. The ins and outs of venous access. Part 2. Nutr Clin Pract 2002; 17:142–155.

30. Barber JR, Miller SJ, Sacks GS. Parenteral feeding formulations. In: Gottschlich MM, Fuhrman MP, Hammond KA, Holcombe BJ, Seidner DL, eds. The Science and Practice of Nutrition Support. A Case-Based Core Curriculum. Silver Spring, MD: American Society for Parenteral and Enteral Nutrition, 2001:251–268.

31. The Veterans Affairs Total Parenteral Nutrition Cooperative Study Group. Perioperative parenteral nutrition in surgical patients. N Engl J Med 1991; 325:525–532.

32. Heyland DK, Montalvo M, MacDonald S, Keefe L, Su XY, Drover JW. Total parenteral nutrition in the surgical patient: a meta-analysis. Can J Surg 2001; 44:102–111.

33. Krzywda EA, Andris DA, Edmiston CE, Wallace JR. Parenteral access devices. In: Gottschlich MM, Fuhrman MP, Hammond KA, Holcombe BJ, Seidner DL, eds. The Science and Practice of Nutrition Support. A Case-Based Core Curriculum. Silver Spring, MD: American Society for Parenteral and Enteral Nutrition 2001:225–250.

34. Beghetto MG, Victorino J, Teixeira L, de Azevedo MJ. Parenteral nutrition as a risk factor for central venous catheter-related infection. JPEN J Parenter Enteral Nutr 2005; 29:367–373.

35. O'Grady NP, Alexander M, Dellinger EP, et al. Guidelines for the prevention and treatment of intravascular catheter-related infections. Infect Control Hosp Epidemiol 2002; 23:759–769.

36. Matarese LE. Metabolic complications of parenteral nutrition therapy. In: Gottschlich MM, Fuhrman MP, Hammond KA, Holcombe BJ, Seidner DL, eds. The Science and Practice of Nutrition Support. A Case-Based Core Curriculum. Silver Spring, MD: American Society for Parenteral and Enteral Nutrition, 2001:269–286.

37. Buchman AL, Iyer K, Fryer J. Parenteral nutrition-associated liver disease and the role for isolated intestine and intestine/liver transplantation. Hepatology 2006; 43:9–19.

38. Taylor EN, Stampfer MJ, Curhan GC. Obesity, weight gain, and the risk of kidney stones. JAMA 2005; 293:455–462.

39. Calvert RC, Burgess NA. Urolithiasis and obesity: metabolic and technical considerations. Curr Opin Urol 2005; 15:113–117.

40. Ferraz RRN, Tiselius H-G, Heiberg IP. Fat malabsorption induced by gastrointestinal lipase inhibitor leads to an increase in urinary oxalate excretion. Kidney Int 2004; 66:676–682.

41. Moe OW. Kidney stones: pathophysiology and medical management. Lancet 2006; 367:333–344.

42. Straub M, Hautmann RE. Developments in stone prevention. Curr Opin Urol 2005; 15:119–126.

43. Pak CYC. Medical management of urinary stone disease. Nephron Clin Pract 2004; 98:c49–c53.

44. Curhan GC, Willett WC, Rimm EB, Stampfer MJ. A prospective study of dietary calcium and other nutrients and the risk of symptomatic kidney stones. N Engl J Med 1993; 328:833–838.

45. Curhan GC, Willett WC, Speizer FE, Spiegelman D, Stampfer MJ. Comparison of dietary calcium with supplemental calcium and other nutrients as factors affecting the risk for kidney stones in women. Ann Intern Med 1997; 126:497–504.

46. Curhan GC, Willett WC, Knight EL, Stampfer MJ. Dietary factors and the risk of incident kidney stones in younger women. Arch Intern Med 2004; 164:885–891.

47. Taylor EN, Stampfer MJ, Curhan GC. Dietary factors and the risk of incident kidney stones in men: new insights after 14 years of follow-up. J Am Soc Nephrol 2004; 15:3225–3232.

48. Borghi L, Schianchi T, Meschi T, et al. Comparison of two diets for the prevention of recurrent stones in idiopathic hypercalciuria. N Engl J Med 2002; 346:77–84.

49. von Unruh GI, Voss S, Sauerbruch T, Hesse A. Dependence of oxalate absorption on the daily calcium intake. J Am Soc Nephrol 2004; 15:1567–1573.

50. Food and Nutrition Board. Dietary Reference Intakes for Energy, Carbohydrate, Fiber, Fat, Fatty Acids, Cholesterol, Protein, and Amino Acids (Macronutrients). Washington, DC: The National Academies Press, 2005.

51. Marcason W. Where can I find information on the oxalate content of foods? J Am Diet Assoc 2006; 106:627–628.

52. National Institute of Diabetes and Digestive and Kidney Diseases. Kidney stones in adults. NIH Publication No. 05–2495. December 2004. (Accessed August 8, 2006, at http://kidney.niddk.nih.gov/kudiseases/pubs/stonesadults/index.htm).

53. Massey LK, Liebman M, Kynast-Gales SA. Ascorbate increases human oxaluria and increases kidney stone risk. J Nutr 2005; 135:1673–1677.

54. Curhan GC, Willett WC, Speizer FE, Stampfer MJ. Intakes of vitamin B6 and C and the risk of kidney stones in women. J Am Soc Nephrol 1999; 10:840–845.

55. Tanrikut C, McDougal WS. Acid-base and electrolyte disorders after urinary diversion. World J Urol 2004; 22:168–171.

56. Roosen A, Gerharz EW, Roth S, Woodhouse CRJ. Bladder, bowel, and bones—skeletal changes after intestinal urinary diversion. World J Urol 2004; 22:200–209.

57. Bostwick DG, Burke HB, Djakiew D, et al. Human prostate cancer risk factors. Cancer 2004; 101(suppl 10):2371–2490.

58. Sonn GA, Aronson W, Litwin MS. Impact of diet on prostate cancer: a review. Prostate Cancer and Prostatic Dis 2005; 8:304–310.

59. Chan JM, Holick CN, Leitzmann MF, et al. Diet after diagnosis and the risk of prostate cancer progression, recurrence, and death (United States). Cancer Causes Control 2006; 17:199–208.

60. Andersson SO, Wolk A, Bergstrom R, et al. Body size and prostate cancer: a 20-year follow-up study among 135006 Swedish construction workers. J Natl Cancer Inst 1997; 89:385–389.

61. Calle EE, Rodriguez C, Walker-Thurmond K, Thun MJ. Overweight, obesity, and mortality from cancer in a prospectively studied cohort of US adults. N Engl J Med 2003; 348:1625–1638.

62. Strom SS, Wang X, Pettaway CA, et al. Obesity, weight gain, and risk of biochemical failure among prostate cancer patients following prostatectomy. Clin Cancer Res 2005; 11:6889–6894.

63. Chan JM, Gann PH, Giovannucci EL. Role of diet in prostate cancer development and progression. J Clin Oncol 2005; 23:8152–8160.

64. Santillo VM, Lowe FC. Role of vitamins, minerals and supplements in the prevention and management of prostate cancer. International Braz J Urol 2006; 32:3–14.

65. Ornish D, Weidner G, Fair WR, et al. Intensive lifestyle changes may affect the progression of prostate cancer. J Urol 2005; 174:1065–1070.

66. Wilkinson S, Chodak GW. Critical review of complementary therapies for prostate cancer. J Clin Oncol 2003; 21:2199–2210.

67. Penniston KL, Tanumihardjo SA. The acute and chronic toxic effects of vitamin A. Am J Clin Nutr 2006; 83:191–201.

68. Vilter RW. Nutritional aspects of ascorbic acid: uses and abuses. West J Med 1980; 133:485–492.

69. Holick MF. Vitamin D. In: Shils ME, Shike M, Ross AC, Caballero B, Cousins RJ, eds. Modern Nutrition in Health and Disease. Baltimore, MD: Lippincott, Williams & Wilkins, 2006:376–395.

70. Traber MG. Vitamin E. In: Shils ME, Shike M, Ross AC, Caballero B, Cousins RJ, eds. Modern Nutrition in Health and Disease. Baltimore, MD: Lippincott, Williams & Wilkins, 2006:396–411.

71. Nichoalds GE. Selenium. In: Baumgartner TG, ed. Clinical Guide to Parenteral Micronutrition. Deerfield, IL: Fujisawa, 1997:387–402.

72. Klepser TB, Klepser ME. Unsafe and potentially safe herbal therapies. Am J Health Syst Pharm 1999; 56:125–138.

73. Saleem M, Adhami VM, Siddiqui IA, Mukhtar H. Tea beverage in chemoprevention of prostate cancer: a mini-review. Nutrition Cancer 2003; 47:13–23.

74. Taylor JR, Wilt VM. Probable antagonism of warfarin by green tea. Ann Pharmacother 1999; 33:426–428.

75. Lagman R, Walsh D. Dangerous nutrition? Calcium, vitamin D, and shark cartilage nutritional supplements and cancer-related hypercalcemia. Support Care Cancer 2003; 11:232–235.

76. Anonymous. Modified citrus pectin-monograph. Altern Med Rev 2000; 5:573–575.

77. Chan JM, Elkin EP, Silva SJ, Broering JM, Latini DM, Carroll PR. Total and specific complementary and alternative medicine use in a large cohort of men with prostate cancer. Urology 2005; 66:1223–1228.

78. Toliusiene J, Lesauskaite V. The nutritional status of older men with advanced prostate cancer and factors affecting it. Support Care Cancer 2004; 12:716–719.
79. van Dijk BAC, Schouten LJ, Kiemeney LALM, Goldbohm RA, van den Brandt PA. Relation of height, body mass, energy intake, and physical activity to risk of renal cell carcinoma: results from The Netherlands Cohort Study. Am J Epidemiol 2004; 160:1159–1167.
80. Pischon T, Lahmann, PH, Boeing H, et al. Body size and risk of renal cell carcinoma in the European prospective investigation into cancer and nutrition (EPIC). Int J Cancer 2006; 118:728–738.
81. Tavani A, La Vecchia C. Epidemiology of renal-cell carcinoma. J Nephrol 1997; 10:93–106.
82. Rashidkhani B, Lindblad P, Wolk A. Fruits, vegetables, and risk of renal cell carcinoma: a prospective study of Swedish women. Int J Cancer 2005; 113:451–455.
83. Hu J, Mao Y, White K, and the Canadian Cancer Registries Epidemiology Research Group. Diet and vitamin or mineral supplements and risk of renal cell carcinoma in Canada. Cancer Causes Control 2003; 14:705–714.
84. van Dijk BAC, Schouten LJ, Kiemeney LALM, Goldbohm RA, van den Brandt PA. Vegetable and fruit consumption and risk of renal cell carcinoma: results from the Netherlands cohort study. Int J Cancer 2005; 117:648–654.
85. Weikert S, Boeing H, Pischon T, et al. Fruits and vegetables and renal cell carcinoma: findings from the European Prospective Investigation into Cancer and Nutrition (EPIC). Int J Cancer 2006; 118: 3133–139.
86. Lee CT, Dunn RL, Chen BT, Joshi DP, Sheffield J, Montie JE. Impact of body mass index on radical cystectomy. J Urol 2004; 172:1281–1288.
87. Radosavljevic V, Sankovic S, Marinkovic J, Dokic M. Diet and bladder cancer: a case-control study. Intern Urol Nephrol 2005; 37:283–289.
88. Schabath MB, Spitz MR, Lerner SP, et al. Case-control analysis of dietary folate and risk of bladder cancer. Nutr Cancer 2005; 53:144–151.
89. Michaud DS, Pietinen P, Taylor PR, Virtanen M, Virtamo J, Albanes D. Intakes of fruits and vegetables, carotenoids and vitamins A, E, C in relation to the risk of bladder cancer in the ATBC cohort study. Br J Cancer 2002; 87:960–965.
90. Holick CN, DeVivo I, Feskanich D, Giovannucci E, Stampfer M, Michaud DS. Intake of fruits and vegetables, carotenoids, folate, and vitamins A, C, E, and risk of bladder cancer among women (United States). Cancer Causes Control 2005; 16:1135–1145.

6 | Complications of Open Renal Surgery

Brian K. McNeil and Robert C. Flanigan
Department of Urology, Loyola University Medical Center, Maywood, Illinois, U.S.A.

INTRODUCTION

Definitive renal surgery has been performed since the mid-19th century when Gustav Simon et al. performed a planned nephrectomy in 1869 for treatment of an ureterovaginal fistula (1). Since then, the indications for open renal surgery have expanded to include management of anatomic abnormalities, renal masses, and ureteropelvic junction obstruction. While the number of laparoscopic procedures performed for conditions once managed by open renal surgery has increased yearly, understanding the complications inherent in open renal surgery remains important.

Complications of open renal surgery can be attributed to numerous factors including, but not limited to, the general medical condition of the patient, failure to recognize anatomic abnormalities, choice of incision, and the relation of the kidney to other intra-abdominal organs (Fig. 1) (2). The goal of this chapter is to explore both common and infrequent complications of open renal surgery, ways to avoid them, and their management.

GENERAL PATIENT CONSIDERATIONS AND UNIQUE CHALLENGES OF RENAL SURGERY

Proper patient selection is paramount in guaranteeing the best outcome for surgical patients. Depending on the surgical approach, open renal surgery can place increased demands on the cardiovascular and pulmonary systems. It is important to perform a thorough preoperative evaluation of patients undergoing open renal surgery.

Pulmonary

Pulmonary function can be significantly impaired during open renal surgery. Ventilation-perfusion mismatch can occur in the flank position, in addition to hypoventilation of the dependent hemithorax as a result of compression (3,4). Trendelenburg positioning can also exaggerate pulmonary hypoventilation, allowing the weight of the abdominal contents to impede diaphragmatic excursion (2). These issues can result in hypoxemia in an individual with moderate to severe chronic obstructive pulmonary disease. Therefore, it is essential to identify patients with pulmonary symptoms preoperatively and have them properly evaluated by a pulmonologist if clinically indicated. An operative incision can then be selected to minimize pulmonary complications.

Cardiovascular

Challenges to the cardiovascular system posed by renal surgery stem from a number of factors. Significant hemodynamic shifts can occur during surgery because of anesthetics, exposed viscera, blood loss, and hypovolemia. Patients should be well hydrated preoperatively. Flank positioning with flexion of the patient can have dramatic effects on cardiac function. Compression of the great vessels can occur during exposure of the kidney and placement of retractors. Compression of the inferior vena cava (IVC) alters cardiac preload, resulting in decreased cardiac output. Aortic compression increases afterload, leading to increased myocardial oxygen consumption. Proper preoperative cardiac evaluation is necessary to identify patients at risk of cardiac complications. Occasionally, operative intervention must to be delayed for cardiac

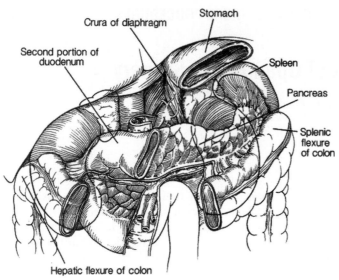

FIGURE 1   The anatomic relationship of the kidneys to surrounding structures in the abdomen. The liver is retracted superiorly. *Source*: From Ref. 1.

revascularization. Fortunately, the slow growth rate (<0.5 cm/yr) of most small (<3.5 cm), incidentally discovered renal lesions, allows cardiac intervention to be accomplished without compromising tumor control (5).

Blood Typing

Because of the kidney's location and vascularity, significant blood loss is possible during surgery. Patients with significant medical comorbidities and those at risk of hemorrhage should be at least typed and screened prior to surgery, with some being cross-matched. Having blood available is paramount in maintaining hemodynamic stability in those who are at risk for a significant loss of blood during renal surgery.

Antibiotics

Antibiotic prophylaxis is recommended for open renal surgery. During some procedures, the collecting system is entered with spillage of urine into the operative field. Although rates of wound infections, subphrenic and intra-abdominal abscesses are relatively low, a perioperative dose of a cephalosporin is generally given. In cases of active infection, culture-specific antibiotics are recommended.

Deep Venous Thrombosis/Pulmonary Embolism Prophylaxis

Venous thromboembolism is a common complication in patients undergoing surgery and one of the most common causes of preventable death in patients hospitalized for surgical procedures (6). Many patients undergoing open kidney surgery have all three risks factors for development of deep venous thrombosis described by Virchow (7). Those with evidence of malignancy may be in a hypercoagulable state. Compression of the IVC during renal surgery can result in a decrease in venous return and increased peripheral venous stasis (2). The use of sequential compression devices can reverse the effect of peripheral venous stasis in patients in the Trendelenburg position (8). It is our institution's preference to use them on all adult patients undergoing open renal surgery.

Wound Infection

Wound infection is a relatively common complication encountered in the postoperative period. Superficial wound infections are best managed with a trial of antibiotics. If erythema persists and a fluid collection is suspected, removal of skin sutures or staples and evacuation of the fluid collection should be performed. The wound should then be allowed to heal through secondary intention with periodic dressing changes. If drainage from the wound is persistent or profuse, the possibility of a retained foreign body or fistulous communication with the urinary tract or intestine should be ruled out.

SPECIFIC COMPLICATIONS RELATED TO SURGICAL APPROACHES TO THE KIDNEY
General Considerations

The kidney can be accessed through a variety of incisions. The choice of incision should be tailored to the operating surgeon's experience and need for exposure. Inadequate exposure can prove disastrous when access to the renal hilum is necessary, making vascular control difficult. One has to balance excellent access with the morbidity of larger incisions. In general, the kidney can be exposed via flank (full flank, rib resection, thoracoabdominal), anterior (chevron, midline transabdominal), or posterior (dorsal lumbotomy) approaches.

Factors to consider in selecting an appropriate incision include the operation to be performed, underlying renal pathology, previous operations, concurrent extra-renal pathology that requires simultaneous management, need for access to both kidneys, and body habitus (1). Other things to consider include the general medical condition of the patient, especially the presence of cardiac or severe pulmonary disease. Each incision places unique stresses on the cardiovascular and pulmonary systems because of changes in ventilatory capacity and cardiac output.

Flank Approaches

An extraperitoneal flank approach minimizes the risk of contamination of the peritoneal cavity with urine, minimizes postoperative ileus, prevents the formation of intraperitoneal adhesions, and allows for direct access to the kidney in obese patients whose pannus falls forward out of the operative field. Disadvantages include the risk of pneumothorax and increased postoperative discomfort secondary to rib removal or fracture. The most common complications of flank incisions are flank bulge, prolonged incisional pain, lumbosacral neuritic pain, and wound herniation (9).

A flank bulge is a common sequela of flank incisions occurring in up to 49% of cases, and is thought to be the result of laxity of the abdominal musculature, caused by intercostal nerve injury as the incision extends laterally toward the intercostal space (10,11). Neurophysiologic studies of Gardener et al. revealed that the affected muscles of patients with flank bulges were denervated, typically from intercostal nerve injury that occurs proximal to the bifurcation of its main trunk (10). Surgical repair of a flank bulge has been described using modified abdominoplasty with plication of the rectus abdominis muscle longitudinally and lateral muscles transversely (12).

Hernia formation, in contrast, is a less common phenomenon after flank renal surgery (9). Patients who are obese have a poor nutritional status, use immunosuppressive medications, experience postoperative wound infection, seroma, or have an increased risk of hernia formation. Flank incisional hernia repairs have been carried out with and without the use of mesh (13,14). In either case, care must be taken to avoid damage to the underlying bowel during exploration. Adhesions can be present, making bowel injury possible during incision and mobilization of the fascia.

Nerve entrapment injuries involving an intercostal nerve can occur resulting in pain and neuralgia (15). In general, nerve entrapment can be managed conservatively with reassurance. If necessary, oral neuroleptics, tricyclic antidepressants, non-steroidal anti-inflammatory agents or local steroid injections can be used to relieve persistent pain (2).

Thoracoabdominal Approaches

A thoracoabdominal incision is desirable for performing radical nephrectomy in patients with large tumors involving the upper portion of the kidney and/or adrenal gland (1). This approach is especially useful for patients with right-sided lesions with vena cava involvement because the great vessels can be visualized up to the level of the diaphragmatic hiatus after division of the triangular and coronary ligaments of the liver (2).

Disadvantages of this approach are the increased operative time necessary to close this incision, postoperative chest tube requirement, and morbidity associated with simultaneous violation of the peritoneal and thoracic cavities (16).

Complications of the thoracoabdominal incision can be divided into those affecting the thoracic and abdominal compartments. Thoracic complications include lung injury with subsequent broncho-pleural fistula formation, empyema, intercostal vessel bleeding, and diaphragmatic paralysis from phrenic nerve injury. Abdominal complications include liver or splenic injury, lumbar vein injury, postoperative adhesion formation, prolonged ileus, and small bowel obstruction (16).

The short- and long-term morbidity of the thoracoabdominal incision for nephrectomy has been compared to the flank approach. Kumar et al. reported comparable morbidity for both incisions with regard to incisional pain, analgesic requirements after discharge home, and return to normal activities (17). Soft tissue injuries can be avoided by refraining from aggressive retraction and proper padding. Care must be taken not to entrap lung parenchyma during closure of the diaphragm. Meticulous closure of the diaphragm, typically using two layers, is required to prevent postoperative diaphragmatic rupture with herniation of abdominal contents into the chest.

Anterior Abdominal Approaches

Anterior transperitoneal approaches may be utilized for large renal masses involving adjacent organs and for patients whose medical status precludes flank exploration. Advantages of the anterior transperitoneal approach include maximum exposure of the renal pedicle, abdominal exploration, management of other intra-abdominal pathology, and less dramatic hemodynamic shifts compared to flank approaches because venous return is not compromised. Disadvantages of the anterior approach are prolonged postoperative ileus and increased risk of intra-abdominal adhesion formation with subsequent small bowel obstruction.

Choices for anterior approaches to the kidney include unilateral subcostal, midline transperitoneal, paramedian, anterior extraperitoneal, and chevron incisions (18). Surgeon experience and need for exposure dictate the choice of anterior approach.

Posterior Approaches

Dorsal lumbotomy provides a less traumatic approach compared to flank and anterior incisions that is useful for removal of small, low-lying kidneys, bilateral nephrectomy in patients with end-stage renal disease, open renal biopsy, pyeloplasty, pyelolithotomy, and upper tract ureterolithotomy to remove an impacted stone (19). The advantages of this technique include avoidance of muscle transection which translates into shorter hospital stays and decreased analgesic requirement (20).

The kidney is accessed by incising the posterior fascial layers. Entry into the peritoneum is avoided and wound complications associated with this incision are rare because of the strength of the lumbodorsal fascia. The main disadvantage of this incision is the limited exposure of the renal hilum, making control of potential bleeding from shearing of the adrenal vessels, renal artery, or renal vein difficult. Complications from this incision are unusual and include dorsolateral nerve rami, subcostal, and iliohypogastric nerve injury. Because injury to these structures can result in significant postoperative discomfort, they should be identified during surgery to avoid inadvertent injury.

COMPLICATIONS OF RENAL EXPOSURE
Pneumothorax

Pneumothorax can result from violation of the pleura during incision, vigorous retraction, or perforation of the pleura by a suture during closure (2). Pneumothorax with accompanying chest tube placement is expected when a thoracoabdominal approach to the kidney is employed.

The reported incidence of pleurotomy during flank surgery ranges from 2% to 29% (21–24). The risk of pleural violation for 12th rib and subcostal approaches is lower than that of 10th or 11th rib approaches. The majority of these injuries are recognized and managed intraoperatively. The injury can be discovered by visual inspection of the operative field or by filling the incision with saline and instructing the anesthesiologist to hyper-expand the lung. Bubbles from the wound suggest the presence of a pleural injury.

If recognized, small pleural defects can be closed with a running 3-0 or 4-0 suture (1). Before complete closure of the incision, a red rubber catheter, cut with extra side holes distally, is inserted into the pleural cavity. The catheter can then be placed under water seal (using a kidney basin or other container), while the anesthesiologist repeatedly hyper-inflates the lung, allowing fluid and air to be drained from the pleural cavity into the basin of water (Fig. 2). Large pleural defects should be managed with closure of the defect and intraoperative chest tube placement.

Although there have been some reports suggesting that routine postoperative plain chest films are not necessary following open flank surgery, it is our preference to obtain routine chest films after flank surgery to rule out the presence of a significant pneumothorax, especially after cases involving pleural violation (21). Minimal pneumothorax (typically <15%) can be managed expectantly with oxygen supplementation until it has resolved on follow-up imaging. Larger pneumothorax, tension pneumothorax, or pneumothorax resulting in respiratory symptoms should be managed with chest tube placement.

Retroperitoneal Hemorrhage and Vascular Injuries

Retroperitoneal hemorrhage can occur during mobilization of the kidney or retraction of the great vessels. There are four predictable bleeding sites in the retroperitoneum (1).

Lumbar veins enter the posterolateral aspect of the vena cava at each vertebral level. Large lumbar veins also course posteriorly from the left renal vein just lateral to the aorta or from the posterior aspect of the vena cava close to the entry of the right renal vein. Undue traction on the vena cava can lead to lumbar vein avulsion. This can be avoided by gentle retraction of the vena cava and careful ligation of these vessels within the operative field. Inadvertent shearing of the venous wall resulting in hemorrhage can also occur during ligation of these

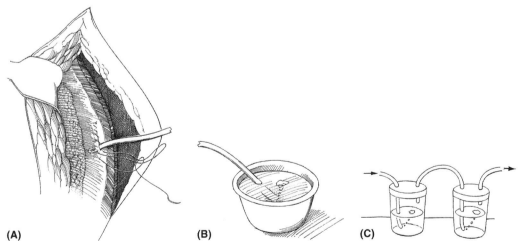

(A) **(B)** **(C)**

FIGURE 2 Repair of a pleural tear. (**A**) Before complete closure of the incision, a red rubber catheter, cut with extra side holes distally, is inserted into the pleural cavity. Use a running 4–0 catgut suture to close the pleural defect, continuing it around the catheter and tying it beyond the end of the defect. (**B**) The catheter can then be placed under water seal (using a kidney basin or other container) while the anesthesiologist repeatedly hyper-inflates the lung, allowing fluid and air to be drained from the pleural cavity into the basin of water. (**C**) If there is a possibility that the lung has been perforated, guide the catheter from the wound and place it under water in a sterile vacuum system (Pleur-Evac). *Source*: From Ref. 14.

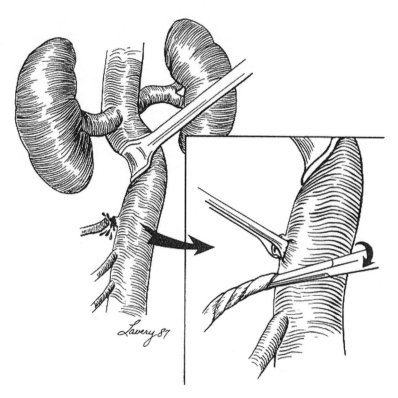

FIGURE 3 Technique for securing ends of a lumbar vein avulsed from the inferior vena cava. *Source*: From Ref. 75.

vessels. If an avulsed lumbar vein is suspected as the source of hemorrhage, the vena cava should be rolled medially with compression above and below the site of bleeding until the posterolateral entry of the vein is exposed and controlled (Fig. 3). Persistent bleeding from the proximal end of an avulsed lumbar can be controlled by securing it with an Allis clamp and ligating it, or placing a figure of eight suture through the psoas muscle overlying the vein if it retracts. Lumbar vein avulsion from the left renal vein can be controlled in a similar fashion (Fig. 4).

Other sources of bleeding encountered during mobilization include the entries of the right gonadal vein, renal veins, and right adrenal vein into the IVC. In all these instances, control of the injured vessel and repair of vena caval lacerations can be accomplished by first gaining proximal and distal control of the vena cava and then closing the defect (Fig. 5).

Vascular injuries to the celiac axis and superior mesenteric artery have also been reported during nephrectomy and are potentially disastrous complications. This injury typically occurs during left radical nephrectomy for large lesions with accompanying adenopathy (25). Failure to recognize these injuries can result in ischemic bowel leading to sepsis and death. If injury to the superior mesenteric artery is suspected, either from transaction or a crush injury, vascular surgery should be consulted immediately to determine the need for repair. Simple visual inspection of the bowel and palpation of pulses is not adequate for determining the severity of injury (26). Blunt et al. reported a case of inadvertent superior mesenteric artery (SMA) injury that was repaired with a native renal vein patch (26).

Mass ligation of the renal pedicle has been described for cases in which the renal artery and vein could not be safely isolated. This technique should be used as a last resort as it may increase the risk of postoperative arteriovenous fistula formation at the stump. Uncontrolled bleeding from the pedicle during dissection can be controlled by compressing the pedicle against the vertebral bodies. A vascular clamp can then be placed across the entire pedicle. Care must be taken not to injure the duodenum, as cases of duodenal injury have been associated

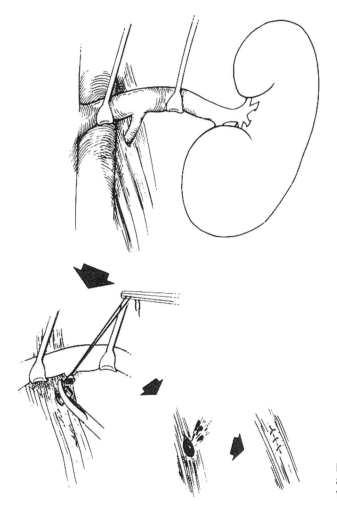

FIGURE 4 Technique for securing ends of a lumbar vein avulsed from the left renal vein. *Source*: From Ref. 75.

with mass ligation of the pedicle. Suture ligatures are more secure than simple mass ligation, but can theoretically augment the risk of arteriovenous fistula formation (2).

Arteriovenous fistula formation is probably an under-reported phenomenon, as it is asymptomatic in most patients. Less than 100 cases have been reported in the literature. Important causative factors include infection and mode of ligation (27). In Lacombe's review of arteriovenous fistulas occurring after nephrectomy, ligation method details were available for 14 patients (27). Approximately 86% (12/14) underwent mass ligation of the pedicle. The interval between nephrectomy and diagnosis of fistula can range from months to decades. Because of this, auscultation of the renal fossa as a component of routine follow-up has been suggested. Clinical symptoms of arteriovenous fistula include high-output congestive heart failure, hypertension, and wide pulse pressure (28). Angiography with embolization or open surgical repair are options available for the management of symptomatic arteriovenous fistulas (29).

Showering of clot or tumor emboli during mobilization of the renal vein and IVC is a severe complication that can result in mortality. Renal vein and IVC involvement should be detected preoperatively using magnetic resonance (MR) or computed tomography (CT) scanning. Two cases have been reported in the literature utilizing a "temporary" vena caval filter to prevent the dispersion of tumor emboli during nephrectomy (30). The authors had temporary suprarenal caval filters placed preoperatively using a jugular vein approach after venography to define the extent of thrombus. In both cases, the thrombus was retrieved two weeks after surgery without complication.

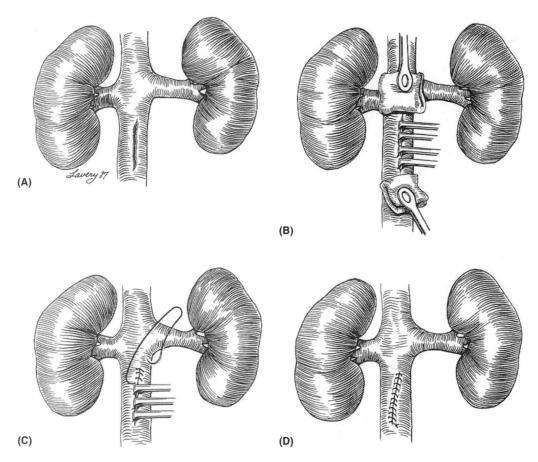

FIGURE 5   Technique for repair of an extensive laceration of the inferior vena cava. *Source*: From Ref. 75.

Temporary renal insufficiency can develop postoperatively, especially after excising tumors with a renal vein or caval thrombus (31,32). This may also occur after temporary occlusion of the left renal vein during procedures for right renal masses with IVC involvement. This is most likely secondary to venous obstruction and typically resolves as venous drainage improves with the development of venous collaterals. Ligation of the right renal vein leads to permanent renal nonfunction because of the lack of collateral circulation (1).

Splenic Injury

Splenic injury is a well recognized complication of open renal surgery, more commonly occurring in cases involving the left kidney. In fact, left nephrectomy has been reported to be the second or third most common cause of splenectomy for iatrogenic reasons (33). While incidence rates as high as 24% have been reported in the literature, contemporary series report an incidence ranging from <1% to 8% depending on the size and location of the renal tumor (34–36). The risk of splenic injury during extraperitoneal flank procedures is less that that associated with anterior transperitoneal approaches. A detailed knowledge of the spleen and its anatomic relationships with adjacent organs is one of the major factors in preventing splenic injury (37).

Direct injury from manual traction and indirect injury from ligament manipulation are the primary sources of splenic injury during open renal surgery. Because of splenic ligamentous attachments, manual retraction on the greater omentum or colon can result in capsular laceration of the spleen. Indirect injuries to the spleen are more common than direct injuries. Cooper et al. reported 18 patients requiring splenectomy from injuries sustained during left radical nephrectomy (38). Avulsion of the splenic capsule was the cause in 12 patients while spleno-renal adhesions (three), retractor injury (two), and splenic laceration (one) were causes in the remaining cases.

Coloepiploic mobilization has been proposed as a way to reduce the risk of iatrogenic splenectomy during left transperitoneal radical nephrectomy (39). Division of the ligaments that attach the spleen to the stomach, colon, kidney, and omentum prior to retraction can also decrease the risk of splenic injury during transperitoneal approaches.

If a capsular tear is suspected intraoperatively, the splenic capsule should be inspected. Although superficial injuries may be controlled with simple packing and re-evaluation of the capsule, mild to moderate injuries are typically managed with splenorrhaphy or non-suture techniques including argon beam coagulation, Neodymium YAG (Nd:YAG) laser coagulation, or the use of fibrin sealant-combined compression (40,41).

For severe lacerations and injuries involving the splenic hilum, splenectomy is indicated. If severe uncontrolled bleeding is encountered, the splenic artery and vein can be compressed to slow the loss of blood by opening the lesser sac and compressing the tail of the pancreas between the thumb and the forefinger (2).

Splenectomy involves division of the attachments of the spleen to the colon, kidney, peritoneum, and diaphragm followed by mobilization of the pancreatic tail away from the splenic hilum. Division of the short gastric vessels facilitates this maneuver. The splenic artery and vein are then dissected, ligated, and divided (2).

Asplenic patients are at increased risk for infection and sepsis caused by encapsulated, gram-positive, and gram-negative bacteria. A pneumococcal vaccine should be given prior to discharge from the hospital. Antibiotic prophylaxis has been recommended for minor surgical and dental procedures after splenectomy (2).

Liver Injury

Liver injuries can result from kidney mobilization, retraction, and accidental laceration. The liver can also be involved by cancerous and/or inflammatory processes extending from the involved kidney (42). Injuries to the liver usually occur during right- sided procedures. Care should be taken to avoid aggressive traction on the liver. All retractors should be well padded.

In cases where large right lesions are present and ready access to the right retroperito-neum is required, liver mobilization should be performed first. Urology and transplant colleagues at the University of Miami have described liver mobilization, beginning with division of the ligamentum teres, followed by division of the falciform ligament (43). This dissection can then be carried around each portion of the divided falciform ligament to the right superior coronary ligament followed by division of the left triangular ligament. Incision of the right inferior coronary ligament, hepatorenal ligament, and ligation of vessels from the bare area of the liver to the diaphragm can provide excellent exposure, minimizing the need for aggressive retraction of the liver. The liver can then be gently rolled to the left side, exposing the right retroperitoneum (Fig. 6).

Superficial laceration of the liver can be managed with fulguration using the bovie, argon-beam coagulation, or horizontal mattress suture placement with a surgical bolster (2). Significant bleeding from the liver can be controlled temporarily by the Pringle maneuver. Intraoperative general surgical consultation should be obtained for deeper injuries as concomitant ductal injury may have occurred. Partial resection of the liver is indicated for tumors involving the liver and significant injuries not controlled with other measures. Closed suction drainage of the area should be considered for all significant liver injuries. Patients with a history of cirrhosis present unique challenges because of their bleeding tendencies, ascites, engorgement of the portal system, and extensive retroperitoneal collateral circulation (44). Careful preoperative imaging is necessary in these patients to define collateral circulation.

Pancreatic Injury

Mobilization of the pancreas may occur because of its anatomic relationship to the kidneys, especially when managing large renal tumors that abut the pancreatic tail. Difficulty may also be encountered in cases of xanthogranulomatous pyelonephritis or other inflammatory

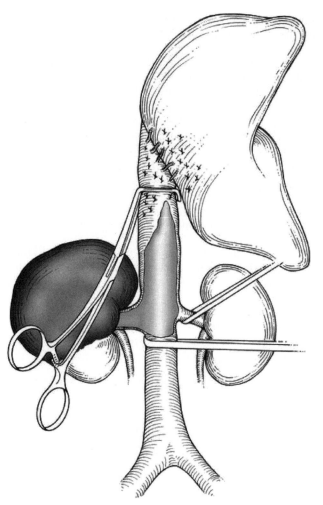

FIGURE 6 Mobilization of the right lobe of the liver to expose the right retroperitoneum and gain control of the inferior vena cava proximal to a caval thrombus. *Source*: From Ref. 76.

processes that result in perirenal inflammation and distorted anatomy. Mobilization of the pancreas during surgery can lead to postoperative pancreatitis, making serum pancreatic enzyme assessment necessary in cases with a prolonged postoperative ileus.

Intraoperative complications involving the pancreas include parenchymal laceration and ductal injuries. Intraoperative recognition of these injuries with immediate repair can limit morbidity. Simple lacerations of the parenchyma can be repaired by closing the capsule with interrupted, nonabsorbable sutures, after inspection to rule out pancreatic duct injury. Reinforcement of the repair with omentum is recommended. A closed suction drain placed near the pancreatic bed allows for detection of postoperative leakage (2). For cases of ductal injury involving the distal two-thirds of the pancreas, resection of the involved parenchyma with exposure and suture ligation of the pancreatic duct is preferred by most surgeons. The capsule can then be reapproximated over this closure.

Postoperative complications of pancreatic injury include pancreatitis, pancreatic fistula, and pseudocyst formation (45). Serial serum pancreatic enzyme levels (amylase and lipase) should be monitored, while the patient remains nothing per mouth (NPO) or is given parenteral nutrition. A diet can be re-instituted after enzymes normalize and the clinical status improves. For cases when enzyme levels remain elevated with bowel rest, a CT scan should be performed to assess inflammation and whether or not a fluid collection is present. If fluid is detected, it should be aspirated and a drain should be left in place. Exploration with debridement should be considered if bacteria are detected, by culture or Gram stain, and necrotic pancreatitis is suspected. Broad-spectrum antibiotic treatment should be instituted until sensitivities are obtained. Octreotide has been shown to decrease pancreatic fistula output leading to spontaneous closure in some cases (46).

Duodenal Injury

Duodenal injury typically occurs during exposure of the right kidney, involves the second portion of the duodenum, and is usually caused by aggressive retraction or inadequate padding of retractors. Accidental punctures and incision of the duodenum can also occur. Small lacerations should be managed with a two-layer closure. An omental flap may be mobilized to cover the repair and minimize the risk of fistula formation.

Trauma to the duodenum can result in sub-serosal hematoma formation. The duodenum should be inspected prior to closure and if a hematoma is discovered, it should be evacuated by incising the overlying serosa. When the source of bleeding is discovered and controlled, sutures can be used to close the serosa followed by omental reinforcement.

Colonic Injury

Complications involving the colon are rare during routine open renal procedures; however, the risk of injury is increased when large masses or an inflammatory process obscures normal anatomy. When large tumors invade the colon, segmental colon resection with primary reanastomosis may be performed. Preoperative bowel preparation is therefore important in any case where bowel resection might be anticipated in order to minimize spillage of bowel contents if injury does occur.

If a thermal injury or laceration of the colon is identified, resection of that segment may be necessary. If a rent in the mesocolon occurs during mobilization of the colon off the anterior surface of Gerota's fascia, it should be closed to prevent internal herniation (2). Injuries altering blood supply to the colon can occur and may be subclinical, not resulting in discoloration of the involved bowel segment.

Adrenal Injury

Injuries to the adrenal gland can occur during mobilization of the kidney. Minor injuries can be controlled by oversewing the bleeding sites. More extensive injuries may require partial or total adrenalectomy, especially if the contralateral adrenal gland is normal.

COMPLICATIONS RELATED TO SPECIFIC RENAL PROCEDURES
Simple Nephrectomy for Inflammatory or Polycystic Kidneys

Simple nephrectomy is indicated for patients with an irreversibly damaged kidney from symptomatic chronic infection, obstruction resulting in renal failure, stone disease, or severe traumatic injury (1). Eventhough simple nephrectomy can be performed through a variety of incisions, the flank extraperitoneal approach is preferred for removal of kidneys involved in infectious processes to avoid peritoneal contamination. Care must be taken not to enter the pleural cavity for similar reasons.

In patients who have severe peri-renal inflammation or have had prior retroperitoneal surgery, a subcapsular technique should be considered. When removing a kidney involved with an infectious process, the operative field should be copiously irrigated and drains should be placed in the renal fossa (1).

Simple nephrectomy is also a viable option for individuals with polycystic kidney disease prior to transplantation. Many patients do not require this but it is considered for individuals with a history of uncontrolled hypertension, intractable pain, bleeding, infection, or those with extremely large polycystic kidneys (2).

Radical Nephrectomy for Complicated Renal Cancers

Renal cell carcinoma is the most commonly diagnosed malignancy of the kidney accounting for approximately 3% of all adult malignancies (47). There are greater than 30,000 newly diagnosed cases and greater than 12,000 deaths that result from this malignancy in the United States annually (48). Radical nephrectomy has been the treatment of choice for patients with localized renal cell carcinoma (49,50). The traditional approach involved early ligation of the renal artery and vein, removal of the kidney outside of Gerota's fascia, removal of the ipsilateral adrenal gland, and performance of a complete regional lymphadenectomy from the crus of the diaphragm to the aortic bifurcation (49). Although lymphadenectomy allows for more accurate pathologic staging, its therapeutic value remains controversial (1). Some have argued that lymph node dissection is not therapeutically useful for most patients (51). Removal of the ipsilateral adrenal gland is not routinely necessary unless the suspected tumor is large or involves the upper pole (52). Reported intraoperative complication rates of radical nephrectomy range from 6% to 20% (34,35). In a series of 656 radical nephrectomies, all performed through a transperitoneal anterior subcostal incision, Mejean et al. reported an intraoperative complication rate of 6.4% and postoperative complication rate of 29.7% (35). Fifteen (2.3%) postoperative complications were treated surgically.

In cases of very large tumors or in cases in which the renal vessels are encased in tumor, preoperative embolization of the renal artery may be used to minimize operative blood loss. Complications associated with preoperative embolization include fever, pain, nausea, and vomiting. Placement of the embolization coils in the renal artery can also occlude the artery, where one wants to tie it off, potentially complicating the operation (2).

Renal neoplasms involve the vena cava in 4% to 15% of patients with renal cell carcinoma (53). Surgical management of these lesions has its own set of inherent complications. In some studies, the incidence of complications increased with higher levels of tumor thrombus (54). Involvement of the supra-diaphragmatic vena cava by tumor thrombus presents a particularly difficult problem. For lesions involving the supra-diaphragmatic vena cava and atrium, we typically prefer a chevron incision combined with a median sternotomy. This approach allows for maximum exposure and easy access to the supra-diaphragmatic vena cava and heart when necessary.

Partial Nephrectomy

Partial nephrectomy is associated with a number of unique complications in addition to those associated with open radical nephrectomy. Complications of partial nephrectomy include bleeding, arteriovenous fistula formation, postoperative urinary leak, fistula formation, ureteral obstruction, renal insufficiency, and infection (1). The reported incidence of complications from partial nephrectomy ranges from 4% to 30% (55–64). In one contemporary review of the literature involving 1129 patients, Uzzo and Novick reported the incidence of postoperative death to be 1.6%, splenic injury 0.6%, urinary fistula formation 7.4%, prolonged acute tubular necrosis 6.3%, infection 3.2%, bleeding 2.8%, and reoperation 1.9% (65).

Profuse intraoperative bleeding during partial nephrectomy can occur when using compression techniques alone or after vascular clamps are removed. Manual compression and suture ligation of bleeding sites is useful in most cases. Combining this technique with occlusion of the pedicle for five minutes is an option in difficult cases yet one must be aware of the risk of reperfusion injury, especially when prior clamping of the vessels has been performed (2). Postoperative delayed bleeding can also occur and is best managed initially with bed rest, serial hemoglobin and hematocrit checks, frequent monitoring of vital signs and transfusion as needed. If bleeding persists, angiography and embolization can be performed. Re-exploration with early control of the pedicle and ligation of active bleeding points may be necessary if embolization is contraindicated or unsuccessful (1).

Prolonged urinary leakage and fistula formation has occurred in 15 to 17% of reported cases (1,58). Prolonged drainage from the flank can be analyzed for creatinine concentration to determine the presence of urine. Another way to confirm the presence of a leak is to inject indigo carmine and monitor the drain output for the appearance of dye (2). The majority of leaks resolve spontaneously. If drainage persists, one should first partially advance the drain because it could be in direct contact with the repair of the collecting system and have a siphoning effect. If this does not alleviate drainage, cystoscopy with retrograde pyelography and ureteral stent placement should be performed. If an indwelling stent is used, concomitant foley bladder drainage should be employed until leakage stops. If this is not possible, a percutaneous nephrostomy tube should be inserted. Fistulas may take several weeks to heal and exploration to close the fistula is rarely necessary (1).

Ureteral obstruction can also occur after surgery because of an obstructing clot. The clot should resolve spontaneously, but in cases when it does not, a ureteral stent should be placed to facilitate antegrade drainage and healing of the collecting system.

Prolonged acute tubular necrosis (ATN) and renal insufficiency after partial nephrectomy have a reported incidence ranging from 0.7% to 15% and are usually the result of removal of substantial renal parenchyma and/or intraoperative renal ischemia. ATN is usually transient and resolves spontaneously with proper fluid and electrolyte management (1). Acute dialysis may be required in up to 5% of cases (65).

Infectious complications after partial nephrectomy have been reported to occur in 0.6% to 6% of patients (65). Infections are typically self-limiting but prolonged drainage and adjuvant antibiotic treatment is necessary for patients with infected urinomas and abdominal abscesses.

Pyeloplasty

While treatment options for congenital and acquired ureteropelvic junction obstruction have expanded with the growing number of urologists comfortable with endourologic and laparoscopic techniques, open pyeloplasty remains the gold standard with success rates greater than 90% (66).

An extraperitoneal approach is preferred for open management of ureteropelvic junction obstruction. This can be accomplished through an anterior, flank, or posterior dorsal lumbotomy approach. Care must be taken to avoid damage to crossing vessels if present. This can result in a devascularized segment of the kidney. At the completion of the procedure, a penrose drain should be placed adjacent to the anastomosis prior to closure.

Complications of open pyeloplasty include devascularization of the ureter, persistent obstruction, anastomotic stricture formation, prolonged leakage with subsequent urinoma and fistula formation, and all other complications associated with renal exposure. Some have debated the utility of internal stenting as a way to minimize complications after open pyeloplasty. Smith et al. found similar outcomes in children undergoing stented versus nonstented repair with complication rates of 12% and 14%, respectively (67).

Anastomotic stricture formation and persistent obstruction are uncommon complications of open pyeloplasty with a published incidence ranging from 2% to 6% (68,69). The risk of both can be minimized by creating a tension-free repair and delicate atraumatic handling of the tissue. Unnecessary manipulation of the ureter can strip the distal segment of its blood supply and compromise healing.

Urinoma formation can occur as a result of prolonged leakage from the anastomosis and inadequate drainage. It should be suspected in patients who experience a prolonged ileus, fever, or complain of significant postoperative pain. CT scanning can confirm the diagnosis and percutaneous drainage should be performed. Broad-spectrum antibiotics should be added until culture results are obtained if infection is suspected. Urinomas are problematic because they can result in an intense inflammatory reaction that can lead to fibrosis and failure of the repair (68).

Surgery on Ectopic and Horseshoe Kidneys

Surgery on ectopic and horseshoe kidneys pose special dilemmas because of variability in their location, blood supply, and proximity to other structures. Many feel that the incidence of surgical complications is greater in individuals with these anatomic abnormalities. In particular, hemorrhage and urinary fistula have been reported in the literature.

Hallmarks of horseshoe kidneys include their low position, multiple and varied arterial supplies, and anteriorly positioned collecting systems (2). The horseshoe kidney characteristically obtains its blood supply from several sources during its incomplete ascent. These sources include the inferior mesenteric artery, aorta, and iliac arteries (70). In approximately 30% of cases, there is one renal artery for each kidney, but there could be duplicate or even triplicate renal arteries supplying one or both kidneys (71,72). The isthmus is sometimes divided during procedures to correct drainage abnormalities and remove renal tumors. Division of the isthmus can lead to further complications because of its vascularity. It should be left intact unless it is an avascular fibrous band, involved with tumor, or the cause of collecting system obstruction. These characteristics augment the risk of surgical complications in these patients.

There have been fewer than 200 cases of malignancy associated with horseshoe kidneys reported in the literature. Malignancy can arise in any portion of a horseshoe kidney and vena caval involvement has been reported in an individual with a tumor located at the isthmus (73). The horseshoe kidney can be approached via midline transperitoneal, thoracoabdominal, extended subcostal transperitoneal, or transverse abdominal incisions depending on the exposure needed.

Thorough preoperative imaging of horseshoe kidneys is imperative to minimize the risk of inadvertent injury to the renal vessels, collecting system and ureters. In 2004, Terrone et al. reported a case of renal cell carcinoma in a presacral ectopic kidney (74). A radical nephrectomy was performed through a median umbilical-pubic laparotomy. They reported no operative or delayed complications nine months after surgery. Because of preoperative MR imaging of the mass and surrounding structures, they were able to avoid damage to the iliac vessels and aorta. The same surgical principles used to avoid complications in patients undergoing normotopic renal surgery should be employed in patients with ectopic kidneys.

Nephron-sparing surgery on horseshoe kidneys can also result in postoperative urine leaks and urinoma formation. Three-dimensional CT angiography can be useful in identifying the anatomic characteristics of these cases.

CONCLUSION

A thorough knowledge of complications of open renal surgery is necessary for all urologists. With the changing scope of urologic training and proliferation of minimally invasive techniques for kidney surgery, residents and fellows may not encounter all of the complications of open renal surgery during their training. An understanding of the etiology of complications and techniques to avoid them will translate into improved peri-operative patient care.

REFERENCES

1. Novick AC. Surgery of the kidney. In: Walsh PC, Retik AB, Vaughan ED, Wein AJ, eds. Campbell's Urology. Philadelphia, PA: Saunders, 2002:3570–3643.
2. Naitoh J, Smith RB. Complications of renal surgery. In: Taneja SS, Smith RB, Ehrlich RM, eds. Complications of Urologic Surgery, Prevention and Management. Philadelphia, PA: Saunders, 2001:299–325.
3. West JB. Mechanics of breathing. In: West JB, ed. Physiologic Basis of Medical Practice. Baltimore, MD: Williams & Wilkins, 1985:580.
4. Borten M. Contraindications. In: Friedman EA, ed. Laparoscopic Complications, Prevention and Management. Toronto, Canada, BC Decker, 1986:139.
5. Bosniak MA, Birnbaum BA, Krinsky GA, et al. Small renal parenchymal neoplasms: further observations on growth. Radiology 1995; 197:589–597.
6. Agnelli G. Prevention of venous thromboembolism in surgical patients. Circulation 2004; 110: IV4–12.
7. Virchow RR. Cellular Pathology as Based Upon Physiological and Pathological istology. London: John Churchill, 1860.
8. Millard JA, Hill BB, Cook PS, et al. Intermittent sequential pneumatic compression in prevention of venous stasis associated with pneumoperitoneum during laparoscopic cholecystectomy. Arch Surg 1993; 128:914–918.
9. Honig MP, Mason RA, Giron F. Wound complications of the retroperitoneal approach to the aorta and iliac vessels. J Vasc Surg 1992; 15:28–33.
10. Gardner GP, Josephs LG, Rosca M, et al. The retroperitoneal incision. An evaluation of postoperative flank "bulge." Arch Surg 1994; 129:753–756.
11. Chatterjee S, Nam R, Fleshner N, et al. Permanent flank bulge is a consequence of flank incision for radical nephrectomy in one half of patients. Urol Oncol 2004; 22:36–39.
12. Hoffman RS, Smink DS, Noone RB, et al. Surgical repair of the abdominal bulge: correction of a complication of the flank incision for retroperitoneal surgery. J Am Coll Surg 2004; 199:830–835.
13. Petersen S, Schuster F, Steinbach F, et al. Sublay prosthetic repair for incisional hernia of the flank. J Urol 2002; 168:2461–2463.

14. Hinman F. Surgical Approaches to the kidney. In: Hinman F, ed. Atlas of Urologic Surgery. Philadelphia, PA: Saunders, 1998:853–910.

15. Foley KM. Posttraumatic neuralgia. In: Berkow R, Fletcher AJ, eds. Merck Manual of Diagnosis and Therapy. Rahway, NJ: Merck, Sharp and Dohme, 1987:1039.

16. Lumsden AB, Colborn GL, Sreeram S, et al. The surgical anatomy and technique of the thoracoabdominal incision. Surg Clin North Am 1993; 73:633–644.

17. Kumar S, Duque JL, Guimaraes KC, et al. Short and long-term morbidity of thoracoabdominal incision for nephrectomy: a comparison with the flank approach. J Urol 1999; 162:1927–1929.

18. Chute R, Baron JA Jr, Olsson CA. The transverse upper abdominal "chevron" incision in urological surgery. J Urol 1968; 99:528–532.

19. Novick AC. Posterior surgical approach to the kidney and ureter. J Urol 1980; 124:192–195.

20. Das S, Egan RM, Amar AD. Dorsal lumbotomy for surgery of the upper urinary tract. J Urol 1987; 137:862–864.

21. Poore RE, Sexton WJ, Hart LJ, et al. Is radiographic evaluation of the chest necessary following flank surgery? J Urol 1996; 155:849–851.

22. Olsson LE, Swana H, Friedman AL, et al. Pleurotomy, pneumothorax, and surveillance during living donor nephroureterectomy. Urology 1998; 52:591–593.

23. Waples MJ, Belzer FO, Uehling DT. Living donor nephrectomy: a 20-year experience. Urology 1995; 45:207–210.

24. Kwik RS. Complications associated with surgery in the flank position for urological procedures. Middle East J Anaesthesiol 1980; 5:485–494.

25. Moul JW, Foley JP, Wind GG, et al. Celiac axis and superior mesenteric artery injury associated with left radical nephrectomy for locally advanced renal cell carcinoma. J Urol 1991; 146:1104–1107.

26. Blunt LW Jr, Matsumura J, Carter MF, et al. Repair of superior mesenteric artery ligation during left nephrectomy with a native renal vein patch. Urology 2004; 64:377–378.

27. Lacombe M. Renal arteriovenous fistula following nephrectomy. Urology 1985; 25:13–16.

28. Maldonado JE, Sheps SG. Renal arteriovenous fistula. Postgrad Med 1966; 40:263–269.

29. Robinson DL, Teitelbaum GP, Pentecost MJ, et al. Transcatheter embolization of an aortocaval fistula caused by residual renal artery stump from previous nephrectomy: a case report. J Vasc Surg 1993; 17:794–797.

30. Wellons E, Rosenthal D, Schoborg T, et al. Renal cell carcinoma invading the inferior vena cava: use of a "temporary" vena cava filter to prevent tumor emboli during nephrectomy. Urology 2004; 63:380–382.

31. Clark CD. Survival after excision of a kidney, segmental resection of the vena cava, and division of the opposite renal vein. Lancet 1961; 2:1015–1016.

32. Pathak IC. Survival after right nephrectomy, excision of infrahepatic vena cava and ligation of left renal vein: a case report. J Urol 1971; 106:599–602.

33. Coon WW. Iatrogenic splenic injury. Am J Surg 1990; 159:585–588.

34. Swanson DA, Borges PM. Complications of transabdominal radical nephrectomy for renal cell carcinoma. J Urol 1983; 129:704–707.

35. Mejean A, Vogt B, Quazza JE, et al. Mortality and morbidity after nephrectomy for renal cell carcinoma using a transperitoneal anterior subcostal incision. Eur Urol 1999; 36:298–302.

36. Stephenson AJ, Hakimi AA, Snyder ME, et al. Complications of radical and partial nephrectomy in a large contemporary cohort. J Urol 2004; 171:130–134.

37. Carmignani G, Traverso P, Corbu C. Incidental splenectomy during left radical nephrectomy: reasons and ways to avoid it. Urol Int 2001; 67:195–198.

38. Cooper CS, Cohen MB, Donovan JF Jr. Splenectomy complicating left nephrectomy. J Urol 1996; 155:30–36.

39. Mejean A, Chretien Y, Vogt B, et al. Coloepiploic mobilization during left radical nephrectomy for renal cell carcinoma is indicated to reduce the risk of iatrogenic splenectomy. Urology 2002; 59:358–361.

40. Vanterpool CC, Alrashedy FH, Gurchumelidze T, et al. Hemostasis and healing of superficial splenic injuries using Nd:YAG laser and nonsuture techniques: preliminary report. Lasers Surg Med 1994; 14:18–22.

41. Canby-Hagino ED, Morey AF, Jatoi I, et al. Fibrin sealant treatment of splenic injury during open and laparoscopic left radical nephrectomy. J Urol 2000; 164:2004–2005.

42. Bennett BC, Selby R, Bahnson RR. Surgical resection for management of renal cancer with hepatic involvement. J Urol 1995; 154:972–974.

43. Ciancio G, Hawke C, Soloway M. The use of liver transplant techniques to aid in the surgical management of urological tumors. J Urol 2000; 164:665–672.

44. Johnston WK III, Montgomery JS, Wolf JS Jr. Retroperitoneoscopic radical and partial nephrectomy in the patient with cirrhosis. J Urol 2005; 173:1094–1097.

45. Spirnak JP, Resnick MI, Persky L. Cutaneous pancreatic fistula as a complication of left nephrectomy. J Urol 1984; 132:329–330.

46. Paran H, Neufeld D, Kaplan O, et al. Octreotide for treatment of postoperative alimentary tract fistu-las. World J Surg 1995; 19:430–433.

47. Dave DS, Lam JS, Leppert JT, et al. Open surgical management of renal cell carcinoma in the era of minimally invasive kidney surgery. BJU Int 2005; 96:1268–1274.

48. Jemal A, Murray T, Ward E, et al. Cancer statistics, 2005. CA Cancer J Clin 2005; 55:10–30.

49. Robson CJ, Churchill BM, Anderson W. The results of radical nephrectomy for renal cell carcinoma. 1969. J Urol 2002; 167:873–875.

50. Skinner DG, Colvin RB, Vermillion CD, et al. Diagnosis and management of renal cell carcinoma. A clinical and pathologic study of 309 cases. Cancer 1971; 28:1165–1177.

51. Wood DP Jr. Role of lymphadenectomy in renal cell carcinoma. Urol Clin North Am 1991; 18:421–426.

52. Sagalowsky AI, Kadesky KT, Ewalt DM, et al. Factors influencing adrenal metastasis in renal cell car-cinoma. J Urol 1994; 151:1181–1184.

53. O'Donohoe MK, Flanagan F, Fitzpatrick JM, et al. Surgical approach to inferior vena caval extension of renal carcinoma. Br J Urol 1987; 60:492–496.

54. Bastian PJ, Haferkamp A, Akbarov I, et al. Surgical outcome following radical nephrectomy in cases with inferior vena cava tumour thrombus extension. Eur J Surg Oncol 2005; 31:420–423.

55. Seveso M, Maugeri O, Taverna G, et al. Incidence and treatment of complications in nephron sparing surgery. Arch Ital Urol Androl 2005; 77:206–210.

56. Lerner SE, Hawkins CA, Blute ML, et al. Disease outcome in patients with low stage renal cell carcinoma treated with nephron sparing or radical surgery. J Urol 1996; 155:1868–1873.

57. Belldegrun A, Tsui KH, deKernion JB, et al. Efficacy of nephron-sparing surgery for renal cell carcinoma: analysis based on the new 1997 tumor-node-metastasis staging system. J Clin Oncol 1999; 17:2868–2875.

58. Thrasher JB, Robertson JE, Paulson DF. Expanding indications for conservative renal surgery in renal cell carcinoma. Urology 1994; 43:160–168.

59. Van PH, Bamelis B, Oyen R, et al. Partial nephrectomy for renal cell carcinoma can achieve long-term tumor control. J Urol 1998; 160:674–678.

60. Duque JL, Loughlin KR, O'Leary MP, et al. Partial nephrectomy: alternative treatment for selected patients with renal cell carcinoma. Urology 1998; 52:584–590.

61. Campbell SC, Novick AC, Streem SB, et al. Complications of nephron sparing surgery for renal tumors. J Urol 1994; 151:1177–1180.

62. Steinbach F, Stockle M, Muller SC, et al. Conservative surgery of renal cell tumors in 140 patients: 21 years of experience. J Urol 1992; 148:24–29.

63. Polascik TJ, Pound CR, Meng MV, et al. Partial nephrectomy: technique, complications and pathologi-cal findings. J Urol 1995; 154:1312–1318.

64. Moll V, Becht E, Ziegler M. Kidney preserving surgery in renal cell tumors: indications, techniques and results in 152 patients. J Urol 1993; 150:319–323.

65. Uzzo RG, Novick AC. Nephron sparing surgery for renal tumors: indications, techniques and out-comes. J Urol 2001; 166:6–18.

66. O'Reilly PH, Brooman PJ, Mak S, et al. The long-term results of Anderson-Hynes pyeloplasty. BJU Int 2001; 87:287–289.

67. Smith KE, Holmes N, Lieb JI, et al. Stented versus nonstented pediatric pyeloplasty: a modern series and review of the literature. J Urol 2002; 168:1127–1130.

68. Lim DJ, Walker RD III. Management of the failed pyeloplasty. J Urol 1996; 156:738–740.

69. Klingler HC, Remzi M, Janetschek G, et al. Comparison of open versus laparoscopic pyeloplasty tech-niques in treatment of uretero-pelvic junction obstruction. Eur Urol 2003; 44:340–345.

70. Stimac G, Dimanovski J, Ruzic B, et al. Tumors in kidney fusion anomalies--report of five cases and review of the literature. Scand J Urol Nephrol 2004; 38:485–489.

71. Glen JF. Analysis of 51 patients with horseshoe kidney. N Engl J Med 1959; 276:684.

72. Bauer SB. Anomalies of the upper urinary tract. In: Walsh PC, Retik AB, Vaughan ED, Wein AJ, eds. Campbell's Urology. Philadelphia: Saunders, 2002:885–924.

73. Pettus JA, Jameson JJ, Stephenson RA. Renal cell carcinoma in horseshoe kidney with vena caval involvement. J Urol 2004; 171:339.

74. Terrone C, Destefanis P, Fiori C, et al. Renal cell cancer in presacral ectopic kidney: preoperative diagnostic imaging compared to surgical findings. Urol Int 2004; 72:174–175.

75. Novick AC, Streem SB, Pontes E, eds. Stewart's Operative Urology. 2nd ed. Baltimore, MD: Williams & Wilkins, 1989

76. Parekh DJ, Cookson MS, Chapman W, et al. Renal cell carcinoma with renal vein and inferior vena caval involvement: clinicopathological features, surgical techniques and outcomes. J Urol 2005; 173:1897–1902.

7 | Complications of Adrenal Surgery

Brian M. Shuch
Department of Urology, David Geffen School of Medicine at UCLA, Los Angeles, California, U.S.A.

Arie S. Belldegrun
Division of Urologic Oncology, Department of Urology, David Geffen School of Medicine at UCLA, Los Angeles, California, U.S.A.

CHANGES IN THE FIELD OF ADRENAL SURGERY

The field of adrenal surgery has undergone drastic changes over the past two decades with technological advancements in the fields of imaging and surgical technology. Adrenal masses have long been known to be very common and have been demonstrated in 9% of the population from post-mortem examination. The incidence of adrenal lesions has increased in the general population from the widespread usage of imaging such as computed tomography (CT) and magnetic resonance imaging (MRI) scans. Most adrenal masses are now found incidentally leading to the advent of the phrase "adrenal incidentaloma."

Whether incidental lesions represent stage migration or tumors that would have remained clinically insignificant is unknown. What is clear is that clinicians' experience with adrenal tumors has changed dramatically. Despite the altered presentation it is important to remain familiar with the classic presentations of the various types of functional tumors. Many patients still present with symptoms secondary to the metabolic effects of increased hormone production. Occasionally large tumors may present with mass effects or secondary to local invasion or venous thrombosis.

It is essential to distinguish tumors that need surgical intervention; hypersecretory lesions or those suspicious for malignancy. The management of asymptomatic lesions without clinical evidence of hypersecretion is challenging as little is known about the clinical progression of these tumors. The natural history of small incidentalomas (median size of 2.5 cm) followed up over a two-year time period demonstrates that less than 10% enlarge and only 2% become hyperfunctional (Table 1) (1). These findings suggest that many small incidentally discovered adrenal masses might be closely followed without adverse effects.

The advent of imaging has coincided with the advancement in laparoscopy and its widespread use within the urologic community. The stage migration of adrenal tumors has allowed the introduction of minimally invasive management of small tumors. The first report of a successful laparoscopic adrenal surgery was performed in 1992 for Conn's syndrome (2). Later that year, additional reports emerged describing laparoscopic adrenalectomy for pheochromocytoma and Cushing's syndrome (3).

Since that time laparoscopy has been performed for all types of adrenal surgery including adrenal cortical carcinoma and isolated metastatic disease (4). Many studies have compared laparoscopic and open adrenal surgery and demonstrated the former's safety and efficacy. Laparoscopic adrenalectomy has resulted in decreased hospital stay, more rapid return to activity, and decreased postoperative pain (5–7). Laparoscopy is now considered by many to be the gold standard for small, benign adrenal lesions. However, the utility of laparoscopy in the setting of adrenal cortical carcinoma or metastatic disease is still in question and most surgeons believe it to be a contraindication.

The indications for adrenal surgery have also changed over the last decade with medical management proving to be efficacious for some hyperfunctional adrenal tumors. With improvements in CT scans and availability of long-term data on adrenal involvement in renal cell carcinoma (RCC), the indications for adrenalectomy in the radical nephrectomy have been revised. Additionally, the long-term complications of adrenal insufficiency have led to the idea of adrenal sparing in patients with hereditary syndromes.

TABLE 1   Change in Size of 229 Incidentally Found Adrenal Tumors
Observed Over a Mean of 25 Months. A Total of 11 Patients were
Excluded as they Underwent Adrenalectomy

Change in size	%
Decrease	5.20
No change	87.40
Change (≥0.5 cm)	7.40
Change (≥1.0 cm)	5.20

Source: From Ref. 1.

UNIQUE TYPES OF COMPLICATIONS

The complications of adrenal surgery can be divided into preoperative errors in planning, operative complications, and those seen in the peri- and postoperative period. While many of the complications of adrenal surgery are not unique to the adrenal gland, several distinct complications are not observed in other urologic procedures. For example, endocrine complications may be related to the metabolic state at the time of surgery secondary to the pathophysiology of the disease. Long-term complications are also observed secondary to the loss of adrenal function and patients may require permanent replacement therapy. With correct preoperative planning, many of these complications can be lessened or ultimately avoided.

A thorough physical examination and detailed history can detect clinical clues for a correct diagnosis. The urologist must be actively involved in pursuing the correct diagnosis, as proper preparation is required for certain tumors. Choosing operative management and surgery is not the end of the urologist's responsibility, since much time is needed for preoperative planning with the anesthesia and endocrinology team to avoid undue complications.

PREOPERATIVE SURGICAL PLANNING
Preoperative Discussion of Adrenal Insufficiency

It is imperative for the surgical team to have a detailed discussion about the morbidity of adrenal insufficiency in addition to the other postoperative complications prior to adrenal surgery. This discussion should not be reserved for patients with a solitary adrenal gland or those in need of a bilateral adrenalectomy. In the setting of a hyperfunctional adenoma, the contralateral gland may be suppressed and the patient may require temporary adrenal support. Additionally, patients undergoing an adrenalectomy may eventually require surgery in the future on the contralateral gland that would lead to permanent adrenal insufficiency.

Adrenalectomy in Hereditary Syndromes

Patients with hereditary syndromes such as multiple endocrine neoplasia type 2 (MEN2) and von Hippel-Lindau disease (VHL) are at risk of developing multiple adrenal pheochromocytomas during the course of their lifetime. The risk of developing contralateral pheochromocytomas is very high and has been demonstrated to develop in 60% of patients with VHL and MEN2 (8). These patients require life-long surveillance to identify surgically amenable disease.

Due to the complications resulting from long-term steroid use, interest developed in the preservation of adrenal cortical function. The partial adrenalectomy or cortical-sparing adrenalectomy was performed to avoid long-term steroid dependence and postoperative Addisonian crisis (9). However, patients and their surgeons must weigh the likelihood of local tumor recurrence against the need for hormonal replacement therapy. Ipsilateral recurrence can occur in up to 60% of patients who undergo cortical-sparing adrenalectomy compared to 20% recurrence associated with total adrenalectomy (10,11). With close surveillance, patients with locally recurrent pheochromocytoma can safely undergo repeat cortical-sparing adrenalectomy (12).

TABLE 2 Adrenal Involvement for Renal Cell Carcinona Based
on T Stage

Stage	Adrenal involvement (%)
T1/T2	0.6
T3	7.8
T4	40.0

Source: From Ref. 14.

Role of Adrenalectomy in Renal Cell Carcinoma

Adrenalectomy was uniformly performed as part of radical nephrectomy for RCC. The surgical technique as described by Robson in 1969 advocated the removal of the ipsilateral adrenal gland to remove any locally invasive or metastatic tumor (13). With the advent of imaging studies and data available from large series, radical nephrectomy has streamlined exenteration. Tsui et al. analyzed a large cohort of 511 patients with localized and advanced RCC that underwent classical radical nephrectomy and demonstrated a low incidence of adrenal involvement (5.7%) (14). Localized T1 and T2 tumors rarely demonstrate adrenal involvement with an incidence of 0.6% (Table 2). Tumors confined to the mid-pole or lower pole were involved 7% and 4% of the time, respectively. Preoperative imaging with abdominal CT scans demonstrated 99.6% specificity and 89.6% sensitivity for detecting adrenal involvement. It is now widely believed that adrenalectomy should not be a routine in radical nephrectomy. Ipsilateral removal of the adrenal gland should be performed only in the setting of advanced disease, guided by preoperative imaging.

Conn's Syndrome—Primary Aldosteronism

Patients with Conn's syndrome may demonstrate hypertension, hypokalemia, and metabolic alkalosis related to hyperaldosteronism. Patients require extensive potassium repletion prior to surgery; however, it may be impossible to restore normal levels (Table 3). Repletion is essential to preoperative planning because hypokalemia and metabolic alkalosis can prolong the action of several neuromuscular blocking agents used by the anesthesia team. Patients with Conn's syndrome also demonstrate hypovolemia related to hypokalemic suppression of the baroreceptor function (15). These patients must be aggressively volume-resuscitated prior to induction. Additionally, these patients should be screened for cardiac dysfunction as hyperaldosteronism and hypokalemia can contribute to cardiomyopathy, myocardial fibrosis, and arrhythmias (15–17). Spironolactone and calcium channel blockers can help in maintaining the preoperative potassium balance and blood pressure control.

Localization of the adrenal lesion must be determined to avoid performing an incorrect surgery. Hyperaldosteronism may result from bilateral adrenal hyperplasia or a solitary adenoma. Both these entities can be surgically treated once the correct diagnosis is determined. To assist localization, CT scans and adrenal vein sampling should be performed.

Cushing's Syndrome

The evaluation of Cushing's syndrome frequently identifies surgically amenable lesions in the pituitary or adrenal gland. To correctly diagnose the etiology, several tests are useful including

TABLE 3 Preoperative Evaluation and Management for
Conn's Syndrome

Adrenal tumor	Mandatary preoperative consideration
Conn's syndrome/primary aldosteronism	Volume expansion Potassium repletion Blood pressure control Cardiac screening Lesion localization

TABLE 4 Preoperative Evaluation and Management for Cushing's
Syndrome Related to Hyperfunctional Adrenal Lesion

Adrenal tumor	Mandatary preoperative consideration
Cushing's syndrome	Possible metyrapone use
	Perioperative steroid administration
	Glucose regulation

urinary cortisol measurements, dexamethasome suppression tests, and measurement of Adreno
corticotropic hormone (ACTH). Up to 10% of patients with Cushing's syndrome are found to
have adrenal lesions including adenomas or adrenocortical carcinomas. Ectopic secretion of
ACTH by tumors can also produce life-threatening hypercortisolism. In the setting of nonre-
sectable tumors, bilateral adrenalectomy can effectively control symptoms (18).

Patients with severe symptoms of hypercorticolism should be treated with the adrenal-
blocking agent metyrapone to minimize metabolic symptoms (Table 4). Diabetes is common in
these patients and blood glucose must be regulated. The addition of preoperative antibiotics
and tight glucose control can limit the incidence of wound infections. Preoperative steroid
administration is important since these patients are at high risk for Addisonian crisis once the
hyperfunctioning adrenal tissue is removed. In the setting of adenoma or carcinoma, the functioning of the contralateral adrenal gland will be suppressed and patients must continue on a
steroid taper.

Adrenal Cortical Carcinoma

Distinguishing adrenal carcinomas from adenomas can be difficult, yet several features should
raise the suspicion for malignancy. A meta-analysis by Belldegrun et al. demonstrated that 92%
of adrenocortical carcinomas were larger than 6 cm (19). Additionally, adrenal carcinomas regularly demonstrate necrosis and calcification on imaging studies (19).

Preoperatively, it is important to identify inferior vena caval involvement or invasion into
adjacent organs to avoid intraoperative surprises (Table 5). Inferior vena caval involvement is
not common but is seen in advanced disease. A recent 2006 review of the literature cited only
106 cases of adrenal cortical carcinoma with inferior vena cava involvement (20). In a series of
60 patients with metastatic adrenal cortical carcinoma, 10% of patients demonstrated caval
invasion (21). Due to the shorter right adrenal vein and its close association with the inferior
vena cava, invasion is more frequently seen in right-sided tumors (22). Imaging of inferior vena
caval invasion has been demonstrated by both CT and MRI scans (22,23).

Despite the best operation, most patients have a recurrence of adrenocortical carcinoma
and five-year disease-specific survival is between 20% and 45% (24). For patients with a high
likelihood of adrenal cortical carcinoma, open surgery may be the best option. The results of 170
patients undergoing open and laparoscopic adrenalectomy for adrenal cortical carcinoma at
M.D. Anderson Cancer Center were reviewed (25). While this series contained only six patients
undergoing laparoscopic surgery, an important statistically significant observation was found.
The risk of peritoneal carcinomatosis as the initial failure was 83% in the laparoscopic group
versus 8% for the open adrenalectomy group. The high rate of carinomatosis may be related to
the standard laparoscopic technique. Direct traction on the friable adrenal cortical carcinoma
during mobilization could potentially contribute to tumor fraction, capsular disruption, and

TABLE 5 Preoperative Evaluation and Management for Adrenal
Cortical Carcinoma

Adrenal tumor	Mandatary preoperative consideration
Adrenal cortical carcinoma	Functional studies
	Presence of metastasis
	Local invasion
	Inferior vena cava involvement

TABLE 6 Preoperative Evaluation and Management for
Pheochromocytoma

Adrenal tumor	Mandatary preoperative consideration
Pheochromocytoma	Blood pressure control
	Cathecholaminc blockage
	Evaluation of cardiomyopathy

peritoneal seeding. The authors concluded that open adrenalectomy remains the standard of care for lesions suspicious for adrenal cortical carcinoma.

Pheochromocytoma

Any patient with an adrenal lesion should be screened for pheochromocytoma to avoid the potential of an operative catastrophe. Patients with incidental pheochromocytomas that undergo general anesthesia for nonrelated surgery frequently have hypertensive crises, which can take the anesthesiology team by surprise. In this setting, the mortality can approach 80% (26). Life-threatening complications frequently observed include cerebrovascular hemorrhage, arrhythmias, and myocardial infarction.

All patients with an adrenal lesion and hypertension must be evaluated with urinary catecholamines to rule out pheochromocytoma. The medication of choice has been phenoxybenzamine, which should be titrated until blood pressure normalizes. Patients should be screened for cardiomyopathy resulting from excessive catecholamine production (Table 6). If present, they require a double blockade with alpha-methyl-para-tyrosine, a hydroxylase inhibitor that blocks the final step in the synthesis of catecholamines (27). These patients require an extensive cardiac evaluation and clearance before surgery.

Patients with pheochromocytoma have a high risk for hemodynamic instability during surgery. To limit complications, they must be volume-resuscitated prior to surgery as their metabolic state causes severe hypovolemia (27). These patients present a challenge to the anesthesia team and frequently require invasive monitoring, including arterial and Swan-Ganz catheters. Transesophageal echocardiograms may be required in cases of dilated cardiomyopathy.

OPERATIVE COMPLICATIONS
Metabolic Complications

Communication between the anesthesiology and surgical team is always important; however, it is vital during an adrenalectomy for a pheochromocytoma (Table 7). Manipulation of the adrenal tumor prior to vascular control of the venous drainage may lead to hypertensive episodes. Insufflation of the peritoneum during laparoscopy frequently contributes to cardiovascular lability. Usually, cessation of manipulation or insufflation is sufficient to improve hemodynamic function. To avoid hypertensive crises from catecholamine release, it is important to ligate the adrenal vein early. However, vascular control of the adrenal vein can also cause hemodynamic instability as a sharp decrease in catecholamine release to the peripheral blood stream can cause a drop in blood pressure. Hemostasis may be difficult for pheochromocytomas since elevated blood pressure can contribute to bleeding. Hypertension should be managed intraoperatively with intravenous medications. Additionally the anesthesia team should be prepared for the development of arrhythmias secondary to catecholamine excess.

TABLE 7 Special Operative Considerations During Adrenalectomy for
Pheochromocytoma to Avoid Metabolic-Related Operative Complications

Close monitoring hemodynamic function during insufflation
Limit manipulation of pheochromocytoma
Early ligation of arenal veins
Tight intraoperative blood pressure control

Hemorrhage and Vascular Injury

Intraoperative hemorrhage represents the most serious and life-threatening complication of adrenal surgery. The adrenal gland has a tremendous vascular supply network despite being a small organ. Even small amounts of bleeding can hinder visualization during laparoscopic adrenalectomy. Bleeding complications necessitate open conversion during laparoscopy in 1.6% of adrenalectomies (28).

To limit complications, it is necessary to fully understand the blood supply and venous drainage to each adrenal gland. Some of the difficulty stems from the gland's rich blood supply and absence of a clearly dominant single artery. The inferior phrenic artery frequently is the main blood supply; however, additional branches from the aorta and the renal artery contribute. The vascular supply feeds the adrenal gland in a circumferential stellate fashion leaving a relatively avascular anterior and posterior surface.

The distinct blood supply and location of the right and left gland lead to variations in the dissection, vascular control, and incidence of vascular complications. The right side has a shorter adrenal vein that enters the inferior vena cava posteriorly. Injury to this vein is a frequent cause of hemorrhage during right-sided adrenalectomy. The inferior vena cava and lumbar veins can be damaged during dissection and must be rapidly controlled and repaired to prevent hemorrhage. A vascular clamp can assist with vascular control while the defect is being repaired. Hepatic veins also drain directly into the inferior vena cava and care must be taken to avoid injury to these vessels during right-sided adrenalectomy. During left-sided adrenalectomy, care must be taken during medial dissection to avoid the left inferior phrenic vein, which typically drains into the left adrenal vein (29).

Vascular Injury

Both adrenal glands are intimately associated with large vascular structures that may be inadvertently clipped or ligated during surgery (Table 8). Any injury to large vascular structures can lead to hemorrhage and require open conversion during laparoscopy. However ischemic complications frequently result from nonhemorrhagic ligation injuries. The mesenteric vessels including the superior mesenteric artery can be damaged during adrenal surgery. While the vascular supply to the mesentery has large amounts of collaterals, acute transection of the superior mesenteric artery can lead to bowel ischemia and a vascular surgeon should be consulted to repair the injury. The upper pole capsular arteries to the kidney may be transected during inferiomedial dissection along the adrenal gland. Ligation can lead to infarction of viable renal parenchyma. These accessory arteries often supply a small portion of the kidney and minimal sequela will result if patients have normal renal function. Finally, during left-sided adrenalectomy, splenic infarction can ensue if a large branch of the splenic artery is injured.

INJURY TO ADJACENT STRUCTURES

The retroperitoneal position of the adrenal glands places specific organs at risk for intraoperative injury (Table 9). The specific incidence of complications varies depending on the side of the adrenal tumor.

Pulmonary Complications

A common complication of open adrenal surgery is entry into the pleural cavity seen during a supra-eleventh rib approach. A chest tube can be placed directly into the chest cavity

TABLE 8   Notable Vascular Injuries Associated with Adrenalectomy

Vascular injury and hemorrhage
Renal vascular injury/parenchymal infarction
Mesenteric vascular injury/mesentreric ischemia
Splenic vascular injury/splenic infarction

TABLE 9   Adjacent Structures that May Be Injured During Adrenalectomy

Diaphragm
Spleen
Pancreas
Liver
Stomach
Colon
Kidney

during closure to protect against pneumothorax. Others advocate closing the diaphragm and suctioning the air with a catheter. A chest tube is placed only if there is a postoperative pneumothorax.

An additional pulmonary complication observed in the laparoscopic approach is injury to the inferior aspect of the diaphragm. Both adrenal glands lie against the posterior surface of the diaphragm. Diaphragmatic injury occurs in 3% of cases and usually results from dissection with the harmonic scalpel (30). These injuries are usually visualized and can be repaired with figure-of-eight sutures and the air suctioned to prevent a postoperative pneumothorax.

Organ Injuries

Due to the close association with many intra-abdominal organs, adjacent organs may be inadvertently injured during adrenalectomy. Injuries to adjacent organs are rare in both the laparoscopic and open approach with the incidence being reported to be less than 1% (28). The specific incidence of injury depends on which side the operation is being performed.

Spleen

The spleen may be damaged during left-sided adrenalectomy. The adrenal gland lies in close proximity to the splenic hilum and can be injured during access or mobilization. The most frequent injury is splenic laceration that occurs with both laparoscopic and open adrenalectomy. Minor splenic lacerations can be repaired by splenorrhaphy with minimal morbidity. Various hemostatic agents and glues have been developed which can aid the repair of minor lacerations. Many of these glues in combination with argon beam have been used during laparoscopic urologic surgery to repair lacerations and avert open conversion (31–33). For large intraoperative lacerations, mesh splenorrhaphy has been described to avoid performing splenectomy and has shown good results (34). In the setting of a major injury to the spleen or splenic hilum, a splenectomy must be performed to control bleeding.

Pancreas

The left adrenal gland lies in close proximity to the tail of the pancreas and can be damaged. A general surgery consult should be called to assess the nature of the injury. Depending on the severity, repair of the pancreatic duct may be possible. However, a distal pancreatectomy may be required in severe cases. These patients should have drains placed to assess for pancreatic leaks. These patients require a prolonged course without oral intake and total parenteral nutrition may need to be instituted.

Liver Injury

The anterior surface of the right adrenal gland is in immediate contact with the inferior–posterior surface of the liver. During right-sided intraperitoneal adrenalectomy, the liver must be retracted to provide access to the adrenal gland. Occasionally, the adrenal gland will adhere to the liver capsule and bleeding will ensue during mobilization of the gland. Injury to the liver may require hepatic resection. However, simple bleeding may be controlled with the argon beam or with topical hemostatic agents.

PERI- AND POSTOPERATIVE COMPLICATIONS

Adrenal cortical function is vital to life and postoperative adrenal insufficiency can be fatal. The acute manifestations of adrenal insufficiency include sepsis, bilateral adrenal hemorrhage, fever, metabolic derangements, severe abdominal pain, and death. To avoid catastrophic complications, patients may require stress dose corticosteroid administration during surgery and a taper postoperatively. Replacement mineralocorticoid therapy is indicated for patients undergoing bilateral adrenalectomy to assist with electrolyte hemostasis. Occasionally, it may be required for patients undergoing unilateral adrenalectomy since temporary hypoadrenalism may occur. Hydrocortisone, which has a modest mineralocorticoid effect, is given intravenously until the patient can tolerate oral medications. Oral fludrocortisone or hydrocortisone can be administered once the patient resumes a diet.

The chronic manifestations of adrenal insufficiency include hyponatremia, hyperkalemia, azotemia, both hyper- and hypothyroidism, diabetes mellitus, and gonadal dysfunction. However, the morbidity associated with long-term complications of steroid replacement is high and potentially life-altering. Steroids are not benign medications and serious side effects are seen with long-term usage. Frequently observed side effects include impaired glucose control, osteoporosis, weight gain, and are associated with poor quality of life (35).

General Complications

Many of the postoperative complications of adrenalectomy are not unique to the field. However, several complications are decreased with laparoscopic surgery, such as the incidence of pneumonia and atelectasis (28). This may be related to decreased postoperative pain and decreased ambulation with laparoscopic surgery. The incidence of wound-related complications including hernia and infection are also diminished with the smaller laparoscopic incisions.

Complications Related to the Specific Disease Entity

Several postoperative complications are seen after resection of hypersecretory tumors that are related to the specific disease entity. After adrenalectomy for Conn's syndrome, patients may suffer from hypoaldosteronism. Thus, it is important to monitor potassium and sodium status postoperatively. During the initial postoperative course a negative balance of potassium and sodium can occur (36). Volume status and urine output must be carefully observed since many of these patients receive large amounts of fluid due to preoperative hypovolemia.

Patients with Cushing's syndrome require corticosteroid replacement since the contralateral adrenal gland has been suppressed by the pituitary access. A steroid taper is required while the contralateral gland regains function. These patients may have poor wound healing and poor glycemic control. Tight monitoring of blood glucose level is required to limit the risk of wound infections. ACTH stimulation tests should be performed to assess return of function prior to cessation of exogenous steroids.

Pheochromocytoma patients may require invasive monitoring in an intensive care unit setting for cardiovascular monitoring. As large amounts of alpha antagonists are used intraoperatively, postoperative hypotension may be observed. These patients may require extensive fluid resuscitation and vasoconstrictive agents to maintain blood pressure (37). Blood glucose must be monitored as life-threatening hypoglycemia has been described (38). Increased insulin production is thought to result from decreased levels of catecholamines due to removal of the gland.

REFERENCES

1. Bulow B, Jansson S, Juhlin C, et al. Adrenal incidentaloma—follow-up results from a Swedish prospective study. Eur J Endocrinol 2006; 154:419–423.
2. Higashihara E, Tanaka Y, Horie S, et al. A case report of laparoscopic adrenalectomy. Nippon Hinyokika Gakkai Zasshi 1992; 83:1130–1133.
3. Gagner M, Lacroix A, Bolte E. Laparoscopic adrenalectomy in Cushing's syndrome and pheochromocytoma. N Engl J Med 1992; 327:1033.

4. Sebag F, Calzolari F, Harding J, Sierra M, Palazzo FF, Henry JF. Isolated adrenal metastasis: the role of laparoscopic surgery. World J Surg 2006; 30:888–892.
5. Winfield HN, Hamilton BD, Bravo EL, Novick AC. Laparoscopic adrenalectomy: the preferred choice? A comparison to open adrenalectomy. J Urol 1998; 160:325–329.
6. Prinz RA. A comparison of laparoscopic and open adrenalectomies. Arch Surg 1995; 130:489–492, discussion 492–494.
7. Thompson GB, Grant CS, van Heerden JA, et al. Laparoscopic versus open posterior adrenalectomy: a case-control study of 100 patients. Surgery 1997; 122:1132–1136.
8. Walther MM, Reiter R, Keiser HR, et al. Clinical and genetic characterization of pheochromocytoma in von Hippel-Lindau families: comparison with sporadic pheochromocytoma gives insight into natural history of pheochromocytoma. J Urol 1999; 162:659–664.
9. Lee JE, Curley SA, Gagel RF, Evans DB, Hickey RC. Cortical-sparing adrenalectomy for patients with bilateral pheochromocytoma. Surgery 1996; 120:1064–1070; discussion 1070–1071.
10. Inabnet WB, Caragliano P, Pertsemlidis D. Pheochromocytoma: inherited associations, bilaterality, and cortex preservation. Surgery 2000; 128:1007–1011; discussion 1011–1012.
11. Neumann HP, Bender BU, Reincke M, Eggstein S, Laubenberger J, Kirste G. Adrenal-sparing surgery for phaeochromocytoma. Br J Surg 1999; 86:94–97.
12. Brauckhoff M, Gimm O, Brauckhoff K, Dralle H. Repeat adrenocortical-sparing adrenalectomy for recurrent hereditary pheochromocytoma. Surg Today 2004; 34:251–255.
13. Robson CJ, Churchill BM, Anderson W. The results of radical nephrectomy for renal cell carcinoma. J Urol 1969; 101:297–301.
14. Tsui KH, Shvarts O, Barbaric Z, Figlin R, de Kernion JB, Belldegrun A. Is adrenalectomy a necessary component of radical nephrectomy? UCLA experience with 511 radical nephrectomies. J Urol 2000; 163:437–441.
15. Stowasser M. New perspectives on the role of aldosterone excess in cardiovascular disease. Clin Exp Pharmacol Physiol 2001; 28:783–791.
16. Struthers AD. Aldosterone escape during ACE inhibitor therapy in chronic heart failure. Eur Heart J 1995; 16(suppl N):103–106.
17. Potts JL, Dalakos TG, Streeten DH, Jones D. Cardiomyopathy in an adult with Bartter's syndrome and hypokalemia. Hemodynamic, angiographic and metabolic studies. Am J Cardiol 1977; 40: 995–999.
18. Hellman P, Linder F, Hennings J, et al. Bilateral adrenalectomy for ectopic Cushing's syndrome-discussions on technique and indication. World J Surg 2006; 30:909–916.
19. Belldegrun A, Hussain S, Seltzer SE, Loughlin KR, Gittes RF, Richie JP. Incidentally discovered mass of the adrenal gland. Surg Gynecol Obstet 1986; 163:203–208.
20. Chiche L, Dousset B, Kieffer E, Chapuis Y. Adrenocortical carcinoma extending into the inferior vena cava: presentation of a 15-patient series and review of the literature. Surgery 2006; 139:15–27.
21. Nader S, Hickey RC, Sellin RV, Samaan NA. Adrenal cortical carcinoma. A study of 77 cases. Cancer 1983; 52:707–711.
22. Wei CY, Chen KK, Chen MT, Lai HT, Chang LS. Adrenal cortical carcinoma with tumor thrombus invasion of inferior vena cava. Urology 1995; 45:1052–1054.
23. Pritchett TR, Raval JK, Benson RC, et al. Preoperative magnetic resonance imaging of vena caval tumor thrombi: experience with 5 cases. J Urol 1987; 138:1220–1222.
24. Roman S. Adrenocortical carcinoma. Curr Opin Oncol 2006; 18:36–42.
25. Gonzalez RJ, Shapiro S, Sarlis N, et al. Laparoscopic resection of adrenal cortical carcinoma: a cautionary note. Surgery 2005; 138:1078–1085; discussion 1085–1086.
26. O'Riordan JA. Pheochromocytomas and anesthesia. Int Anesthesiol Clin 1997; 35:99–127.
27. Kinney MA, Narr BJ, Warner MA. Perioperative management of pheochromocytoma. J Cardiothorac Vasc Anesth 2002; 16:359–369.
28. Brunt LM, Doherty GM, Norton JA, Soper NJ, Quasebarth MA, Moley JF. Laparoscopic adrenalectomy compared to open adrenalectomy for benign adrenal neoplasms. J Am Coll Surg 1996; 183:1–10.
29. Loukas M, Louis RG Jr, Hullett J, Loiacano M, Skidd P, Wagner T. An anatomical classification of the variations of the inferior phrenic vein. Surg Radiol Anat 2005; 27:566–574.
30. Del Pizzo JJ, Shichman SJ, Sosa RE. Laparoscopic adrenalectomy: the New York-Presbyterian Hospital experience. J Endourol 2002; 16:591–597.
31. Biggs G, Hafron J, Feliciano J, Hoenig DM. Treatment of splenic injury during laparoscopic nephrectomy with BioGlue, a surgical adhesive. Urology 2005; 66:882.
32. Canby-Hagino ED, Morey AF, Jatoi I, Perahia B, Bishoff JT. Fibrin sealant treatment of splenic injury during open and laparoscopic left radical nephrectomy. J Urol 2000; 164:2004–2005.
33. Hedican SP. Complications of hand-assisted laparoscopic urologic surgery. J Endourol 2004; 18:387–396.
34. Berry MF, Rosato EF, Williams NN. Dexon mesh splenorrhaphy for intraoperative splenic injuries. Am Surg 2003; 69:176–180.

35. Telenius-Berg M, Ponder MA, Berg B, Ponder BA, Werner S. Quality of life after bilateral adrenalectomy in MEN 2. Henry Ford Hosp Med J 1989; 37:160–163.
36. Winship SM, Winstanley JH, Hunter JM. Anaesthesia for Conn's syndrome. Anaesthesia 1999; 54:569–574.
37. Williams DT, Dann S, Wheeler MH. Phaeochromocytoma—views on current management. Eur J Surg Oncol 2003; 29:483–490.
38. Allen CT, Imrie D. Hypoglycemia as a complication of removal of a pheochromocytoma. Can Med Assoc J 1977; 116:363–364.

8 | Complications of Radical Retropubic Prostatectomy

Travis L. Bullock, Elizabeth R. Williams, and Gerald L. Andriole, Jr.
Division of Urologic Surgery, Washington University School of Medicine, St. Louis, Missouri, U.S.A.

INTRODUCTION

Prostate cancer is the most common malignant neoplasm in men. In 2007, it is estimated that 218,890 will be diagnosed and 27,050 will die of the disease (1). Moreover, autopsy studies have revealed the presence of prostate cancer in 25% of men aged 65 and 40% aged 85 (2). Treatment options for prostate cancer include watchful waiting, hormonal ablation, cryotherapy, external beam radiation, brachytherapy, and surgery. All treatment modalities have certain inherent risks, benefits, implications on cancer control, and complications. The widespread application of prostate cancer screening using prostate-specific antigen (PSA) and digital rectal examination (DRE) coupled with advances in surgical technique as described by Walsh has significantly increased the number of men diagnosed with clinically localized prostate cancer and likewise an increase in the number of patients choosing surgery.

Surgery is regarded by many as the optimal treatment choice for localized prostate cancer. Complete surgical removal of the prostate was once a procedure with unacceptable morbidity only employed by highly specialized surgeons in a minority of cases. The introduction of the anatomical approach to radical retropubic prostatectomy (RRP) by Walsh brought several advantages including better control of the dorsal venous complex, decreased intraoperative blood loss, preservation of the neurovascular bundles (NVBs), and decreased incontinence rates (3). More recently the explosion of minimally invasive laparoscopic and robotic procedures has also led to an increase in the number of patients choosing surgery.

Although the technique of radical prostatectomy has evolved considerably and urologists have become more facile performing the procedure significant morbidity still exist as well as the potential for patients living with the long-term side effects of surgery. Morbidity following radical prostatectomy is dependent upon many factors including surgeon experience, patient characteristics (such as concomitant medical comorbidities, pelvic anatomy), use of neoadjuvant therapies, and extent of cancer. The following sections will highlight the potential intraoperative, perioperative, and postoperative complications in detail.

INTRAOPERATIVE COMPLICATIONS
Hemorrhage

The highly vascularized anatomy of the pelvis coupled with deep dissection can result in significant blood loss during radical prostatectomy. The majority of the blood loss is incurred during the first half of the operation, namely during the pelvic lymph node dissection, opening of the endopelvic fascia along with division of the puboprostatic ligaments, and especially during division of the dorsal vein complex. In recent years, the decline in mean blood loss has plateaued as most urologists employ the nerve-sparing approach to radical prostatectomy. The increased blood loss with nerve-sparing is secondary to preservation of the NVBs, which were previously ligated for hemostasis. This trend is evident in results from more recent large series (Table 1).

One of the most important factors in limiting blood loss during prostatectomies is the experience of the surgeon. A number of case series have demonstrated decreased mean blood loss and fewer units of blood transfused with increasing experience of the surgeon. Dash et al. noted that the main predictor for homologous blood transfusion in their series was the surgeon's expertise (11). One surgeon's series of 620 radical prostatectomies showed a 50% decrease in blood loss (700–300 mL) when comparing his first 100 cases to the last 220 cases

TABLE 1   Reported Blood Loss During Radical Retropubic Prostatectomy

Investigator	Year	Number of patients	Mean blood loss (mL)
Igel et al. (4)	1987	692	1018
Leandri et al. (5)	1992	620	530
Keetch et al. (6)	1994	810	1200–1500
Hautmann et al. (7)	1994	418	900
Zincke et al. (8)	1994	1728	600
Lerner et al. (9)	1995	1000	844
Catalona et al. (10)	1999	1870	1500

along with a decrease in mean transfusion rate from 3 units to 0.2 units (5). With time and experience, surgeons have also increased the threshold for transfusion, discharging patients with lower hemoglobins than were seen earlier in the series. In the Mayo Clinic experience, 69% of patients were transfused from 1985 to 1986 whereas only 7.1% were transfused in 1999, and the mean hemoglobin at discharge decreased from 12 to 10.9 g/dL during the same time period (12).

Despite improved surgical technique and experience, hemorrhage requiring intraoperative transfusion remains the primary intraoperative complication of radical prostatectomy (13). Therefore, recent studies have focused on the use of autologous blood transfusions, preoperative erythropoietin injections, and acute normovolemic hemodilution (ANH) as alternatives to allogenic transfusions. The primary objective of these techniques is to limit the risk of transfusion reactions, clerical errors, and blood-borne pathogen exposure associated with allogenic transfusions. Initial studies showed decreased rates of allogenic transfusions when autologous blood donation was utilized. One 1994 study reported an allogenic transfusion decrease from 70% to 9% with the use of autologous units (6). A later study suggested autologous units were unnecessary due to the declining transfusion rate over time (14).

Injection of recombinant human erythropoietin has been shown to correct anemia in patients with chronic renal failure, cancer therapy, as well as the human immunodeficiency virus (HIV) stimulating competitive erythropoiesis. It has more recently been approved in the United States and Canada in combination with autologous blood donation for patients where perioperative blood transfusion is likely (15). However, in the orthopedic surgery literature erythropoietin therapy has failed to show any clinical benefit compared to autologous donation alone in those patients who are not anemic (hematocrit >39%) (15).

ANH is a technique that involves the removal of fresh whole blood with simultaneous infusion of crystalloid immediately before surgery. The blood is stored in the operative room, at room temperature, and is reinfused after major blood loss. Since blood is transfused before the completion of surgery there are no associated costs of storage and the risk of clerical error is negligible (15). A study by Monk et al. in patients undergoing radical prostatectomy found ANH to be as effective as autologous blood donation with a 60% reduction in transfusion-associated costs. ANH alone was associated with a 21% allogenic transfusion rate; however, the concomitant use of one or two units of autologous blood donation reduced allogenic exposure rates to 6% and 0%, respectively (16).

Rectal Injury

Rectal injury is a recognized, but unlikely complication of radical prostatectomy. Most large series report a 1% to 5% incidence (Table 2) (4–7,10,17–19). There are three primary risk factors for rectal injury during prostatectomy: previous radiation therapy, prior rectal surgery, and previous transurethral resection of the prostate (TURP). The preferred method for rectal injury repair is a two-layer closure with the use of an omental flap to minimize the risk of fistula or abscess formation (20,21). Most series agree that small defects should be closed primarily. However, if the patient has had previous pelvic irradiation, gross fecal contamination, or no preoperative bowel preparation, a colostomy is often necessary to prevent infectious complications (4,5,21,22). Borland and Walsh reported a 1% rectal injury rate in 1000 cases. Nine out of the ten injuries were discovered intraoperatively and were repaired with a two-layer closure

TABLE 2 Intraoperative Complications of Radical Retropubic Prostatectomy

Investigator	Year	Number of patients	Rectal injury (%)	Ureteral injury (%)	Nerve injury (%)
Igel et al. (4)	1987	692	1.3	0.3	NR
Leandri et al. (5)	1992	620	0.5	NR	NR
Hautmann et al. (7)	1994	418	2.9	0.2	NR
Keetch et al. (6)	1994	810	0.1	0.1	0.1
Catalona et al. (10)	1999	1870	0.05	0.05	0.3
Lepor et al. (17)	2001	1000	0.5	0.1	0.1
Maffezzini et al. (18)	2003	300	0.3	0.3	0.3
Augustin et al. (19)	2003	1243	0.2	0.3	0.1

Abbreviation: NR, none reported.

with interposition of an omental flap. They reported no cases of abscesses, urethrorectal fistulas, or wound infections (22).

Urethrorectal fistula is the primary complication after missed or inadequately repaired rectal injury. If small, these fistulas can initially be managed conservatively with bladder decompression and bowel rest; however, many cases may eventually require surgical repair (21). This is particularly true if the operative field has previously been irradiated.

Ureteral Injury

Intraoperative injury to the ureter is rare during RRP with a reported incidence of 0.05% to 1.6% is most large series (Table 2) (4,6,7,10,17–19,23). Ureteral injury may occur during the pelvic lymphadenectomy if an extended dissection is performed above the level of the iliac bifurcation, while creating a plane between the bladder base and seminal vesicles, or during ligation of the lateral pedicels of the prostate. However, injury most commonly occurs while dissecting the posterior bladder neck, especially in large prostates, where benign prostatic hyperplasia (BPH) often leads to J-hooking of the ureters (6,23).

To aid in avoidance of injury many advocate the use of intravenous indigo carmine or methylene blue for identification of the ureteral orifices intravesically. The most important factor in the management of ureteral injury is prompt intraoperative recognition. If injury is suspected the ureter should be intubated with a 5-french feeding tube and if injury confirmed one should proceed with immediate ureteroneocystostomy in either a refluxing or nonrefluxing manner (24). It may be necessary to leave a ureteral stent in place for several weeks to facilitate healing.

Noncavernous Nerve Injury

The most common nerve-related injury during RRP is transection of the obturator nerve during pelvic lymph node dissection or stretch injury from retractor positioning. Obturator nerve injury manifests itself as weakness of ipsilateral thigh adduction (23). Other reported mononeuropathies involving pelvic surgery are injuries to the femoral, sciatic, and peroneal nerves (17,25).

Femoral neuropathy has been reported in the gynecologic, renal transplantation, and urologic literature. Injury most commonly occurs secondary to direct nerve compression, indirect compression between the bodies of the psoas and iliacus muscles, or ischemia by compromising the iliolumbar artery from misplaced self-retaining retractor blades. The femoral nerve supplies motor innervation to the quadriceps, pectineal and sartorius muscles, and sensory innervation to the anterior and medial thigh thus symptoms of femoral neuropathy include weakness of hip flexion, knee extension, and paresthesias over the anteromedial thigh. Treatment involves physiotherapy and pain management, and patients should be assured that the injury is short lived with most resolving within six months from surgery (26).

PERIOPERATIVE COMPLICATIONS
Medical Complications

Medical complications are a major part of any major pelvic surgery. Myocardial infarction is a relatively rare complication of RRP with the reported incidence ranging from 0.1% to 0.7%

TABLE 3 Perioperative Complications of Radical Retropubic Prostatectomy

Investigator	Year	Number of patients	Myocardial infarction (%)	Pulmonary embolus (%)	Deep vein thrombosis (%)	Wound infection (%)
Igel et al. (4)	1987	692	NR	2.7	1.2	1
Leandri et al. (5)	1992	620	0.2	0.8	2.3	0.1
Ahearn et al. (25)	1994	1324	0.7	1.7	0.6	0.1
Hautmann et al. (7)	1994	418	NR	2.6	NR	2.6
Keetch et al. (6)	1994	810	0.4	2.3	0.8	0.4
Catalona et al. (10)	1999	1870	0.1	2	NR	0.8
Lepor et al. (17)	2001	1000	0.5	0.3	0.1	NR
Maffezzini et al. (18)	2003	300	NR	0.3	NR	0.3
Augustin et al. (19)	2003	1243	0.1	0.2	1	0.1

Abbreviation: NR, none reported.

(Table 3). Much more frequent and potential serious are thromboembolic complications in the form of pulmonary embolus (PE) and deep venous thrombosis (DVT) seen in up to 3% of patients (Table 3) (5,6,10,17,19,27).

Symptoms of DVT usually include calf pain or swelling with PE manifested as acute drop in oxygen saturations, fever, tachycardia, pleuritic chest pain, or new-onset atrial fibrillation. DVT is usually diagnosed on physical examination with the use of bilateral lower extremity Doppler ultrasound. In the diagnosis of PE a nuclear medicine ventilation perfusion scan or spiral chest computed tomography is employed. Factors thought to reduce the incidence of DVT are shorted anesthesia time, early postoperative ambulation, and the use of sequential compression devices (SCD) or subcutaneous heparin preparations. It is likely that most significant DVTs occur intraoperatively. Therefore, it is recommended that SCDs be placed at the induction of anesthesia and maintained until the patient is ambulating regularly (22).

Wound Complications

Wound-related problems are relatively unusual, occurring in 1% to 3% of individuals undergoing RRP (Table 3) (4–7,10,18,19,23,24,27). Wound infection generally occurs in patients with excessive subcutaneous fat or large amounts of urinary extravasation. A urine culture should be obtained preoperatively and if necessary the patient should be placed on appropriate antibiotics to sterilize the urine. An antiseptic solution should be used to clean the skin before incision and perioperative antibiotics should be broad spectrum, aimed at skin flora, and maintained for at least 24 to 48 hours postoperatively. If wound infection does occur the incision should be opened and allowed to heal by secondary intention.

Delayed Hemorrhage

Significant postoperative hemorrhage after RRP has been reported to occur in 0.5% to 1.7% of patients with the resulting bleeding often leading to pelvic hematoma formation (4,7,17,28). Small hematomas usually require no intervention, but larger ones may result in anastomotic disruption with potential urinary morbidity and formation of pelvic abscess. Hedican and Walsh reported on their series of 7 of 1350 patients undergoing RRP who experienced significant bleeding in the postoperative period requiring acute transfusion. Four patients were explored while three were managed conservatively.

Overall the patients who were explored had a shorter hospital course and experienced fewer postoperative complications. Specifically, the three patients managed expectantly were all found to have evacuation of the pelvic hematoma through the vesicourethral anastomosis (VUA) leading to symptomatic bladder neck contraction (BNC) versus only one patient who was explored suffering BNC. Furthermore, two of three patients who were not explored suffered significant prolonged urinary incontinence compared to one patient experiencing mild incontinence who was explored with hematoma evacuation. It was concluded that significant postoperative hemorrhage should be managed surgically to minimize long-term urinary complications (28).

TABLE 4 Reported Incidence of Lymphoceles After Radical Retropubic Prostatectomy

Investigator	Year	Number of patients	Lymphocele formation (%)
Igel et al. (4)	1987	692	0.9
Leandri et al. (5)	1992	620	2.3
Keetch et al. (6)	1994	810	0.4
Hautmann et al. (7)	1994	418	6.6
Lerner et al. (9)	1995	1000	0.1
Catalona et al. (10)	1999	1870	0.4
Gheiler et al. (29)	1999	1129	0.6

Lymphocele

Lymphocele formation is a recognized complication of pelvic surgery. Lymphoceles occur when afferent lymphatic channels have been transected without complete occlusion with hemoclips. Since an inflammatory reaction within the adjacent peritoneum prevents resorption of the lymph, the extravasated lymph organizes into a cystic collection. The extent of surgical dissection and experience of the surgeon are directly related to the incidence of lymphocele formation. With the advent of earlier detection of prostate cancer, the pelvic lymph node dissection performed during the prostatectomy has become more anatomically selective, decreasing the incidence of reported lymphoceles after RRP (Table 4) (4–7,9,10,29).

Lymphocele formation is a frequent but often insignificant complication of lymphadenectomy during radical prostatectomy. Most lymphoceles are subclinical and resolve without recognition or intervention. Pepper et al. reviewed the charts of 260 patients undergoing open prostatectomies at one institution. Of the 260 patients, nine patients (3.5%) developed clinically significant lymphoceles. Eight of these were radiographically confirmed, and four required ultrasound-guided percutaneous drainage. Fifty percent of the symptomatic lymphoceles regressed without intervention (30). Similarly, a prospective study from Norway reported a 2.3% incidence of clinically significant lymphoceles after RRP (31).

Relative indications for treatment of a lymphocele include infection, size greater than 5 cm, pain, or compression on adjacent structures such as ureter, bladder, or iliac vein (32). Symptomatic lymphoceles are confirmed radiographically with either a pelvic ultrasound or computed tomography (Fig. 1). The primary treatment modality is percutaneous drainage with radiographic manipulation. If infection is suspected based on clinical symptoms or the presence of bacteria in the drained sample, antibiotics are initiated. In cases of prolonged drainage,

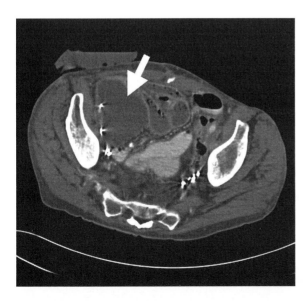

FIGURE 1 Computed tomography imaging showing postoperative lymphocele in right obturator fossa (*white arrow*).

sclerotherapy with tetracycline, ethanol, or povidine-iodine solution cures 90% of persistent lymphoceles (33–35). Open or laparoscopic marsupialization of the lymphocele is employed for those who fail sclerotherapy (6).

Anastomotic Leak

The VUA is one of the most technically-challenging aspects of RRP and the rate of anastomotic leakage after surgery is directly related to the quality of the anastomosis (23). The incidence of anastomotic leakage is difficult to assess since most institutions recommend foley catheter drainage for 7 to 14 days, during which time most small urinary leaks resolve without recognition. Thus, the reported incidence of prolonged anastomotic leakage ranges from 0.1% to 22.3% in most large series.

Continued elevated output from the surgical drain beyond postoperative day three is suggestive of an anastomotic leak. The fluid should be analyzed for creatinine and if elevated relative to the serum creatinine, a urine leak is confirmed. A cystogram is then obtained to evaluate the exact leakage site relative to the foley catheter and the surgical drain (Fig. 2). If the drain is in close proximity to the leak, it is withdrawn slightly and changed from bulb suction to gravity. The foley catheter may need repositioning and possibly traction to allow maximal drainage from the bladder. Additionally, the foley catheter can be exchanged for a catheter with side fenestrations to optimize drainage (36). The majority of anastomotic leaks will resolve with continued catheter drainage (6).

Catheter Dislodgment

After RRP, most practitioners advocate drainage via urethral catheter for 7 to 14 days. On occasion, catheter malfunction or injury can lead to dislodgment. In the early postoperative period, blind passage of a urethral catheter is discouraged due to the risk of anastomotic disruption. The preferred technique is the usage of flexible cystoscopy with placement of a 18-french council-tip catheter over a floppy tipped guide wire. If there is doubt as to the position of the catheter, a cystogram should be performed to confirm its location. If this maneuver is unsuccessful, suprapubic cystotomy may be required as a temporary measure.

In rare occasions, reoperation with anastomotic revision may be required. Some surgeons prefer cystotomy and antegrade catheter passage to reconstruction of the anastomosis (24).

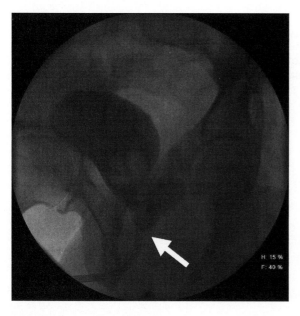

FIGURE 2   Cystography showing posterior anastomotic leak (*white arrow*).

In the late postoperative period (>5 days) consideration can be given to blind passage of a catheter versus leaving the catheter out as long as the patient is able to void.

LONG-TERM COMPLICATIONS
Bladder Neck Contracture
Etiology
BNC is a well-known complication of prostate surgery and may lead to both patient and physician dissatisfaction. The area of scar most often forms between the bladder neck and membranous urethra and may result in significant voiding dysfunction. The primary goals of the vasourethral anastomosis (VUA) during radical prostatectomy are the formation of an anastomosis that is tension free, highly vascular, and water tight. The use of a catheter or sound to identify the urethral lumen and techniques of bladder neck eversion are advocated to create a mucosa-to-mucosa apposition to maximize healing. The failure to achieve any or all of these goals may lead to potential anastomotic stricturing. The reported incidence of vesicourethral stricture following RRP is between 0.5% and 32% (Table 5) (4,10,37–45). Symptoms of BNC include weakening of urinary stream, frequency, urgency, incomplete emptying, and acute urinary retention (AUR). The majority of patients who develop BNC present within the first year from surgery (40,42–44). Park et al. reported that the time to diagnosis in their series ranged from 1 to 15.25 months with 72% presenting within the first six months of surgery (43). This is similar to reports by Surya et al. and Besarani et al. where 94% and 66%, respectively, presented within the first six months from surgery (37,44).

Predisposing factors to the development of anastomotic stricture are not entirely understood. Currently excepted risk factors include prior TURP, increased intraoperative blood loss, and the presence of urinary extravasation (37,42,45,46). Excessive blood in the operative field may lead to poor visualization and failure of apposition. Mass ligation of pelvic bleeders may lead to devascularization of the bladder neck and proximal urethra and resultant fibrosis. Ineffective hemostasis may produce postoperative pelvic hematoma formation with subsequent disruption of the anastomosis. Previous transurethral resection may lead to poor vascularity at the bladder neck and subsequent fibrosis and scaring resulting in stricture formation (37).

In a series of 156 radical prostatectomies by Surya et al., 13 of 72 patients who had had previous TURP developed anastomotic strictures compared to 5 of 84 who had not undergone transurethral prostatectomy (P < 0.05). Of 26 patients who had extravasation on retrograde urethrogram (RUG), 14 developed strictures compared to 4 of 130 who had an intact anastomosis (P < 0.005). Patients who developed BNC also had significantly higher mean operative blood loss (9.5 units vs. 1.8 units) (37).

The caliber of the reconstructed bladder neck may play a role as well. Keetch et al. reported that their incidence of BNC decreased from 7.8% to 0.6% when the bladder neck was tailored to 22–24 French (Fg) rather that 18 Fg (6). Contact by suction drainage tubes at the anastomosis way also bring about or worsen extravasation leading most to advocate placement of these

TABLE 5   Reported Incidence of BNC

Investigator	Year	Number of patients	BNC (%)
Igel et al. (4)	1987	692	5.4
Surya et al. (37)	1990	156	9.4
Levy et al. (38)	1994	143	14.1
Geary et al. (39)	1995	481	17.5
Popken et al. (40)	1998	340	7
Catalona et al. (10)	1999	1870	4
Kao et al. (41)	2000	863	20.5
Borboroglu et al. (42)	2000	467	11.1
Park et al. (43)	2001	753	4.8
Besarani et al. (44)	2004	510	9.4

Abbreviation: BNC, bladder neck contractions.

tubes at a reasonable distance from the anastomosis. Previously many promoted urinary diversion via suprapubic tube or ureteral catheters to decrease extravasation and resultant scar formation. However, a review of the literature fails to show that this strategy protects one from the complications of BNC. Surya et al. reported a 14.7% incidence of stricture in those diverted with additional drains versus 9.4% in those with foley catheter alone and Veenema et al. noted a 17% incidence of BNC in those with diversion via suprapubic tube or ureteral catheters (37,47).

Although widely held as an etiology of BNC, the role that urinary extravasation plays in anastomotic stricture has been debated. Surya et al. 1994 reported a positive correlation between extravasation and BNC. In his series of 156 patients undergoing RRP all underwent retrograde urethrogram (RUG) and voiding cystourethrogram (VCUG) at postoperative days 12 to 16 to evaluate the integrity of the anastomosis. Of the 26 patients with extravasation 14 were found to have stricture compared to 4 of 130 with a water-tight anastomosis (37). Levy et al. reported their series of 128 patients undergoing RRP and 15 treated with radical perineal prostatectomy (RPP). Of note, direct mucosa-to-mucosa apposition was performed in 93 RRP patients while a modified Vest anastomosis with traction sutures placed next to the bladder neck and anchored at the perineum was performed in 35 cases. All patients underwent imaging three weeks postoperatively. Urinary extravasation was seen in 14.1%. The highest rates of extravasation, were seen in the RPP group (33.3%) with the RRP and vest anastomosis groups having an 18.1% and 6.1% rate of extravasation, respectively. At follow-up anastomotic strictures occurred in 27.3% of patients who underwent vest anastomosis, 14% with direct anastomosis, and 0% in the RPP group. Of patients with extravasation on VCUG, only one patient in the RRP group and one patient in the Vest group experienced BNC (38). Findings from this and other studies support the technique of direct mucosa-to-mucosa apposition over Vest technique and suggest the possibility that if appropriate drainage is maintained until healing is complete, then BNC can be avoided despite the presence of urinary extravasation at the VUA.

Borboroglu et al. hypothesized that the presence of microvascular disease may lead to impaired healing and resultant stricturing. In their series of 467 patients treated with RRP vesicourethral stricture occurred in 11.1%. Recognized factors leading to microvascular disease such as cigarette smoking, hypertension, diabetes mellitus, and coronary artery disease were significantly higher in patients suffering from BNC. In addition, similar to previous reports, average operative time was longer (271 minutes vs. 249 minutes) and average blood loss was greater (1639 mL vs. 1093 mL) in those with BNC (42). Park et al. found that men with an average maximal scar width of 10 mm were eight times more likely to suffer anastomotic stricturing suggesting a generalized tendency in some men to form hypertrophic scars (43).

Management

There is no clear consensus on the management of anastomotic strictures. Possible strategies include dilation (urethral sounds, filiforms and followers, balloon dilation), cold knife urethrotomy, transurethral bladder neck incision or resection, and rarely open surgical repair (37,40,42–44). Often patient continence and quality of life (QOL) is altered by the stricture and subsequent corrective procedure. Park et al. reported their incidence of BNC in 753 patients undergoing RRP where 36 patients (4.8%) developed anastomotic stricture. The investigators treated these patients with a regimen of in-office dilation to 18 Fg and a schedule of three-month clean intermittent catheterization (CIC). 92.3% of men were managed by this protocol requiring dilation and CIC alone and 26.9% required more than one dilation. Direct vision internal urethrotomy was performed if greater than three dilations were needed in a nine-month period. The mean time to stricture recurrence was 2.75 months and it was felt that if there was no clinical recurrence by six months one could consider the stricture cured. Men who underwent a procedure to dilate or incise the stricture were significantly more likely to suffer urinary incontinence and require pad usage. Ninety-two percent of men in the control group became totally continent after RRP versus 62% in the stricture group who underwent dilation (43).

Yurkanin et al. reported their results of cold knife urethrotomy as primary treatment for BNC. Sixty-one patients who underwent one to three urethrotomies (87%, 10%, and 3%) were analyzed compared to similar patients without anastomotic stricture. The investigators found no difference from the control patients in terms of flow rate, post void residual urine (PVR), American Urological Association symptom scores (AUA-SS), QOL, or continence (45). Surya et al. found that dilation alone was ineffective in roughly half of the patients. They advocated cold knife incision in those in whom dilation failed and showed 37% efficacy with maintenance of continence. Transurethral incision of the BNC is associated with a very high rate of incontinence in many reports. Surya et al. reported a 75% incidence in their series of four patients (37). In contrast, Popken et al. advocate transurethral incision or resection as first-line treatment of BNC. High rates of efficacy were reported with a 0% incontinence rate. Meticulous attention must be paid to keeping the resection margin proximal to the sphincter mechanism (40).

Wessells et al. reported their series of open urethral reconstruction of obliterated VUA after radical prostate surgery. In their series, patients underwent a variety of procedures including primary end-to-end anastomosis, fasciocutaneous flap, free-graft urethroplasty with rectus muscle flap, and anterior bladder tube with omental flap. Urethral patency was established in all patients at 33 months follow-up, but no patient remained continent. They showed that with an obliterated anastomosis no one procedure is applicable in all cases, patency is the primary goal of surgery, and continence is rarely achievable (48). Another study of patients with obliterative strictures showed that patency can be obtained with a series of antegrade and retrograde approaches and a regimen of long-term intermittent catheterization (49).

In conclusion, it is important to counsel all patients undergoing RRP about the possible incidence of BNC and its effect on voiding function. Dilation and cold knife incision are effective for most strictures and are the most common initial methods of management. Refractory or recurrent strictures often respond to transurethral incision or resection, but do so often at the expense of continence. With more complex and obliterative strictures, patency is attainable but often results in complete urinary incontinence secondary to destruction of the sphincter mechanism.

Urinary Incontinence

Postprostatectomy urinary incontinence is one of the most troubling side effects of prostate surgery and can have great impact on QOL. Many patients report mild stress incontinence related to activity, but others may suffer severe uncontrollable leakage. With the introduction of the anatomic technique by Walsh and improvements in methods of handling the prostatic apex and urethra incontinence rates have improved, but in most large series from high volume academic centers the reported incidence of persistent incontinence still ranges from 6% to 20% with severe incontinence reported in 0.5% to 12.5% (Table 6) (4,6,7,10,18,39,50–57).

Urinary incontinence impacts patients on a medical, social, and psychological level. Medical complications such as irritation and skin breakdown can become a chronic debilitating problem. Patients may limit social activities and become isolated and many report feelings of anger, loss of dignity, and depression secondary to the social stigma associated with incontinence.

TABLE 6   Reported Incidence of Urinary Incontinence

Investigator	Year	Number of patients	Mean follow-up (mo)	Continent (%)
Igel et al. (4)	1997	692	33	75
Steiner et al. (50)	1991	593	12	92
Ramon et al. (51)	1993	484	6	90
			12	95
Geary et al. (39)	1994	481	3	71
			6	93
			12	97
Hautmann et al. (7)	1994	418	12	80
Keetch et al. (6)	1994	810	18	94
Shelfo et al. (52)	1998	365	<6	70
			>6	88
Catalona et al. (10)	1999	1870	50	92
Poon et al. (53)	2000	220	24	95
Maffezzini et al. (18)	2003	300	29	89
Lepor and Kaci (54)	2004	500	24	98.5

The true rate of urinary incontinence is difficult to calculate secondary to variability in the definition of continence, the lack of consensus on the optimal time of evaluation, and non-standardized methodology of incontinence assessment. In addition, patient verus physician-reported incontinence rates vary, possibly secondary to patients minimizing outcomes when speaking to their physician, lack of understanding of the impact of urinary leakage, or an unconscious bias of the surgeon toward adverse outcomes. One study, which compared physician-reported versus patient-reported outcomes of continence showed only 19% to 67% correlation depending on the definition of continence used (58).

As mentioned previously, the reported incidence of urinary incontinence in most large series from high volume centers is less than 20%. Fowler et al. reported a series of 757 Medicare patients undergoing prostatectomy between 1988–1990. In all 47% of patients self-reported that they drip urine on a daily basis, with over 30% reporting wearing protective pads, diapers, or clamps (2). A similar study examining self-reported questionnaires in 1069 men revealed that 65.6% of men reported some degree of postprostatectomy leakage of urine; however, protective measures were only required in 33% (41). In contrast, studies report results from self-administered questionnaires showing very high rates of continence with 93% and 98.5% of patients reporting either no usage, or usage of one protective pad daily (54,59).

In conclusion, incontinence is a troubling side effect of radical prostatectomy; however, in most large series its incidence is relatively low. In addition, it is clear that there is no one universally excepted definition of continence and physicians and patients do not always apply the same definition in their rating or urinary leakage. There is a need to develop a standardized measure of urinary incontinence following prostatectomy focusing on its impact on patient QOL rather than just on the presence of leakage.

Pathophysiology

The pathophysiologic explanation for incontinence following radical prostatectomy is likely multifactorial with detrusor instability (DI), loss of bladder compliance, damage to pelvic diaphragm musculature, and intrinsic sphincter deficiency all implicated as playing potential causative roles. The urethral sphincteric unit is composted of an intrinsic smooth muscle component at the bladder neck and a skeletal muscle component termed the external sphincter both of which contribute to the functional length of the urethra and its ability to coapt and maintain continence (57). It is likely that damage to both of these sphincter mechanisms affects postoperative continence status. The external sphincter has broad fascial attachments and is innervated by the pudendal nerves and autonomic nerves from the pelvic plexus anatomically located near the apex of the prostate (60,61). The internal sphincter is located at the bladder neck and proximal urethra. Its tonicity is under autonomic control and this disruption may also contribute to the degree of postoperative incontinence experienced.

Mechanical damage to the musculature of the sphincter mechanism or its innervation can occur during ligation of the dorsal venous complex, urethral division, apical dissection, or VUA and is likely the prime derangement responsible for postprostatectomy incontinence. Therefore, it is generally believed that during surgical dissection great care should be taken to preserve as much of the urethra and surrounding musculature and neurovascular tissue during the apical dissection, while still performing adequate cancer excision.

The roles of detrusor factors such as reduced compliance and DI also seem to have some impact on postprostatectomy incontinence, especially in the early postoperative period, leading to an urge component superimposed upon prominent stress urinary incontinence. Chao and Mayo examined videourodynamics in 64 incontinent patients following RRP. In their study, 96% of incontinent men had sphincteric weakness as a contributing factor with 57% as the sole source of their incontinence. Twenty-eight percent had associated DI as a coexistent abnormality. Only 4% of patients had DI as a sole source of incontinence. Other detrusor abnormalities such as decreased compliance, reduced bladder capacity, and areflexia occurred in a smaller number of patients (62).

In another study, Presti et al. evaluated urodynamic parameters in 24 patients presenting with moderate or severe postprostatectomy incontinence and compared them to 13 continent controls. Statistically significant differences were found between continent and incontinent men in mean functional profile length, maximal urethral closure pressure, and maximal urethral closure pressure during voluntary contraction of the external sphincter, indicating that sphincteric efficiency was the primary determinant of postoperative continence status. Differences in maximal detrusor pressure, volume at initial contraction, maximum cystometric capacity, and residual urine volume were not statistically significant. In contrast to previous studies, bladder dysfunction did not seem to play a prominent role with rates of DI present equally in 25% and 23% of incontinent and continent patients, respectively (57).

In conclusions it is evident that the etiology of postprostatectomy incontinence is multifactorial and complex. DI likely plays a role in initial incontinence, which may be improved with pharmacotherapy and pelvic floor exercises. Persistent incontinence is mainly stressful in nature and caused by sphincter dysfunction. In this situation, more invasive surgical treatment may be needed to provide an adequate level of dryness for the postprostatectomy patient.

Prevention

Surgical techniques for prevention of postoperative incontinence have been implemented and debated in multiple studies. While meticulous dissection of the prostatic apex seems to improve continence status, the benefits of other procedural modifications such as preservation of the NVBs, bladder neck sparing, puboprostatic ligament ligation, and the effects of anastomotic stricture have been debated. In a series by Eastman et al. the investigators examined the outcomes of 581 radical prostatectomies performed between 1983 and 1994 by chart review and patient questionnaires. At 24-months, follow-up, 91% of patients had regained continence with the vast majority achieving dryness by 12 months. On multivariate analysis risk factors for incontinence were patient age, surgical technique, NVB preservation, and incidence of BNC (55).

The role of sparing the NVBs and their effect on the return of continence is controversial and has been examined in a number of studies. Anatomic dissections have shown that both pudendal and pelvic nerves give intrapelvic branches that course at the 5 and 7 o'clock position on the prostate toward the external urethral sphincter (61). As previously discussed, Eastman et al. reported NVB resection as a risk factor for postsurgical incontinence in their series of 581 men undergoing RRP. A retrospective review of a similar cohort of 593 patients at Johns Hopkins Medical Center found no significant difference in postoperative incontinence based upon excision of one or both NVBs. Of the 328 patients where both NVBs were preserved continence was achieved in 94%. Ninety-two percent of 228 with preservation of one NVB and 81% of 37 patients where both bundles were excised reported continence. Although there was a trend toward increased rates of incontinence in the later group this difference was not statistically significant (50). Ramon et al. confirmed these finding in a series of 484 men in which continence was achieved in 96% with preservation of both bundles versus 94% with excision of both bundles (51). Lepor and Kaci in their series of 500 men undergoing prostatectomy also failed to show improved continence in men receiving bilateral nerve-sparing procedures; however, in this study most patients were young (<65) and continence rates were very high (98.5%) (53).

The impact of bladder neck preservation has been debated. In this technique, care is taken to preserve the circular muscle fibers at the bladder neck so as to minimize injury to the sphincteric mechanism (63). Shelfo et al. reported early return of continence with a bladder neck preservation technique with 67%, 70%, and 88% achieving continence at three months, less than six months, and greater than six months, respectively (52). In addition, Lowe showed that there was a significantly decreased time to continence of 62.4% versus 44.3% at three months in 91 patients with bladder neck-sparing procedure and in 99 patients where bladder neck resection was performed. However, excellent outcomes were obtained at one year in both groups with 89.4% and 86.3% of patients continent (63). In contrast, Poon et al. found no statistically significant differences in early or delayed urinary incontinence between bladder neck preservation and bladder neck resection techniques with similar results and all time points and with 93% and 96% dry at one year (53).

Preserving the puboprostatic ligaments has also been advocated to improve early continence rates by providing maximal urethral length and leaving its anterior support undisturbed. Poore et al. assessed this in 43 men undergoing radical prostatectomy. Standard apical dissection was performed in 25 while a puboprostatic ligament-sparing technique was performed in 18. Median time to achieve continence was significantly shorter in the puboprostatic ligament-sparing group when compared with the standard dissection (6.5 weeks vs. 12 weeks). However, much like in the literature regarding bladder neck-sparing techniques, equivalent continence rates were seen at one year (100% vs. 94%) (64).

In conclusion, the exact etiology of postprostatectomy incontinence is complex and not fully understood. It is imperative to communicate with the patient before surgery the inevitability of early leakage, the time course of its recovery, realistic expectations of long-term continence, and the possible need for surgical intervention to achieve desired dryness. From a surgical standpoint meticulous dissection of the prostatic apex, careful bladder neck reconstruction, and a water-tight VUA appear to be of paramount importance in preventing prolonged postoperative urine leakage. Sphincter inefficiency is likely the major contributor to incontinence, but detrusor factors such as decreased compliance and DI must be taken into account. It is also clear that symptoms perceived by the patient do not always correlate with pathophysiology making urodynamic evaluation an indispensable tool to formulate an accurate diagnosis and an individualized treatment plan for a given patient.

Treatment Options for Postprostatectomy Urinary Incontinence
Behavioral Methods
A variety of treatment methods are available for the patient with postprostatectomy incontinence including pharmacotherapy, pelvic floor exercises with or without biofeedback, penile clamps, external collection devices, urethral bulking agents, bulbourethral suspension procedures, and implantation of an artificial urinary sphincter (AUS). Due to its benign nature and potential efficacy The Agency for Health Care Policy and Research Guidelines recommends the use of behavioral methods as first-line therapy for stress and urge urinary incontinence, but specific treatment recommendations regarding postprostatectomy incontinence are limited (60,65).

The return of urinary continence seems to be a time-related process. In a study by Geary et al. of patients that regained complete urinary continence 71% did so by three months, an additional 22% at six months, and another 4% at one year. Very few (3%) showed recovery after one year (39). Lepor and Kaci showed similar results with 70.9%, 87.2%, 92.1%, and 98.5% continent at 3, 6, 12, and 24 months postoperatively (54). Therefore, it is widely agreed upon that any more invasive intervention for postprostatectomy incontinence should be delayed for at least one year to give the patient adequate time to regain continence. During that time patients should be taught to focus on pelvic muscle exercises (PME), and certain behavioral strategies, such as timed voiding, fluid limitation, and possibly biofeedback in order to improve or regain continence.

The existing literature on the treatment of postprostatectomy incontinence is mainly centered on surgical therapy such as collagen injection, bulbourethral slings, and AUS. While effective, these treatments are subject to failure and need for repeat procedures or surgical revision leading to patient and physician dissatisfaction. Research into behavioral therapies for postoperative incontinence is limited, but has shown promising results.

The use of PMEs in the treatment of incontinence was first described by Kegel in the 1940s and early studies showed significant improvements in both stress and urge incontinence in those treated. The goal of PMEs is to isolate and contract the pubococcygeus muscle thus increasing its strength and with it urethral resistance (60). Meaglia, evaluated PMEs in 24 incontinent men after radical or perineal prostatectomy in which men were given detailed instruction on how to perform PMEs and were prescribed a home schedule of 51 repetitions daily. Overall incontinence episodes decreased by 56.6% at six months follow-up. 8.3% achieved total continence, 42% improved greatly, and 33% showed no change in incontinence severity (66). In a similar study, Burgia et al. treated 20 men with postprostatectomy incontinence with PMEs, timed voiding, inhibition techniques, and biofeedback. At six months, follow-up stress and urge incontinence were decreased by an average of 78.3% and 80.7%, respectively, unfortunately there was little improvement in patients with severe leakage (67). Because several techniques were used, it is difficult to interpret which effected continence the most, but does point to the fact that multiple behavioral methods may lead to better outcomes than PMEs alone.

In biofeedback abdominal electromyography or rectal instrumentation is used to provide the patient with a visual or auditory response and assist in isolation of the correct pelvic muscles to contract. Franke et al. evaluated whether the addition of behavioral therapies enhanced the return of continence in 30 patients randomized to a regimen of PMEs and biofeedback versus control where no specific instructions were given. Treated patients received 45-minute biofeedback behavior training sessions at 6, 7, 9, 11, and 16 weeks postoperatively and were prescribed a regimen of 20 PMEs three times daily. Overall 87% of patients were pad free at six months, including 86% in the treatment and 88% in the control group. The investigators concluded that intensive biofeedback was not effective in increasing the rate of postoperative incontinence (68). The lack of statistical significance could be secondary to the high rate of continence achieved and low patient population masking any potential difference.

In conclusion, due to its potential efficacy, minimally invasive nature, and lack of side effects, PMEs should be considered first line in the treatment of postprostatectomy incontinence. Biofeedback can be added for the highly motivated patient or those with difficulty isolating their perineal musculature, but its role in increasing efficacy is unknown. Additionally, there is some controversy in the literature whether PMEs can be taught by verbal instruction alone or whether formal biofeedback training with a physiotherapist is need to ensure that the patient performs the maneuvers correctly.

Urethral Bulking Agents

Another method proposed in the treatment of postprostatectomy incontinence is the injection of bulking agents into the submucosa of the bladder neck and proximal urethra in order to provide added resistance. A variety of agents have been investigated including autologous fat, polytetrafluoroethylene (Teflon, Polytef), and collagen preparations. Politano et al. showed efficacy with Polytef paste cystoscopically injected in a retrograde manner in 720 incontinent males following prostate surgery. Sixty-seven percent of patients incontinent after RRP were improved or cured at follow-up with no major complications reported (69). However, concerns over safety, durability, and migration of particles to the lungs, lymph nodes, brain, and kidneys in laboratory animals led to its removal from the market by the Federal Food and Drug Administration (FDA) (70,71). Studies of the use of autologous fat have been disappointing with one report only showing 16% efficacy in men with postprostatectomy incontinence (72).

Glutaraldehyde cross-linked bovine collagen was approved by the FDA for use in intrinsic sphincter deficiency in October 1993 (73,74). Since then collagen injection has emerged as the mainstay of injectable bulking agents for postprostatectomy incontinence secondary to its efficacy, minimally invasive application, lack of migration, and safety. The implanted material is derived from highly purified bovine dermal collagen containing 95% type I and 5% type III collagen cross-linked with 0.0075% glutaraldehyde to prevent degradation. The material is suspended in a phosphate-buffered saline solution and is packed in a syringe containing 2.5 mL of material (71).

The implantation procedure is begun with a skin test to document lack of hypersensitivity to the compound. If allergy is excluded a standard rigid cystoscope is used under sedation, local, general, or spinal anesthesia to visualize the bladder neck and urethra. A specially designed needle is used to implant the material in the submucosa at the targeted area at the bladder neck and proximal urethra (Fig. 3). An attempt is made to produce visual obstruction of the urethra and once achieved the cystoscope should not be passed beyond the collagen as not to disrupt its coaptation. Injections can be repeated at several week intervals until satisfaction in terms of dryness is achieved. The optimal amount to inject or the absolute number of injection to perform before labeling a patient a failure has not been clearly defined.

Cummings et al. examined their initial results with retrograde collagen injection in 19 men with postprostatectomy stress urinary incontinence. Most men had mild (one to two pads daily) and moderate (three to four pads daily) incontinence. At one year follow-up good results (dry or wearing only an occasional pad) were obtained in 21%. Improvement (decreased leakage by 75%) was observed in an additional 37% with 42% classified as treatment failures. The overall treatment satisfaction rate was 58%. Of those achieving success the average number of injections performed was 1.8 (range 1–3) with a mean of 13.8 mL (range 3–32.5) of collagen implanted. Severity of leakage and bladder neck scarring were shown to negatively affect the success rate (75).

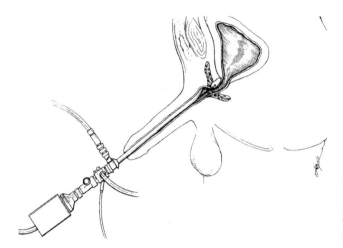

FIGURE 3 Line drawing of technique of retrograde collagen injection using a rigid cystoscope and a specially designed needle to implant the material at the bladder neck and proximal urethra.

Smith et al. examined the long-term success rates of collagen injection in 62 men with postprostatectomy incontinence followed for a median of 29 months. Of those treated 38.7% achieved social continence, but only 8.1% became dry. The median duration of success was 17.5 months. Of the patients who obtained social continence 60.9% maintained it at one year and 42.8% of two years, follow-up. On average, four injection procedures and 20.0 mL of collagen were required to achieve social continence. As in previous studies outcomes correlated with the severity of incontinence and poorer results were seen in patients with intense scaring at the region of the sphincter and in those with BNC. Complications were minimal with transient urinary retention and self-limiting hematuria reported in 11.3% (73). Griebling et al. associates evaluated a series of 25 men incontinent after prostatectomy treated with transurethral collagen implantation with a disappointing 8% achieving significant improvement, 32% with minimal improvement, and 60% with no appreciable change in leakage. These results may have been skewed secondary to the high percentage of patients (44%) with severe stress or total urinary incontinence. At follow-up five patients (20%) eventually underwent placement of an AUS. It was noted that previous collagen injection did not interfere with surgical dissection, placement, or function of the prosthesis (71).

To maximize the implantation of collagen into the desired area at the bladder neck and proximal urethra, Klutke et al. developed an antegrade method of collagen injection through a percutaneous suprapubic tract (Fig. 4). At a follow-up of 8.5 months, 9 of 20 patients (45%) had significant subjective improvement and five (25%) were dry after one injection procedure. At a longer follow-up of 28 months only 35% remained improved with only two patients (10%) with durable cure. It was felt by the investigators that antegrade collagen implantation showed similar long-term efficacy to retrograde collagen injection and allowed the procedure to be performed with one instillation by minimizing technical failures due to inappropriate site of implantation (74,76).

In conclusion, the use of transurethral bulking agents, mainly collagen, shows some efficacy in mild to moderate post-prostatectomy incontinence. Patients should be counseled that multiple injections are often necessary and complete dryness may not be attainable in a substantial number of patients. In addition, the efficacy may be of short duration requiring repeat injection or progression to other surgical procedures.

Bulbourethral Sling Procedures
In more severe cases of postprostatectomy incontinence minimally invasive therapies such a Kegal exercises and collagen injection do not provide adequate relief of symptoms. In these cases many patients opt for more invasive surgical procedures, once such option is the placement of a urethral sling. Numerous sling procedures have been developed and employed in the treatment of women with stress urinary incontinence with efficacy approaching 90% (77). Based on these techniques various procedures have been developed to treat men with stress incontinence after prostate surgery.

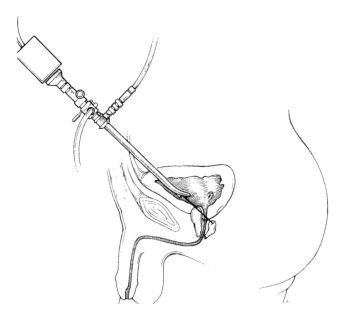

FIGURE 4 Line drawing of technique of antegrade collagen injection into the bladder neck and proximal urethra using a rigid cystoscope through a suprapubic tract.

In 1998 Schaeffer et al. reported their initial results of 64 men with severe post-prostatectomy incontinence treated between 1992 and 1996 with a modified version of a Stamey suspension sling used in female patients with stress urinary incontinence. In the procedure, the bulbourethra was suspended from the rectus fascia by a series of bolsters thereby increasing urethral resistance with increasing abdominal pressure. The goal of the procedure was to render patients dry and provide physiologic voiding with complications and cost less than that of the AUS. At a mean follow-up of 22.4 months 64% of patients were reported to be dry or improved. Secondary procedures were need to tighten the sling in 17 patients (27%) increasing the success rate to 75%. Two patients (3%) developed wound infection requiring device removal and there was a 6% rate of erosion into the urethra. Urinary retention was reported in one patient and perineal numbness and pain lasting four to six weeks was reported in 19% (77). A follow-up study was published in 2005 reporting the long-term results of 95 patients treated with this procedure. At a mean follow-up of four years, the efficacy was durable with 38% completely dry and 68% of patients requiring two or less pads daily. Patients with previous pelvic radiation were found to have inferior results with only 43% improved versus 72% of paints without prior radiation (78).

In recent years, a variety of slings anchored to the pubic bone have been described. The advantage of these procedures is that only one perineal incision is required and resistance is maintained by attaching the sling to a fixed structure. Madjar et al. reported 16 men with postprostatectomy incontinence treated with a gelatin-coated polyethylene terephthalate sling or cadaveric fascia lata tied to the pubic bone with four pairs of sutures attached to bone anchors. Of 14 patients with urodynamically confirmed stress urinary incontinence, 12 were considered cured, defined as dry or one pad daily. Two patients were improved with a 50% or greater reduction in pad usage. The remaining two patients had an urge component to their incontinence and became dry with the addition of anticholinergic medication. One patient reported urinary retention that resolved spontaneously and no patients suffered urethral erosion, wound infection, or osseous complications (79).

Recently a bone-anchored sling has become commercially available, termed the InVance (American Medical Systems, Minnetonka, Minnesota, U.S.A.). This modification of the bulbourethral sling hopes to provide efficacy with lower complication and mechanical failure rates when compared with the AUS. Through this minimally invasive procedure, a midline perineal incision is made and the bulbar urethra is exposed. After the dissection a compressive polypropylene mesh sling is anchored to the descending pubic rami bilaterally (Fig. 5). Early studies

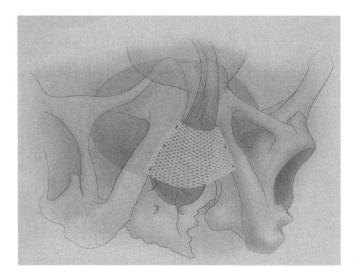

FIGURE 5 Schematic of bulbourethral sling anchored to descending pubic ramus. *Source*: Courtesy of American Medical Systems, Minnetonka, Minnesota, U.S.A.

were published by Comiter on 21 men undergoing the procedure to correct stress urinary incontinence, 18 of whom underwent previous radical prostatectomy. Of patients with postprostatectomy incontinence 72% were considered cured. This group included patients that had failed other surgical procedure such as previous AUS and collagen injection. At one year follow-up there were no reports of infection, erosion, prolonged pain, or de novo urinary urgency (80). Recently the same group has published their 24 month follow-up in 36 patients undergoing the male sling procedure. Overall 67% of patients were pad free, 14% used one pad daily, 11% used three pads daily, and 8% used three or more pads daily. The most frequent complication was transient urinary retention reported in 19%. There were no reports of prolonged urinary retention, erosion, infection, or need for device revision. It is believed that the lower incidence of erosion over the AUS is secondary to only the ventral rather than circumferential compression of the urethra which may avoid venous constriction and lessen urethral atrophy (81).

Castle et al. had less favorable results in 42 patients undergoing male sling secondary to postoperative stress incontinence. At a mean follow-up of 18 months only a 39.5% success rate was achieved, defined as using one thin pad daily, and only 15.8% were completely dry. Infection was seen in three patients (7.9%) with urethral erosion in one patient. Results were likely affected by the high number of patients with adverse prognostic factors such as severe incontinence in 32%, previous radiation in 21%, and prior AUS in 10.5% (82). In general, it is believed that the male sling is most appropriate for the patient with mild to moderate stress incontinence who has not received previous pelvic irradiation.

Artificial Urinary Sphincter
The AUS, first introduced in 1972, is a mechanical device composed of an inflatable cuff, placed around the bulbar urethra, a reservoir, pump, and a series of interconnecting tubes to carry fluid to the urethral cuff (Figs. 6 and 7). Reported efficacy is as high as 75% to 90% in some series (83–85). While efficacious, the procedure requires an open operation under general or spinal anesthesia, a substantial recovery period is often necessary, and a certain amount of strength and manual dexterity is needed to operate the device. In addition, infection and erosion, requiring device removal, and the need for surgical revision secondary to recurrent incontinence remain substantial drawbacks of the AUS. Reported revision and explantation rates range from 10.8–44.6% to 2.8–17% respectively (86). One long-term report by Fulford et al. showed only 13% of patients were continent with their original device at 10 year follow-up (87).

Initial reports on the use of the AS 800 AUS (American Medical Systems, Minnetonka, Minnesota, U.S.A.) were from Goldwasser et al. at Mayo Clinic. In their series of 109 patients (both male and female) with urinary incontinence of various etiologies, continence was achieved in 83.5% after AUS placement. Various degrees of leakage recurred in 9.2% and 7.3% remained

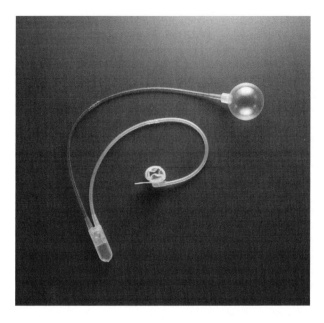

FIGURE 6 Photograph of artifical urinary sphincter. *Source*: Courtesy of American Medical Systems, Minnetonka, Minnesota, U.S.A.

incontinent. Nearly 25% of patients required at least one surgical revision, most common indications being loss of cuff compression (nine), tubing kink (three), cuff erosion (three), and infection (two) (83).

Litwiller et al. published results of 50 men treated with AUS for severe postprostatectomy incontinence. Initially 44% of patients were completely continent after surgery, but at a median of 23.4 months follow-up only 20% continued to be dry. Onset of leakage varied from one month to seven years. Of those who reported leakage, 55% reported only a few drops daily and 22% less than a teaspoon. Patient satisfaction was uniformly high with 90% of patients reported as

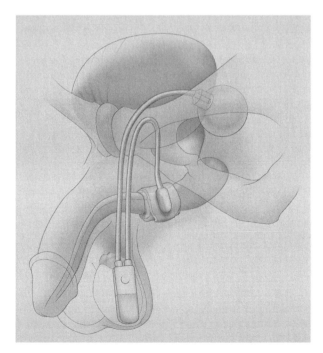

FIGURE 7 Depiction of in situ placement of artificial urinary sphincter. *Source*: Courtesy of American Medical Systems, Minnetonka, Minnesota, U.S.A.

satisfied with the device, 96% would recommend it to a friend, and 92% would in retrospect have the procedure performed again. Satisfaction correlated with experienced efficacy in terms of amount of leakage, no negative effect was seen in those patients needing surgical revision (88). Gundian et al. had slightly better results in their series of 117 men undergoing AUS for postprostatectomy incontinence with 90% of patients significantly improved and a 90% overall satisfaction rate. In the series, 37 patients underwent 64 surgical revisions secondary to inadequate cuff compression (33%), tubing kinks (16%), cuff erosion (13%), scrotal hematoma (9%), and cuff leaks (4%) (84).

The common causes of recurrent leakage in previously dry patients are mechanical failure manifested as fluid leak in the system and urethral atrophy secondary to the circumferential pressure exhibited by the activated cuff. To combat the problem of urethral atrophy Brito et al. reported on the addition of a second cuff, or tandem cuff, around the urethra, which in their series increased the success rate of the AUS to over 95% (89). Another option is replacement of the reservoir to a larger size, thus providing a higher pressure gradient for coaptation of the urethra.

Since the introduction of the AUS in 1972 advances in product design and improved surgical techniques has resulted in decreased complication rates and increased product durability. The AMS 800 was introduced in 1983 to replace the previous AMS 791 model and in 1987 the design was again changed to a narrow backed cuff providing more even pressure distribution on the urethra leading to a decreased incidence of cuff erosion and reoperation rates (86,90). One of the largest series of AUS implantations comes from the Mayo Clinic in which 400 patients with urinary incontinence of various etiologies treated with AUS placement over 11 years. The investigators reported results in 323 patients, 160 of whom were incontinent after radical prostatectomy, with a mean follow-up of 68.8 months. A total of 139 prenarrow backing cuff sphincters and 184 narrow backing cuff sphincters were placed. Overall 27% of patients required surgical revision for various reasons including device malfunction, recurrent incontinence, erosion, or infection. Overall 42% of patients with the pre-narrow backing cuff and 17% with the narrow backing cuff required reoperation. Kaplan–Meier analysis revealed a five year expected device survival of 67%. Taken as a whole, at last contact 90.4% had a property functioning device (90).

It was hoped that with device improvements, such as narrow backing cuff, that the AUS would prove to be efficacious and durable with fewer patients requiring reoperation. To test this Clemens et al. reported 70 patients, only five of whom had an AUS with the prenarrow back design. Overall 54 revisions were performed in 24 patients for a reoperation rate of 36.4%. One revision was required in 12 patients, two in five, and three or more in seven patients. The majority of revisions (42.5%) were secondary to recurrent incontinence in the form of increased reservoir size, decreased cuff size, or the addition of a tandem cuff. Overall 27.7% of procedures were for replacement or removal of infected or eroded components and 9% of revisions were due to mechanical failure. Available data showed that at a median follow-up of 29.3 months 34% were completely dry, 20% required one to two pads daily, and 20% required three or more pads daily (85). Differences in reported revision rates are likely multifactorial, including variations in patient characteristics, surgical techniques, and differences in the threshold for reoperation. However, most studies show that the device is durable with most surgical revisions secondary to patient factors, such as urethral atrophy, rather than mechanical failure.

In conclusion, the AUS remains the gold standard treatment for men with postprostatectomy incontinence. Reported success and patient satisfaction rates are high with many patients stating that they would have the procedure performed again. Both patient and physician should be aware of the risks of infection, erosion, and the high surgical revision rate, and many patients continue to have minimal leakage even with a properly functioning device.

Impotence

Impotence has been a major complication of the RRP since its introduction in 1947. With the advent of PSA and the public awareness regarding prostate cancer, this is no longer a disease of the aged. Younger men, many of whom are potent prior to surgery, undergo RRP in an attempt to eradicate cancer and find that their sexual function has been compromised postoperatively.

QOL studies have quantified the subjective decline in sexual function, noting that almost no patients return to their baseline level of sexual functioning (91).

There have been numerous advances in the past 20 years to limit the percentage of patients rendered impotent after RRP. These include the nerve-sparing approach to RRP and a broader range of medical and surgical treatments for those with postprostatectomy impotence. The introduction of the nerve-sparing RRP (NSRRP) in the early 1980s by Walsh revolutionized the approach to prostate cancer (92). By defining the neuroanatomy of the pelvis including the innervation of the corpora cavernosa, it is no longer necessary to sacrifice sexual function for cancer cure.

The potency rates reported in the literature after the introduction of NSRRP range from 40% to 80% (Table 7) (2,4–6,10,39,59,93,94). It is difficult to compare potency rates among the series since there is no universal definition of potency, the method of assessment (self-assessment vs. physician questioning) varies among the studies, and some series span the pre- and postnerve-sparing technique era.

Anatomical Approach to Radical Retropubic Prostatectomy

The most significant surgical advancement in potency preservation was the development of the NSRRP. Impotence was almost a universal postoperative complication of the original RRP introduced by Millin in 1947. In 1981, Walsh and Donker collaborated in an effort to define the innervation to the corpora cavernosa. Previous studies had suggested that the innervation necessary for erection originated from the pelvic plexus. However, the course of the pelvic plexus from its origin to its innervation of the corpora had not yet been delineated. Using stillborn males and fetuses as a model, the pelvic plexus was identified along the lateral aspects of the rectum with branches to the corpora running between the rectum and prostate in an extracapsular plane. Adult cadaveric dissections by Walsh demonstrated that the cavernous nerves traveled in close proximity to the prostatic capsular vasculature along the dorsolateral surface of the prostatic capsule (13).

Understanding the relationship between the nerve plexus and the bladder, rectum, seminal vesicles, and prostate is essential to a nerve-sparing approach to radical prostatectomy. The preservation of the NVBs begins with apical dissection to free both bundles from the apex, avoiding inadvertent traction on the contralateral nerve. After careful division off of the anterior surface of the rectum, the lateral pelvic fascia is divided posterior to the NVB on the posterolateral surface of the rectum. The dissection stops at the tip of the seminal vesicle (13).

Nonsurgical Factors Affecting Postoperative Erectile Function

There are several nonsurgical factors, which help predict the return of potency postoperatively. Stanford et al. evaluated 1291 community-based patients postoperatively and noted that age

TABLE 7 Reported Potency After Radical Retropubic Prostatectomy

Investigator	Year	Number of patients	Impotence (%)	Definition of potency
Igel et al. (4) (non-nerve sparing)	1987	692	97.5	Functional potency
Quinlan et al. (93)	1991	503	32	AFI
Leandri et al. (5)	1992	620	29	AFI
Nerve sparing		106	28	
Keetch et al. (6)	1994	295	42	AFI
Geary et al. (39)	1995	459	44.4	AFI
Bilateral nerve sparing		69	68.1	
Unilateral nerve sparing		203	86.7	
Catalona et al. (10)	1999	858	33.5	AFI
Bilateral nerve sparing		798	32	
Unilateral nerve sparing		60	53	
Fowler et al. (2)	1993	739	79	Erection after surgery
Walsh et al. (59)	2000	70	14	Unassisted intercourse
Stanford et al. (94)	2000	1291	59	AFI

Abbreviation: AFI, adequate for intercourse.

and baseline sexual function were the primary predictors of postoperative potency, though race, education, and access to a partner also influenced potency after surgery (94). Young, African-American males without sexual dysfunction preoperatively were the most likely to regain potency after surgery. Rabbani et al. concurred that preoperative sexual functioning was a statistically significant predictor of postoperative potency. Those with complete preoperative erectile function had a 54% recovery of potency postoperatively. In comparison, there was a 37% recovery if patients had recently experienced diminished function prior to surgery and only a 22% recovery in patients experiencing partial preoperative erections (95).

Psychological factors related to the diagnosis of prostate cancer also affect postoperative potency rates. Many men experience fear and depression related to the cancer diagnosis. The diagnosis of prostate cancer and slow recovery of erectile function can create a dysfunction in sexual relationship between the patient and his partner. Patients often withdraw emotionally and sexually because of their inability to engage in sexual activity, and their partners avoid initiating sexual activity to prevent the patient from experiencing anxiety over his inability to perform (96).

Surgical Factors Affecting Postoperative Erectile Function

The surgical factors influencing postoperative potency include patient selection (particularly age), use of unilateral versus bilateral nerve-sparing approach, and time since surgery (3,10,97). Age of the patient at the time of surgery is a major predictor of potency return. In the Quinlan and Walsh series, potency rates were directly related to age. They reported a 91% potency rate in patients less than 50, which declined with age to only 25% potency in those over 70 years of age (93). Stanford et al. reported a similar trend with younger age correlating with higher return of potency rates. Of those less than 60 years old, 39% were able to achieve an erection and engage in sexual intercourse compared with only 19% in those greater than 75 years of age (94). Data from the Catalona series confirm these findings, stating that a man less than 50 years old is twice as likely to regain potency as someone greater than 70 years old (10).

Studies evaluating potency rates over a time continuum show that erectile function is often impaired for the first 6 to 12 months after surgery as the nerves regenerate from the trauma incurred during surgery. Burnett (98) proposed that the time-dependent recovery of nerve function has several possible surgical etiologies: intraoperative trauma as the nerve is stretched during traction, thermal damage from electrocautery, ischemic injury while attempting to gain hemostasis, and an inflammatory reaction. Walsh concluded that a period of at least 18 months is necessary to comprehensively evaluate the postoperative potency rates (99). Catalona et al. noted an overall 59% return of potency by two years with 73% return by 4 years, supporting the time-dependent nature of return of potency (10).

Treatment Options for Postprostatectomy Impotence

Though much attention has been focused on preserving potency after RRP, a significant portion of patients are rendered impotent postoperatively. Multiple investigations have examined QOL indices in patients dealing with postoperative erectile dysfunction (ED) (100,101). Though many return to general baseline health shortly after RRP, sexual dysfunction remains an area of concern after the other parameters are corrected.

There are several medical and surgical treatment options for ED. Stephenson et al. evaluated the treatment options utilized along with outcomes in a sample of 1977 men included in the surveillance, epidemiology, and end results prostate cancer outcomes study (PCOS). Sixty-eight percent of the subjects had undergone RRP and overall, 50% of subjects tried one or more ED treatment methods. The study concluded after 60 months, follow-up. The major factors predisposing patients to seek out ED treatment include: younger age, presence of a sexual partner, and frequent sexual encounters prior to RRP. Of all the treatment options available, penile prosthesis was viewed as the best option (52%) though relatively few patients had a prosthesis (1.9%). Of note, sildenafil was introduced three years into the study. The number of patients seeking ED treatment increased from about one-third to 50% after the introduction of sildenafil, though only 12% reported that it dramatically improved sexual function. Overall, less than half of the subjects were able to achieve a full erection with the various therapies, suggesting that a wider variety and more selective therapies are necessary (102).

Timing of Treatment After Prostatectomy

The concept of prophylaxis against penile atrophy and ED has been suggested as a reason to initiate ED therapy in the immediate postoperative period. The belief that penile atrophy occurs postoperatively is derived from a study by Klein et al in which rats undergoing bilateral cavernous nerve neurotomy demonstrated histologic evidence of penile apoptosis (103). Penile apoptosis is a plausible explanation for reported decreased penile length after RRP. Fraiman et al. evaluated penile morphometrics after RRP and reported an 8% decrease in length and 9% decrease in circumference after NSRRP (in both the erect and flaccid state). Additionally, it was found that the greatest reduction in penile volume occurred in the first four to eight months postoperatively. The proposed etiology was smooth muscle atrophy caused by denervation (104). Gontero and Kirby clarified that the atrophy and resulting ED was likely due to cavernosal damage. Therefore, vacuum devices and intracorporal injections (ICIs) would likely provide increased early postoperative sexual rehabilitation rather than sildenafil, which requires functional neural tissue for effect (105). In contrast, Padma-Nathan et al. cited the neuroprotective and neuroregenerative properties of sildenafil as support for daily sildenafil usage as prophylaxis against ED (106). The conflicting options and lack of evidence-based medicine are a testament to the experimental nature of ED prophylaxis after RRP.

Erectile Dysfunction Therapeutic Modalities

Therapeutic modalities and efficacy for post-prostatectomy ED are outlined in Table 8.

Oral Therapy.   Oral therapy is considered to be the first-line agent of choice for ED after RRP. It has a high response rate, is minimally invasive, and has few side effects. The primary class of medications utilized is the phosphodiesterase-5 (PDE5) inhibitors. The PDE5 inhibitors promote erectile function by inhibiting the enzyme PDE5, resulting in increased levels of cyclic GMP (cGMP). cGMP promotes smooth muscle relaxation, allowing increased blood flow to the penis with resultant erections. The increased concentration of cGMP provides smooth muscle relaxation to achieve and maintain erections (107).

After the introduction of sildenafil as an effective treatment for ED in 1998, studies have examined the efficacy of sildenafil in the postprostatectomy cohort. In the sildenafil study group a 40% response rate was reported following prostatectomy, which was dependent on age and nerve preservation (107). Zippe et al. evaluated potency with sildenafil in patients who had undergone bilateral versus unilateral NSRRP using the International Index of erectile function (IIEF) questionnaire. 71.7% of patients undergoing bilateral NSRRP responded to therapy compared with 50% for unilateral NSRRP (108,109). Lowentritt et al. demonstrated similar results with better response to sildenafil with those undergoing bilateral NSRRP (110).

The use of sildenafil in patients who have had both nerves transected during RRP is debatable. Zippe et al. reported that 4 out of 26 (15.4%) undergoing non-NSRRP responded to sildenafil, suggesting that there is possible residual nerve tissue that is not identified during surgery (109). In contrast, Zagaja et al. demonstrated no improvement in sexual function in all 33 patients undergoing non-NSRRP (111).

TABLE 8   Medical and Surgical Therapies for Postprostatectomy Erectile Dysfunction

Therapeutic modality	Role	Efficacy % (ability to have sexual intercourse)	Comment
Oral phosphodiesterase-5 inhibitors	First line	70–80 (nerve-sparing prostatectomy) 0–15 (non-nerve-sparing prostatectomy)	Function of "nitric oxide-producing" penile nerves essential; sexual stimulation required
Intraurethral medications (penile suppository)	Second line	20–40	In-office instruction and titration recommended
Intracavernosal injections	Second line	85–90	In-office instruction and titration recommended
Vacuum constriction device	Second line	90–100	Basic instruction sufficient
Penile implants (malleable and inflatable)	Third line	95–100	Surgical expertise required

The timing of sildenafil after RRP is controversial with multiple studies reporting conflicting results. Zippe et al. showed that the duration from surgery (3–6, 6–12, or greater than 12 months) was not a statistically significant predictor of response to sildenafil (109). Conversely, in a similar study, Hong et al. reported increasing patient satisfaction over time with peak satisfaction at 18–24 months. Eight patients were included in this study, and their sexual satisfaction was assessed postoperatively with sildenafil using the Erectile Dysfunction Inventory of Treatment Satisfaction (EDITS) questionnaire. Only 26% of patients were satisfied with their erectile function using sildenafil during the first six months after surgery. Over time this satisfaction rate improved, peaking at 60% after 18 months postoperatively. This delayed effect of sildenafil is thought to be caused by neuropraxia in the immediate postoperative period which resolves with time (112).

Some studies advocate starting sildenafil almost immediately after surgery as a form of penile rehabilitation. The idea of penile rehabilitation is based on the premise that erections promote tissue oxygenation and suppress smooth muscle fibrosis. Therefore, increasing the number and duration of nocturnal erections should promote better overall erectile function. Fraiman et al. had previously shown that nocturnal tumescence is dramatically decreased after RRP (113).

Montorsi et al. later demonstrated that nocturnal erections increase in frequency and duration in those using sildenafil (114). These studies provide theoretical evidence for the use of sildenafil in the immediate postoperative period. Definitive long-term evidence that nightly PDE5 inhibitors are a statistically significant therapy in the recovery of erectile function after RRP is still lacking.

In addition to being an efficacious drug, the PDE5 inhibitors have a relatively benign side effect profile. The major side effects include, headache, flushing, gastroesophageal reflux, nasal congestion, and visual symptoms (abnormal-colored vision). Moreira et al. reviewed the side-effect profile of sildenafil. 31.6% of the participants experienced one or more side effects, though none of which caused participants to withdraw from the study. The most common adverse reaction was flushing at 30.8%. The study also demonstrated a dose-related increase in the severity of the side effects experienced (115). The main contraindication to PDE5 use is patients who are currently taking nitrates as the combination of the two drugs can lead to a dramatic decrease in systolic blood pressure (116).

Intracorporal Injection Therapy.   Intracorporal injection (ICI) therapy is a second-line agent for treatment of postprostatectomy ED given the invasive nature of the therapy and the need for visual acuity and manual dexterity to execute the procedure. Patients with the following afflictions are not considered candidates for ICI: hemoglobinopathies, bleeding disorders, Peyronie's disease, inability to tolerate periods of hypotension, or idiopathic priapism (116). The advantages of ICI include its use in patients who have failed oral therapy, who are take nitrates, or who desire a therapy with a more rapid onset of action. Another major advantage of ICI is that it can be utilized in patients without any cavernosal nerve function. Injection therapy works by releasing vasoactive chemicals directly into the corpora, allowing for vascular smooth muscle dilation and subsequent erection.

ICI was first presented to the urologic community in the early 1980s. The first drugs used for ICI were papaverine and phentolamine. Papaverine is a synthetic opium alkaloid, which acts primarily as a phosphodiesterase inhibitor, increasing the intracavernosal levels of cAMP and cGMP. The elevated levels of cyclic adenosine monophosphate (cAMP) and cGMP relax the vascular smooth muscle of the corpora, facilitating an erection. Virag reported the first use of papaverine as an ICI in 1982. It is a relatively inexpensive drug with priapism and fibrosis being the primary side effects, both of which are dose dependent. Barada and McKimmy reported up to 35% incidence of priapism and 33% incidence of corporal fibrosis (117). Phentolamine is a nonselective, competitive alpha-adrenergic blocker. By relaxing arterial and venous smooth muscle, it allows increased blood flow to the penis. Most of the side effects of phentolamine are related to its inhibition of serotonin receptors and subsequent histamine release. These include hypotension, tachycardia, nasal congestion, and dyspepsia. These two drugs have been combined to increase the spectrum of action and limit the dose of each agent necessary for erectile function. Multiple studies quote a 70% to 87% efficacy rate with the combination compared with about a 40% efficacy rate for a single agent (118,119). Additionally, the combination therapy allowed for lower doses of each agent, limiting the side effect profile. The studies reported a 1% to 23% incidence of priapism and 1.4% to 16% incidence of fibrosis.

Alprostadil (prostaglandin E1) was later introduced for intracavernosal therapy. Prostaglandin E1 is a vasodilator, relaxing the vascular smooth muscle of the corpora. Multiple studies examined the efficacy of papaverine and phentolamine versus alprostadil. Lee et al. reported a modest superiority of alprostadil to the combination therapy (120). Lui and Lin showed that 67% of participants achieved an erection with papaverine and phentolamine while 79% did with alprostadil (121). The most frequent side effects reported were pain with injection/erection, fibrosis, and hematomas. Priapism (1.3%) was less frequent than with papaverine and phentolamine (122).

In the early 1990s, a trimix of papaverine, phentolamine, and alprostadil was introduced. By combining three agents with different mechanisms of action, the goal was to decrease the doses needed to achieve similar results and limit the side effect profile, particularly pain with injection and erection. Studies by Bennett et al. reported satisfaction rates of 89% with 65% consistently using ICI. The incidence of priapism was similar to rates with alprostadil alone though many series reported decreased injection pain (123).

Intraurethral Suppository. The vascular communications between the corpora spongiosum and cavernosa provide another route by which to administer therapies for ED (124). The FDA approved intraurethral alprostadil in 1997, providing a noninjectable route to administering prostaglandins to the corpora. Once alprostadil is absorbed from the spongiosum to the cavernosa, it exhibits the same mechanism of action as with ICI. Patients use the medicated transurethral system for erection (MUSE) to deposit the alprostadil in the urethra for absorption.

In one study, intraurethral alprostadil was administered to 384 patients who had undergone a prostatectomy. Seventy percent of the participants were able to achieve an erection when alprostadil was administered in the office, of which 57% were able to achieve an erection with alprostadil at home. The most frequent complaint was urethral burning (18.3%). Additional side effects include penile pain and hypotension (125).

Vacuum Constriction Device. Vacuum constriction devices (VCD) were developed almost a century ago but have gained popularity in the past two decades. VCD is a relatively inexpensive and noninvasive treatment for ED, and it was the first-line therapy for postprostatectomy impotence until sildenafil was introduced on the market. VCD can be used by most ED patients. Those with hematologic/bleeding disorders, who are taking anticoagulant medications, who have a history of idiopathic priapism, who have decreased penile sensation, or who have Peyronie's disease are not candidates for this therapy. The major side effects of this therapy include penile pain, penile numbness, inability to ejaculate with preservation of orgasm, bruising, and skin breakdown (126,127).

The device consists of a plastic cylinder with a vacuum pump device that is used to create an erection by applying negative pressure to the penis and engorging the corpora with blood. Once the erection is achieved, a constrictive band is placed at the base of the penis for up to 30 minutes to maintain the erection. Color Doppler ultrasound reveals no arterial inflow to the penis once the constrictive band is secured, suggesting that the erection created with this device mimics an ischemic, low-flow priapism state (128).

Penile Prosthesis. Penile prosthesis was introduced as an alternative therapy to VCD for ED in the 1970s. This is the most invasive and one of the most expensive treatments for ED. Prostheses are the treatment of choice for those who have failed other less invasive therapies, particularly in the setting of a non-NSRRP, and those who are not candidates for other therapies, especially those with scarring from recurrent priapism or Peyronie's disease (96). There are few contraindications to prosthesis therapy. These include an inability to operate the device secondary to comorbidities and active infections, which increases the risk of seeding the device (129).

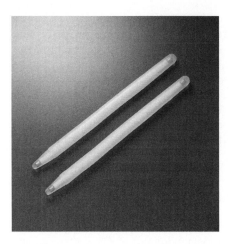

FIGURE 8   Photograph of malleable/semi-rigid penile prosthesis. *Source*: Courtesy of American Medical Systems, Minnetonka, Minnesota, U.S.A.

There are two primary prosthetic models—the malleable or semi-rigid and the inflatable. Each has advantages and disadvantages, and patient comorbidities, surgeon's expertise, cost, and patient preferences should all be evaluated prior to choosing a model. The malleable/semi-rigid prosthesis is less expensive, requires minimal manual dexterity, is less surgically challenging to place, and has a lower incidence of failure (Figs. 8 and 9). The major disadvantages include higher erosion risk, difficulty in concealing the implant, and an inability to change the erectile dimensions. The inflatable prosthesis is advantageous in that it is allows for rigidity and flaccidity, mimicking normal erectile function. Thus, it is easier to conceal and has a lower rate of erosion than the malleable device. The inflatable prosthesis is available in a two-piece and three-piece model. The two-piece model consists of inflatable corporal cylinders and a pump/reservoir mechanism in the scrotum (Figs. 10 and 11). This is the preferred inflatable device in patients in whom an abdominal reservoir (necessary in the three-piece

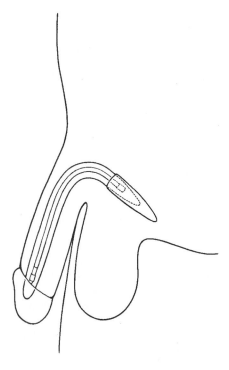

FIGURE 9   Line drawing of in situ placement of malleable/semi-rigid penile prosthesis. *Source*: Courtesy of American Medical Systems, Minnetonka, Minnesota, U.S.A.

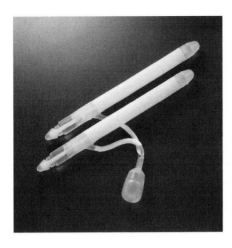

FIGURE 10 Photograph of two-piece inflatable penile prosthesis. *Source*: Courtesy of American Medical Systems, Minnetonka, Minnesota, U.S.A.

implant) is contraindicated. These patients include those with extensive abdominal and pelvic dissection such as pelvic exenteration, significant retroperitoneal scarring from the retropubic dissection of RRP, and those on peritoneal dialysis. When compared with the three-piece inflatable implant, the two-piece device has less adaptability in girth, length, and rigidity, resulting from a lower fluid volume in the reservoir (Figs. 12 and 13). Thus, the major advantage of the three-piece device is that it most closely mimics natural erections in its rigidity and flaccidity capabilities (129).

The primary complications of penile prostheses are infection, erosion, and mechanical failure. Infection has been reported in 0.6% to 8.9% of all prostheses placed (129,130). Patient with uncontrolled diabetes, frequent urinary tract infections, and spinal cord injuries are the most likely to become infected (131). Infection can be minimized by perioperative antibiotics,

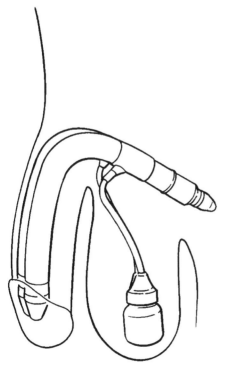

FIGURE 11 Line drawing of in situ placement of two-piece inflatable penile prosthesis. *Source*: Courtesy of American Medical Systems, Minnetonka, Minnesota, U.S.A.

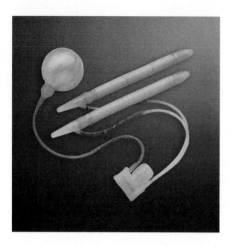

FIGURE 12   Photograph of three-piece inflatable penile prosthesis. *Source*: Courtesy of American Medical Systems, Minnetonka, Minnesota, U.S.A.

strict sterile technique, and avoidance of indwelling foreign bodies (early catheter removal). Erosion of the prosthesis can result from incorrect sizing, failure to deflate the device when not in use, aggressive corporal dilation, and infection. Mechanical failure requiring reoperation, particularly for leakage of fluid, defective pump, or breaks in the tubing, is reported in up to 5% of all prosthesis in place for 5 to 10 years (129,131).

Penile prosthesis is an efficacious and well-tolerated treatment for ED. Of all the therapeutic modalities, it was perceived to have the most drastic improvement in erectile function (102). There is an overall 85% patient satisfaction rate after implantation (132). Sexton et al. assessed satisfaction with various ED modalities by comparing the long-term use of ICI therapy and penile prostheses for the treatment of ED. After five years, only 41% of participants were still using the ICI compared with 70% who reported frequent use of the implant (133).

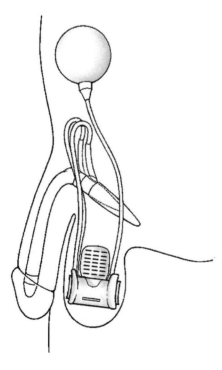

FIGURE 13   Line drawing of in situ placement of three-piece inflatable penile prosthesis. *Source*: Courtesy of American Medical Systems, Minnetonka, Minnesota, U.S.A.

REFERENCES

1. American Cancer Society. Cancer Facts and Figures 2007. Atlanta, GA: American Cancer Society, 2007.
2. Fowler FJ, Barry MJ, Lu-Yao G, et al. Patient reported complications and follow-up treatment after radical prostatectomy. The national Medicare experience: 1988–1990. Urology 1993; 42:622–628.
3. Walsh PC. Anatomic radical prostatectomy: evolution of the surgical technique. J Urol 1998; 160:2418–2424.
4. Igel TC, Barrett DM, Segura JW, et al. Perioperative and postoperative complications from bilateral pelvic lymphadenectomy and radical retropubic prostatectomy. J Urol 1987; 137:1189.
5. Leandri P, Rossignol G, Gautier JR, et al. Radical retropubic prostatectomy: morbidity and quality of life. Experience with 620 consecutive cases. J Urol 1992; 147:883.
6. Keetch DW, Andriole GL, Catalona WJ. Complications of radical retropubic prostatectomy. AUA Updates 1994; 13:46–51.
7. Hautmann RE, Sauter TW, Wenderoth UK. Radical retropubic prostatectomy: morbidity and urinary continence in 418 consecutive cases. Urology 1994; 43(suppl 2):47–51.
8. Zincke H, Bergstralh EJ, Blute ML, et al. Radical prostatectomy for clinically localized prostate cancer: long term results of 1143 patients from a single institution. J Clin Oncol 1994; 12: 2254–2263.
9. Lerner SE, Blute ML, Lieber MM, et al. Morbidity of contemporary radical retropubic prostatectomy for localized prostate cancer. Oncology 1995; 9:379.
10. Catalona WJ, Carvalhal GF, Mager DE, et al. Potency, continence and complication rates in 1,870 consecutive radical retropubic prostatectomies. J Urol 1999; 162:433–438.
11. Dash A, Dunn RL, Resh J, et al. Patient, surgeon, and treatment characteristics associated with homologous blood transfusion requirement during radical retropubic prostatectomy: multivariate nomogram to assist patient counseling. Urology 2004; 64:117–122.
12. Nuttall GA, Cragun MD, Hill DL, et al. Radical retropubic prostatectomy and blood transfusion. Mayo Clin Proc 2002; 77:1301–1305.
13. Walsh PC. Anatomic radical retropubic prostatectomy. In: Walsh PC, Retik AB, Vaughan ED, Wein AJ, eds. Campbell's Urology. Vol. 4. 8th ed. Philadelphia, PA: Saunders, 2002:3107–3129.
14. Goad JR, Eastham JA, Fitzgerald KB, et al. Radical retropubic prostatectomy: limited benefit of autologous blood donation. J Urol 1995; 154:2103.
15. Goodnough LT, Monk TG, Andriole GL. Erythropoietin therapy. N Engl J Med 1997; 336:933–938.
16. Monk TG, Goodnough LT, Brecher ME, et al. Acute normovolemic hemodilution can replace preoperative autologous blood donation as a stand of care for autologous blood procurement in radical prostatectomy. Anesth Analg 1997; 85:953–958.
17. Lepor H, Nieder AM, Ferrandino MN. Intraoperative and postoperative complications of radical retropubic prostatectomy in a consecutive series of 1,000 cases. J Urol 2001; 166:1729–1733.
18. Maffezzini M, Seveso M, Taverna G, et al. Evaluation of complications and results in a contemporary series of 300 consecutive radical retropubic prostatectomies with the anatomic approach at a single institution. Urology 2003; 61:982–986.
19. Augustin H, Hammerer P, Graefen M, et al. Intraoperative and perioperative morbidity of contemporary radical retropubic prostatectomy in a consecutive series of 1243 patients: results of a single center between 1999 and 2002. Eur Urol 2003; 43:113–118.
20. McLaren RH, Barrett DM, Zincke H. Rectal injury occurring at radical retropubic prostatectomy for prostate cancer: etiology and treatment. Urology 1993; 42:401.
21. Harpster LE, Rommel FM, Sieber PR, et al. The incidence and management of rectal injury associated with radical prostatectomy in a community based urology practice. J Urol 1995; 154:1435.
22. Borland RN, Walsh PC. The management of rectal injury during radical retropubic prostatectomy. J Urol 1992; 147:905.
23. Shekarriz B, Upadhyay J, Wood DP. Intraoperative, perioperative, and long-term complications of radical prostatectomy. Urol Clin North Am 2001; 28(3):639–653.
24. Taneja SS, deKernion JB. Complications of radical retropubic prostatectomy. In: Taneja SS, Smith RB, Ehrlich RM, eds. Complications of Urologic Surgery: Prevention and Management. 3rd ed. Philadelphia, PA: Saunders, 2001:411–418.
25. Ahearn GS, Bedlack RS, Price DT, et al. Transient lumbosacral polyradiculopathy after prostatectomy: association with spinal stenosis. Southern Med J 1999; 92:809–811.
26. Burnett AL, Brendler CB. Femoral neuropathy following major pelvic surgery: Etiology and prevention. J Urol 1994; 151:163–165.
27. Andriole GL, Smith DS, Rao G, et al. Early complications of contemporary anatomical radical retropubic prostatectomy. J Urol 1994; 152:1858–1860.
28. Hedican SP, Walsh PC. Postoperative bleeding following radical retropubic prostatectomy. J Urol 1994; 152:1181–1183.
29. Gheiler EL, Lovisolo JA, Tiguert E, et al. Results of a clinical care pathway for radical prostatectomy patients in a open hospital metaphysician system. Eur Urol 1999; 35:210.

30. Pepper RJ, Pati J, Kaisary AV. The incidence and treatment of lymphoceles after radical retropubic prostatectomy. BJU Int 2005; 95:772–775.
31. Solberg A, Angelsen A, Bergan U, et al. Frequency of lymphoceles after open and laparoscopic pelvic lymph node dissection in patients with prostate cancer. Scand J Urol Nephrol 2003; 37:218–221.
32. Yablon CM, Banner MP, Ramchandani P, et al. Complications of prostate cancer treatment: spectrum of imaging findings. Radiographics 2004; 24:181–194.
33. McDowell GC, Babaian RJ, Johnson DE. Management of symptomatic lymphocele via percutaneous drainage and sclerotherapy with tetracycline. Endourology 1991; 37:237–240.
34. Gilliland JD, Spies JB, Brown SB, et al. Lymphoceles: percutaneous treatment with povidone-iodine sclerosis. Radiology 1989; 171:227–229.
35. Sun GH, Fu YT, Wu CJ, et al. Povidone-iodine instillation for management of pelvic lymphocele after pelvic lymphadenectomy for staging prostate cancer. Arch Androl 2003; 49:463–466.
36. Kylmala T, Kaipia A, Matikainen M. Management of prolonged urinary leakage at the urethrovesical anastomosis. Urol Int 2005; 74:298–300.
37. Suyra BV, Provet J, Johanson KE, et al. Anastomotic strictures following radical prostatectomy: risk factors and management. J Urol 1990; 143:755–758.
38. Levy JB, Ramchandani P, Berlin JW, et al. Vesicourethral healing following radical prostatectomy: is it related to surgical approach? Urology 1994; 44:888–892.
39. Geary ES, Dendinger TE, Freiha FS, et al. Incontinence and vesical neck strictures following radical retropubic prostatectomy. Urology 1995; 45:1000–1006.
40. Popken G, Sommerkamp H, Schultze-Seemann W, et al. Anastomotic stricture after radical prostatectomy: incidence, findings, and treatment. Eur Urol 1998; 33:382–386.
41. Kao TC, Cruess DF, Garner D, et al. Multicenter patient self-reporting questionnaire on impotence, incontinence, and stricture after radical prostatectomy. J Urol 2000; 163:858–864.
42. Borboroglu PG, Sands JP, Roberts JL, et al. Risk factors for vesicourethral anastomotic stricture after radical prostatectomy. Urology 2000; 56:96–100.
43. Park R, Martin S, Goldberg JD, et al. Anastomotic strictures following radical prostatectomy: insights into incidence, effectiveness of intervention, effect on continence and factors predisposing to occurrence. Urology 2001; 57:742–746.
44. Besarani D, Amoroso P, Kirby R. Bladder neck contracture after radical retropubic prostatectomy. BJU Int 2004; 94:1245–1247.
45. Yurkanin JP, Dalkin BL, Cui H. Evaluation of cold knife urethrotomy for the treatment of anastomotic strictures after radical retropubic prostatectomy. J Urol 2001; 165:1545–1548.
46. Eastham JA, Scardino PT. Radical prostatectomy. In: Walsh PC, Retik AB, Vaughan ED, Wein AJ, eds. Campbell's Urology. Vol. 4. 8th ed. Philadelphia, PA: Saunders, 2002:3080–3106.
47. Veenema RJ, Gursel EO, Lattimer JK. Radical retropubic prostatectomy for cancer: a 20 year experience. J Urol 1977; 117:330–331.
48. Wessells H, Morey AF, McAnich JW. Obliterative vesicourethral strictures following radical prostatectomy for prostate cancer: reconstructive armamentarium. J Urol 1998; 160:1373–1375.
49. Carr LK, Webster GD. Endoscopic management of the obliterative anastomosis following radical prostatectomy. J Urol 1996; 156:70–72.
50. Steiner MS, Morton RA, Walsh PC. Impact of anatomical radical prostatectomy on urinary continence. J Urol 1991; 145:512–515.
51. Ramon J, Leandri P, Rossignol G, et al. Urinary continence following radical retropubic prostatectomy. Br J Urol 1993; 71:47–51.
52. Shelfo SW, Obek C, Soloway MS. Update on bladder neck preservation during radical retropubic prostatectomy: impact on pathologic outcome, anastomotic strictures, and continence. Urology 1998; 51:73–78.
53. Poon M, Ruckle H, Bamshad BR, et al. Radical retropubic prostatectomy: bladder neck preservation versus reconstruction. J Urol. 2000; 163:194–198.
54. Lepor H, Kaci L. The impact of open radical retropubic prostatectomy on continence and lower urinary tract symptoms: a prospective assessment using validated self-administered outcome instruments. J Urol 2004; 171:1216–1219.
55. Eastman JA, Kattan MW, Rogers E, et al. Risk factors for urinary incontinence after radical prostatectomy. J Urol 1996; 156:1707–1713.
56. Narayan P, Konety B, Aslam K, et al. Neuroanatomy of the external urethral sphincter: implications for urinary continence preservation during radical prostate surgery. J Urol 1995; 153:337–341.
57. Presti JC, Schmidt RA, Narayan PA, et al. Pathophysiology of urinary incontinence after radical prostatectomy. J Urol 1990; 143:975–978.
58. Wei JT, Montie JE. Comparison of patients' and physicians' ratings of urinary incontinence following radical prostatectomy. Semin Urol Oncol 2000; 18:76–80.
59. Walsh PC, Marschke P, Ricker D, et al. Patient reported urinary continence and sexual function after anatomic radical prostatectomy. Urology 2000; 55:58–61.
60. Harris J. Treatment of post prostatectomy urinary incontinence with behavioral methods. Clin Nurse Spec 1997; 11:159–166.

61. Peyromaure M, Ravery V, Boccon-Gibod L. The management of stress urinary incontinence after radical prostatectomy. BJU Int 2002; 90:155–161.

62. Chao R, Mayo ME. Incontinence after radical prostatectomy: detrusor or sphincter causes. J Urol 1995; 154:16–18.

63. Lowe BA. Comparison of bladder neck preservation to bladder neck resection in maintaining post prostatectomy urinary incontinence. Urology 1996; 48:889–893.

64. Poore RE, McCullough DL, Jarow JP. Puboprostatic ligament sparing improves urinary continence after radical retropubic prostatectomy. Urology 1995; 51:67–72.

65. Moore KN, Griffiths D, Hughton A. Urinary incontinence after radical prostatectomy: a randomized controlled trial comparing pelvic muscle exercises with or without electrical stimulation. BJU Int 1999; 83:57–65.

66. Meaglia JP, Joseph AC, Chang M, et al. Post-prostatectomy urinary incontinence: response to behavioral training. J Urol 1990; 144:674–676.

67. Burgia KL, Stutzman RE, Engel BT. Behavioral training for post-prostatectomy urinary incontinence. J Urol 1989; 141:303–306.

68. Franke JJ, Gilbert WB, Grier J, et al. Early post-prostatectomy pelvic floor biofeedback. J Urol 2000; 163:191–193.

69. Politano VA. Transurethral polytef injection for post-prostatectomy urinary incontinence. Br J Urol 1992; 69:26–28.

70. Malizia AA, Reiman HM, Myers RP, et al. Migration and granulomatous reaction after periurethral injection of polytef (Teflon). JAMA 1984; 251:3277–3281.

71. Griebling TL, Kreder KJ, Williams RD. Transurethral collagen injection for treatment of post prostatectomy urinary incontinence in men. Urology 1997; 49:907–912.

72. Santarosa RP, Blaivas JG. Periurethral injection of autologous fat for the treatment of sphincteric incontinence. J Urol 1994; 151:607–611.

73. Smith DN, Appell RA, Rackley RR, et al. Collagen injection therapy for post-prostatectomy incontinence. J Urology 1998; 160:364–367.

74. Klutke JJ, Subir C, Andriole GL, et al. Long-term results after antegrade collagen injection for stress urinary incontinence following radical retropubic prostatectomy. Urology 1999; 53:974–977.

75. Cummings JM, Boullier JA, Parra RO. Transurethral collagen injections in the therapy of post-radical prostatectomy stress incontinence. J Urol 1996; 155:1011–1013.

76. Klutke CG, Nadler RB, Tiemann D, et al. Early results with antegrade collagen injection for post-radical prostatectomy stress urinary incontinence. J Urol 1996; 156:1703–1706.

77. Schaeffer AJ, Clemens JQ, Ferrari M, et al. The male bulbourethral sling procedure for post-radical prostatectomy incontinence. J Urol 1998; 159:1510–1515.

78. Stern JA, Clemens JQ, Tiplitsky SI, et al. Long-term results of the bulbourethral sling procedure. J Urol 2005; 173:1654–1656.

79. Madjar S, Jacoby K, Gilberti C, et al. Bone anchored sling for the treatment of post-prostatectomy incontinence. J Urol 2001; 165:72–76.

80. Comiter CV. The male sling for stress urinary incontinence: a prospective study. J Urol 2002; 167:597–601.

81. Ullrich NF, Comiter CV. The male sling for stress urinary incontinence: 24-month followup with questionnaire based assessment. J Urol 2004; 173:207–209.

82. Castle EP, Andrews PE, Itano N, et al. The male sling for post-prostatectomy incontinence: mean followup of 18 months. J Urol 2005; 173:1657–1660.

83. Goldwasser B, Furlow WL, Barrett DM. The model AS 800 artificial urinary sphincter: Mayo clinic experience. J Urol 1987; 137:668–671.

84. Gundian JC, Barrett DM, Parulkar BG. Mayo clinic experience with use of the AMS800 artificial urinary sphincter for urinary incontinence following radical prostatectomy. J Urol 1989; 142:1459–1461.

85. Clemens JQ, Schuster TG, Konnak JW, et al. Revision rate after artificial urinary sphincter implantation for incontinence after radical prostatectomy: actuarial analysis. J Urol 2001; 166:1372–1375.

86. Gousse AE, Madjar S, Lambert MM, et al. Artificial urinary sphincter for post-radical prostatectomy urinary incontinence: long-term subjective results. J Urol 2001; 166:1755–1758.

87. Fulford SC, Sutton C, Bales G, et al. The fate of the "modern" artificial urinary sphincter with a follow-up of more than 10 years. Br J Urol 1997; 79:713–716.

88. Litwiller, SE, Kim KB, Fone PD, et al. Post-prostatectomy incontinence and the artificial urinary sphincter: a long-term study of patient satisfaction and criteria for success. J Urol 1996; 156:1975–1980.

89. Brito CG, Mulcahy JJ, Mitchell ME, et al. Use of a double cuff AMS800 urinary sphincter for severe stress urinary incontinence. J Urol 1993; 149:283–285.

90. Elliott DS, Barrett DM. Mayo clinic long-term analysis of the functional durability of the AMS 800 artificial urinary sphincter: a review of 323 cases. J Urol 1998; 159:1206–1208.

91. Jayadevappa R, Bloom BS, Fomberstein SC, et al. Health related quality of life and direct medical care cost in newly diagnosed younger men with prostate cancer. J Urol 2005; 174:1059–1064.

92. Walsh PC, Donker PJ. Impotence following radical prostatectomy; insight into etiology and prevention. J Urol 1982; 128:492.

93. Quinlan DM, Epstein JI, Carter BS, et al. Sexual function following radical prostatectomy: influence of preservation of neurovascular bundles. J Urol 1991; 145:998.

94. Stanford JL, Feng Z, Hamilton HS, et al. Urinary and sexual function after radical prostatectomy for clinically localized prostate cancer: the Prostate Cancer Outcomes Study. JAMA 2000; 283: 354–360.

95. Rabbani F, Stapleton AM, Kattan MW, et al. Factors predicting recovery of erections after radical prostatectomy. J Urol 2000; 164:1929–1934.

96. McCullough AR. Prevention and management of erectile dysfunction following radical prostatectomy. Urol Clin North Am 2001; 28:1–18.

97. Hollenbeck BK, Dunn RL, Wei JT, et al. Determinants of long-term sexual health outcome after radical prostatectomy measured by a validated instrument. J Urol 2003; 169:1453–1457.

98. Burnett AL. Erectile dysfunction following radical prostatectomy. JAMA 2005; 21:2648–2653.

99. Walsh PC. Radical prostatectomy for localized prostate cancer provides durable cancer control with excellent quality of life: a structured debate. J Urol 2000; 163:1802–1807.

100. Potosky AL, Harlan C, Stanford JL, et al. Prostate cancer practice patterns and quality of life: the Prostate Cancer Outcomes Study. J Natl Cancer Inst 1999; 91:1719.

101. Litwin MS, Melmed GY, Nakazon T. Life after radical prostatectomy: a longitudinal study. J Urol 2001; 166:587–592.

102. Stephenson, RA, Mori M, Hsieh YC, et al. Treatment of erectile dysfunction following therapy for clinically localized prostate cancer: patient reported use and outcomes from the Surveillance, Epidemiology, and End Results Prostate Cancer Outcomes Study. J Urol 2005; 174:646–650.

103. Klein LT, Miller MI, Buttyan R, et al. Apoptosis in the rat penis after penile denervation. J Urol 1997; 158:626–630.

104. Fraiman MC, Lepor H, McCullough AR. Changes in penile morphometrics in men with erectile dysfunction after nerve-sparing radical retropubic prostatectomy. Mol Urol 1999; 3:109–115.

105. Gontero P, Kirby R. Proerectile pharmacological prophylaxis following nerve-sparing radical prostatectomy (NSRP). Prostate Cancer Prostatic Dis 2004; 7:223–226.

106. Padma-Nathan H, McCullough A, Forest C. Erectile dysfunction secondary to nerve-sparing radical retropubic prostatectomy: comparative phosphodiesterase-5 inhibitor efficacy for therapy and novel prevention strategies. Curr Urol Rep 2004; 5:467–471.

107. Goldstein I, Lue T, Padma-Nathan H, et al. Oral sildenafil in the treatment of erectile dysfunction. N Engl J Med 1998; 339:59.

108. Zippe CD, Kedia AW, Kedia K, et al. Treatment of erectile dysfunction after radical prostatectomy with sildenafil citrate (Viagra). Urology 1998; 52:963–966.

109. Zippe CD, Jhaveri FM, Klein AE, et al. Role of Viagra after radical prostatectomy. Urology 2000; 55:241–245.

110. Lowentritt BH, Scardino PT, Miles BJ, et al. Sildenafil citrate after radical retropubic prostatectomy. J Urol 1999; 162:1614–1617.

111. Zagaja GP, Mhoon DA, Aikens JE, et al. Sildenafil in the treatment of erectile dysfunction after radical prostatectomy. Urology 2000; 56:631–634.

112. Hong EK, Lepor H, McCullough AR. Time dependent patient satisfaction with sildenafil for erectile dysfunction (ED) after nerve sparing radical retropubic prostatectomy. Int J Impot Res 1999; 11:15–22.

113. Fraiman MC, Lepor H, McCullough AR. Nocturnal penile tumescence activity in 81 patients presenting with erectile dysfunction after nerve sparing radical prostatectomy. J Urol 1999; 161:179.

114. Montorsi F, Maga T, Salonia A, et al. Sildenafil taken at bedtime significantly increases nocturnal erectile activity. Results of a prospective Rigiscan study. J Urol 2000; 164:148.

115. Moreira SG Jr, Brannigan RE, Spitz A, et al. Side-effect profile of sildenafil citrate (Viagra) in clinical practice. Urology 2000; 56:474–476.

116. Montorsi F, Salonia A, Deho F, et al. Pharmacological management of erectile dysfunction. BJU Int 2003; 91:446–454.

117. Barada JH, McKimmy RM. Vasoactive pharmacotherapy. In: Bennett AH, ed. Importence. Philadelphia, PA: Saunders, 1994:229.

118. Stief CG, Wetterauer U. Erectile responses to intracavernous papaverine and phentolamine: comparison of single and combined delivery. J Urol 1988; 140:1415.

119. Zorgniotti AW, Lefleur RS. Auto-injection of the corpus cavernosum with a vasoactive drug combination for vasculogenic impotence. J Urol 1985; 133:39.

120. Lee LM, Stevenson RW, Szasz G. Prostaglandin E1 versus phentolamine/papaverine for the treatment of erectile impotence: a double-blind comparison. J Urol 1989; 141:549.

121. Lui SM-C, Lin JS-N. Treatment of impotence: comparison between the efficacy and safety of intracavernous injection of papaverine plus phentolamine (Regitine) and prostaglandin E1. Int J Impot Res 1990; 1:147.

122. Linet OK, Neff LL. Intracavernous prostaglandin E1 in erectile dysfunction. Clin Invest 1994; 72:139.

123. Bennett AH, Carpenter AJ, Barada JH. An improved vasoactive drug combination for a pharmacological erection program. J Urol 1991; 146:1564.
124. Vardi Y, Saenz de Tejada I. Functional and radiologic evidence of vascular communication between the spongiosal and cavernosal compartments of the penis. Urology 1997; 49:749–752.
125. Costabile RA, Spevak M, Fishman IJ, et al. Efficacy and safety of transurethral alprostadil in patients with erectile dysfunction following radical prostatectomy. J Urol 1998; 160:1325–1328.
126. Broderick GA, Lue TF. Evaluation and nonsurgical management of erectile dysfunction and priapism. In: Walsh PC, Retik AB, Vaughan ED, et al. Campbell's Urology. Vol. 2. 8th ed. Philadelphia, PA: Saunders, 2002:1619–1671.
127. Jarow J. Non-oral therapy for erectile dysfunction. Phoenix5 2000.
128. Broderick GA, McGahan JP, Stone AR, et al. The hemodynamics of vacuum constriction erections: assessment by color Doppler ultrasound. J Urol 1992; 147:57–61.
129. Chang YJ, Santucci R. Penile prosthesis implantation. EMedicine; 2004.
130. Carson CC. Management of penile prosthesis infection. Probl Urol 1993; 7:368–380.
131. Lewis RW, Jordan GH. Surgery for erectile dysfunction. In: Walsh PC, Retik AB, Vaughan ED, Wein AJ, et al., eds. Campbell's Urology. Vol. 2. 8th ed. Philadelphia, PA: Saunders, 2002:1673–1709.
132. Goldstein I, Bertero EB, Kaufman JM, et al. Early experience with the first pre-connected 3-piece inflatable penile prosthesis: the Mentor Alpha 1. J Urol 1993; 150:1814–1818.
133. Sexton W, Benedict J, Jarow J. Comparison of long-term outcomes of penile prostheses and intracavernosal injection therapy. J Urol 1998; 159:811–815.

9 | Modern Complications of the Radical Perineal Prostatectomy

Jeffrey M. Holzbeierlein and J. Brantley Thrasher
Department of Urology, University of Kansas Medical Center, Kansas City, Kansas, U.S.A.

INTRODUCTION

Radical perineal prostatectomy (RPP) is the oldest approach for the removal of the prostate gland due to cancer. Unlike many of the newer forms of prostatectomy namely the robotic and laparoscopic prostatectomies, the complications of perineal prostatectomy are well described and relatively predictable. In light of this, the patient should be both properly counseled and prepared for RPP. With proper preparation, many of the complications during RPP can be either prevented or effectively treated during the procedure.

PREOPERATIVE PREPARATION

One of the unique aspects of RPP is the rather exaggerated positioning required for the procedure (Fig. 1). In morbidly obese patients this may increase the ventilatory pressures to >40 cmH$_2$O resulting in poor oxygenation and inability to perform the procedure. A simple test that demonstrates the patient's ability to tolerate the exaggerated lithotomy position from a respiratory standpoint involves having the patient lie supine on the examination table and bringing his knees to his chest. If the patient is able to tolerate this test, then he will likely tolerate the positioning required for RPP. At the beginning of the procedure when the patient is placed in the exaggerated lithotomy position, the surgeon should check with the anesthesiologist to make sure that the patient is able to be adequately ventilated at reasonable pressures. In our practice, carefully selected patients of even 400 to 500 pounds in weight have been successfully managed with RPP.

One of the indications for RPP is significant abdominal obesity. However, if the patient's body habitus is such that the base of the prostate gland is not palpable on digital rectal examination, this may make dissection during RPP very difficult due to the depth of the wound. Therefore, it is critical to perform a rectal examination prior to the procedure to make sure that the base of the prostate gland is palpable. Although we have successfully completed RPPs in this situation, as a rule of thumb this makes the perineal approach much more difficult. Furthermore, if the patient has a narrow distance between his ischial tuberosities such that the prostate gland is wider than this distance, then perineal removal of the prostate becomes very difficult. Prostate glands more than 100 g are difficult to remove through the perineal approach, and generally should not be selected for this approach or should be considered for downsizing using an luteinizing hormone-releasing hormone (LH-RH) agonist prior to removal.

It should be mentioned that those patients with high-risk features such as prostate-specific antigen (PSA) >20, Gleason score >8, or T3 disease have a higher probability of positive nodes. Pelvic lymph nodes are not routinely removed during RPP, since it requires a second incision. More recently, the lymph nodes have been removed laparoscopically and then the RPP performed. With the predictive models, such as the Partin tables and the Kattan nomogram, patients at low risk for pelvic lymph node metastases can be identified, thus allowing for the safe exclusion of a pelvic lymph node dissection. In addition, with the stage migration of prostate cancer seen in the United States, fewer and fewer patients have lymph node involvement.

COMPLICATIONS DURING SURGERY
Rectal Injury

Rectal injuries have been shown to occur more frequently in cases of RPP than in radical retropubic prostatectomy (RRP) (1). A recent study comparing RPP with RRP showed a

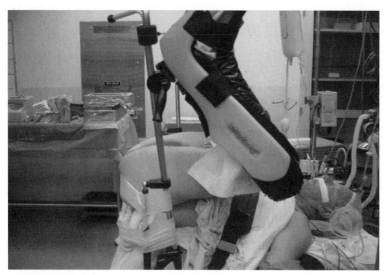

FIGURE 1   Exaggerated lithotomy position in yellow fin stirrups.

statistically significant increase in rectal injuries in the perineal compared to the retropubic approach (2). The experience of the surgeon plays a role in the frequency of rectal injuries, with very low rectal injury rates being reported by surgeons experienced in RPP (3). Rectal injuries that usually occur as the rectourethralis is divided or as the plane of dissection changes from vertical to horizontal just before the apex of the prostate. Moreover, if the posterior retractor is pulled down too vigorously this may also lead to a rectal laceration. Rectal injuries are best prevented by placing a finger in the rectum during the division of the rectourethralis to help identify the rectum. Careful padding of the rectum and paying attention to the tension on the retractor (Thompson retractor) (Fig. 2) can minimize the risk of a retractor-induced rectal injury. In our own series of approximately 200 RPPs, we have experienced seven cases of (3.5%) rectal injuries, with all except one being managed by primary closure without sequelae.

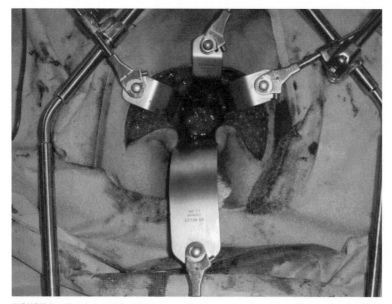

FIGURE 2   Thompson retractor.

Management of Rectal Injuries

Management of rectal injuries requires several things. First is adequate preparation of the bowel prior to surgery. At our institution on the day prior to surgery, patients are asked to consume only clear liquids and undergo a full mechanical and antibiotic preparation. The second most important aspect is the recognition of the rectal injury. Patients who have unrecognized rectal injuries suffer the greatest consequences of this complication. We evaluate for possible rectal injury by several means. First, a finger is placed in the rectum and the integrity of the rectal wall inspected both by tactile and visual inspection. Furthermore, a clean glove is placed and a finger inserted in the rectum. If any blood is noted on the finger then a vigilant search for a rectal injury is performed with a high index of suspicion. If any doubt persists, then the rectum is irrigated by using a bulb syringe with betadine to look for any accumulation in the wound. Rectal injuries when recognized and in patients properly prepared are relatively easily treated. The rectal injury is typically closed in two layers, with absorbable suture (we prefer 3-O braided absorbable polyglactin suture) for the first layer followed by 3-O silk sutures in a Lembert fashion for the second layer. The surgical field is then copiously irrigated with 1 L of antibiotics and then a two-finger anal dilation performed to reduce sphincter tone. Broad-spectrum antibiotics are given for 48 hours and a low-residue diet encouraged for five days postoperatively.

Bleeding

Blood loss during RPP is usually minimal. In essentially all comparative studies done between RPP and RRP, the most significant difference across all series is the decreased blood loss associated with RPP. If blood loss does occur it usually occurs in one of two areas. First, in the initial plane of dissection if the surgeon is too anterior, the perineal muscles, bulb of the penis or corporal bodies may be dissected. This may result in a significant amount of blood oozing out that obscures vision. The best way to avoid this is to stay underneath the external anal sphincter and keep the dissection to the anterior wall of the rectum. The second is during the dissection of the anterolateral fascia (which contains the dorsal venous complex) of the anterior portion of the prostate. If the dissection is too anterior the surgeon may encounter the dorsal venous complex (Santorini's plexus), which may result in significant bleeding. If this is encountered, usually the best management practice is to place a laparotomy tape anteriorly on the venous complex and put ventral pressure on it by using either a retractor held by an assistant or Thompson retractor until the prostate is removed. In most cases when the pack and retractor are removed the bleeding stops. If there is continued bleeding it is usually easily ligated with a suture. We prefer using a 3-O chromic suture on UR-6 needles, using a Haney needle driver to suture ligate any bleeding vessels.

Ureteral Injuries

As with all forms of radical prostatectomy, the division of the bladder neck too proximally may result in injury to the ureter or ureteral orifice. This is particularly true for the patient with a large intravesical component of a median lobe. Identification of the ureteral orifices by the administration of indigo carmine, methylene blue, or placement of 5 Fr feeding tubes is helpful in preventing ureteral injury particularly in patients with large median lobes. Moreover, during RPP, it is important when dissecting in the plane between the bladder and prostate that the plane of the dissection of the scissors to the bladder be at a right angle. We have found that the use of Thorek scissors facilitates this. Careful attention to close a large bladder neck defect is also necessary in order to avoid injuring a ureter. Again identification of the ureters by one of the above means is usually effective in reducing this complication. If a ureteral injury occurs and is recognized at the time of RPP, a ureteroneocystotomy may be performed through the perineal incision, or a double-J ureteral stent may be placed in the ureter and the bladder mucosa and ureteral orifice inverted by incorporating more seromuscular tissue during the bladder neck reconstruction. The stents are removed six weeks postoperatively using flexible cystoscopy.

EARLY POSTOPERATIVE COMPLICATIONS
Lower Extremity Neuropraxia

A unique morbidity to RPP is lower extremity neuropraxia. The etiology is presumed to be undue pressure on the peroneal nerve due to positioning. Price et al. reported that 43 of 111 patients (38.7%) undergoing RPP experienced some degree of lower extremity neuropraxia (4). Fortunately, these cases of neuropraxia were of short duration (two to three days) and were resolved in all cases. We also experienced this problem at our institution until we began using the Yellofins Stirrups™ and subsequently we have not seen this complication again. This is due to the fact that the stirrups support the entire leg from the calf down to the foot in a boot-like support. This minimizes any pressure on the fibular head and ankle, which prevents the neuropraxia. Candy cane stirrups will also prevent the neuropraxia, but in our experience are too unstable.

Urinary Leak

Urinary leak after perineal prostatectomy is an uncommon complication. This is due to the direct visualization of the urethrovesical anastomosis and the tying of these sutures under direct vision. A penrose drain usually diverts the urine and prevents the development of a sub-cutaneous fluid collection, which may become infected. As in the retropubic approach, traction on the catheter will bring the bladder down to the urethra typically resulting in sealing of the leak within 24 hours. Prolonged urinary drainage more than two to three days should be a cause for concern. Possibilities include an unrecognized ureteral injury or a disruption of the anastomosis. Treatment should be based on the recognized cause of the leak, with placement of a Foley catheter and percutaneous nephrostomy tubes if necessary.

Wound Problems

Wound problems, particularly infection, after RPP are distinctly uncommon probably due to the dependent drainage of the wound, which does not usually allow fluid to accumulate. The penrose drain is typically removed postoperatively on day 1 unless a significant amount of drainage on the perineal dressing is noted. Patients are advised to clean the area by showering. Postoperative antibiotics are given until catheter removal. Patients do not typically complain of significant pain and are usually easily managed by oral analgesics. It is important when closing the skin, to leave the tails of the 2-O chromic sutures approximately 2 inches long (Fig. 3). This minimizes the cut ends from poking the patient and increasing patient discomfort. It is also important to avoid constipation by keeping patients on a stool softener and more aggressive measures as necessary.

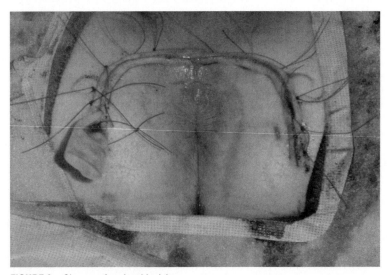

FIGURE 3   Closure of perineal incision.

LATE COMPLICATIONS
Rectovesical or Rectourethral Fistula

Most late rectovesical fistulas are the result of an unrecognized rectal injury at the time of RPP. Fortunately, this significant side effect is very uncommon. This complication may be more problematic and common in the patient who has had pelvic irradiation prior to RPP. Conservative attempts consisting of bowel rest and urinary diversion through a catheter may be successful particularly in the nonirradiated patient. For patients who fail conservative measures, closure of the fistula and fecal diversion is usually required.

Fecal Incontinence

Fecal incontinence after radical prostatectomy is a particular complication that was not reported until relatively recently. In 1998, Bishoff et al. reported a significant rate of fecal incontinence in patients after prostatectomy (5). Patients were mailed a questionnaire asking about both fecal and urinary incontinence. From these questionnaires, 3%, 9%, 3%, and 16% reported daily, weekly, monthly, or less than monthly fecal incontinence, respectively, after RPP. This was less although still present in the RRP group who reported rates of 2%, 5%, 3%, and 8% daily, weekly, monthly, or less than monthly fecal incontinence, respectively. This experience is different from the authors' experience as well as the experience of other experienced surgeons employing RPP. Furthermore, this study did not employ a validated quality of life questionnaire for prostate cancer, once again calling into question the validity of the data. A review of the cancer of the prostate strategic urologic research endeavor (CaPSURE) database, with an emphasis on bowel dysfunction after RRP or RPP found no difference between the two procedures. Furthermore, for those patients who had significant bowel bother or bowel dysfunction after radical prostatectomy, most improved greatly within the immediate postoperative period. Another study examining quality of life after one year found no difference in bowel function between RRP and RPP (2).

BLADDER NECK CONTRACTURE

Most series examining the rates of bladder neck contractures show no difference between RRP and RPP. Two studies, one by Haab et al. (6) and one by Parra (7), found a slightly higher incidence in the RRP group versus the RPP group (4% for RRP vs. 2% for RPP). Fortunately, most bladder neck contractures are easily treated by passage of a sound, or filiforms and followers, without a significant impact on continence. More aggressive measures such as direct visual internal urethrotomy are occasionally required but may result in significant incontinence.

CONCLUSIONS

RPP remains a viable option for the treatment of localized prostate cancer. Its advantages include decreases in pain, blood loss, and convalescence, which are, the same arguments currently being made in favor of laparoscopic prostatectomy. In addition, it is the optimal approach for many obese patients, patients with prior pelvic surgery, or those with prior pelvic radiation. Proper patient selection, preparation, and counseling are critical to the success of the procedure and the minimization of complications. It cannot be stressed enough that a detailed understanding of the perineal anatomy as well as surgeon experience are important factors in keeping complications minimal. Most complications when recognized can be treated simply and effectively and only rarely result in prolonged debilitation.

REFERENCES

1. Lassen PM, Kearse WS Jr. Rectal injuries during radical perineal prostatectomy. Urology 1995; 45:266–279.
2. Lance RS, Freidrichs PA, Kane C, et al. A comparison of radical retropubic with perineal prostatectomy for localized prostate cancer within the uniformed services urology research group. BJU Int 2001; 87:61–65.

3. Paulsen DF. Impact of radical prostatectomy in the management of clinically localized disease. J Urol 1994; 152:1826–1830.
4. Price DT, Vieweg J, Roland F, et al. Transient lower extremity neuropraxia associated with radical perineal prostatectomy: a complication of the exaggerated lithotomy position. J Urol 1998; 160:1376–1378.
5. Bishoff JT, Motley G, Optenberg SA, et al. Incidence of fecal and urinary incontinence following radical perineal and retropubic prostatectomy in a national population. J Urol 1998; 160:454–458.
6. Haab F, Boccon-Gibbod L, Delmas V, Boccon-Gibod L, Toublanc M. Perineal versus retropubic radical prostatectomy for T1, T2 prostate cancer. Br J Urol 1994; 74:626–629.
7. Parra RO. Analysis of an experience with 500 radical perineal prostatectomies in localized prostate cancer. J Urol 1997; 158:1470–1475.

10 | Complications of Open Prostate Surgery

Stephen S. Connolly
Department of Urology, Mater Misericordiae Hospital, University College, Dublin, Ireland

John M. Fitzpatrick
Academic Department of Surgery, Mater Misericordiae Hospital and University College, Dublin, Ireland

INTRODUCTION

Open prostate surgery is the oldest definitive surgical therapy for benign prostatic hyperplasia (BPH). From its infancy it became rapidly established in the early part of the 20th century and reached the peak of its popularity by the middle of the century. Transurethral surgery was perceived as less invasive and rose to prominence in the United States from the 1950s. It quickly displaced open surgery and became the gold-standard surgical therapy for the majority of men requiring prostatectomy for BPH in the later part of the century. The additional development of alternative medical therapies for BPH has resulted in further reduction in the number of men undergoing open surgery to the relatively low levels seen today.

Despite this move toward the less invasive option, open prostatectomy for benign obstructing disease remains very necessary in select circumstances. Recent studies have shown that open prostatectomy currently continues to comprise 3% and 14% of surgeries for BPH in the United States and France, respectively (1,2). One contemporary multi-center Italian series found open prostatectomy to account for 32% of all surgical treatment for BPH (3). Logically, one could assume this percentage to be higher in less technologically advanced countries. In this context, a thorough understanding of the complications of the surgery remains essential for all practicing urologists.

CHOICE OF OPEN SURGERY

While remaining at the discretion of the individual urologist, open prostatectomy is most commonly reserved to situations where the patient is unsuitable for transurethral prostatectomy, most commonly with a large gland volume. Arbitrarily a volume greater than 100 cc, "large" may be considered any volume that would require a transurethral resection time in excess of 60 minutes. Concomitant pathology requiring open surgery, such as bladder calculi, diverticula, or even inguinal hernia, and conditions that prevent adequate lithotomy positioning for transurethral surgery may also make open surgery preferable. Previous urethral stricture disease or complex urethroplasty of any form may also be considered a relative indication for the avoidance of transurethral surgery.

The technique of open prostatectomy can be broadly categorized into transvesical or retropubic, each described in turn by notable Irish surgeons. Peter Freyer, originally from County Galway, described a series of four cases managed by a transvesical, suprapubic approach while working in St. Peters Hospital in London in 1901 (4). This method may be preferential for procedures involving the bladder, such as concomitant diverticulectomy or removal of stones. The procedure has been well described and involves opening the bladder above the level of the prostate and enucleating the adenoma after a sharp incision of the overlying bladder mucosa. Alternatively, retropubic prostatectomy involves dissection of the space of Retzius with transverse prostatic capsulotomy to facilitate complete enucleation of the adenoma. This approach was described by Terence Millin, native of County Down, when he was working in London in 1945, and provided an anatomic basis for the radical retropubic prostatectomy described by Walsh later (5,6).

MORTALITY DATA AND OVERVIEW OF STUDIES

The vast majority of data used to compare the outcome of open prostatectomy with transurethral resection of the prostate (TURP) is retrospective and must be considered to be of poor quality. There is an appreciable lack of randomized trials comparing TURP with open surgery, and control for prostate size and comorbidity is notably absent although likely to be a very significant factor in predicting complications, such as postoperative hemorrhage and mortality. A number of reports over the past two decades have specifically addressed the mortality rates associated with open prostatectomy in comparison with transurethral surgery, albeit in a retrospective fashion (7–10). Despite the more invasive aspect of open surgery, interestingly all such series have suggested that it is marginally beneficial in terms of long-term survival. Critics have suggested that such studies are deeply flawed by a retrospective bias, which failed to identify that the less invasive option may logically have been preferred for those men with greater co-morbidities (11). The largest series of over 65,000 men in Scotland found an increased risk of late mortality after TURP, seemingly attributable to increased deaths from respiratory conditions and cancer, but confusingly not due to ischemic heart disease or cardiovascular problems (7). In a further study of over 40,000 men undergoing prostatectomy in Denmark, Canada, and England, analysis to support the previous finding was found, with relative risks for mortality and myocardial infarction of 1.45 and 2.5, respectively, following TURP (8). This multinational series further highlighted the increased risk of retreatment in men undergoing TURP (17% vs. 7% with eight years of follow-up) and implied that this fact may contribute to the apparent negative impact on outcome (9). By contrast, smaller series directly examining the incidence of myocardial infarction found that no increased risk could be specifically attributed to the type of prostatectomy, however, the rate of myocardial infarction of 6% far exceeded what one would expect to see in the general population controlled for age ($\approx$2.5%) (10). Preoperative co-morbidity may be the key aspect in relation to an increased mortality risk postprostatectomy, but this is exceedingly difficult to adequately control in a retrospective fashion (12–14).

An overview of the principal complications of open prostatectomy is presented in Table 1, and large-scale transurethral prostatectomy series of Mebust et al. (15) and Horninger et al. (16) are included for comparison. Varkarakis et al. reported on 232 men undergoing open transvesical prostatectomy in Athens, Greece. All men with prostate cancer or resection weight less than 75 g were excluded from analysis in an attempt to present useful data applicable to modern practice (17). The largest contemporary series has been reported by Serretta et al. is of 1804 men in the Sicily and Calbria regions of Italy (3). The retropubic approach was undertaken in only 202 (11.2%) men, and mean prostate volume was preoperatively calculated to be 75 cc although the weight of the resected mass was not reported. A further Italian series by Mearini et al. reported a survey of the combined experience of 47 urology units in north Italy with comparison to their unit with 342 cases in Perrugia (18). Suprapubic prostatectomy (a modification of the Hryntschak prostatectomy) was again most popular, and the weight of tissue removed was not reported (19). From developing nations, Condie et al. reported 200 consecutive suprapubic prostatectomies in a rural community in Pakistan over a three-year period (20). Data in this series were limited by social and financial factors, and minimal follow-up with almost no routine pathological analysis further limits the value of this series. Meier et al. reported 240 men undergoing suprapubic prostatectomy, all having presented with acute urinary retention in sub-Saharan Africa (21). With a mean weight of 61 g of the resected mass, Meier et al. reported low morbidity and mortality comparing very favorably with other reports despite the lack of technology and resources.

EARLY COMPLICATIONS

Anesthetic complications for all forms of surgery have reduced steadily over the past decades as advances in anesthetic technology and therapeutics are being furthered. Regional anesthesia is as possible for open prostatectomy as for TURP, however, avoidance of irrigation and thus TUR syndromes makes the choice of anesthesia for the simple open procedure less important.

Hemorrhage remains a dominant early complication in all types of prostate surgery, open or transurethral. Mebust et al. showed that intraoperative hemorrhage during TURP was more common with larger glands, but prospective randomization of large glands to different surgical

TABLE 1 Percentage Complications of Open and Transurethral Prostatectomy in Contemporary Series

Series	Mortality	Blood transfusion	Persistent incontinence	Bladder neck stricture	Urethral/meatal stricture	Need for re-treatment
Open surgery						
Varakakis et al. (17) (n = 232)	0	6.8	n/r	3.3	1.8	3.9
Condie et al. (20) (n = 200)	1	1	0.5	1	n/r	n/r
Mearini et al. (18) (n = 380)	0.5	26.5	1.7	3.5	2	n/r
Serretta et al. (3) (n = 1804)	0.06	8.2	1.2	4.8		3.6
Meier et al. (21) (n = 240)	0	4.6	0.4	1.7	n/r	n/r
Transurethral surgery						
Mebust et al. (15) (n = 3885)	0.2	6.4	n/r	n/r	n/r	n/r
Horninger et al. (16) (n = 1211)	0	4.2	0	1.9	3.7	2.5

Abbreviation: n/r, not reported.

techniques has never been performed (15). Various intraoperative steps to optimize vascular control of Santorinis' plexus during open prostatectomy have been detailed by numerous authors and may include dorsal venous complex control, ligation of the inferior vesical pedicles, and temporary occlusion of the internal iliac arteries (22,23). The concept of minimizing hemorrhage through use of an absorbable bladder neck suture was popularized after modification by Hryntschak, and has been subsequently revised (19). The use of a purse-string suture at the bladder neck was later labeled as the modified Denis technique (24,25). An extracapsular prostatectomy performed by applying lateral capsular transfixing sutures, and even a combined suprapubic–retropubic prostatectomy has been proposed with the advantage of maximizing exposure and hemostasis (26,27). Postoperative hemorrhage may be encountered despite the best precautions and may not respond to the initial steps of bed-side bladder irrigation. Innovative measures such as simple digital rectal pressure have been anecdotally described (28). Historically, medical therapies such as epsilon amino-caproic acid and arteriographic embolization procedures have been examined, but never accepted (29,30). Severe persistent postoperative hemorrhage may necessitate a return to the operating room. Although packing of the pelvis is a well-described maneuver for uncontrollable ongoing hemorrhage, this should only very rarely be required and truly reflects the most severe end of the spectrum of hemorrhage.

Wound-related problems are intrinsic to all open surgery. In general, wound-related problems are reported in less than 5% of men undergoing open prostatectomy (17,21). The reduced morbidity, however, associated with avoiding any skin incision remains an undisputable advantage of TUR surgery and remains a major factor for physician and patient preference for the less invasive surgery. Urinary tract infection complicating prostatectomy has been difficult to clearly define, however, it is clear that the rare deaths occurring with prostatectomy most commonly follow sepsis (15). Perioperative administration of antibiotics has been reported to be routine in 60% of those audited as part of a British national study by Emberton et al. (31). Of the series presented in Table 1, only Varkarakis et al. (17) and Meier et al. (21) reported data on wound problems, 4.3% and 2.9%, respectively, with the latter author also reporting epididymitis in 1.3%. Similarly, the TURP series of Mebust et al. (15) and Horninger et al. (16) reported urinary tract infections in 2.9% and 2.4%, respectively. The highest risk of infection continues to be in those men with preoperative catheterization or positive urine cultures, however, no universally accepted regime for antibiotic administration has yet been devised.

Hospitalization may be prolonged for open surgery when compared with transurethral surgery. Emberton et al.'s audit of TURPs in Britain showed a mean postoperative length of stay of 5.2 days, while Mebust et al. found that 80% were discharged by postoperative day 5 (15,31). By contrast, open prostatectomy series (3,17,21) report mean hospitalization as six, seven, and nine days, respectively, but again no control for prostate size or comorbidity is provided.

DELAYED PROBLEMS

Incontinence is not uncommon in the age category of men undergoing prostatectomy, and continence status prior to any prostatectomy should always be recorded. Persistent incontinence following open prostatectomy is uncommon and at worst an infrequent complication. Careful resection of apical tissue remains the principal operative means of avoiding damage to the rhabdosphincter and during open surgery, sharp incision of apical tissue under direct vision may reduce risk of damage. Significant bladder overactivity may precede TURP and men with preoperative incontinence or features raising a doubt over the presence of obstruction should have preoperative urodynamic analyses of urodynamics to clarify the issue. All men with persistent problematic postprostatectomy incontinence should be evaluated by urodynamic analyses and endoscopic examination of their lower urinary tract.

Urodynamic investigation of postprostatectomy incontinence in 68 men has shown that sphincter damage plays a role in 69% of men with incontinence, but is the sole factor in only 27% (32). The same study, in which 31% of prostatectomies were open, found bladder dysfunction (detrusor instability) to be a factor in 66%, with the most common cause of incontinence being a combination of sphincter dysfunction and detrusor instability in 41% (28 men). Residual obstruction was documented in 15% and a normal micturating videocystography and synchronous pressure-flow measurements study was found in 4% of men complaining of postprostatectomy incontinence. Management is dictated by the underlying cause. Detrusor overactivity may be treated appropriately with anticholinergic therapy. Conservative management for sphincter damage may include nothing other than simple lifestyle changes, such as absorbent undergarments, or alternatively pelvic floor muscle training, biofeedback techniques, compression devices such as penile clamps, or a combination of methods (33). Duloxetine now provides a medical alternative for sphincter incompetence, but no reports of its efficacy in this setting have yet made reported (34). Collagen injection and male slings have also been described, and may provide alternatives to insertion of an artificial urethral sphincter for severely problematic cases (35–39).

Urethral stricture disease is probably the most common long-term complication of prostatectomy and can occur following either an open or transurethral procedure, however, no proper studies have been performed to allow a direct comparison. The multiple series presented in Table 1 show bladder neck contracture or urethral stricture to be uncommon following open prostatectomy, but to occur in a small definite number approximating 5%. The urethral instrumentation involved in transurethral surgery logically may make stricture disease more common. The largest review of TURP-related urethral stricture disease was undertaken by Lentz et al. retrospectively reporting 2223 TURPs (40). They reported a 6.3% incidence of new strictures, unrelated to race, presence of prostate carcinoma, preoperative urine infection, length of postoperative catheterization, or experience of the surgeon, although resident staff did have higher levels of meatal and postnavicular strictures. The association of larger postoperative catheters (26F) with strictures was not statistically significant. Jorgensen et al. reviewed 417 TURPs with a high incidence of urethral stricture (9%), and found that the only factor to correlate with postoperative stricture was the presence of an indwelling catheter within the month prior to surgery (41). Hammarsten et al. expanded on this by randomizing 205 men to urethral or suprapubic catheterization following TURP and found that postoperative transurethral catheter was perhaps the most important factor in stricture formation (42). A number of studies have randomized men to internal urethrotomy (Otis urethrotome) prior to TURP and have demonstrated significant benefit in reducing the incidence of stricture (43,44). Resection via perineal urethrostomy has been suggested as a means of avoidance, but has never been widely accepted (45). Bladder neck incision is a relatively simple procedure for contracture located at the site of the prostatectomy, but does carry increased risks in this often aging population. Meatotomy, urethral dilatation, or internal urethrotomy each provide an alternative to more formal urethroplasty, based on the type of stricture encountered. However, many of these strictures are long and are prone to recurrence. These affected patients may be best served by early formal repair to maximize chances of success.

Erectile dysfunction is common in the group of older men most commonly undergoing this surgery and all postprostatectomy problems can clearly not be attributed automatically to the surgery. Retrograde ejaculation is inherently associated with prostatectomy due to the anatomic disruption of the bladder neck that occurs with prostatectomy of either form, and adequate preoperative counseling regarding this fact makes patient dissatisfaction unlikely. Given our now detailed understanding of the anatomy of the neurovascular bundles, it is clear that following correct enucleation of the prostate adenoma during open prostatectomy, impotence directly related to the prostatectomy should be a rare occurrence (6). Libman et al. reviewed the topic of prostatectomy and sexual function, and found that the incidence of impotence post-prostatectomy increases with age (46). Additionally, no major differences between transurethral, retropubic, or suprapubic prostatectomy were found, but radical and perineal prostatectomies did have worse outcome. Prospective studies evaluating the specific impact of TURP on potency have been performed. One such study found that 88% of men with erectile function sufficient for intercourse retained the capability post-TURP compared with 97% following a more general surgical procedure (47). No prospective randomized comparative studies in relation to open prostatectomy have been performed. There have been suggestions that transmitted heat may damage the neurovascular structures responsible for potency and this may be related to the copious use of diathermy during TURP (48). Other studies have further highlighted the occurrence of small nerve fiber damage following TURP, supporting the suggestion that neurogenic postoperative erectile dysfunction is in fact a very real issue post-TURP, but may be less of an issue following open prostatectomy (49).

Re-treatment rates following both open and transurethral prostatectomy are comparable with each being less than 5%. Lack of adequate length of follow-up remains the most difficult obstacle to satisfactory reporting of re-treatment rates. Emberton et al.'s national audit reported 12% of prostatectomies as being a second or subsequent procedure. Unsurprisingly less tissue was resected endoscopically during this revision procedure than during the first operation (31). Horninger et al. reported that 2.5% required re-operation within three years (16). Revision rates for both open and transurethral surgery should be low, but data to compare are again deficient.

SUMMARY

No prospective randomized data has ever permitted a direct comparison of open prostatectomy with TURP, and the level of bias produced by patient selection and prostate size remains unquantifiable by the independent critic. The few contemporary series analyzing open prostatectomy in developed nations do so retrospectively and with relatively small volume analysis, however, there is currently only very scant data to suggest any increased morbidity or mortality with the open surgical option when compared with transurethral surgery. Open prostatectomy continues to constitute a very reasonable treatment strategy for men with large-volume prostates and those unsuited for transurethral surgery. This surgery should be considered safe, with complication rates comparable to the transurethral alternative. Detailed knowledge of the indications, techniques, and complications should be acquired by all trained urologists.

REFERENCES

1. Bruskewitz R. Management of symptomatic BPH in the US: who is treated and how? Eur Urol 1999; 36:7–13.
2. Lukacs B. Management of symptomatic BPH in France: who is treated and how? Eur Urol 1999; 36:14–20.
3. Serretta V, Morgia G, Fondacaro L, et al. Open prostatectomy for benign prostatic enlargement in southern Europe in the late 1990s: a contemporary series of 1800 interventions. Urology 2002; 60:623–627.
4. Freyer P. Suprapubic prostatectomy. Report of 4 cases. BMJ 1901.
5. Millin T. Retropubic prostatectomy: new extravesical technique. Report on 20 cases. Lancet 1945; 2:693–696.
6. Walsh PC, Donker PJ. Impotence following radical prostatectomy: insight into aetiology and prevention. J Urol 1982; 128:492–497.
7. Hargreave TB, Heynes CF, Kendrick SW, et al. Mortality after transurethral and open prostatectomy in Scotland. BJU Int 1996; 77:547–553.
8. Roos NP, Wennberg JE, Malenka DJ, et al. Mortality and reoperation after open and transurethral resection of the prostate for benign prostatic hyperplasia. N Engl J Med 1989; 320:1120–1124.
9. Roos NP, Ramsey EW. A population-based study of prostatectomy: outcome associated with differing surgical approaches. J Urol 1987; 137:1184–1188.
10. Shalev M, Richter S, Kessler O, et al. Long-term incidence of acute myocardial infarction after open and transurethral resection of the prostate for benign prostatic hyperplasia. J Urol 1999; 161:491–493.

11. Klotz L. Re: Mortality and reoperation after prostatectomy for benign prostatic hyperplasia. Letter to the Editor. N Engl J Med 1989; 321:1122–1123.

12. Crowley AR, Horowitz M, Chan E, Macchia RJ. Transurethral resection of the prostate versus open prostatectomy: long term mortality comparison. J Urol 1995; 153:695–697.

13. Concato J, Horwitz RI, Feinstein AR, et al. Problems of comorbidity in mortality after prostatectomy. JAMA 1992; 267:1077–1082.

14. Taylor Z, Karkauer H. Mortality and reoperation following prostatectomy: outcomes in a Medicare population. Urology 1991; 38:27–31.

15. Mebust WK, Holtgrewe HL, Cockett AT, Peters PC. Transurethral prostatectomy; immediate and postoperative complications. A cooperative study of 13 participating institutions evaluating 3885 patients. J Urol 1989; 141:243–247.

16. Horninger W, Unterlechner H, Strasser H, Bartsch G. Transurethral prostatectomy: mortality and morbidity. Prostate 1996; 28:195–200.

17. Varkarakis I, Kyriakakis Z, Delis A, et al. Longterm results of open transvesical prostatectomy from a contemporary series of patients. Urol 2004; 64:306–310.

18. Mearini E, Marzi M, Mearini L, et al. Open prostatectomy in benign prostatic hyperplasia: ten year experience in Italy. Eur Urol 1998; 34:480–485.

19. Hyrntschak T. Suprapubic Prostatectomy: With primary Closure of the Bladder by an Original Method. Springfield, IL: Charles C. Thomas, 1955.

20. Condie JD Jr, Cutherell L, Mian A. Suprapubic prostatectomy for benign prostatic hyperplasia in rural Asia: 200 consecutive cases. Urology 1999; 54:1012–1016.

21. Meier DE, Tarpley JL, Imediegwu OO, et al. The outcome of suprapubic prostatectomy: a contemporary series in the developing world. Urology 1995; 46:40–44.

22. Walsh PC, Oesterling JE. Improved haemostasis during simple retropubic prostatectomy. J Urol 1990; 143:1203–1204.

23. Shaheen A, Quinlan D. Feasibility of open simple prostatectomy with early vascular control. BJU Int 2004; 93: 349–352

24. Overgaard Nielsen H, Hojsgaard A, Larsen A, et al. The haemostatic effect of purse-string suture in transvesical prostatectomy: a controlled clinical trial. Urol Int 1979; 34:147–152.

25. Lezrek M, Ameur A, Renteria JM, et al. Modified Denis technique: a simple solution for maximum haemostasis in simple retropubic prostatectomy. Urology 2003; 61:951–955.

26. Amen-Palma JA, Arteaga RB. Haemostatic technique: extracapsular prostatic adenomectomy. J Urol 2001; 166:1364–1367.

27. Firfer R, Birkson BM, Lipshitz S, Hseih WH. The combined prostatectomy. J Urol 1984; 132:687–689.

28. Kirollos MM. Bleeding following retropubic prostatectomy. Simple digital rectal pressure could be life saving. J Urol 1998; 160:477–478.

29. Sack E, Spaet TH, Gentile RL, Hudson PB. Reduction of postprostatectomy bleeding by epsilon-aminocaproic acid. N Engl J Med 1962; 266:541–543.

30. Pereiras RV Jr, Meier WL, Katz ER, Viamonte M Jr. Arteriographic embolization treatment for post-prostatectomy haemorrhage. Urology 1977; 9:705–707.

31. Emberton M, Neal DE, Black N, et al. National prostatectomy audit: the clinical management of patients during hospital admission. Br J Urol 1995; 75:301–316.

32. Fitzpatrick JM, Gardiner RA, Worth PH. The evaluation of 68 patients with post-prostatectomy incontinence. Br J Urol 1979; 51:552–555.

33. Hunter KF, Moore KN, Cody DJ, Glazener CM. Conservative management for post-prostatectomy urinary incontinence. Cochrane Database Syst Rev 2004; 2:CD001843.

34. Chapple CR. Duloxetine for male stress incontinence. Eur Urol 2006; 49:958–960.

35. Cespedes RD, Leng WW, McGuire EJ. Collagen injection therapy for postprostatectomy incontinence. Urology 1999; 54:597–602.

36. Cespedes RD, Jacoby K. Male slings for postprostatectomy incontinence. Tech Urol 2001; 7:176–183.

37. Petrou SP. Treatment of postprostatectomy incontinence: is the bulbourethral sling a viable alternative to the artificial urinary sphincter? Curr Urol Rep 2002; 3:360–364.

38. Singh G, Thomas DG. Artificial urinary sphincter for post-prostatectomy incontinence. Br J Urol 1996; 77:248–251.

39. Elliott DS, Barrett DM. Mayo Clinic long-term analysis of the functional durability of the AMS 800 artificial urinary sphincter: a review of 323 cases. J Urol 1998; 159:1206–1208.

40. Lentz HC Jr, Mebust WK, Foret JD, Melchior J. Urethral strictures following transurethral prostatectomy: review of 2223 resections. J Urol 1977; 117:194–196.

41. Jorgensen PE, Weis N, Bruun E. Etiology of urethral stricture following transurethral prostatectomy. A retrospective study. Scand J Urol Nephrol 1986; 20:253–255.

42. Hammarsten J, Lindqvist K, Sunzel H. Urethral strictures following transurethral resection of the prostate. The role of the catheter. Br J Urol 1989; 63:397–400.

43. Bailey MJ, Shearer RJ. The role of internal urethrotomy in the prevention of urethral stricture following transurethral resection of the prostate. Br J Urol 1979; 51:28–31.

44. Schultz A, Bay-Nielson H, Bilde T, et al. Prevention of urethral stricture formation after transurethral resection of the prostate: a controlled randomized study of Otis urethrotomy versus urethral dilation and the use of polytetrafluoroethylene coated versus the uninsulated metal sheath. J Urol 1989; 141:73–75.
45. Nielsen KK, Nordling J. Urethral stricture following transurethral prostatectomy. Urology 1990; 35:18–24.
46. Libman E, Fichten CS. Prostatectomy and sexual function. Urology 1987; 29:467–478.
47. Bolt JW, Evans C, Marshall VR. Sexual dysfunction after prostatectomy. Br J Urol 1987; 59:319–322.
48. Schou J, Holm Christensen NE, Nolsoe C, Lorentzen T. Prostatectomy and impotence: can temperature variations around the prostate during TURP explain post-prostatectomy impotence? Scan J Urol Nephrol 1996; 179:123–127.
49. Lefaucheur JP, Yiou R, Salomon L, et al. Assessment of penile small nerve fibre damage after transurethral resection of the prostate by measurement of penile thermal sensation. J Urol 2000; 164:1416–1419.

11 | Complications of Urethral Stricture Surgery

Ehab A. Eltahawy
Ain Shams University, Cairo, Egypt

Ramon Virasoro
Department of Urology, Eastern Virginia Medical School, Norfolk, Virginia, U.S.A.

Gerald H. Jordan
Urology of Virginia and Department of Urology, Eastern Virginia Medical School, Norfolk, Virginia, U.S.A.

INTRODUCTION

Surgery for urethral stricture can be accomplished, in most cases, with minimal morbidity and complication. The most common complication of surgery for urethral stricture is recurrence of stricture. One must certainly also consider the potential complications of hematoma and/or infection. As many of these surgeries require tissue transfer, donor site issues must be considered. In many cases, surgery for urethral stricture can be accomplished with the patient in a supine or frog-leg/split-leg supine position. However, much of the surgery also requires lithotomy position. The distribution of complications with regard to the lithotomy position varies in accordance with the degree of lithotomy. These issues along with others will comprise the body of this Chapter.

RECURRENCE OF STRICTURE

It is trite to say, but clearly accurate to say, that recurrence of stricture occurs because of the surgeon's failure to identify the extent of the stricture, or in many cases, the surgeon's inability to do so.

Factors such as poor graft take, poor flap survival, and poor technique of primary anastomosis, can contribute to the failure of reconstruction for stricture (1–5). However, it is the failure or lack of ability to identify the true extent of the stricture process, which is, in our opinion, the true downfall of the urethral reconstructive surgeon.

We have found the pneumonic length, location, depth, and density of stricture to be helpful. It is a thinking mechanism. Contrast studies and endoscopy very accurately identify the length and location of the apparent stricture. What is never accurately defined is the true length of spongiofibrosis and in many cases its depth and density. Ultrasound has been proposed as an adjuvant to contrast studies and endoscopy. Certainly ultrasound very accurately identifies the length of narrow caliber areas of stricture; however, it has failed to be more accurate in identifying the extent of spongiofibrosis. The staining of the urethral epithelium with methylene blue has also been proposed as a way of identifying those portions of the urothelium that are involved in the stricture process; however, in our opinion, that technique also fails in its goal. Magnetic resonance has been suggested as an adjuvant study for the evaluation of the patient with pelvic fracture urethral distraction defect (PFUDD). It is proposed to address malalignment of the proximal and distal urethral lumena (6). Thus, much of the identification of the length of spongiofibrosis is left to gestalt. It is left to the surgeon's understanding of the nature of stricture disease. For example, abnormal urethra proximal to a narrow caliber anterior urethral stricture can be and will be hydrodilated. When the narrow caliber area is dealt with, the proximal area becomes a loose cannon. The authors have resorted to reconstruction of these areas. One possible mechanism for identification of these areas is to divert the patient in advance of reconstruction, the concept being that the true nature of that portion of the urethra, when deprived of hydrodilation, will declare itself. We have found that in some cases this is true and in some cases it is not. Thus, recurrence of stricture is a reality of our inabilities, with the techniques and technologies we have available to us at present. In the authors' opinion, the true advancement in surgery for reconstruction of anterior urethral stricture disease will come with the identification of some biomarker, easily applied, which truly identifies the potential of the urothelium and corpus spongiosum with regard to tendency to fibrose and contract.

The membranous urethral distraction defect, however, is much more predictable. Here the trauma, while devastating in its truest extent, is relatively localized in its involvement of the urethra (7). Normal urethra is truly pulled apart from normal urethra. The scar process does extend very slightly proximally and distally, but in the uninstrumented patient, one can reanastomose normal proximal urethral lumen to a normal distal urethral lumen (7,8). This is also the case in the anterior urethral stricture associated with straddle trauma. Unfortunately, many of these patients have been instrumented chasing the ill-conceived process of believing that these strictures respond to "minimally invasive techniques." Thus, the length of the stricture is no longer predictable, it is no longer an isolated area of scar, which can be excised, dealt with in unifocal fashion, and reliably reanastomosed, normal to normal.

The entities of tissue handling, elevation and transposition of flaps, and issues of ischemia of the corpus spongiosum must all be considered; however, they play a minor role in the big picture of urethral restenosis (9,10). In the case of posterior urethral strictures, the entity of ischemic necrosis/stenosis cannot be underestimated in the authors' opinion (11). Ischemic stenosis is a manifestation of poor perfusion of the proximal corpus spongiosum, once elevated in the process of primary anastomotic reconstruction (8). The authors have spent a great deal of time studying this issue and it would appear that the patients who are at risk for this phenomenon are predictable. They appear to be predictable using the entities of duplex ultrasound and in some occasions the entity of pudendal angiography. If a patient has reconstitution of a single side of the common penile arterial system, our experience would suggest that these patients can be reliably reconstructed without fear for ischemic necrosis/stenosis. In the case of the patient with a normal common penile arterial system, demonstrable either by the entities of duplex ultrasound, or directly identified by pudendal angiography can also be reliably reconstructed. Thus, it is the patient with bilateral obliteration of the common penile arterial system who seems to be at risk. The authors, however, are not prepared to say that all patients with bilateral disruption, will in every case, fail primary anastomotic urethral reconstruction.

Another entity contributing to restricture is the inappropriate use of techniques of urethral reconstruction (2). The literature would support that primary anastomosis is clearly the most reliable technique of reconstruction, with the best durability record (E.A. Eltahawy, R. Virasoro, S.M. Schlossberg, K.A. McCammon and G.H. Jordan, Department of Urology, Sentara Norfolk General Hospital, Norfolk, Virginia, U.S.A.). Thus, if a patient inappropriately undergoes a technique that requires tissue transfer, indeed, then it is that inappropriate use of tissue transfer that would contribute to urethral restricture. This can be avoided by accurately identifying the true length of the urethral stricture and then as accurately as possible applying the technique of reconstruction best suited to each individual patient. A reconstructive surgeon cannot have a "favored technique;" the urethral reconstructive surgeon must have a full toolbox that allows him to accurately best reconstruct the stricture.

Certainly postoperative care contributes. In the authors' opinion, urinary diversion should be optimized, and in our hands that means suprapubic diversion. There are, however, many surgeons who feel comfortable using only a urethral catheter for many cases of anterior urethral reconstruction. The length of diversion is a matter of personal surgeon's preference. In the case of graft reconstruction, we divert patients at our center for 28 days. This is based on the observation of superficial grafts, in which one sees the graft becoming somewhat mature at about 28 days postoperatively. Prior to that, grafts have certainly taken; however, their physical characteristics may be truly tenuous. In the case of primary reconstruction, it is our practice to divert patients for a period of 14 to 21 days. Webster's study would certainly suggest diversion in the range suggested (12), but what is proposed is our preference, and in most centers it is the preference of the surgeon, which dictates the length of diversion.

HEMATOMA

Urethral surgery is not attended with massive hemorrhage. The blood vessels that are encountered are usually easily controlled with cautery, either monopolar or bipolar. There are some vessels that require ligation, and there are times when vessels will retract requiring suture ligation.

In the authors' opinion, the problems with hematoma arise in the patient who is anticoagulated, and in whom anticoagulation has not been properly dealt with. In the patient who is on warfarin, one can easily test prothrombin time, partial prothrombin time/international normalized ratio. One would expect those patients with normal variables to coagulate normally. However, the antiplatelet medications are less predictable. Certainly one could do bleeding times on all these patients. In the authors' opinion, the patient who will develop a hematoma will be the patient who is on aspirin, who has not been advised to refrain from taking aspirin, who does not accurately report to the surgeon his time off of aspirin, or in whom his taking of aspirin has not been considered. In the case of the patient with paraurethral hematoma, these are usually easily drained and should be promptly drained.

At our center, for anterior urethral reconstruction as well as posterior urethral reconstruction, the space beneath the midline fusion of the closed ischiocavernosus musculature is drained with a small suction drain, and the space superficial to the closed Colles' fascia but deep to the closed subcuticular tissues is also drained with a suction drain. These drains are removed as drainage allows. As will be discussed later, many patients who need urethral reconstruction may also require prophylactic low dose anticoagulation, which we virtually never see as a problem leading to bleeding or hematoma.

INFECTION

Urethral reconstruction is usually performed with few concerns about infection. In the authors' experience, those patients most at risk for infection are those in whom the colonization of the bladder, because of either the stricture or attendant antecedent diversion, has not been taken into account (13). At our center, it is our custom to make every effort to sterilize the urine in advance of urethral reconstruction. In the patients with suprapubic cystostomy tubes, this is done by obtaining preoperative cultures, and treating with culture-specific antibiotics—IV antibiotics in the hospital if required. In most cases, the patients can be treated with oral antibiotics. Particularly problematic are those patients in whom suprapubic diversion has been placed, and patients have then had treatment of positive urine cultures, with the false concept that one's urine can be permanently sterilized using antibiotics in the face of colonization with intubation. At our center, we choose to place patients on suppressive antibiotics, to monitor their colonization, and to treat the colonization only when it becomes symptomatic (i.e., infection), or immediately prior to urethral reconstruction. In patients in whom we have been deprived accurate culture information preoperatively, we use broad-spectrum antibiotics. The combination of an aminoglycoside as well as Zosyn (combination of Piperacillin and tazobactam) has been very effective. Certainly the combination of an inadequately treated urine culture, along with a hematoma/seroma, is a sure recipe for a closed tissue space infection. Thus as mentioned, drains at our institution are liberally used, and their use we believe contributes to our very low rate of infection.

ERECTILE DYSFUNCTION

The entity of erectile dysfunction (ED) has to be addressed with any urethral reconstructive surgery (14–17). As the anterior perineal triangle is dissected, particularly proximally, the dissection is carried close to the nerves that govern erection. Additionally, there appear to be vascular factors, which are equally involved in the creation of posturethral reconstruction ED. In the case of posterior urethral reconstruction, it is easy to believe that one's dissection has interfered with the function of the nerves that govern erection (18,19). However, in the anterior urethra that concept becomes a little bit more difficult to accept. It is in this area that vascular factors have been implicated. It has been said that the rate of ED following urethral reconstruction approximates the rate of ED following circumcision (16). Unfortunately, ED following urethral reconstruction is mentioned usually as an aside in many series.

With regard to the avoidance of ED, the only information that can be provided is that one needs to limit dissection strictly to the anatomic planes (13). In the case of posterior urethral reconstruction, incisions or excisions of scar need to be very strictly limited to the midline where possible. Additionally, patients need to be counseled that the operation of urethral reconstruction is associated with a finite rate of ED, and that is a risk that the patient must be willing to accept if the patient is to undergo urethral reconstruction. In our recent analysis of primary anastomosis for bulbous urethral strictures, the rate of ED was 2% in a series that analyzed over 250 patients (E.A. Eltahawy, R. Virasoro, S.M. Schlossberg, K.A. McCammon, and G.H. Jordan, Department of Urology, Sentara Norfolk General Hospital, Norfolk, Virginia, U.S.A.). The patients who had suffered significant straddle trauma leading to their urethral stricture seem to be those most at risk, but they were not the only patients at risk. Thus, in summary, there are two factors that surgeons must consider in the case of ED. First is that one's dissection needs to be as accurately planned as possible, and second one's counseling of patients must accurately reflect this risk, before the time of urethral reconstruction.

DONOR SITE CONSIDERATIONS

Donor site issues can be those attendant to flap elevation, or attendant to graft harvest. The considerations are different. There is little in the literature that deals with consideration of donor site morbidity. In the case of local flaps used for urethral reconstruction, the entities of penile tethering with erection, and foreshortening of the penis, have all been mentioned. In the authors' opinion, the best way to avoid a flap donor site issue is to select the location of the skin island, as much as possible, in accordance with areas of redundancy of the genital skin, provided that the skin has acceptable physical characteristics. For example, in the case of reconstruction for hypospadias, the issue is very straightforward. The patients have redundancy of skin dorsally, the blood supply is most reliable dorsally, and techniques exist for the transposition of the fascial flap with the skin island ventrally for the use of urethral reconstruction. In the case of anterior stricture not associated with hypospadias, the issue is not necessarily so straightforward. However, accurate preoperative survey of the genitalia, and in particular, the hairless areas of the genital skin, will, in most cases, allow the patient to undergo reconstruction, using flap techniques, without significant morbidity. There are some patients in whom the urethral reconstruction takes precedence, and donor site considerations have to be adapted. In the case of the patient who needs tubed long segment reconstruction of the proximal urethra, then the donor site consideration may be as simple as planning for a graft reconstructive coverage of the penile shaft, once the flap has been transposed.

In the case of graft morbidity, the most commonly used donor sites are skin, bladder epithelium, oral mucosa, and in some cases rectal mucosa. There is very little in the literature that discusses donor site considerations when one has used a rectal mucosal graft. It would appear, however, that effective repair of the bowel is paramount, and if there is any doubt, then one should resort to diversion. It would make sense to the authors that these grafts would be taken only in the scenario where the patient has been both mechanically and antibiotic bowel prepped.

With regard to the oral mucosa, several subdonor sites have been proposed: the lingual graft taken from the undersurface of the tongue, the cheek donor site, and the lip donor site (20). Problems with the lip donor site have been referred to in the literature in passing; one has to worry about the entity of lip contracture, following the taking of a buccal mucosal graft from the lip. It is the authors' preference to leave that site as one of last resort, and when used, patients are very candidly counseled with regard to the potential of the use of that donor site and the possibility of a lip contracture postoperatively (21).

With regard to cheek donor site, again there are certain issues which are raised in passing, but the literature is relatively silent with regard to complication. If a Stensen's duct is injured and the injury is not recognized, then one certainly could imagine that a significant complication could arise. I (G.H. Jordan, personal communication) have discussed this situation with other reconstructive surgeons (22); one in particular was involved in a case in which Stensen's duct was injured. I was told that this is a large duct, which is very easily repaired, and which the repairs do well because of the large volume of secretions that pass through the duct. We have no experience with complications involving Stensen's duct. Fortunately, Stensen's duct is usually very accurately identified as adjacent to the upper second molar, and hence the way to avoid the complication is to accurately identify the duct and avoid it with the dissection. Hemostasis is usually not a problem, occasionally with leaving a cheek donor site open; one can encounter some bleeding. Again, anecdotally these are dealt with either suture ligation at the bedside or with select cautery (20,21; G.H. Jordan, personal communication). Again the authors have no personal experience with the management of bleeding complications from buccal mucosal donor sites. The lingual mucosa is not a donor site that is closed. Hemostasis is achieved with cautery and the use of epinephrine. The literature is again silent on the potential complications associated with the use of that graft and the authors have no experience with management of complications associated with that graft donor site.

In the case of full thickness skin, the best way to avoid a donor site complication is to align the axis of excision with the Langer's lines. This is the way that all excisional areas should be designed, the potential then for donor site contracture is thus minimized. In most cases, full thickness skin graft donor sites can be closed per primum, achievement of hemostasis prior to closure is important.

With regard to split-thickness skin graft donor sites, the body is essentially one big split-thickness skin graft donor site. For the use of staged urethral reconstruction, grafts are harvested at approximately 14 to 16 thousandth of an inch. Grafts harvested are usually not associated with significant donor site considerations. We manage the donor site initially with an occlusive dressing, a fine mesh gauze placed on the donor site, and that creates a "synthetic scab," which then is "sloughed" from the donor site as epithelialization occurs from the donor site edges. By and large, these donor sites take care of themselves. Occasionally, a donor site can be super colonized with Staph and treatment with an appropriate Staph-sensitive antibiotic would be appropriate.

POSITIONING

Complications of positioning are, for the most part, related to how extreme a lithotomy position is used. Neither the low lithotomy position nor the exaggerated lithotomy position are free of complication (22). The complications are just different (23). Many of the series that report complications preceded the advent of modern style stirrups. In the older series, neurapraxia, compartment syndrome, and persistent neurologic injury were not infrequently seen. With the use of more modern stirrups, the low lithotomy position is used by many with very few complications. The exaggerated lithotomy position is likewise attended with morbidity. In the authors' experience, the most frequently encountered morbidity is that of some numbness of the feet, which resolves quickly, completely, and spontaneously. Whether this is a peroneal nerve stretch injury, or merely a pressure phenomena because of the weight of the legs being supported on the instep, is not clear.

More severe neuropraxias can evolve, however. These are probably due to sciatic nerve injury and it has been proposed that these injuries may be aggravated due to the anatomy of the sciatic nerve through the space of Gowell. This has never been proved, it is merely proposed. Classically these patients will complain of buttocks pain, they often times will go to the recovery room neurologically intact, and then will evolve a rather dense neurapraxia in the early postoperative course. It has been proposed that perhaps this represents a compartment syndrome of the space of Gowell or an aberrant path or high bifurcation of the sciatic nerve. We have aggressively treated these patients with steroids; and to date, all have resolved their neurapraxia without persistent sequelae. What must be paramount in the surgeon's mind, when he is positioning the patient, is that the only good padding is air. All other paddings are double-edged in nature, and the boot stirrup that is packed full of egg-crate, or even gel pads, is just as dangerous as having the boot itself applying pressure to the patient's lower extremity (22,23). A number of series have looked at the complications of the exaggerated lithotomy position. The only variable that seems uniform in those studies is that the longer a patient is in lithotomy, the more prone that patient is to developing problems (23,24). Exaggerated lithotomy position clearly results in impaired oxygenization and increased cardiac-filling pressures, but these levels are acceptable in healthy individuals (24,25). In high-risk individuals, more invasive monitoring must be used. Additionally the legs are placed at a significant distance above the heart, and in the older individual where perfusion pressures are not as great, certainly it is possible to have hypoperfusion of the lower extremities while the patient is in lithotomy, and a reperfusion phenomena when the patient is returned flat to the table. These issues can be minimized by putting the table in reverse Trendelenburg, limiting the column height to perfuse the lower legs. However, it cannot be emphasized how time in lithotomy can ruin a well done urethral reconstruction because of an unacceptable positioning complication.

In patients who might have a compartment syndrome of the space of Gowell, none elevated their creatine phosphokinase (CPK) and none developed myoglobinuria. Thus, we would assume that there was no significant rhabdomyolysis. The literature indicates that the incidence of positioning complications is directly related to time in position. Five hours seems to be a critical time, although, "the shorter the better." Fortunately, the vast majority of urethral reconstruction can be done with the patient in position for less than three hours. Thus, positioning complications are quite unusual.

MORBIDITY FACTORS PARTICULAR TO OPERATING ON THE OLDER PATIENT

A recent analysis suggests that the results of urethral reconstruction in the older patient are equal to those in the younger patient (26). This certainly is somewhat counterintuitive, and only one analysis has looked at the issue. However, it is the authors' opinion that the older patient can be successfully operated on. However, the opportunity for comorbidity is much greater. These patients must be cleared by their primary care physician and in many cases by their cardiologist. If there are any pulmonary issues, then those need to be resolved preoperatively and pulmonary function testing may be indicated.

Many older patients tend to have had a number of vascular issues, and many are on chronic anticoagulation of some form or another. The suspension of anticoagulation therapy surrounding the time of surgery must be very carefully coordinated in order to minimize bleeding while also minimizing the occurrence of complication resulting from suspension of anticoagulation therapy. Additionally, as mentioned, many older patients do not regard low-dose aspirin as an anticoagulant and will fail to mention the fact that they take that therapy. It is the authors' experience that the older patient does not "bounce back from surgery" as quickly as the younger patient. However, we have, in the older patient, enjoyed equal success with regard to the issues of urethral reconstruction.

Certainly one must worry about small vessel vascular disease, and the potential for ischemic necrosis or stenosis should the corpus spongiosum be divided, and some form of primary or augmented anastomosis be performed. We have not routinely subjected the older patients to the same vascular testing that we do in the patient referred with PFUDD, but it may indeed be warranted. It is probably safe to assume that no older patient is indeed absolutely healthy, and extreme caution must be taken with regard to clearing all possible potentials for comorbidity. The older patient does seem to be prone to thromboembolic complications, and thus, while the patient is off of formal anticoagulation therapy, low-dose therapy, we feel, is probably warranted.

ASSORTED OTHER PROBLEMS

In the hypospadias patient, the fistula rate may be as high as 30% (27; G.H. Jordan, personal communication). The patient undergoing redo surgery following complications of prior urethral reconstruction seems to be particularly at risk. The patient's tissues have been operated on previously, and there is a paucity of tissues available for interposition.

We have used the tunica dartos flap carrying a tunica vaginalis island rather extensively in these patients and have enjoyed a significant diminished rate of fistula. In patients undergoing second-stage graft reconstruction, prior to employing this flap interposition, our fistula rate was approximately 30%. Upon employing these flaps, the fistula rate has become almost nil.

If one does end up with a fistula following urethral reconstruction, the tissues must be allowed to settle and a reoperation should not be performed for at least six months. Urethral diverticula have been attributed to the use of a number of techniques of urethral reconstruction. These would include the use of bladder epithelial grafts, and the use of penile skin islands mobilized on a tunica dartos flap. It is our opinion, that these diverticula are actually errors on the part of the surgeon with regard to tailoring of the transferred tissue.

It has been proposed that ventral onlay is more prone to diverticula, because of the "lack of support" of the transferred tissue. The incidence of ventral diverticula associated with ventral onlay varies significantly from one surgeon to another, or from one report to another.

Dorsal onlay is felt to have a lesser rate of development of urethral diverticulum in that the graft or flap is supported by the triangular ligament and the corpora cavernosa. However, the literature has not examined this issue in any detail and thus all that is proposed with regard to iatrogenic urethral diverticula should be regarded as anectodal.

Incontinence has been proposed as a complication of urethral reconstruction and also the entity of pelvic fracture. Indeed, we would maintain that incontinence following posterior urethral reconstruction has nothing to do with the surgery, but rather due to injury to the more proximal sphincter mechanism. It is clear that the patient who has had reconstruction for PFUDD may lose his ability to voluntarily recruit sphincter activity, but with regard to passive continence, either the problem is caused by injury and scarring of the proximal sphincter mechanism, and/or denervation of the bladder and hence poor storage on the part of the bladder. The distal external sphincter is destroyed in some patients who suffer PFUDD. However, what is regarded by most as the external sphincter is the mechanism of voluntary continence, and in most patients who have suffered a PFUDD, the involuntary or involuntary continence mechanism is usually intact (28–31). Webster and Iselin's analysis would suggest that the endoscopic appearance of the bladder neck is not predictive of eventual continence (32). We find the scarred bladder neck, however, to be a useful finding, in that if present, we counsel the patients that they may have less than optimal passive continence and further procedures may be required. With regard to incontinence following anterior urethral reconstruction on closer inquiry that usually is shown to be postvoid dribbling. Following anterior urethral reconstruction, particularly in the bulbous urethra, the urethra becomes somewhat less elastic, hence the emptying of the anterior urethra following voiding is not as efficient. Additionally, if the midline of the ischial cavernosus musculature has been opened during the approach to the bulbous urethra, then that mechanism will obviously be less efficient. Patients must be counseled with regard to these sequelae preoperatively, and if they are, they will recognize that an element of postvoid dribbling is a consequence of a successful anterior urethral reconstruction in many, if not most, cases.

SUMMARY

In summary, the most frequently encountered complications of urethral reconstructive surgery for stricture have been addressed in this chapter. Fortunately they are few in number, and their incidence is low. In most patients, urethral reconstruction can be accomplished with minimal morbidity and minimal opportunity for complication.

REFERENCES

1. Kizer WS, Morey AF. Proximal bulbar urethroplasty via extended anastomotic approach: what are the limits? J Urol 2005; 173(Suppl):a316.
2. Secrest CL, Jordan GH, Winslow BH, et al. Repair of the complications of hypospadias surgery. J Urol 1993; 150:1415–1418.
3. Wessells H, McAninch JW. Current controversies in anterior urethral stricture repair: free-graft versus pedicled skin-flap reconstruction. World J Urol 1998; 16:175–180.
4. Bhargava S, Chapple CR. Buccal mucosal urethroplasty: is it the new gold standard? BJU Int 2004; 93:1191–1193.
5. Barbagli G, Palminteri E, Guazzoni G, et al. Bulbar urethroplasty using buccal mucosa grafts placed on the ventral, dorsal or lateral surface of the urethra: are results affected by the surgical technique? J Urol 2005; 174:955–958.
6. Narumi Y, Hircak H, Armenakas NA, McAninch JW. MR imaging of traumatic posterior injury. Radiology 1993; 188:439–443.
7. Latini J, Stoffel JT, Zinman L. The acute posterior urethral injury. In: Schreiter F, Jordan J, eds. Reconstructive Urethral Surgery. Heidelberg: Springer, 2006:70–76.

8. Webster GD, Mathes GL, Selli C. Prostatomembranous urethral injuries: a review of the literature and a rational approach to their management. J Urol 1983; 130:898–902.

9. Andrich DE, Mundy AR. Substitution urethroplasty with buccal mucosa free grafts. J Urol 2001; 165:1131–1134.

10. McAninch JW, Morey AF. Penile circular fasciocutaneous skin flap in 1 stage reconstruction of complex anterior urethral strictures. J Urol 1998; 159:1209–1213.

11. Jordan GH. Management of membranous urethral distraction injuries via the perineal approach. In: McAninch JW, Carroll PR, Jordan GH, eds. Traumatic and Reconstructive Urology. Philadelphia, PA: W.B. Saunders Co., 1996:393–415.

12. Jordan GH. Management of anterior urethral stricture disease. In: Webster GD, ed. Vol. 1. Problems in Urology. Philadelphia: JB Lippincott Co., 1987:199–226.

13. Berger B, Sykes Z, Freedman M. Patch graft urethroplasty for urethral stricture disease. J Urol 1976; 115:681–684.

14. Anger JT, Sherman ND, Webster GD. The effect of bulbar urethroplasty on erectile function [Abstr]. J Urol 2005; 173(Suppl):331.

15. Coursey JW, Morey AF, McAninch JA, et al. Erectile function after anterior urethroplasty. J Urol 2001; 1666:2273–2276.

16. Andrich DE, O'Malley K, Holden F, et al. Erectile dysfunction following urethroplasty [Abstr]. J Urol 2005; 173(Suppl):329.

17. Wright JL, Wessells HB, Nathens AB, et al. Sexual and excretory dysfunction one year after pelvic fracture [Abstr]. J Urol 2005; 173(Suppl):330.

18. Shenfeld OZ, Kiselgorf ON, Verstandig AG. The incidence and causes of erectile dysfunction after pelvic fractures associated with posterior urethral disruption. J Urol 2003; 169:2173–2176.

19. Mark SD, Keane TE, Vandemark RM, Webster GD. Impotence following pelvic fracture urethral injury: incidence, etiology and management. BJU Int 1995; 75:62–64.

20. Jang TL, Erickson B, Medendrop A, Gonzales CM. Comparison of donor site intraoral morbidity after mucosal graft harvesting for urethral reconstruction. Urology 2005; 66:716–720.

21. Kamp S, Knoll T, Osman M, et al. Donor site morbidity in buccal mucosa urethroplasty: lower lip or inner cheek. BJU Int 2005; 96:619–623.

22. Eltahawy EA, Schlossberg SM, McCammon KM, Jordan GH. Long term follow up for excision and primary anastomosis in anterior urethral strictures [Abstr]. J Urol 2005; 173(Suppl):315.

23. Angermier KW, Jordan GH. Complications of the exaggerated lithotomy position: a review of 177 cases. J Urol 1994; 151:866–868.

24. Anema JG, Morey AF, McAninch JW, et al. Complications related to the high lithotomy position during urethral reconstruction. J Urol 2000; 164:360–363.

25. Ryniak S, Brannstedt S, Blomqvist H. Effects of exaggerated lithotomy position on ventilation and haemodynamics during radical perineal prostatectomy. Scan J Urol Nephrol 1998; 32:200–203.

26. Santucci RA, McAninch JW, Mario LA, et al. Urethroplasty in patients older than 65 years: indications, results, and suggested treatment modifications. J Urol 2004; 172:201–203.

27. McCammon KA, Shenfeld OZ, Schlossberg SM, Jordan GH. Mesh split-thickness skin graft urethroplasty in the treatment of complex anterior urethral strictures. J Urol 1999; 161(Suppl 379):101.

28. Mourtzinos A, Smith JJ, Barrett DM. Treatments for male urinary incontinence: a review. AUA update series 2005; 24:122–131.

29. Jordan GH, Schlossberg SM. Surgery of the penis and urethra. In: Walsh PC, Retik AB, Vaughan ED Jr, Wein A, eds. Campbell's Urology. Vol. 4, 8th ed. Philadelphia, PA: WB Saunders, 2002:3917–3918.

30. Mouraviev VB, Santucci RA. Cadaveric anatomy of pelvic fracture urethral distraction: most injuries are distal to the external urinary sphincter. J Urol 2005; 173:869.

31. Koraitim MM, Atta MA, Ismail HR. Mechanism of continence after repair of posttraumatic posterior urethral strictures. Urology 2003; 61:287–290.

32. Iselin CE, Webster GD. The significance of the open bladder neck associated with pelvic fracture urethral distraction defects. J Urol 1999; 162:34–51.

12 | Complications of Radical Cystectomy

Erik Pasin, Maurizio Buscarini, and John P. Stein
*Department of Urology, University of Southern California, Norris Comprehensive
Cancer Center, Los Angeles, California, U.S.A.*

INTRODUCTION

In the United States, bladder cancer is the fourth most common cancer in men and the eighth
most common in women, with transitional cell carcinoma (TCC) compromising nearly 90% of
all primary bladder tumors (1). Although the majority of patients present with superficial
bladder tumors, 20% to 40% of patients will present with or ultimately develop muscle-invasive
disease. Invasive bladder cancer is a lethal malignancy. If untreated, over 85% of patients die of
their disease within two years of the diagnosis (2). Furthermore, a certain percent of patients
with high-grade bladder tumors without involvement of the lamina propria will recur/progress
and/or fail intravesical management, and may best be treated with an earlier cystectomy when
survival outcomes are optimal (3). The rationale for an aggressive treatment approach employing radical cystectomy for high-grade, invasive bladder cancer is based on several clinical
observations.

1. The best long-term survival rates, coupled with the lowest local recurrences, are seen
   following definitive surgery including removal of the primary bladder tumor and regional
   lymph nodes (4,5).
2. The morbidity and mortality of radical cystectomy has significantly improved over the past
   several decades.
3. TCC tends to be a tumor resistant to radiation therapy, even at high doses.
4. Chemotherapy alone, or in combination with bladder-sparing protocols, has not demonstrated long-term local control and survival rates equivalent to those with cystectomy (6).
5. Radical cystectomy provides accurate pathologic staging of the primary bladder tumor
   (p stage) and regional lymph nodes, thus selectively determining the need for adjuvant
   therapy based on precise pathologic evaluation.

For the aforementioned reasons, radical cystectomy has become a standard and arguably the
ideal form of therapy for high-grade, invasive bladder cancer today.

The evolution and improvements in lower urinary tract reconstruction, particularly orthotopic diversion, has been a major component in enhancing the quality of life of patients requiring
cystectomy. Currently, most men and women can safely undergo orthotopic lower urinary tract
reconstruction to the urethra following cystectomy (7). Orthotopic reconstruction most closely
resembles the original bladder in both location and function, provides a continent means to
store urine, and allows volitional voiding via the urethra. The orthotopic neobladder eliminates
the need for a cutaneous stoma, urostomy appliance, and the need for intermittent catheterization
in most cases. These efforts have been directed to improve the quality of life of patients who
must undergo bladder removal, and have stimulated patients and physicians to consider radical
cystectomy at an earlier, more curable stage (8).

At the University of Southern California (USC), a dedicated effort has been made to
improve upon the surgical technique of radical cystectomy and to provide an acceple form of
urinary diversion, without compromise of a sound cancer operation (9–11). Radical cystectomy
is a technically challenging operation, often performed in elderly patients with associated
comorbidities that require diligent attention to pre-, intra-, and postoperative details. Despite
this, complications do occur. Therefore, it is prudent for all surgeons to be familiar with the
presentation, prevention and treatment of the major causes of morbidity and mortality associated
with this surgical procedure. The complications of radical cystectomy can be categorized as
those specific to the removal of the anterior pelvic organs and associated lymphadenectomy,

and those specific to the form of urinary diversion. This chapter will focus on the early and delayed complications associated with radical cystectomy and intestinal urinary diversion.

COMPLICATIONS OF CYSTECTOMY
Mortality

With improvements in surgical technique and perioperative anesthetic care, the early mortality from radical cystectomy has decreased from nearly 20% before 1970 (12) to 1% to 5% in most contemporary series (4,5,13–16). In a retrospective analysis of 1359 patients following radical cystectomy at USC, the most common cause of death in the perioperative period was cardiovascular, with septic complications from resulting urine and bowel leaks the second most common (Table 1) (12).

Hemorrhage

Hemorrhage is a common complication of radical cystectomy that can occur acutely intraoperatively and in the delayed setting. The bladder, prostate, uterus, and vagina are vascular organs and drained by a rich venous supply that necessitate careful and secure vascular control. While several patient characteristics may affect intraoperative blood loss and the need for transfusion, a sound understanding of pelvic anatomy and adherence to proper surgical technique remain the cornerstone in preventing significant bleeding in the intraoperative and delayed settings.

The blood supply to the anterior pelvic organs is derived primarily from the anterior branches off the internal iliac vessels (Fig. 1). The anterior division of the hypogastric artery gives off seven branches supplying the pelvic viscera (superior vesical, middle rectal, inferior vesical, uterine, internal pudendal, obturator, and inferior gluteal arteries) that collectively form the lateral pedicle. At our institution, the lateral vascular pedicle is isolated and each individual branch clipped and divided after dissecting the obturator fossa and ligating the obturator vessels. Isolation and development of this pedicle is crucial for proper vascular control and to help minimize bleeding during radical cystectomy.

TABLE 1 Perioperative Mortalities from Radical Cystectomies from 1971 to 2001[a]

Category	No. of perioperative mortalities	Median age (years) at surgery (range)	Median time (days) to death (range)	Total number of patients with type of complication	Complications resulting in perioperative mortality (%)
Cardiovascular	8	65 (47–72)	13 (0–28)	34	24
Acute myocardial infarction	4				
Arrythmia	2				
Cerebrovascular accident	1				
Arterial thrombosis (superior mesenteric artery)	1				
Infectious/sepsis	8	71 (58–78)	33 (23–47)	212	4
Primary contributing factor					
Urine leak	3			72	4
Bowel leak/fistula	3			24	13
Small bowel obstruction	1				
Hematoma	1				
Pulmonary embolus	4	69 (66–77)	20 (0–28)	25	16
Hepatic failure	3	73 (62–78)	38 (5–48)	34[b]	15[b]
Upper gastrointestinal bleeding	2				
Hemorrhage, surgical site	1				
Hemorrhage	2	72 (66–77)	23 (1–44)	34[b]	15[b]
Hemophilia B	1				
Conduit-arterial fistula	1				
Unknown	2	62 (57–67)	64 (47–80)		
Total	27	67 (47–78)	28 (0–80)		

[a]N = 1359 patients.
[b]All hemorrhagic complications regardless of primary etiology considered collectively.

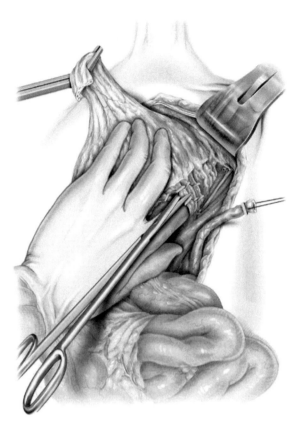

FIGURE 1 Technique for isolation and ligation of the lateral pedicle. All anterior branches of the hypogastric vessels are isolated and divided between hemoclips down to the endopelvic fascia.

With the lateral pedicle entrapped between the left index and middle fingers, firm traction is applied vertically and caudally (Fig. 1). This facilitates identification and allows individual branches of the anterior portion of the hypogastric artery to be isolated. The posterior trunk of the hypogastric artery, including the superior gluteal, ilio-lumbar, and lateral sacral arteries, is preserved to avoid gluteal claudication. All anterior branches of the hypogastric artery are isolated and divided between hemoclips down to the endopelvic fascia. The proximal aspect of each vessel is doubly clipped. We prefer right angle hemoclips, with care ensuring that 0.5 to 1 cm of tissue projects between each clip when the pedicle is divided. This prevents the clips from becoming dislodged during the operation, resulting in unnecessary bleeding.

After control of the lateral pedicle, attention is directed toward the posterior pedicle. The posterior pedicle is developed after entry into Denonvilliers' space is made. The pouch of Douglas is incised slightly on the rectal side and the plane between the posterior sheath of Denonvilliers' fascia and the rectum (Denonvilliers' space) is developed. A combination of sharp and blunt dissection will allow the rectum to be carefully swept off the seminal vesicles, prostate and bladder in men and the posterior vaginal wall in women. This sweeping motion, when extended laterally, helps to thin and develop the posterior pedicle, which appears like a collar emanating from the lateral aspect of the rectum (Fig. 2). Once the posterior pedicles have been defined, they are clipped and divided down to the endopelvic fascia in the male patient. In women, the posterior pedicles, including the cardinal ligaments are divided 4 to 5 cm beyond the cervix. Again, proper hemoclip placement and technique are essential to minimize blood loss.

While it is standard practice at USC to dissect and ligate the individual vessels of the lateral and posterior pedicles between carefully placed hemoclips, it has been proposed that staple ligation of these pedicles contributes to significantly lower estimated blood loss and transfusion requirements compared to suture ligation alone (17). We have not found this useful, and in fact strongly encourage individual vessel ligation to ensure vascular control.

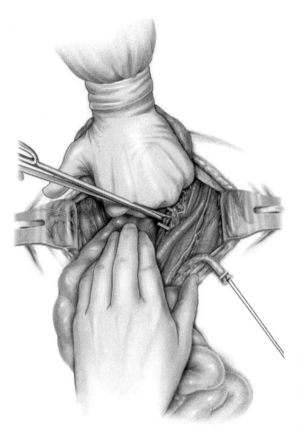

FIGURE 2 Technique for isolation and ligation of the posterior pedicle. The posterior pedicle is developed after entry into Denonvillier's space with a combination of blunt and sharp dissection, appears like a collar emanating from the lateral aspect of the rectum.

The third major vascular structure that must be controlled prior to removal of the cystectomy specimen is the dorsal venous complex (DVC). Although several methods have been described, we utilize one of two methods of securing the DVC, both of which offer excellent vascular control. An angled clamp can carefully be passed beneath the DVC, anterior to the urethra. The venous complex can then be ligated with a 2–0 absorbable suture, and divided close to the apex of the prostate. Any additional bleeding after transection of the venous complex, should it occur, can be oversewn with the previously placed absorbable 2–0 suture. Alternatively, the venous complex may be gathered at the apex of the prostate with a long Allis clamp. This technique may help to better define the plane between the DVC and the anterior urethra. A figure-of-eight 2–0 absorbable suture can then be placed under direct vision anterior to the urethra and distal to the apex of the prostate around the gathered venous complex. This maneuver not only affords secure vascular control, but avoids the passage of instruments between the DVC and the rhabdosphincter, which could potentially injure these structures and compromise the continence mechanism.

Several patient characteristics reported in the literature predispose to greater estimated blood loss and a higher transfusion rate. Increased body mass index (BMI) has been shown to correlate with a larger estimated blood loss in several retrospective analyses (18,19). In one analysis, BMI was the only preoperative variable on a multivariate analysis to independently predict increased blood loss during radical cystectomy (18). Gender differences have been thought to affect transfusion requirements in patients undergoing radical cystectomy. One study found that the transfusion rate and the median number of units transfused were greater in women compared to men, owing to the rich lateral vascular pedicles unique to the female pelvis (cardinal and uterosacral ligaments) (20).

Controlled hypotensive anesthesia as a means to reduce blood loss in radical cystectomy has been studied and remains the standard surgical practice in selected individuals at our institution (21). The anesthesiologist titrates intravenous nitroglycerin to lower mean arterial pressure until the cystectomy specimen is removed, at which time the blood pressure returns to normal range. Return to normotension facilitates identification of any bleeding vessels that may not have been identified or properly secured during the hypotensive period, thus allowing further pelvic hemostasis. Despite obtaining secure vascular control during the intraoperative period, postoperative bleeding may occur that requires return to the operating room. In our series of 1359 cystectomy patients, 11 patients (0.8%) experienced surgically related postoperative hemorrhage, eight of whom (72%) required return to the operating room. We routinely place a large hemovac drain in the pelvis to drain any blood for the first 24 hours postoperatively. An undrained pelvic hematoma may predispose to abscess formation, delayed return of bowel function, or disruption of urethral–intestinal anastomoses in orthotopic neobladders.

Rectal Injury

Rectal injury as a complication of radical cystectomy remains an entity with potentially grave consequences if not recognized intraoperatively. Contemporary series report an incidence of rectal injury ranging from 0.3% to 9.7% (4,5,14–16,22). Factors predisposing to intraoperative rectal injury include prior pelvic surgery, colonic inflammatory disease, extensive prior transurethral resection of a posterior bladder mass, direct extension of a posterior bladder mass into Denonvilliers' space, and, most importantly, prior pelvic radiotherapy (22). Morbidity can be minimized by prospectively identifying those patients at increased risk and employing primarily sharp dissection of the posterior bladder off the anterior rectal wall in patients with an obliterated posterior plane. Furthermore, recognition of a rectal injury intraoperatively, appropriate repair, adequate decompression of the injured rectum, eslishment of sufficient pelvic drainage, and aggressive nutritional and antimicrobial support are all critical to prevent the potential for significant sequelae.

The advent of preoperative bowel preparation over three decades ago has led to numerous clinical trials that have clearly shown a therapeutic advantage with respect to lowering the incidence of infectious postoperative complications in modern elective colorectal surgery (23). Proper bowel prep is also important to minimize the infectious sequelae following a rectal injury. A three-tier regimen is standard practice when performing surgery where breach of the distal intestinal tract is anticipated. This includes (*i*) preoperative mechanical cleansing to decrease the fecal load and facilitate the efficacy of orally administered antibiotics, (*ii*) preoperative oral antimicrobial bactericidal therapy targeting both aerobic and anaerobic organisms, and (*iii*) perioperative parenteral antimicrobial therapy (23). All patients at our institution undergoing radical cystectomy are admitted the day prior to surgery for antibacterial bowel preparation and intravenous hydration. A clear liquid diet may be consumed until midnight, at which time the patient is to consume nothing orally thereafter. A standard Nichols bowel preparation (23) consisting of 120 mL of castor oil orally at 09.00 hours, 1 g of neomycin orally at 10.00, 11.00, 12.00, 13.00, 16.00, 20.00, and 24.00 hours, and 1 g of erythromycin base orally at 12.00, 16.00, 20.00, and 24.00 hours. We have found that this regimen is generally well tolerated, obviates the need for enemas, and maintains nutritional and hydrational support.

Key to minimizing the risk of rectal injury is a sound understanding of the fascia layers between the bladder and the rectum. The anterior and posterior peritoneal reflections converge in the cul-de-sac to form Denonvilliers' fascia, which further extends caudally to the urogenital diaphragm (Fig. 3). This important anatomic boundary in the male separates the prostate and seminal vesicles from the rectum posteriorly. The plane between the prostate and seminal vesicles and the anterior sheath of Denonvilliers' fascia will not develop easily. However, the plane between the rectum and the posterior sheath of Denonvilliers' fascia (Denonvilliers' space) should develop easily with sharp and blunt dissection. Therefore, the peritoneal incision in the cul-de-sac should be made slightly on the rectal side, rather than on the bladder side. This facilitates proper and safe entry and development of Denonvilliers' space. Occasionally, patients with an invasive posterior bladder tumor or those who have undergone previous pelvic radiotherapy may have this plane obliterated, increasing the risk of rectal injury.

As the majority of rectal injuries are created as a result of the shearing forces produced during blunt dissection of Denonvilliers' space, patients with obliterated posterior planes

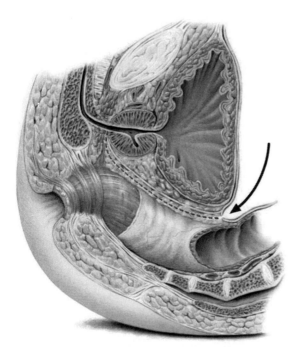

FIGURE 3 The peritoneal incision in the cul-de-sac should be made slightly on the rectal side for safe entry into Denonvillier's space and should develop easily with sharp and blunt dissection. Knowledge of the fascial layers between the bladder and rectum facilitates the posterior dissection and minimizes the risk of rectal injury.

necessitate entry into this space sharply. If rectal injury does occur, it is crucial that it be identified intraoperatively. Often a small rectal laceration can be missed, and in patients at high risk for rectal injury, diligent intraoperative inspection of the anterior and lateral rectal walls is essential. In patients where visualization is inconclusive and rectal injury is suspected, delineaion of the site of injury can be accomplished by insufflating the rectum with air while the pelvis is filled with saline.

Once identified, it is recommended that the injury be closed in layers. In previous reviews, it had been advocated that proctotomies be closed at the time of initial injury in three layers (24); however, most literature now regards a two-layer closure to be sufficient (25). A running absorbable suture is used to close the mucosa after the wound edges are debrided. Care should be taken to invert the mucosal edges into the bowel lumen when closing this layer. The second layer of interrupted silk sutures in a Lembert's fashion is used to complete the closure. If possible, the interposition of a greater omental apron is advised to discourage fistula formation (26), particularly if rectal injury occurred in the setting of orthotopic neobladder construction, where fresh suture lines of the neobladder and urethral anastomosis are vulnerable.

Diversion of the fecal stream by means of a sigmoid loop colostomy should be performed when the rectal defect is considerable, the contamination is great, or impaired healing from previous pelvic radiation or colonic inflammatory disease is expected (22).

Venous Thromboembolism

It lingers in the mind of every surgeon that after such a dedicated intraoperative effort, acute pulmonary events developing from insidious venous clots may complicate the patient's perioperative outcome. A wealth of information has been gathered regarding the etiology, risk factors, treatment, and prevention of venous thromboembolism since Virchow first reported on the factors, which predispose to thrombosis in 1856.

Thromboembolism accounts from 1% to 4% of all perioperative complications reported in contemporary cystectomy series (4,5,14–16). Several risk factors have been identified that predispose patients to a higher incidence of venous thromboembolism than that of the general population (Table 2). Indisputable evidence has accumulated over the years in the form of randomized clinical trials that demonstrates the effect of primary thromboprophylaxis in the

TABLE 2   Risk Factors for Venous Thromboembolism

Obesity
Smoking
Advanced age
Previous venous thromboembolism
Prolonged immobility/paresis
Trauma (major or lower extremity)
Central venous catheterization
Estrogen-containing oral contraceptives
Heart or respiratory failure
Myeloproliferative disorders
Acute medical illness
Inherited or acquired thrombophilia

reduction of deep venous thrombosis (DVT), pulmonary embolism and fatal pulmonary embolism (27). To prevent such complications, it is common practice amongst surgical patients to be covered with some form of thromboprophylaxis during their hospital stay.

The evidence-based guidelines of the seventh american college of chest physicians conference on antithrombotic and thrombolytic therapy reported that the absolute risk of DVT in hospitalized patients who undergo major urologic surgery (defined as open urologic procedures) and who received no form of thromboprophylaxis is 15% to 40% (27). Additionally, the conference reported that the ratio between asymptomatic DVT and symptomatic thromboembolism is approximately 5–10:1. The conference thus recommended based on strong evidence (28) that patients undergoing major, open urologic procedures, routine prophylaxis with low-dose unfractionated heparin twice or three times daily is the preferred thromboprophylaxis regimen. Low molecular weight heparin (LMWH) or prophylaxis with intermittent pneumatic compressions (IPC) and/or graduated compression stockings (GCS) are acceple alternatives. For patients with multiple risk factors, the conference recommended combining GCS and/or IPC with either low-dose unfractionated heparin or LMWH. For those patients who are actively bleeding or at high risk of bleeding, the conference recommended the use of mechanical thromboprophylaxis with IPC and/or GCS at least until the bleeding decreases (27).

As the majority of venous thromboembolic events are diagnosed several weeks after hospital discharge, the duration of thromboprophylactic therapy necessary to prevent thromboembolism while negligibly affecting the rate of hemorrhage in postoperative cancer patients remains unclear. One study found that enoxaparin prophylaxis for four weeks after surgery for abdominal or pelvic cancer is safe and significantly reduces the incidence of venographically demonstrated thrombosis, whom compared with enoxaparin prophylaxis for one week (29). This suggests that some form of thromboprophylaxis for one month postoperatively may be important.

At our institution, coumadin, together with IPC devices are used as thromboprophylaxis in the postoperative hospitalization period. It has been our experience that excellent prophylaxis from thromboembolic events while minimally affecting the postoperative hemorrhage rate can be achieved with an initial coumadin load of 10 mg given via a gastrostomy tube immediately in the postanesthesia recovery unit, followed by daily dosing of coumadin while monitoring the patients protime to keep within a range of 18 to 22 seconds. For patients who are particularly sensitive to coumadin, smaller doses are commonly used and any dangerous elevation of the protime can be effectively and immediately reversed with the administration of intravenous vitamin K. As seen in Table 1, 25 of 1359 patients (1.8%) receiving radical cystectomy in our series developed pulmonary embolism occurring a mean of 20 days after surgery. Sixteen percent of these proved fatal, emphasizing the significance of this complication after major pelvic exenterative surgery for malignancy. It has been our experience that the rate of hemorrhage and need for transfusion in patients receiving low-dose unfractionated heparin or LMWH has been greater compared with the use of coumadin, and as such, coumadin administration in the postoperative period as a mean of thromboprophylaxis for the radical cystectomy patient has been standard practice at the USC.

Ileus

Postoperative ileus is the delay in the coordinated movements of the gastrointestinal tract. This common complication of intra-abdominal surgery is often responsible for a prolonged hospital stay and significant perioperative morbidity. Several factors responsible for the pathogenesis of postoperative ileus have been elucidated, which involve imbalance between the sympathetic, parasympathetic, and intrinsic nervous system of the small intestine and the colon, and the role of inflammatory mediators in the development of a postoperative ileus. While a complete discussion of this extensive topic is beyond the scope of this chapter, the reader is referred to an excellent review for more detail regarding the etiology and pathogenesis of postoperative ileus (30).

Prolonged ileus after radical cystectomy is a common complication ranging from 7% to 23% in recent series (4,5,14–16,31). In one report, this is the most common complication resulting in a prolonged hospital stay in patients undergoing radical cystectomy (31). Chang et al. defined ileus as delayed return of bowel function beyond postoperative day 4. As such, a larger number of patients from their retrospective series were regarded as having ileus compared to other series (31). The definition of ileus is debale; however, the delay in recovery of coordinated intestinal movements from surgical trauma typically resolves after three to four postoperative days, with the colon being the last of the intestinal segments to regain function (30).

Because postoperative ileus prolongs hospital stay, and longer time spent in the hospital places patients at increased risk for nosocomial-acquired infections and other complications, it seems prudent for physicians to tailor the standard perioperative care toward the evidence-based strategies shown to help resolve postoperative ileus in the safest and most expeditious manner. While concluding that the best method of reducing the duration of postoperative ileus is difficult as much of the published literature is skewed by differences in study protocols, several general conclusions can be made.

Some authors recommend placement of a thoracic epidural and the use of local anesthetic to reduce the possibility of a postoperative ileus (30). Epidural anesthesia with bupivicaine has been shown to be superior to systemic and epidural opioid with respect to reduction in postoperative ileus in patients undergoing abdominal surgery without significantly affecting pain relief (30). Limiting the use of intravenous opioids and supplementing narcotics with nonsteroidal anti-inflammatory drugs (NSAIDs) may also be helpful. In addition to reducing the total amount of narcotic use, the use of NSAIDs decreases the amount of local inflammatory mediators in the intestinal wall and may minimize the duration of postoperative ileus via this mechanism as well (30). There are no prospective, randomized trials that validate the use of prokinetic agents, including erythromycin or metoclopromide, in the resolution of postoperative ileus. Cisapride did show promise in previous years; however, the discovery of its arrythmiagenic effect as a consequence of its prolongation of the Q-T interval has led to its current unavailability in the United States (30). Contrary to popular belief, early ambulation has no demonstrable effect at expediting the resolution of postoperative ileus. Early ambulation is to be encouraged, however, as it is beneficial primarily in the prevention of atelectasis, pneumonia, and DVT (30).

Ileus that fails to resolve by the 10th to 14th postoperative day may warrant investigation as to its cause. Correction of the electrolyte imbalances, particularly hyponatremia, hypokalemia, and hypomagnesemia, which may occur in the perioperative period, is important to restore bowel function. A search for additional causes such as abscess from intestinal anastomotic or urine leak should also be considered.

Bowel decompression is advised to prevent the sequelae of an ileus including nausea, vomiting, abdominal distention, and pain. Poorly decompressed bowel in the setting of unresolved ileus may cause significant fluid shifts and potentially stress enteric anastomoses predisposing to anastomotic leaks. Traditionally, nasogastric decompression has been the method of choice as conservative management of postoperative ileus. In addition to the general discomfort associated with nasogastric tubes, recent literature has suggested postoperative nasogastric intubation to be the single most important variable associated with the development of postoperative pulmonary complications (32). It is standard practice at our institution to place an operative gastrostomy tube at the time of cystectomy in a modified Stamm fashion, where greater omentum is interposed between the stomach and the abdominal wall, to facilitate resolution of the postoperative ileus (33), without the need for a nasogastric tube.

Bowel Leak/Enterocutaneous Fistula

The development of a bowel leak after radical cystectomy is a devastating complication associated with a significant morbidity and mortality. Up until the 1960s, the mortality rate of patients with gastrointestinal fistulae was 43% (34). While the advent of improved methods of critical care and artificial nutrition steadily decreased the mortality rate of postoperative bowel leaks, they continue to pose a great deal of patient anxiety, discomfort and negative self image during the course of disease and remain a considerable source of elevated hospital cost (34).

The finding of fever, wound infection, and elevation of white blood cell count occurring at the fifth to seventh postoperative day or delayed return of bowel function persisting and temporally associated with these events should raise suspicion of an intra-abdominal abscess from a potential bowel leak or an unrecognized enterotomy. Patients are often extremely ill and may display signs of sepsis, including hypotension, tachycardia, and organ system failure requiring an intensive care setting. The finding of enteric contents from a surgically placed drain confirms the diagnosis. A computed axial tomography (CT) scan with water soluble oral contrast in those patients with no external evidence of fistula is prudent and typically reveals extravasation of contrast from the bowel lumen into an intra-abdominal or pelvic fluid collection. A CT scan is also necessary to rule out any distal intestinal obstruction that may have contributed to the formation of, and will invariably prevent the closure of, the enteric fistula.

Once diagnosed, management of a bowel leak from an unrecognized enterotomy or breakdown of intestinal anastomosis is a clinical dilemma. Two schools of thought exist, emergent laparotomy or conservative management. The decision to choose one or the other is not always obvious given the lack of clear evidence-based guidelines in dealing with this complication. The decision to begin a trial of conservative management is largely dependent on the presence or absence of peritonitis or sepsis (35). If the patient is well drained, or there is a controlled fistula and in the absence of clinical peritonitis or multiple intra-abdominal abscesses refractory to percutaneous drainage, a trial of conservative management is warranted. (35). Maximal drainage of any intra-abdominal or pelvic fluid collections from radiographically placed drains is mandatory to treat the septic patient. Every attempt to aggressively control intra-abdominal infection is essential as the major cause of death in this group of patients is a result of a neglected intra-abdominal or pelvic abscess (36). The abdominal incision, if displaying signs of infection, should be opened and left to heal by secondary intention. Cultures should be obtained and broad-spectrum antibiotic therapy should be employed and tailored to organism sensitivity. The patient should be made to take nothing by mouth, proximal decompression and drainage by means of a nasogastric or gastrostomy tube should be begun and hyperalimentation instituted. Total parenteral nutrition (TPN) is classically indicated in patients with enterocutaneous fistulas. TPN has been shown to increase the spontaneous closure rate by inducing bowel hypoactivity, and better prepare the patient from a nutritional perspective for reoperation after a defined period of nutritional support if the fistula fails to spontaneously close (37).

The data regarding the use of somatostatin analogs in the conservative management of enterocutaneous fistula are debate. While somatostatin and its analogs have been shown to decrease fistula output thus making it easier to manage fluid, electrolyte and protein imbalances, the therapeutic advantage with regard to reducing the time to fistula closure has not been consistently shown in clinical trials (38–41).

With aggressive attention to detail and patience, when treated conservatively, only 50% of postoperative bowel fistulas close spontaneously within four to six weeks in the absence of distal obstruction or the loss of bowel continuity. If nutritionally anabolic and free of sepsis, the remainder of patients usually respond favorably to elective reoperation to repair the fistula and restore intestinal continuity (35). Reoperation is best delayed for at least three to four months after surgery.

The decision for acute emergent laparotomy is warranted in patients displaying peritonitis or signs of sepsis with proven or suspected intraperitoneal abscesses, which have failed, or are not amenable to percutaneous drainage (35). The goal of laparotomy is to cleanse the abdominal cavity and pelvis of any loculated abscesses utilizing copious amount of irrigation, to provide adequate drainage of the pelvis and peritoneum by means of surgically placed drains, and to control the source of contaminating infection, typically through the creation of a proximal enterostomy, irrespective of the level of injury (35).

It may be possible to resect the affected bowel segment and primarily reanastomose in a patient who presents with a fistula within the first two postoperative days. These occurrences are usually the result of technical error and may afford a cure in a minimally compromised patient with insignificant peritonitis and a normal serum albumin (35). However, intestinal diversion should be performed if the quality of bowel is suspect or if the patient has a history of radiation therapy, as these patients often fail primary repair.

Strict attention to surgical detail when performing the intestinal anastomosis is crucial to avoid the development of an enterocutaneous fistula. At our institution, a two-layered, hand-sewn, interrupted, end-to-end anastomosis utilizing a series of 3–0 silk sutures is performed to reeslish intestinal continuity after the appropriate segment of bowel is gathered to form the urinary reservoir. Adequate exposure to the anastomosing segments, maintenance of excellent blood supply to the severed ends, avoidance of local spillage of enteric contents, which may facilitate a focal septic environment, accurate serosa to serosa apposition, and avoidance of tissue strangulation by sutures tied too tightly are all important details that, when methodically adhered to, allow for successful intestinal anastomosis (42).

Lymphocele

A series of studies published in the last decade emphasize the importance of pelvic lymph node dissection during cystectomy for invasive bladder cancer. Most investigators advocate lymph node dissection not only as a staging procedure but also as an integral part of the curative intent of radical surgery of invasive bladder cancer (43–45). Although most patients undergoing radical cystectomy are elderly and have significant comorbidities, a proper lymphadenectomy may still be beneficial. Recent studies have shown that removing more lymph nodes increased survival in both node-negative and node-positive bladder cancer (43,46,47). However, there continues to be a divergence of opinion about how the lymphadenectomy should be carried out and about the minimum number of nodes that should be removed.

The incidence of lymphocele with limited or extended lymph node dissection is 1% to 4% according to the major published series (44,48). The vast majority of these cases can be managed expectantly. In our series with an extended lymphadenectomy, only two patients required percutaneous CT-guided drainage of the lymph collection, which promptly resolved the problem in both cases.

In a recent study, Brossner et al. reported the events during and after radical cystectomy in a series of 92 consecutive patients, in terms of major and minor complications, comparing a minimal with an extended lymphadenectomy (45). The authors found that extended lymphadenectomy in patients receiving radical cystectomy does not increase the morbidity within 30 days of surgery. Most investigators advocate lymph node dissection as an integral part of the curative intent of radical surgery for invasive bladder cancer, and not only as a staging procedure. Multiple studies demonstrated that, despite prolonging the operation, extended lymphadenectomy causes no significant increase in complications during and after surgery.

Wound Infection/Fascial Dehiscence

Surgical site infections and wound and tissue dehiscence are well-known postoperative complications in gastrointestinal and urologic surgery. The severity of these complications embraces mild cases needing local wound care and antibiotics to serious cases with multiple re-operations and a high mortality rate. In most cases, such complications may prolong hospitalization, with a substantial increase in cost of care (49,50).

The reported incidence of wound infection and fascial dehiscence after radical cystectomy in the reported series is 3% to 6% and 1% to 3%, respectively. Several patient characteristics increase the risk of wound infection and fascial dehiscence in major abdominal operations. Extensive prior smoking history, diabetes mellitus, and cardiopulmonary disease are associated with increased risk of surgical site infections and abdominal wall dehiscence (51–56) by a variety of proposed mechanisms. Smoking, microvascular disease as a result of long-standing diabetes mellitus, and severe lung disease are known causes of peripheral tissue hypoxia (57,58), which increases the risk of wound infection and dehiscence (59). In addition, some studies suggest that hypoxia, smoking, and diabetes reduce collagen synthesis and oxidative killing mechanisms of neutrophils (60–64), resulting in impaired wound healing. The association between elevated perioperative blood loss and postoperative tissue and wound complications in elective operations suggests that hypovolemia and reduction in tissue oxygenation by loss of red blood cells is detrimental to healing and increases the risk of infection and tissue dehiscence (65–70). Common for all tissues subject to surgery is disruption of the local vascular supply, thrombosis of vessels, and tissue hypoxia (71). Once the blood supply is restored, several factors may complicate healing. The most important seems to be proliferation of bacteria in the wound and tissue, which affects the processes involved in wound healing and increases the risk of wound infection and dehiscence. Fascial dehiscence is invariably associated with previous wound infection (72), and represents a serious postoperative problem that often necessitates immediate operative exploration and repair. Occasionally, in the case of minor fascial separation, it may be possible to delay immediate repair for several months in the absence of frank evisceration or incarceration of bowel. However, immediate return to the operating room is usually mandatory in eviscerated or obstructed individuals. In our cohort of cystectomy patients, we observed 17 fascial dehiscences (1.2%), 12 of whom (70.5%) underwent reoperation.

COMPLICATIONS OF URINARY DIVERSION
Urine Leak

Persistent leak of urine from the pouch occurs in the early postoperative period in 3% to 9% of cases (4,5,14–16). Diagnosis can be eslished by testing the high fluid output from the drain for creatinine or via a pouchogram. Urine leaks can be managed conservatively in a majority of cases with adequate proximal diverting drainage. Some patients with prolonged urinary leakage may need temporary nephrostomy tube placement. Occasionally, the drains may be responsible for maintaining the leak sitting along a suture line. In these situations it is helpful to advance the drain ("crack") to resolve the situation. Spontaneous perforation of a continent urinary diversion is extremely rare. Several case reports have illustrated this complication (73,74). It is more common in spinal cord injury patients who lack that sensation of abdominal fullness often described by patients after continent urinary diversion (75). Unlike leaks that occur in the early postoperative period, perforations invariably require formal open surgical repair.

Ureteroenteric Anastomotic Stricture

Lower urinary tract reconstruction following radical cystectomy complicated by ureteroenteric anastomotic stricture ranges from 0.3% to 9% in recent series (4,5,14–16). It is a difficult complication that may result in pain, urosepsis, and compromised renal function in a patient population that often requires a sufficient renal reserve to prevent the various metabolic complications frequently associated with the intestinal-urinary diversion. Additionally, many patients with advanced bladder cancer may require an adjuvant course of chemotherapy, further necessitating preservation of renal function. While the majority of ureteroenteric strictures can be managed by endoscopic means, there is a substantial failure rate and many necessitate open reoperation. Careful radiographic surveillance of the upper tracts of patients with ureteroenteric anastomoses is essential to identify this problem early, and to preserve kidney function.

The key to reducing the incidence of ureterointestinal stricture is the surgical harvest of the ureter with preservation of the blood supply and delicate handling of the ureter during the anastomosis. After mobilization and packing of the bowel, the ureters are easily identified in the retroperitoneum just cephalad to the common iliac vessels and are dissected into the pelvis several centimeters distal to the common iliac vessels. They are then divided between two large hemoclips, placed approximately 2 cm apart, with the interposing piece of ureter being sent off for frozen section. The proximal hemoclip is left in place on the divided ureter during the exenteration. This allows the occluded ureter to hydrostatically dilate, and facilitates the ureteroenteric anastomosis.

It is of utmost importance to maintain adequate ureteral blood supply during mobilization of the ureter. Often, an arterial branch from the common iliac artery or the aorta medially requires division to provide adequate ureteric mobilization. However, every effort should be made to maintain the integrity of the laterally emanating gonadal vessels. These attachments are an important blood supply to the ureter and ensure adequate vascular supply for the ureteroenteric anastomosis at the time of diversion. In the irradiated patient who is more prone to the development of anastomotic stricture, we tend to divide the ureter higher (above the common iliac vessels) to help reduce the portion of the ureter that may be affected by the radiation.

An additional intraoperative effort should be made to create a large enough window through the sigmoid mesentery that allows the free and unobstructed passage of the left ureter for the enteric anastomosis. We develop this mesenteric window cephalad, to approximately the level of the inferior mesenteric artery, to prevent any undue angulation that may impede blood flow to the area of anastomosis. This concept may be one reason why ureteroenteric anastomotic strictures more commonly affect the left renal unit (76). It is not uncommon to find a stenotic area at the level of angulation away from the anastomosis for this same reason, providing further explanation why left-sided strictures are observed more frequently following urinary diversion.

The type of ureteral anastomosis performed may also impact the stricture rate. One prospective study found the stricture rate to be 13% for nonrefluxing or tunneled techniques, compared to 1.7% for direct, end-to-side refluxing methods in patients receiving continent urinary diversion (77). This study further suggested that the risks of reflux nephritis are outweighed by that of obstructing nephropathy and as such the authors recommend that a refluxing anastomosis be the method of choice in eslishing ureterointestinal continuity.

The fact that the ureteroenteric anastomosis is at risk for stricture throughout the life of the anastomosis mandates that these patients be followed indefinitely (42). At USC, patients receiving radical cystectomy and continent urinary diversion receive both an intravenous pyelogram or an abdominal/pelvic CT scan and gravity cystogram at the four month mark, the one year mark and annually thereafter. For patients with an elevation in serum creatinine, an ultrasound may be used to evaluate the upper tracts for new or changing hydronephrosis (Table 3).

New-onset hydronephrosis or delayed excretion of contrast into the urinary reservoir from a functioning renal unit at the level of the anastomosis is suggestive of obstruction from either a benign or malignant source. We recommend that obstructed kidneys be diverted with a nephrostomy tube and urine cytology and accurate radiographic images be performed to clearly delineate the site of obstruction and potential etiology. Often times, an absent or delayed nephrogram on intravenous pyelogram (IVP) may be the initial abnormality to warrant further investigation (Fig. 4). Once diagnosed, the "gold standard" method of treatment includes open surgical repair with identification and excision of the stenosed segment and spatulated reimplantation to the reservoir. This method of treatment typically yields long-term patency rates approaching 90% (78). If the stricture proves to be malignant, nephroureterectomy with a cuff of intestine

TABLE 3 University of Southern California Surveillance Regimen Postradical Cystectomy

	4 mo	1 yr	Years 2–5 (annually)	After 5 yr (annually)
Orthotopic neobladder, continent cutaneous diversion[a], ileal conduit[b,c]	Intravenous pyelogram (ultrasound if creatinine >1.8) Gravity cystogram Comprehensive metabolic panel Liver function tests Chest radiograph	Intravenous pyelogram (ultrasound if creatinine >1.8) Gravity cystogram Comprehensive metabolic panel Liver function tests Chest radiograph Urine cytology	Intravenous pyelogram (ultrasound if creatinine >1.8) Gravity cystogram Comprehensive metabolic panel Liver function tests Chest radiograph Urine cytology	Intravenous pyelogram (ultrasound if creatinine >1.8) Gravity cystogram Comprehensive metabolic panel Liver function tests Chest radiograph Urine cytology Vitamin B12 every other year

[a]Same as orthotopic neobladder with annual urethral washings in male patients.
[b]Same as orthotopic neobladder, may use loopogram to assess upper tracts.
[c]Consider CT abdomen/pelvis at 6, 12, and 24 months in pT3 or pT4 disease.

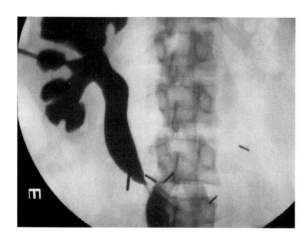

FIGURE 4 Ureteroileal anastomotic stricture as seen from an antegrade study after nephrosotomy tube drainage.

excised at the anastomosis should be performed at the time of intended repair. As open surgery in an elderly population, often with a prior history of radiation, is not without morbidity, a variety of minimally invasive techniques have been developed and are available that provide satisfactory long-term patency rates while avoiding the morbidity of a repeat open operation for the ureterointestinal stricture. Various minimally invasive techniques and their associated patency rates in the treatment of ureteroenteric anastomotic stricture are well documented (79). Balloon dilation techniques yield the worst long-term patency rates as this technique fails to incise the scar. Balloon dilation appears to be most successful in non-ischemic, short, benign strictures away from the anastomosis (79). Endoureterotomy should be reserved for those strictures with a compromised vascular supply (80), as is the case for strictures that develop at the ureteroenteric anastomosis. Despite the large amount of data on endoureterotomy, no universal agreement has been reached regarding the best cutting modality, postoperative time to continue stent diversion, or cutoff of stricture size (79). It is known, however, that shorter strictures (<2 cm) and those of nonischemic origin respond more favorably to endoureterotomy (79). The use of the holmium laser to create a ureterotomy under direct visualization has shown promising long-term patency rates with minimal morbidity, which has led many investigators to recommend this technique as the method of choice in the initial treatment of ureteroenteric anastomotic stricture disease (76,79). Regardless of the method, the technique of choice should only be employed after a malignant cause of ureterointestinal stricture has been excluded.

Pouch Stones

The varying incidence of pouch stones occurring in patients with lower urinary tract reconstruction is largely a result of the type of intestinal reservoir created and whether it is orthotopic or cutaneous in location. Urinary stasis and mucus production are inherent to all types of continent reservoirs and are known predisposing factors to pouch stones (81). Urine from continent cutaneous reservoirs is chronically contaminated with bacteria resulting from the need to empty the pouch by means of intermittent catheterization, and thus predispose this form of diversion to a higher incidence of calculi. Urease-producing bacteria such as *Proteus*, which break down urea into ammonia and carbon dioxide provide the necessary alkaline microenvironment for the production of struvite stones, and together with calcium phosphate, account for the majority of stones seen within continent reservoirs. Additional risk factors for the formation of pouch stones include metabolic derangements such as metabolic acidosis, hypocitraturia, hypercalciuria, hyperoxalauria and the presence of non-absorbable foreign bodies within the reservoir (81). The Kock ileal reservoir, for example, with its staple line used to secure the afferent nipple valve often exposed to urine, has the highest rate of pouch stones of any ileal reservoir. This complication has been reported in 5% to 6% of patients with this type of lower urinary tract reconstruction and its incidence is reported to be three-fold higher in those-patients with continent cutaneous versus orthotopic Kock pouches (82).

The majority of patients with pouch stones present incidentally with a calcification found on routine imaging studies. Some may present with signs and symptoms of urinary tract infection, while others, rarely, present after spontaneous passage of a stone per urethra (82). Some patients may present with gross hematuria, incontinence or sense of fullness or pressure within the pouch with episodes of incontinence. The common identification of this complication on routine imaging studies however further emphasizes the importance of long-term radiographic surveillance in patients with lower urinary tract reconstruction (Table 3).

Several different modalities have been utilized to achieve a stone-free state in the continent reservoir. Endoscopic methods of stone removal provide a highly effective and minimally invasive means at achieving this end. Stones found in an orthotopic neobladder can typically be treated in a similar manner as stones in a native bladder. For continent cutaneous reservoirs, while small stone burdens can be easily extracted with the use of endoscopic basket devices through a 16 F flexible cystoscope via the efferent limb. Fear of disrupting the continence mechanism has led investigators to attempt alternative methods of stone removal. Boyd et al. described the success of extracorporeal shock wave lithotripsy in the treatment of obstructive small stone burden within the afferent limb staple line of the continent cutaneous Kock pouch (83). While this method was successful in fragmenting the stone burden, endoscopy with retrieval of the fragmented pieces was often necessary to completely remove the stone burden. Huffman, in his series of 45 patients with a continent cutaneous Kock ileal reservoir and stones reported no injury to the efferent limb continence mechanism with the utilization of a 24.5 F rigid nephroscope and a 9 F electrohydrolic lithotripsy probe for fragmentation (84). An Amplatz sheath can be passed over the nephroscope and left in position in the efferent limb to facilitate reentry into the pouch throughout the operation while any of the stone fracturing devices (electrohydrolic, ultrasonic, or laser) can be used to completely fragment the stone.

Still, potential injury to the continence mechanism exists, particularly in small caliber efferent limbs such as seen with the appendix. This has led to the development of percutaneous approaches at stone removal performed in much the same way as a percutaneous nephrolithotomy. In this approach, after preoperative evaluation with a CT scan to assure an area above the pouch free of overlying bowel, the pouch is distended to bring it closer to the anterior abdominal wall. Under ultrasound and fluoroscopic guidance, a wire is passed through a needle into the pouch and the cutaneous tract and fascia are dilated to a size that is able to negotiate the appropriate instruments. Postoperatively, a large caliber malencot tube or similar catheter should be left to drain the pouch at the percutaneous access site. At about the one week mark, this tube can be removed after placing a small caliber Red Robinson catheter (16 F) into the cutaneous stoma to provide adequate pouch decompression for the percutaneous access site to seal.

A novel method (85) described to percutaneously remove pouch stones involves placing a 16 F flexible cystoscope through the cutaneous stoma for visualization of the stones. Under ultrasound guidance and direct vision, a laparoscopic trocar can be placed into the pouch using a small skin incision. Through this trocar, a specimen retrieval laparoscopic bag is used to capture the stone burden and bring the retrieval bag neck to the level of the skin, through which standard ultrasonic or electrohydrolic devices can be placed into the bag through a nephroscope to fragment the stones. The stones and bag can then be removed intact. If minimally invasive means of stone removal are not feasible or the stone burden is too great, open surgical removal may be required.

Patient compliance with catheterization schedules and irrigation protocols is necessary in the prevention of recurrent reservoir stones. Additionally, chronic metabolic acidosis occurring from urine exposed to bowel mucosa and perpetuated by underlying renal insufficiency places patients with intestinal reservoirs at high risk of stone formation. Urinary alkalinizing agents used to minimize metabolic academia and resulting hypercalciuria and hypocituria may be effective in the prophylaxis of intestinal reservoir stones.

SUMMARY

Radical cystectomy has become a standard and arguably the best definitive form of therapy for high-grade, invasive bladder cancer. Lower urinary tract reconstruction, particularly orthotopic diversion, has been a major component in enhancing the quality of life of patients requiring cystectomy. As with any major surgery, however, complications do arise. It is important for all surgeons to be familiar with the presentation, prevention, and treatment of the major causes of morbidity and mortality associated with radical cystectomy and lower urinary tract reconstruction. The complications discussed are among the most common of the complications seen with cystectomy and urinary-intestinal diversion. There are, in fact, many others that may be encountered, as the published literature testifies, and a thorough understanding as to their presentation, prevention, and treatment is equally essential for a successful patient outcome. Adherence to proper surgical technique, familiarization with recent data regarding the most successful treatment methods, and attention to detail in the perioperative period are crucial for minimizing complications in any surgical undertaking.

REFERENCES

1. Jemal A, Thomas A, Murray T, et al. Cancer Statistics 2002. CA Cancer J Clin 2002; 52:23–47.
2. Prout G, Marshal VF. The prognosis of untreated bladder tumors. Cancer 1956; 9:551–558.
3. Stein JP. Indications for early cystectomy. Urology 2003; 62:591–595.
4. Stein JP, Lieskovsky G, Cote R, et al. Radical cystectomy in the treatment of invasive bladder cancer: long-term results in 1054 patients. J Clin Oncol 2001; 19:666–675.
5. Ghoneim MA, El-Makresh MM, El-Baz MA, et al. Radical cystectomy for carcinoma of the bladder: critical evaluation of the results in 1026 cases. J Urol 1997; 158:393–399.
6. Montie JE. Against bladder sparing surgery. J Urol 1999; 162:452–455.
7. Stein JP, Skinner DG. Orthotopic bladder replacement. In: Walsh PC, Retik AB, Vaughan ED, Wein AJ, eds. Campbell's Urology. 8th ed. Philadelphia, PA: WB Saunders, 2002:3835–3867.
8. Hautmann RE, Paiss T. Does the option of ileal neobladder stimulate patient and physician decision toward earlier cystectomy? J Urol 1998; 159:1845–1850.
9. Stein JP, Skinner DG. Radical cystectomy in the female. Atlas Urol Clin North Am 1997; 5:37–64.
10. Stein JP, Skinner DG, Montie JE. Radical cystectomy and pelvic lymphadenectomy in the treatment of infiltrative bladder cancer. In: Droller MJ, ed. Bladder Cancer: Current Diagnosis and Treatment. Totowa, NJ: Humana Press, 2001:267–307.
11. Stein JP, Quek MD, Skinner DG. Contemporary surgical techniques for continent urinary diversion: continence and potency preservation. Atlas Urol Clin North Am 2001; 9:147–173.
12. Glantz GM. Cystectomy and urinary diversion. J Urol 1966; 96:714–717.
13. Rosario DJ, Becker M, Anderson JB. The changing pattern of mortality and morbidity from radical cystectomy. BJU Int 2000; 85:427–430.
14. Frazier HA, Robertson JE, Paulson DF. Complications of radical cystectomy and urinary diversion: a retrospective review of 675 cases in 2 decades. J Urol 1992; 148:1401–1405.
15. Chang SS, Cookson MS, Baumgartner RG, et al. Analysis of early complications after radical cystectomy: results of a collaborative care pathway. J Urol 2002; 167:2012–2016.
16. Hautmann RE, Gschwend JE, de Petriconi RC, et al. Cystectomy for transitional cell carcinoma of the bladder: results of a surgery-only series in the neobladder era. J Urol 2006; 176(2):486–492.
17. Chang SS, Smith JA, Cookson MS. Decreased blood loss in patients treated with radical cystectomy: a prospective randomized trial using a new stapling device. J Urol 2003; 169:951–954.
18. Chang SS, Jacobs B, Wells N, et al. Increased body mass index predicts increased blood loss during radical cystectomy. J Urol 2004; 171:1077–1079.
19. Lee CT, Dunn RL, Chen BT, et al. Impact of Body mass index on radical cystectomy. J Urol 2004; 172:1281–1285.
20. Lee KL, Freiha F, Presti JC, et al. Gender differences in radical cystectomy: complications and blood loss. Urology 2004; 63:1095–1099.
21. Ahlering TE, Henderson JB, Skinner DG. Controlled hypotensive anesthesia to reduce blood loss in radical cystectomy for bladder cancer. J Urol 1983; 129:953–954.
22. Flechner SM, Spaulding JT. Management of rectal injury during cystectomy. Urology 1982; 19:143–147.
23. Nichols RL, Choe EU, Weldon CB. Mechanical and antibacterial bowel preparation in colon and rectal surgery. Chemotherapy 2005; 51(suppl 1):115–121.
24. Winter CC, Gluesenkamp EW. Management of intraoperative proctotomy incidental to total cystectomy for bladder carcinoma. J Urol 1973; 109:62–63.
25. Kozminski M, Konnak JW, Grossman HB. Management of rectal injuries during radical cystectomy. J Urol 1989; 142:1204–1205.
26. Walsh PC. Anatomic Radical Retropubic Prostatectomy. In: Walsh PC, Retik AB, Vaughan ED, Wein AJ, eds. Campbell's Urology. 8th ed. Philadelphia, PA: WB Saunders, 2002:3107–3129.
27. Geerts WH, Pineo GF, Hett JA, et al. Prevention of venous thromboembolism: the seventh ACCP conference on antithrombotic and thrombolytic therapy. Chest 2004; 126:338S–400S.

28. Guyatt G, Schunemann HJ, Cook D, et al. Applying the grades of recommendation for antithrombotic and thrombolytic therapy: the seventh ACCP conference on antithrombotic and thrombolytic therapy. Chest 2004; 126:S79–S87.

29. Bergqvist D, Angelli G, Cohen AT, et al. Duration of prophylaxis against venous thromboembolism with enoxaparin after surgery for cancer. N Engl J Med 2002; 346:975–980.

30. Baig MK, Wexner SD. Postoperative ileus: a review. Dis Colon Rectum 2004; 47:516–526.

31. Chang SS, Baumgartner RG, Wells N, et al. Causes of increased hospital stay after radical cystectomy in a clinical pathway setting. J Urol 2002; 167:208–211.

32. Mitchell CK, Smoger SH, Pfeifer MP, et al. Multivariate analysis of factors associated with postoperative pulmonary complications following general elective surgery. Arch Surg 1998; 133:194–198.

33. Buscarini M, Stein JP, Lawrence MA, et al. Tube gastrostomy after radical cystectomy and urinary diversion: surgical technique and experience in 709 patients. Urology 2000; 56:150–152.

34. Falconi M, Pederzoli P. The relevance of gastrointestinal fistula in clinical practice: a review. Gut 2002; 49(suppl 4):iv2–iv10.

35. Schein M. Postoperative small bowel leak. Br J Surg 1999; 86:979–980.

36. Schein M, Decker GA. Postoperative external alimentary tract fistulas. Am J Surg 1991; 161:435–438.

37. Smith SJ, Austen WG Jr, Souba WW. Nutrition and meolism. In: Greenfield LJ, Mulholland MW, Oldham KT, Zelenock GB, Lillemoe KD, eds. Surgery: Scientific Principles and Practice. 3rd ed. Philadelphia, PA: Lippincott Williams and Wilkins, 2001:43–68.

38. Munawar J, Umair A, Humaira S, Sobia. Role of somatostatin analogues in the management of enterocutaneous fistulae. J Coll Physicians Surg Pak 2004; 14:237–240.

39. Allivizatos V, Felekis D, Zorbalas A. Evaluation of the effectiveness of octreotide in the conservative treatment of postoperative enterocutaneous fistulae. Hepatogastroenterology 2002; 49:1010–1012.

40. Memon AS, Siddiqui FG. Causes and management of postoperative enterocutaneous fistulas. J Coll Physicians Surg Pak 2004; 14:25–28.

41. Martineau P, Shwed JA, Dennis R. Is octreotide a new hope for enterocutaneous and external pancreatic fistula closure? Am J Surg 1996; 172:386–395.

42. McDougal WS. Use of intestinal segments and urinary diversion. In: Walsh PC, Retik AB, Vaughan ED, Wein AJ, eds. Campbell's Urology. 8th ed. Philadelphia, PA: WB Saunders, 2002:3745–3788.

43. Leissner J, Hohenfellner R, Thuroff JW, et al. Lymphadenectomy in patients with transitional cell carcinoma of the urinary bladder: significance for staging and prognosis. BJU Int 2000; 85:817–823.

44. Lerner SP, Skinner DG, Lieskovsky G, et al. The rationale for en bloc pelvic lymph node dissection for bladder cancer patients with nodal metastases: long-term results. J Urol 1993; 149:758–764.

45. Brossner C, Pycha A, Toth A, et al. Does extended lymphadenectomy increase the morbidity of radical cystectomy? BJU Int 2004; 93:64–66.

46. Herr HW, Bochner BH, Dalbagni G, et al. Impact of the number of lymph nodes retrieved on outcome in patients with muscle invasive bladder cancer. J Urol 2002; 167:1295–1298.

47. Stein JP, Cal, J, Groshen S, et al. Risk factors for patients with pelvic lymph node metastases following radical cystectomy with en bloc pelvic lymphadenectomy: concept of lymph node density. J Urol 2003; 170:35–41.

48. Herr HW, Donat SM. Outcome of patients with grossly node positive bladder cancer after pelvic lymph node dissection and radical cystectomy. J Urol 2001; 165:62–64.

49. Collins TC, Daley J, Henderson WH, et al. Risk factors for prolonged length of stay after major elective surgery. Ann Surg 1999; 230:251–259.

50. Taylor GD, Kirkland TA, McKenzie MM, et al. The effect of surgical wound infection on postoperative hospital stay. Can J Surg 1995; 38:149–153.

51. Sorensen LT, Jorgensen T, Kirkeby LT, et al. Smoking and alcohol abuse are major risk factors for anastomotic leakage in colorectal surgery. Br J Surg 1999; 86:927–931.

52. Dunne JR, Malone DL, Tracy JK, et al. Abdominal wall hernias: risk factors for infection and resource utilization. J Surg Res 2003; 111:78–84.

53. Sorensen LT, Horby J, Friis E, et al. Smoking as a risk factor for wound healing and infection in breast cancer surgery. Eur J Surg Oncol 2002; 28:815–820.

54. Myles PS, Iacono GA, Hunt JO, et al. Risk of respiratory complications and wound infection in patients undergoing ambulatory surgery: smokers versus nonsmokers. Anesthesiology 2002; 97:842–847.

55. Ghorra SG, Rzeczycki TP, Natarajan R, et al. Colostomy closure: impact of preoperative risk factors on morbidity. Am Surg 1999; 65:266–269.

56. Fawcett A, Shembekar M, Church JS, et al. Smoking, hypertension, and colonic anastomotic healing; a combined clinical and histopathological study. Gut 1996; 38:714–718.

57. Jensen JA, Goodson WH, Hopf HW, et al. Cigarette smoking decreases tissue oxygen. Arch Surg 1991; 126:1131–1134.

58. Willis N, Mogridge J. Indicators of histohypoxia. Acta Anaesthesiol Scand Suppl 1995; 107:45–48.

59. Hopf HW, Hunt TK, West JM, et al. Wound tissue oxygen tension predicts the risk of wound infection in surgical patients. Arch Surg 1997; 132:997–1004.

60. Jorgensen LN, Kallehave F, Christensen E, et al. Less collagen production in smokers. Surgery 1998; 123:450–455.

61. Black E, Vibe-Petersen J, Jorgensen LN, et al. Decrease of collagen deposition in wound repair in type 1 diabetes independent of glycemic control. Arch Surg 2003; 138:34–40.

62. Allen DB, Maguire JJ, Mahdavian M, et al. Wound hypoxia and acidosis limit neutrophil bacterial killing mechanisms. Arch Surg 1997; 132:991–996.

63. Tan JS, Anderson JL, Watanakunakorn C, et al. Neutrophil dysfunction in diabetes mellitus. J Lab Clin Med 1975; 85:26–33.

64. Sørensen LT, Nielsen HB, Kharazmi A, et al. Effect of smoking and abstention on oxidative burst and reactivity of neutrophils and monocytes. Surgery 2004; 136:1047–1053.

65. Riou JP, Cohen JR, Johnson H Jr. Factors influencing wound dehiscence. Am J Surg 1992; 163: 324–330.

66. Alves A, Panis Y, Trancart D, et al. Factors associated with clinically significant anastomotic leakage after large bowel resection: multivariate analysis of 707 patients. World J Surg 2002; 26:499–502.

67. Yasuda K, Shiraishi N, Adachi Y, et al. Risk factors for complications following resection of large gastric cancer. Br J Surg 2001; 88:873–877.

68. Hartmann M, Jonsson K, Zederfeldt B. Effect of tissue perfusion and oxygenation on accumulation of collagen in healing wounds: randomized study in patients after major abdominal operations. Eur J Surg 1992; 158:521–526.

69. Esrig BC, Frazee L, Stephenson SF, et al. The predisposition to infection following hemorrhagic shock. Surg Gynecol Obstet 1977; 144:915–917.

70. Hunt TK, Zederfeldt BH, Goldstick TK, et al. Tissue oxygen tensions during controlled hemorrhage. Surg Forum 1967; 18:3–4.

71. Niinikoski J. Tissue oxygenation in hypovolaemic shock. Ann Clin Res 1977; 9:151–156.

72. De Haan BB, Ellis H, Wilks M. The role of infection on wound healing. Surg Gynecol Obstet 1974; 138:693–700.

73. Singh S, Choong S. Rupture and perforation of urinary reservoirs made from bowel. World J Urol 2004; 22:222–226.

74. Hensle TW, Dean GE. Complications of urinary tract reconstruction. Urol Clin North Am 1991; 18:755–764.

75. Razi SS, Bennett CJ. Selecting the appropriate urinary diversion procedure in the spinal cord injured: a poignant reminder. J Spinal Cord Med 1996; 19:197–200.

76. Watterson JD, Sofer M, Wollin TA, et al. Holmium:Yag laser endoureterotomy for ureterointestinal strictures. J Urol 2002; 167:1692–1695.

77. Pantuck AJ, Han K, Perrotti M, et al. Ureteroenteric anastomosis in continent urinary diversion: long-term results and complications of direct versus nonrefluxing techniques. J Urol 2000; 163:450–455.

78. Kramolowsky EV, Clayman RV, Weyman PJ. Management of ureterointestinal anastomotic strictures: comparison of open surgical and endourological repair. J Urol 1988; 139:1195–1198.

79. Laven BA, O'Connor C, Steinberg GD, et al. Long-term results of antegrade endoureterotomy using the holmium laser in patients with ureterointestinal strictures. Urology 2001; 58:924–929.

80. Richter F, Irwin RJ Jr, Watson RA, et al. Endourologic management of benign ureteral strictures with and without compromised vascular supply. Urology 2000; 55:652–657.

81. Razvi HA, Martin TV, Sosa ER, et al. Endourological management of complications of urinary intestinal diversion. AUA Update Ser 1996; 25:174–179.

82. Stein JP, Freeman JA, Esrig D, et al. Complications of the afferent antireflux valve mechanism in the Kock ileal reservoir. J Urol 1996; 155:1579–1583.

83. Boyd S, Everett RW, Schiff MM, et al. Treatment of unusual Kock pouch urinary calculi with extracorporeal shock wave lithotripsy. J Urol 1988; 139:805.

84. Huffman JL. Endoscopic management of complications of continent urinary diversion. Urology 1992; 39:145–149.

85. Jarrett TW, Pound CR, Kavoussi LR. Stone entrapment during percutaneous removal of infection stones from a continent diversion. J Urol 1999; 162:775–776.

13 | Complications of Urinary Diversion

Gregory S. Adey
Division of Urologic Surgery, Mercy Hospital, Portland, Maine, U.S.A.

Robert C. Eyre
Division of Urologic Surgery, Beth Israel Deaconess Medical Center, Boston, Massachusetts, U.S.A.

INTRODUCTION

Diversion of urine following radical cystoprostatectomy has a long history in the urologic literature. Although the first orthotopic urinary reconstruction was proposed in 1888 (1), it was not until the 1950s when this idea was reactivated. In 1935, Seiffert was the first to introduce the ileal conduit (2). In the 1950s, Bricker and others popularized the ileal conduit urinary diversion (3). Since that time, urinary diversions have expanded to include conduits, continent catheterizable reservoirs (CCR), and orthotopic bladder substitutions (OBS). In this chapter, we will examine the complications associated with each type of urinary diversion.

ILEAL CONDUIT

The ileal conduit has been the gold standard for urinary diversion following cystectomy for bladder carcinoma. Short- and long-term complications include stomal problems, anastomotic stricture, loop stricture, entero-loop fistula, bowel obstruction, urinary tract infection, metabolic derangements, and urolithiasis. In 2003, Madersbacher et al. (4) analyzed their series of 131 patients who had undergone ileal conduit urinary diversion with at least five years of follow-up (median 98 months, range 60–354 months). They found an astounding overall complication rate of 66%, including both short- and long-term complications. Most conduit-related morbidity is related to stomal problems, including parastomal hernia and stomal stenosis. Bringing the conduit through the rectus muscle and attaching it to the anterior rectus sheath will reduce the likelihood of developing a parastomal hernia (5). Parastomal hernias occur in 10% to 15% of patients (6). These almost always require surgical revision, as they can cause bowel obstruction as well as problems with appliance sealing to skin. Larger or recurrent parastomal hernias may require stomal relocation to the opposite side of the abdominal wall in order to properly repair the hernia. In all cases, the use of prosthetic graft materials should be avoided because of a high risk of graft infection.

The reported incidence of stomal stenosis is between 2% and 19%, and was 6% in the large series from Switzerland (4). Stomal stenosis often requires abdominal exploration in order to free the conduit at the level of the fascia. As the loop tends to lengthen with time, there is generally enough excess length to advance a fresh segment through the fascia to create a new, healthy everted stoma. Hyperkeratosis of the peristomal skin and mucosal surface of the stoma is rare. It is caused by excessive alkalinity of the urine, which is often associated with a loop infection with a urea-splitting organism. Vinegar soaks on the surface of the stoma generally resolve the problem, and patients should be encouraged to use urine-acidifying agents.

The skin site for placement of the stoma is very important and requires preoperative planning. The patient should be evaluated in the supine, seated, and standing positions in order to find the ideal right lower quadrant site that will maintain the stomal appliance properly. Many of the stomal problems occur within the first two years following urinary diversion. Most stomal problems can be avoided by careful attention at the time of original diversion to meticulous preservation of loop vascularity, avoiding tension on the loop, and creating a generous eversion of the stoma.

Anastomotic stricture is perhaps the most troubling of the complications associated with urinary conduit diversion. The incidence of stricture of the ureterointestinal junction is reported to be 4% to 8% of those patients with refluxing anastomoses (7). The development of stricture can occur at any point after ileal conduit diversion. In the early postoperative period, it is usually caused by technical errors during diversion surgery. Late strictures are usually caused by ischemic changes in the ureter caused by less than meticulous ureteral dissection, tension on the ureter, or radiation effect. The mean interval from conduit to treatment in a series of 23 patients from Canada was 45 months (range 1–432) (8).

Traditional treatment of these strictures involves open exploration with excision of the stenotic segment and reconstruction. Alternatively, one can bypass the stricture by doing a side-to-side anastomosis of the proximally dilated ureter to another site in the loop, which may reduce the risk of ischemic tissue at the distal edge of the divided ureter. More recently, there has been interest in less invasive means of intervention. Minimally invasive techniques include high-pressure balloon dilation or endoureterotomy using laser energy, cold-knife, or electrocautery. The results of high-pressure balloon dilation of anastomotic stricture are dismal and most centers have discontinued its use as a single modality of treatment (8). Mayo clinic evaluated their experience with initial open repair, and found an average operative time of 320 minutes and 86% patency rate at three years of follow-up (9). The three-year patency rate decreased to 76% when including those patients who had previously failed balloon dilation.

Endoureterotomy has received attention in the past decade. The principle is based on that of the Davis intubated ureterotomy, as described in the 1940s (10). Proponents of the laser endoureterotomy favor the direct-vision, controlled incision provided by the Holmium YAG (yttrium-aluminum-garnet), laser. The ability to directly observe surrounding arterial pulsation is one main advantage. The Holmium:YAG laser has a thermal injury zone of 0.5 to 1.0 mm, much smaller than the injury zone from standard electrocautery (11). Laser endoureterotomy is performed with a pulsed 80 W Holmium:YAG laser and a 365-micron end-firing quartz laser fiber, using settings of 0.6 to 2.0 J per pulse, and a pulse rate of 8 to 15 Hz. The incision is made until retroperitoneal fat is visualized, and an indwelling stent is left in place for six weeks. In a series of 24 laser endoureterotomies, the patency rate was 70.8% at a mean follow-up of 22.5 months (range 3–68), and there were no major complications (8).

Success rates vary for endoureterotomy performed with the Acucise cutting balloon catheter, with reports ranging from 30% (12) to 68% (13) at a mean follow-up of 18 and 25 months, respectively. The primary disadvantage of the Acucise balloon involves risk of injury to surrounding structures. Published case reports have described ureteroenteric fistula development and iliac artery injury with this technique (14). Some investigators are avoiding the use of transmittable energy with the cold-knife application. A series of 43 anastomotic strictures treated with cold-knife endoureterotomy in Germany showed promising results, with a patency rate of 60.5% at three years, follow-up (15). This particular technique involved multiple incisions made circularly around the stenotic segment (range 3–6), done with a flexible, wire-mounted cold-knife.

Irrespective of the technique chosen to repair the stricture, long-term follow-up is mandatory to ensure that failures are recognized. Wolf et al. (16) examined factors linked to endoureterotomy outcome, and they found that renal function greater than 25% correlated with increased success of endoureterotomy. These results have been substantiated by others (12,15). Should the stricture recur following endoscopic repair, subsequent treatment must consist of open revision, or continuous anastomotic stent changes. Success rates of all repeat endoscopic techniques are poor.

Bowel problems occur frequently after ileal conduit diversion. In the large series from Switzerland, 12% of patients developed small bowel obstruction. This can occur because a loop of small bowel may get stuck to the raw pelvic surface from the cystectomy or pelvic lymph node dissection site, from radiation changes to the bowel, or from an internal hernia, usually related to inadequate closure of the small bowel mesentery when developing the diversion segment. Half of these patients required operative adhesiolysis at a median of 22 months following diversion (4). Once recovered from the perioperative period, problems with fat and vitamin absorption, diarrhea, and other motility problems are quite rare. Anatomic knowledge in selecting a segment of ileum for diversion has all but eliminated these problems.

Colonization of the ileal conduit is usually the rule following diversion. The symptoms of urinary tract infection (UTI) after ileal conduit can be elusive, and often empiric treatment is necessary. One should be suspicious of changes in urine odor, generalized abdominal or back pain, hematuria, increased mucus production, or stomal tenderness. It is important that a culture specimen never be taken from the collection bag. It is mandatory that the appliance be removed, the stoma cleansed with betadine or chlorhexidine solution, and a sterile catheterized specimen be obtained from the conduit. In the patient with ileal conduit diversion and recurrent UTI, radiographic evaluation must be completed to look for nephrolithiasis, as well as loopography to ensure there is not stasis of urine within the conduit, anastomotic strictures, or loop strictures. Strictures of the conduit segment can be treated with an add-on ileal segment sutured to the proximal stump of the conduit distal to the ureteral anastomoses, with the new segment of bowel creating a new stoma.

Metabolic derangements after urinary diversion are related to the type and length of bowel used. Hyperchloremic metabolic acidosis is the most common disturbance after ileal conduit diversion. Mild acidosis is reported to occur in up to 15% of patients following ileal conduit diversion, with persistent acidosis requiring treatment in up to 10% (17). In the authors' experience, patients who present with ueteral obstruction prior to cystectomy and diversion are particularly at risk for persistent acidosis secondary to renal tubular acidosis. Treatment involves alkalizing agents, such as oral sodium bicarbonate. Chronic metabolic acidosis after urinary diversion is a very important complication to recognize, because if left untreated it will lead to debilitating bone demineralization (18). Patients who have an unexplained decline in renal function after diversion (increased creatinine from baseline) are often found to have metabolic acidosis. Correction of the acidosis often produces a rapid improvement in renal function. The clinician must maintain a high index of suspicion for metabolic acidosis when the patient with urinary diversion presents with nonspecific illness.

Upper urinary tract calculi following ileal conduit represent a challenge to the urologist. The risk of developing upper tract calculi is not well established. Studer et al. found a lifetime risk of 9% in their cohort (4). The risk increased with time from diversion as no patient developed an upper tract calculus during the first two years following diversion. The rate of stone formation increased to 20% within the first five years after conduit formation, and then increased to 38% after 10 years following diversion. Traditionally these calculi are treated with either extracorporeal shock wave lithotripsy or antegrade endoscopic techniques, because obtaining retrograde access through the conduit can be rather difficult. Wallace-type ureteral reimplantation at the time of ileal conduit creation makes subsequent attempts at retrograde ureterorenoscopy more feasible.

Entero-conduit fistulae are quite rare, and generally occur in the presence of a bowel anastomotic leak, poor external drainage during the initial postoperative period, and ureterointestinal anastomoses that are in direct proximity to the bowel anastomosis. This complication should be avoidable by careful inspection of the bowel anastomotic staple or suture line for leaks, closure of the bowel mesentery in a way that maximizes the separation of the reconstructed bowel from the conduit, and good drainage postoperatively. Initial management of this complication should include a period of total parenteral nutrition for at least two weeks coupled with continued external drainage. Re-exploration is necessary only if the bowel leak fails to resolve after an appropriate period of conservative management.

Many urologists counsel patients that the ileal conduit urinary diversion has a lower complication rate than the continent-type diversions. There are certain circumstances in which continent diversion is to be avoided and ileal conduit is the correct choice by default. These include, but are not limited to advanced age, compromised baseline renal function (creatinine >2.5), compromised manual dexterity that would complicate self catheterization, and diminished mental acuity. Specific contraindications to neobladder surgery include prior lower urinary tract surgery that might affect continence or the need for an en bloc urethrectomy. One must be careful to recognize, however, that even the gold standard ileal conduit carries a very high complication rate over the lifetime of the patient. Thus, follow-up for the patient with urinary diversion must continue indefinitely, and the urologist must remain vigilant for the development of late complications.

CONTINENT CATHETERIZABLE RESERVOIRS

Urinary diversion in the form of a CCR takes many different names. The original Indiana and Mainz pouches have been modified numerous times by several surgeons (19). The inadequacies of the ileal conduit have fueled the search for more effective means of urinary diversion.

The complications related to CCR are similar to those previously discussed with ileal conduit urinary diversion. This section of the chapter will be devoted to examining how the rates of these complications differ with CCR compared to ileal conduit diversion.

The use of CCR for urinary diversion has decreased in recent years as the use of OBS has increased. The most common type of CCR uses the right colon and terminal ileum to construct the reservoir. Some surgeons will detubularize the colonic portion (20), but the majority leave the bowel intact. The most common complications after CCR relate to the loss of the ileocecal valve and terminal ileum within the intestinal tract, and stomal problems.

All patients with urinary diversions are at risk for developing chronic metabolic acidosis. The risk of developing metabolic acidosis with CCR was 37% in a group of 94 patients followed for a median 9.0 years (21). The terminal ileum is the only site of vitamin B12 absorption in the gastrointestinal tract, and vitamin B12 levels need to be followed in patients with CCR. It may take years for signs of a vitamin B12 deficiency to develop, and approximately one-third of patients with CCR will require B12 supplementation (21). The loss of the terminal ileum may also cause decreased absorption of bile salts and fats. The combination of these with resection of the ileocecal valve can lead to chologenic diarrhea and steatorrhea in approximately one-third of patients with CCR. These problems are usually easily treatable with loperamide or cholestyramine.

As the CCR involves storage of urine, some were concerned that reservoir-filling pressures might pose an additional risk to the upper urinary tracts. Several studies have addressed this issue. Berglund and Kock found that baseline pressure is slightly higher inside cecal reservoirs when compared with the ileum (22). Goldwasser et al. determined the incidence of clinically significant contractions within different bowel CCRs. They found contractions exceeding 40 cmH$_2$O at volumes smaller than 200 mL in 70% of patients when tubularized ileum was used, 36% for tubularized right colon, 10% for detubularized colon, and 0% for detubularized ileum (23).

The use of antireflux procedures for ureteral reimplantation has been controversial when performing urinary diversion given concerns about upper tract deterioration from higher reservoir pressures and ascending infection. The risk of ureteral obstruction using nonrefluxing techniques is double the rate seen using refluxing anastomoses (24). The use of antirefluxing procedures dates back to an era when the use of tubularized colon was common and there was a valid concern about reservoir pressures. As described in the previous paragraph, the majority of CCRs created today are low-pressure. The reported obstruction rate after refluxing anastomosis varies between 1.7% and 3%, and between 10% and 13% for the nonrefluxing technique (25). Many surgeons have found a much higher rate of obstruction when using previously irradiated ureters and bowel, since continent diversions (particularly neobladders) require a longer length of ureter for construction. Webster et al. experienced a 28% anastomotic obstruction rate in those patients having previous pelvic radiation (20). The repair of ureteral anastomotic strictures was discussed in the previous section on ileal conduit diversion, and the same techniques and issues apply to all types of urinary diversion.

Difficulty with catheterization can occur after CCR. In a large series with long follow-up, stomal stenosis was seen in 4% of patients, while another 1.4% of their study group had difficulty with catheterization (20). When stomal stenosis occurs, it requires careful dilation. If this does not solve the problem, the stenosis can often be remedied with skin Y-V plasty. Retrograde contrast study and endoscopy of the channel must be utilized early in the treatment process. A flexible ureteroscope is often the best instrument for clear visualization of the entire channel. False passages, diverticula, and proximal stenoses are easily diagnosed by this technique.

Ischemic damage to the catheterizable segment may be seen if the appendix (Mitrofanoff technique) has inadequate vascular supply or is brought through the abdominal wall under tension, producing stomal retraction. Prolonged postoperative intubation of the catheterizable segment or excessive plication of an ileal catheterizable segment may also produce tissue necrosis. The ultimate result of ischemia may be severe stomal stenosis or necrosis that requires reconstruction of the segment, including an intussuscepted continent nipple valve.

Persistent incontinence of a CCR may have many causes, including inadequate capacity, high filling pressures, or inadequate nipple length and resistance. Occasionally, such situations may be remedied by injection of bulking agents into the ileal stomal segment of the junction with the reservoir, or by circumferential plication of the ileal segment at the level of the rectus fascia. One can also consider placing a prosthetic sleeve circumferentially around the stomal bowel segment at the level of the rectus fascia, although these have been associated with an increased risk of erosion, false passage, and infection.

ORTHOTOPIC BLADDER SUBSTITUTIONS

In the past decade, neobladders have established themselves as a safe, reliable form of urinary diversion for the appropriate patient. General principles of patient selection and exclusion criteria have been widely published. Complications of neobladders are similar to those already outlined, although one can avoid some of the issues of vitamin B12 deficiency, bile salt and fat malabsorption by preserving the terminal ileum and colon, using only an ileal segment for the neobladder. Several reconstructive techniques yield a high-capacity reservoir with good emptying capability, although all neobladders require a longer length of ureter in order for the segment to reach the urethral stump without tension.

The most troublesome issue with neobladders is an approximately 50% incidence of nocturnal incontinence. This can usually be managed with an external drainage device, clamp, or pad. It is important to instruct patients to empty their neobladder at bedtime, limit fluids after dinner, and get up at least once per night to void. Infection should be ruled out. Patients who incompletely void may benefit from self-catheterization at bedtime. Desmopressin (DDAVP) may also reduce the volume of nocturnal urine output. For patients with unacceptable stress incontinence, artificial urinary sphincters can be very beneficial.

REFERENCES

1. Tizzoni G, Foggi A. Die wiederherstellung der harnblase. Zentralb Chir 1888; 15:921–924.
2. Seiffert L. Die darm-siphonblase. Arch Klin Chir 1935; 183:569–573.
3. Bricker EM. Bladder substitution after pelvic eviseration. Surg Clin North Am 1950; 30:1511–1521.
4. Madersbacher S, Schmidt J, Eberle JM, et al. Long-term outcome of ileal conduit diversion. J Urol 2003; 169:985–990.
5. Killeen KP, Libertino JA. Management of bowel and urinary tract complications after urinary diversion. Urol Clin North Am 1988; 15:183–188.
6. Willams O, Vereb MJ, Libertino JA. Noncontinent urinary diversion. Urol Clin North Am 1997; 24:735–744.
7. Sullivan JW, Grabstald H, Whitmore WF. Complications of ureteroileal conduit with radical cystectomy: review of 336 cases. J Urol 1980; 124:797–801.
8. Watterson JD, Sofer M, Wollin TA, et al. Holmium:YAG laser endoureterotomy for ureterointestinal strictures. J Urol 2002; 167:1692–1695.
9. DiMarco DS, LeRoy AJ, Thieling S, et al. Long-term results of treatment for ureteroenteric strictures. Urology 2001; 58:909–913.
10. Davis D, Strong G, Drake W. Intubated ureterotomy: experimental work and clinical results. J Urol 1948; 59:851–859.
11. Johnson DE, Cromeens DM, Price RE. Use of the holmium:YAG laser in urology. Lasers Surg Med 1992; 12:353–363.
12. Lin DW, Bush WH, Mayo ME. Endourological treatment of ureteroenteric strictures: efficacy of Acucise endoureterotomy. J Urol 1999; 162:696–698.
13. Cornud F, Chretien Y, Helenon O, et al. Percutaneous incision of stenotic uroenteric anastomoses with a cutting balloon catheter: long-term results. Radiology 2000; 214:358–362.
14. Chandhoke PS, Clayman RV, Stone AM, et al. Endopyelotomy and endoureterotomy with the Acucise ureteral cutting balloon device: preliminary experience. J Endourol 1993; 7:45–51.
15. Poulakis V, Witzsch U, DeVries R, Becht E. Cold-knife endoureterotomy for nonmalignant ureterointestinal anastomotic strictures. Urology 2003; 61:512–517.
16. Wolf JS, Elashry OM, Clayman RV. Long-term results of endoureterotomy for benign ureteral and ureteroenteric strictures. J Urol 1997; 158:759–764.
17. Schmidt JD, Hawtrey CE, Flocks RH, Culp DA. Complications, results, and problems of ileal conduit diversions. J Urol 1973; 109:210–216.
18. Mills RD, Studer UE. Metabolic consequences of continent urinary diversion. J Urol 1999; 161:1057–1066.
19. Rowland RG, Mitchell ME, Bihrle R. The cecoileal continent urinary reservoir. World J Urol 1985; 3:185–190.

20. Webster C, Bukkapatnam R, Seigne JD, et al. Continent colonic urinary reservoir (Florida Pouch): long-term surgical complications (greater than 11 years). J Urol 2003; 169:174–176.
21. Pfitzenmaier J, Lotz J, Faldum A, et al. Metabolic evaluation of 94 patients 5 to 16 years after ileocecal pouch (Mainz pouch 1) continent urinary diversion. J Urol 1884; 170:1884–1887.
22. Berglund B, Kock NG. Volume capacity and pressure characteristics of various types of intestinal reservoirs. World J Surg 1987; 11:798–803.
23. Goldwasser B, Madgar I, Hanani Y. Urodynamic aspects of continent urinary diversions. Review. Scand J Urol Nephrol 1987; 21:245–253.
24. Hautmann RE, De Petriconi E, Gottfried H-W, et al. The ilealneobladder: complications and functional results in 363 patients after 11 years of followup. J Urol 1999; 161:422–428.
25. Hautmann RE. Urinary diversion: ileal conduit to neobladder. J Urol 2003; 169:834–842.

14 | Complications of Retroperitoneal Lymphadenectomy

Stephen D. W. Beck, Richard Bihrle, and Richard S. Foster
Department of Urology, Indiana University School of Medicine, Indianapolis, Indiana, U.S.A.

INTRODUCTION

The role of retroperitoneal lymph node dissection (RPLND) in the management of germ cell cancer is both staging and therapeutic. In low volume disease (clinical stage A/B1) primary RPLND defines the pathologic stage and is curative in the setting of metastatic disease allowing for the avoidance of chemotherapy. In larger volume metastatic disease primary therapy is cisplatin-based chemotherapy. Approximately 70% of patients are expected to obtain a complete response with resolution of radiographic disease and normalization of serum tumor markers. Postchemotherapy RPLND is performed for patients with residual retroperitoneal tumor with the final pathology revealing teratoma or active cancer in 50% to 60% of patients. The surgical technique for RPLND has evolved over the last 30 years with an associated decline in acute morbidity. In this chapter we will review the complications related to RPLND.

WOUND COMPLICATIONS

Though considered a minor complication, superficial wound infection is the most common complication with an incidence of 5% (1). The morbidity of superficial wound infection is low and treatment consists of wet to dry dressing changes. Incisional hernias are rare in this population with an incidence of less than 1%.

PULMONARY COMPLICATIONS

In the Indiana series, atelectasis was observed in 10 of 478 patients undergoing primary RPLND (1). This complication was largely minor with treatment being aggressive respiratory physiotherapy. In the postchemotherapy setting, atelectasis/pneumonia was observed in 34 of 603 patients with 15 considered minor and 19 major (2). Of patients with fever and leukocytosis the average hospital stay was 9.2 days (range 6–30) (Table 1–3).

Though atelectasis is a minor pulmonary complication, the most morbid complication in the postchemotherapy population was pulmonary related. In the Indiana series, 12 patients had severe pulmonary complications. Six patients had respiratory failure due to adult respiratory distress syndrome, which was also the cause of death in two. Five patients needed prolonged postoperative ventilation beyond 24 hours (range 2–5 days). A pulmonary embolism was diagnosed in one patient and treated successfully with systemic anticoagulation.

Severe pulmonary complications after RPLND are fortunately rare, and likely secondary to bleomycin toxicity. Bleomycin is known for producing acute interstitial pneumonia and chronic fibrotic changes in the lung. It exerts its cytotoxic effect by induction of free oxygen radicals, resulting in DNA breaks and cell death, as well as the inhibition of tumor angiogenesis. Due to the lack of the bleomycin-inactivating enzyme, bleomycin hydrolase in the lungs and skin, bleomycin-induced toxicity occurs predominantly in these organs. A multi-institutional study involving 812 testis cancer patients performed serial pulmonary function tests to define pulmonary toxicity related to bleomycin administration (3). This study revealed a median acute decline in carbon monoxide diffusion capacity (DCLO) of 19% in men who received a cumulative dose of 270 units. Chronic decline in DCLO has not been shown. The toxic death rate at this dose is less than 0.2%, with no long-term clinically significant impaired pulmonary function. At doses of 360 units, the toxic death rate increased to 1% to 2%.

Prior bleomycin exposure has been associated with an increased risk of postoperative pulmonary complications including fatal acute respiratory distress syndrome (ARDS). The

TABLE 1 Total Number of Complications in 1081 Patients Undergoing Retroperitoneal Lymph Node Dissection at Indiana University from 1982 to 1992

	No. minor	No. major	Total no. (%)
Wound infection	24	28	52 (4.8)
Pulmonary			
Pneumonia/atelectasis	16	28	44 (4.0)
Acute respiratory diseases syndrome	—	6	6 (0.5)
Prolonged ventilation		5	5 (0.4)
Pulmonary embolism	—	1	1 (0.01)
Small bowel obstruction	2	23	25 (2.3)
Chylous ascites	—	13	13 (1.2)
Lymphocele	—	11	11 (1.0)
Neural injury	—	7	7 (0.5)
Pancreatitis	—	7	7 (0.5)
Ureteral injury	4	4	8 (0.7)
Urinary tract infection	5	3	8 (0.7)
Renal infarction	—	3	3 (0.3)
Gastrointestinal bleed	2	1	3 (0.3)
Retroperitoneal bleed	—	2	2 (0.2)
Colon necrosis	—	1	1 (0.1)

Source: From Refs. 1 and 2.

TABLE 2 Total Number of Complications in 478 Patients Undergoing Primary Retroperitoneal Lymph Node Dissection at Indiana University from 1982 to 1992

	No. minor	No. major	Total no. (%)
Wound infection	11	12	23 (4.8)
Pneumonia/atelectasis	1	9	10 (2.0)
Small bowel obstruction	1	10	11 (2.3)
Chylous ascites	1	—	1 (0.2)
Lymphocele	1	—	1 (0.2)
Pancreatitis	1	—	1 (0.2)
Ureteral injury	1	—	1 (0.2)
Urinary tract infection	1	2	3 (0.6)
Ventral hernia	1	—	1 (0.2)

Source: From Ref. 1.

TABLE 3 Total Number of Complications in 603 Patients Undergoing Postchemotherapy Retroperitoneal Lymph Node Dissection at Indiana University from 1982 to 1992

	No. minor	No. major	Total no. (%)
Wound infection	13	16	29 (4.8)
Pulmonary			
Pneumonia/Atelectasis	15	19	34 (5.6)
Acute respiratory diseases syndrome	—	6	6 (1.0)
Prolonged ventilation	—	5	5 (0.8)
Pulmonary embolism	—	1	1 (0.2)
Small bowel obstruction	1	13	14 (2.3)
Chylous ascites	—	12	12 (2.0)
Lymphocele	—	10	10 (1.7)
Neural injury	—	7	7 (1.0)
Pancreatitis	—	6	6 (0.9)
Ureteral injury	3	3	6 (0.9)
Urinary tract infection	4	1	5 (0.8)
Renal infarction	—	3	3 (0.5)
Gastrointestinal bleed	2	1	3 (0.5)
Retroperitoneal bleed	—	2	2 (0.3)
Colon necrosis	—	1	1 (0.1)

Source: From Ref. 2.

etiology of postoperative ARDS in testis patients previously exposed to bleomycin is felt to be a combination of high inspired oxygen concentrations and large volumes of fluid. A hypervolemic state due to liberal intravenous fluid administration may cause interstitial edema and increase the diffusion defect in the presence of fixed pulmonary artery resistance. The result would require increasing levels of inspired oxygen potentially reaching toxic levels. In the 1980s and early 1990s at our institution, the postoperative management of such patients involved the judicious administration of postoperative fluid, preferring oliguria and prerenal creatinine rise to the potential morbidity of ARDS. In that era, fluid replacement was administered with caution, typically keeping maintenance fluid at 75 cc per hour accepting an hourly urine output of 10 to 15 cc. In a comparison of 150 postchemotherapy RPLND performed at Indiana University between 2000 and 2002 to 79 patients who underwent the same procedure between 1990 and 1992 there were fewer pulmonary complications in the contemporary group (4). With clinical experience, improved surgical technique with decrease blood loss and operative time, we no longer severely restrict postoperative hydration nor do we obtain pulmonary function tests. Massively obese patients, those who have received salvage chemotherapy, or have extensive surgical dissections are at higher risk of postoperative pulmonary complications and we would recommend judicious fluid administration with accurate monitoring of volume status in this select population.

LYMPHATIC COMPLICATIONS

After RPLND, lymphoceles can occur in 1% to 2% of patients (1). These are typically asymptomatic and do not warrant treatment, though can be misdiagnosed as recurrent retroperitoneal tumor.

Chylous ascites is rare after RPLND occurring in 2% of patients. Indiana University reported on 18 (1.1%) patients developing chylous ascites after 1520 RPLND from 1965 to 1992 (5). Chylous ascites is the accumulation of chylomicron-laden lymphatic fluid in the peritoneal cavity. Chylous ascites can occur secondary to obstruction or disruption of the abdominal lymphatic channels. The cisterna chyli drains the lower body and liver and represents the confluence of the right and left lymphatic trunks of the retroperitonuem. The cisterna is located on the body of the second lumbar vertebra, medial and posterior to the aorta, by the side of the right crus of the diaphragm. It then continues through the aortic hiatus as the thoracic duct and ascends into the venous system at the junction of the left internal jugular and subclavian vein. Damage to the thoracic duct may lead to chylousthorax.

Long-chain triglycerides are absorbed in the intestine by the omental lymphatics and empty into the cisterna chyli. After a fatty meal lymph flow can increase from 1–200 mL/kg/hr and if the lacteals are disrupted lymph may accumulate in the abdomen (6). Lymph is a transparent, colorless, or slightly yellow watery fluid with a specific gravity of 1.015, closely resembling plasma, and contains about 5% protein and 1% salt and other extracts. In contrast, chyle is an opaque, milky-white fluid, absorbed by the villi of the small intestines and carried to the lymphatics by vessels name lacteals. Chyle differs from lymph in its chemical properties in that it contains a large quantity of fats, soaps, lecithin, and cholesterin.

Risk factors for developing chylous ascites after RPLND include extensive, high volume disease, suprahilar dissection, and vena cava resection (5). Abundant lymphatic vessels and the cisterna chyli are located above the renal vessels and supra hilar dissection may lead to inadvertent transection, and without appropriate ligation, the development of chylous ascites. Six of the 18 patients developing chylous ascites reported in the Indiana series underwent simultaneous vena cava resection. The association between chylous ascites and cava resection is probably secondary to the interruption of venous return. Lymphatic vessels communicate with the venous system and with the interruption of venous return a high lymphatic pressure may develop with subsequent leakage.

Clinical signs and symptoms of chylous ascites include abdominal distention, increase abdominal girth, weight gain, and dyspnea. Dyspnea may be secondary to poor inspiratory volumes or chylothorax. Paracentesis is the primary means of diagnosis and can be therapeutic. Diagnosis is confirmed in identifying fluid that is milky, stains positive for fat, has an alkaline pH and leukocytes on cytology. Triglyceride content is higher while the protein level is lower than observed in the serum (7). With removal of fluid via paracentesis, symptoms may improve; however, this is typically transitory and not curative. Multiple paracentesis, while capable of temporarily relieving symptoms, can lead to peritonitis, protein wasting, and malnutrition.

Definitive management of chylous ascites includes dietary modifications to decrease mesenteric lymphatic flow, peritoneovenous shunts, and reoperation. Long-chain triglycerides are transported through the mesenteric lymphatics and into the cisterna. Median-chain triglycerides bypass the mesenteric lymphatics and drain directly into the liver via the portal vein. As such, a low fat diet restricted to median-chain triglycerides with the addition of diuretics may be curative in up to 50% of patients with mild to moderate symptoms.

For more severe symptoms or if conservative therapy fails, total parenteral nutrition should be considered, which will decrease mesenteric lymph flow and provide nutrition for healing. These patients are often treated with an indwelling percutaneous drain to alleviate symptoms while on hyperalimentation for several weeks. We feel it is better for interventional radiology to anchor a permanent drain versus repeated paracentesis.

In refractory cases, somatostatin has been shown to be effective in closing lymphatic fistulas (8–13). Somatostatin is a naturally occurring peptide present in the central nervous system, the pancreas, and the gastrointestinal tract. The somatostatin analog, octreotide, has been shown to decrease intestinal absorption of fats, lower triglyceride concentration in the thoracic duct, and decrease lymph flow in the major lymphatic channels (11). Shapiro et al. reported resolution of chylous ascites after a liver transplantation within two days of starting hyperalimentation and octreotide (10). Similarly, Leibovitch et al. reported a case of refractory chylous ascites after radical nephrectomy and inferior vena cava (IVC) thrombectomy with drainage of 1000 to 2000 cc on hyperalimentation decreasing to 150 cc after two days of starting octreotide 100 µg three times a day (9). The addition of octreotide with total parenteral nutrition should be considered in patients failing more conservative therapy.

Placement of peritoneovenous shunts (LeVeen shunts) should be considered for patients who have continued chylous leak despite hyperalimentation. LeVeen et al. originally reported the use of such shunts in eight adults and two children with chylous ascites (14). The patency rate was 80% in this report while others have reported a higher occlusion rate (50%) and other complications including sepsis and compartmentalization secondary to adhesions (7). Shunt placement remains controversial, though it should be at least considered for patients failing more conservative therapy.

To avoid the potential lengthy time (weeks to months) conservative therapy requires for chylous ascites to resolve, or for refractory cases, some authors have advocated surgery. The rationale is that at reoperation any leaking lymphatic can be ligated. The leak is often identified by locating the milky discharge, if not an injection of lipophilic sudan black into the bowel mesentery can aid in identifying the leak. Others report a high rate of failure in identifying and controlling the lymphatic channels (7,15). As conservative therapy is successful in the majority of patients, we feel that re-operation has a minimal role in the management of chylous ascites.

In populations at high risk of chylous ascites (large volume disease, suprahilar dissection, and vena caval resection) we now anchor an intraperitoneal drain to prevent the accumulation of chlyi. The drain is removed when output is less than 100 cc per 24 hours. As postchemotherapy patients are discharged typically by postoperative day 4 or 5, these patients often go home with the drain in place and are removed when the output decreases. They are placed on no special diet. The vast majority of patients do not have a drain placed at surgery and do not develop chylous ascites. If this does occur, our typical recommendation is to first place an intraperitoneal drain and follow output for four to six weeks, if output remains high then hyperalimentation is started. It is unusual for these conservative measures to fail.

GASTROINTESTINAL COMPLICATIONS

Intraoperative bowel injury is uncommon during RPLND and when recognized has little morbidity. Subserosal injury to the duodenum may occur during mobilization of the second and third portion of the duodenum off the vena cava and area often densely adherent. Duodenal leak and fatal aortoduodenal fistula has been reported (16). Small bowel ileus is the most common postoperative bowel complication typically seen in 2% to 3% of patients (1). Morbidity from this is little, with therapy being bowel rest and at times temporary placement of a naso-gastric tube. Similarly, small bowel obstruction is seen in 2% to 3% of patients and usually can be managed conservatively. With the nerve-sparing technique, this is the single long-term morbidity after RPLND.

In the majority of postchemotherapy surgery, the inferior mesenteric artery (IMA) is ligated in order to mobilize the left colon laterally to obtain exposure to the para aortic space. Due to the dual blood supply of the distal colon via the marginal artery the IMA can be ligated with little concern for any sequelae. A potential exception to this is in older men with compromised vascularity resulting from age, chemotherapy, or radiotherapy. One of 603 patients undergoing postchemotherapy RPLND from 1982 to 1992 at Indiana University developed postoperative sepsis with an acute abdomen (2). At surgical exploration a necrotic left colon was identified. This patient had received extensive abdominal radiotherapy possibly affecting the mesenteric blood supply to the colon.

GENITOURINARY COMPLICATIONS

Ureteral injury is uncommon and typically occurs in the postchemotherapy setting. At primary RPLND, one ureteral injury occurred in 478 cases at Indiana University. At postchemotherapy surgery, there were six (0.9%) ureteral injuries in 603 patients (Tables 1–3). In two of these six patients, the ureters were resected primarily due to tumor involvement without renal obstruction and four were inadvertently damaged during dissection. These four ureteral lacerations were repaired by primary anastamosis and stenting at time of the RPLND. Two patients had delayed diagnosis of a ureteral leak which ultimately required ileal ureter for repair (2). Memorial Sloan Kettering reported a 3% rate of ureteral injury in 57 patients undergoing "redo" postchemotherapy surgery (17). Ureters densely adhered to the tumor requiring close dissection may lead to ischemic ureteral stricture requiring reoperation.

The need for nephrectomy to ensure tumor clearance is typically dictated by encasement of the renal vein or the renal artery. Renal artery injury or aggressive manipulation may occur and impair renal function. In the Indiana series of 603 postchemotherapy surgeries, two patients were diagnosed with postoperative renal infarction. These patients presented with hypertension one to two months postoperatively with renal scan revealing absent perfusion. Progressive hypertension nonresponsive to conservative therapy in this population has been treated with nephrectomy, though this is uncommon. The German Testicular Cancer Study Group reported one (0.4%) renal artery laceration requiring nephrectomy in 239 patients undergoing primary RPLND (18).

Lower pole renal arteries are present in 10% to 15% of renal units and are at risk of transection during RPLND. Treatment options include repair with primary vascular anastamosis or formally transecting the lower pole renal artery. While the former may preserve renal parenchyma (roughly 10% for small lower pole renal arteries) it carries the risk of hypertension. Though injury to a lower pole renal artery is rare, in such instances, we feel it is less morbid to sacrifice the lower pole renal artery, which will have little or no effect on overall renal function than risk renal vascular hypertension in this young population.

NEUROLOGIC COMPLICATIONS

Neurologic sequelae after RPLND are uncommon and if present are typically transitory. In 603 postchemotherapy surgeries in the Indiana series, seven patients experienced a peripheral neurologic injury. Three patients had femoral neuropraxia, three had brachial nerve injury, and one had Horner's syndrome postoperatively. Two patients had early recovery of all neurologic deficits while the remaining five patients had prolonged recovery. The primary cause of peripheral neuropraxia, not unique to retroperitoneal surgery, is secondary to a compression or stretch injury to the nerve. Nerve compression or stretch can be caused by patient positioning or inappropriate placement of abdominal retractors. Patient positioning for a thoracoabdominal incision may place stretch on the brachial plexus and care must be taken to ensure the arm is not overextended and the axilla in supported. Currently we rarely use the thoracoabdominal incision. Inappropriate retractor placement with prolonged pressure to the psoas muscle may result in femoral nerve injury. Risk factors for femoral neuropraxia include thin patients and pelvic surgery.

Spinal cord ischemia with resultant permanent paraplegia is a feared complication of RPLND. The arterial blood supply to the spinal cord consists of three interconnected arterial systems. The outer extraspinal system is the primary blood supply consisting of interconnecting multiple branches including the vertebral, costocervical, intercostal, lumbar, and sacral arteries. The innermost arterial system comprises three arteries lying along the surface of the spinal cord and include two posterior spinal arteries and one anterior spinal artery. The single anterior spinal artery supplies two-thirds of the cord and is fed by the third arterial system, the anterior radicular branches (one or two cervical, one or two thoracic, and one or two lumbarsacral).

The great anterior radicular artery (the artery of Adamkiewicz) is the most significant radicular artery and is often the major artery supplying the lumbosacral cord. The origin of this artery is variable with 80% arising off the left side of the aorta as either a lower intercostal or higher lumber artery. Seventy-five percent arise between T9 and T12, 15% at L1–L2, and 10% at T4–T8 (19,20). Interruption of the great anterior radicular artery is commonly felt to be the primary cause of spinal cord ischemia after aortic surgery but the exact mechanisms remain unclear and are likely multifactorial.

The incidence of spinal cord ischemia after aortic aneurysm repair is 0.3% and increases to 1.4% to 2.0% for emergent cases (19–23). Leibovitch et al. reported a 0.56% incidence of spinal cord ischemia identified in 4 of 712 patients undergoing RPLND at Indiana University (24). Motor neuralgic deficits in all four patients included flaccid paraparesis in one or both lower extremities with decrease strength and hypo or areflexia. Three patients had loss of light touch below the level of T10/L1. All patients developed urinary retention. Treatment consisted of physical therapy and corticosteroids with improvement of motor and sensory function by six days. These four patients all had extensive nodal dissection above the level of the renal vessels and/or retrocrural dissection.

Risk factors for spinal cord ischemia include older age, extensive retroperitoneal disease requiring suprahilar, retrocrural, or posterior mediastinal dissection, previous RPLND, prolonged aortic cross clamping, and history of abdominal radiation. Though the development of spinal cord ischemia is both uncommon and unpredictable, the routine ligation of all lumbar arteries at RPLND should be reconsidered in high-risk patients, specifically those requiring bilateral retrocrural dissection. In such patients, preservation of an upper lumbar artery or lower intercostal artery should be at least entertained as long as tumor resection is not compromised.

FERTILITY

Thirty to fifty percent of men presenting with testicular cancer have some degree of underlying impairment of spermatogenesis. Pre-orchiectomy gonadal function was evaluated by Petersen et al. in 71 patients and semen analysis in 63 (25). Sperm concentration (15 million/mL) and total sperm count (29 million) in patients with testicular cancer prior to any therapy were significantly lower than that found in the control group (48 million/mL and 162 million, respectively). Follicular-stimulating hormone levels were increased in men with testicular cancer at a median of 5.7 IU/L compared to a median of 4.1 IU/L for controls (P = 0.001). Luteinizing hormone levels, however, were significantly lower in the testis cancer group compared to the control with a median of 3.6 and 4.7 IU/L, respectively (P = 0.01). Also noted was a significant decrease in sperm concentration, total count, and motility compared to controls (26). Of 51 patients, 45% had sperm concentrations less than 20 million/mL and 23% had counts less than 10 million/mL. Fertility may be further impaired with treatment including cisplatin-based chemotherapy affecting spermatogenesis or retroperitoneal surgery with transection of postganglionic lumbar sympathetic fibers with loss of emission and antegrade ejaculation.

In managing clinical stage A nonseminomatous germ cell tumor, the major impetus behind surveillance strategies was the loss of antegrade emission after full bilateral RPLND. With modified templates more patients maintained antegrade ejaculation but some continued to suffer loss of emission. With better understating of the anatomy of the postganglionic sympathetic nerve fibers, nerve-sparing techniques were developed initially in low-stage testis cancer in an attempt to preserve ejaculation. On the right side, the postganglions sympathetic chain is posterior to the vena cava with nerve fibers (L2, L3, L4) coursing medially to join the condensed sympathetic trunk in the ventral preaortic tissue. The left sympathetic chain is dorsolateral to the aorta. The nerve fibers L2–L4 can be recognized and preserved along the anterolateral aspect of the lower aorta.

Jewett et al. reported outcomes of 20 patients undergoing nerve-sparing surgery of whom 18 (90%) maintained antegrade ejaculation (27). Donohue et al. subsequently reported on 75 patients undergoing nerve-sparing RPLND, of whom all 75 maintained ejaculation (28). Foster et al. evaluated pregnancy rates in patients undergoing nerve-sparing surgery (26). A fertility questionnaire was sent to 289 patients of whom 201 (69%) responded. Ninety patients did not attempt pregnancy and were excluded. Of 66 patients attempting pregnancy after nerve-sparing RPLND, 50 (76%) were successful. Wahle et al. reported on 38 patients undergoing postchemotherapy nerve-sparing RPLND (29). At a minimum follow-up of 12 months there were no reported retroperitoneal relapses with 34 of 38 reporting normal ejaculation. In a subsequent report from Indiana University, Coogan et al. reviewed 472 patient charts undergoing postchemotherapy RPLND of whom 93 (19.7%) had a nerve-sparing procedure (30). Of the 93 patients, two died and ejaculatory status could not be confirmed in 10. Of the remaining 81 patients, 76.5% retained antegrade emission with 10 pregnancies. There were six recurrences all outside of the retroperitoneum.

While patients with testicular cancer may have some degree of underlying impairment of spermatogenesis, surgery in clinical stage A disease is a viable option in young men were fertility remains important. First, if the patient has pathologic stage B disease, RPLND is therapeutic with a high likelihood of avoiding systemic chemotherapy and secondly, with nerve-sparing techniques, antegrade emission will be preserved in 99% of patients. Likewise, in the postchemotherapy setting, in select patients, nerve-sparing technique can be performed without compromising cure.

VASCULAR COMPLICATIONS

Major vascular injuries after primary RPLND are uncommon. The German testicular cancer study group reported clinical outcomes of 209 patients undergoing primary RPLND (18). The mean blood loss was 150 cc (range 80–1800). Only two patients required blood transfusions. Vascular injuries to the renal artery, superior mesenteric artery, and the IVC were noted in six cases (2.5%). In a consecutive series of 75 patients at Indiana University undergoing primary RPLND, the mean blood loss was 207 cc (range 20–500) with no patient requiring a blood transfusion (31).

In the postchemotherapy setting vascular injuries and significant hemorrhage is more common but not well reported. In the Indiana series, 2 of 603 patients undergoing postchemotherapy surgery experienced a postoperative bleed. Both were on anticoagulation, one for a pulmonary embolism and one with a deep venous thrombosis. One patient was managed conservatively while one underwent exploratory laparotomy with no obvious site of bleeding identified.

An important technical aspect in postchemotherapy surgery is dissection of the retroperitoneal tumor away from the great vessels in the correct plane. Subadvantitial dissection, though often an easier dissection, weakens both the aorta and vena cava. Jaeger et al. reported a death from postoperative aortic rupture after postchemotherapy surgery (32). Babaian et al. described a case of fatal postoperative aortic rupture after inadvertent enterotomy following RPLND (33). Skinner et al. suggested the use of aortic sleeve graft to prevent aneurysm formation after extensive aortic dissection (34). From the same institution, Carter et al. later reported a postoperative aortoduodenal fistula (35). Donohue et al. described three patients requiring postoperative aortic grafts after postchemotherapy RPLND (36). One patient had an aortic rupture nine hours postoperatively and underwent emergent aortic graft placement. He died of recurrent disease 42 months later. In two patients, an aorto-enteric fistula presented 9 and 24 days postoperatively. Each operation involved bowel resection and extensive aortic dissection. One patient died two days after aortic replacement, while the other survived after an extended hospital stay. These series demonstrate the potential complications of subadvantitial aortic dissection. In this clinical situation or when the tumor cannot be safely peeled off the aorta, aortic replacement should be performed. In a review of 1250 cases at Indiana University from 1970 to 1998, 15 patients underwent aortic replacement (37). Eleven patients underwent 15 additional procedures including nephrectomy in seven, vena caval resection in three, pulmonary resection in one, small bowel resection in two, hepatic resection in one, and L4 vertebrectomy in one. Of the 15 patients, 12 received first and second-line chemotherapy prior to surgery. There were no graft-related complications with an overall survival of 33%.

Similarly, subadvantitial dissection along the vena cava can significantly weaken the caval wall making suturing of any cavotomy difficult. The involvement of the IVC by tumor necessitating resection occurs in 6% to 11% patients (38). In a retrospective review of the Indiana University database from 1973 to 1996, 955 patients were identified with bulky (B2/B3) postchemotherapy residual disease (39). Of this cohort, 65 (6.8%) underwent vena cava resection. Twenty-four of the sixty five patients remained alive at a median follow-up of 89 months. These 24 patients all responded to a written or verbal survey to assess long-term morbidity of IVC resection. The IVC had intraluminal thrombus in 16 of 24 patients with pathology revealing active cancer in four, teratoma in three and fibrosis in nine. Long-term morbidity was assessed via the american venous forum international consensus form. Long-term disability was absent or mild (disability score of 0 or 1) in 75% of patients. Two patients had moderate disability and one patient alive at 149 months had chronic calf ulceration, abdominal varicosities, and lifestyle limitations. The university of southern california reported on 11 of 19 patients surviving longer than six months after postchemotherapy RPLND and IVC resection (40). With a follow-up of 9 to 120 months, four (36%) patients continued to have lower extremity edema, three (27%) complained of chronic lower extremity pain and paresthesia, one had varicose veins, and one had thrombophlebitits.

Dissection along the great vessels can cause significant morbidity if performed in the incorrect plane. When tumor clearance demands subadvantitial dissection or even resection, though uncommon, both aortic replacement and vena cava resection can be performed safely with acceptable long-term morbidity.

SEMINOMA

Approximately 25% of patients with pure seminoma present with metastatic disease and are treated with systemic chemotherapy. Management of residual masses in this population is controversial. The desmoplastic reaction and fibrosis encountered makes the surgery technically demanding, with incomplete resections and high patient morbidity (41–44). Even seminomatous elements in the retroperitoneum in patients with metastatic non-seminomatous disease increases patient morbidity at postchemotherapy surgery. Mosharafa et al. evaluated the morbidity of 97 patients with elements of seminoma in the dissected specimen compared to 1269 patients with no component of seminoma (45). Of the 97 patients in the seminoma group, 37 (38.1%) required a total of 47 additional intraoperative procedures including 25 nephrectomies, nine IVC resections, five arterial grafts, five bowel resections, and three hepatic resections/biopsies, compared with 340 of the 1269 patients (26.8%) in the group without seminomatous elements (P = 0.02). Postoperative complications occurred in 24 of 97 patients (24.7%) in the seminoma group versus 257 of 1269 (20.3%) in the group without seminomatous elements (P = 0.29).

Fortunately, with the introduction of positron emission tomography (PET scan), the controversy regarding residual masses in patients with pure seminoma is largely over. In the European study evaluating PET imaging in metastatic pure seminoma, 51 patients with 56 masses underwent PET scan after chemotherapy (46). In this study, the positive predictive value of PET scan was 100% and the negative predictive value was 96% for residual masses greater than 3 cm.

QUALITY OF LIFE

RPLND over the last 30 years has maintained its therapeutic benefit while reducing patient morbidity. Quality of life is difficult to quantitate. The reduction in patient morbidity is largely observed in low stage disease with the introduction of nerve-sparing techniques preserving emission and antegrade ejaculation. With improved surgical technique and anesthesia, morbidity after both primary and postchemotherapy surgery has declined. In a consecutive series of 75 patients undergoing primary RPLND at Indiana University, the mean operative time was 132 minutes (range 81–246), mean blood loss was 207 cc (range 50–500 cc). Nasogastric tubes were placed in only two (2.7%) patients. Clear liquids were started on day 1 and the mean hospital stay was 2.8 days (range 2–4) (31). Likewise in the postchemotherapy setting, comparing a contemporary group of 150 patients from July 2000 to July 2002 to 79 patients undergoing postchemotherapy surgery from 1990 to 1992, Mosharafa et al. demonstrated fewer intraoperative complications and additional procedures in the contemporary group versus historical controls (29.3% vs. 51.9%, respectively, P = 0.0008) (4). Average hospital stay also decreased with a mean hospital stay of 5.6 days in the contemporary group versus 8.4 days in the 1992 group (P=0.0001). As with primary RPLND we no longer routinely place nasogastric tubes and typically start clear liquids on postoperative day 1 or 2.

CONCLUSIONS

Complications from RPLND are infrequent and usually minor and self-limiting. In the primary group, with the adoption of the nerve-sparing technique, the long-term morbidity is limited to small bowel obstruction. In the postchemotherapy group, additional intraoperative procedures, postoperative complications, and hospital stay have continued to decline. In centers devoted to the management of testicular cancer, RPLND can be performed safely, offering therapeutic benefit with little morbidity. At times a more aggressive surgical approach is necessary to ensure tumor clearance and include aortic replacement and IVC resection, both of which have acceptable long-term morbidity.

REFERENCES

1. Baniel J, Foster RS, Rowland RG, Bihrle R, Donohue JP. Complications of primary retroperitoneal lymph node dissection. J Urol 1994; 152(2 Pt 1):424–427.
2. Baniel J, Foster RS, Rowland RG, Bihrle R, Donohue JP. Complications of post-chemotherapy retroperitoneal lymph node dissection. J Urol 1995; 153(3 Pt 2):976–980.
3. de Wit R, Roberts JT, Wilkinson PM, et al. Equivalence of three or four cycles of bleomycin, etoposide, and cisplatin chemotherapy and of a 3- or 5-day schedule in good-prognosis germ cell cancer: a randomized study of the European Organization for Research and Treatment of Cancer Genitourinary Tract Cancer Cooperative Group and the Medical Research Council. J Clin Oncol 2001; 19:1629–1640.
4. Mosharafa AA, Foster RS, Koch MO, Bihrle R, Donohue JP. Complications of post-chemotherapy retroperitoneal lymph node dissection for testis cancer. J Urol 2004; 171:1839–1841.
5. Baniel J, Foster RS, Rowland RG, Bihrle R, Donohue JP. Management of chylous ascites after retroperitoneal lymph node dissection for testicular cancer. J Urol 1993; 150(5 Pt 1):1422–1424.
6. Meinke AH III, Estes NC, Ernst CB. Chylous ascites following abdominal aortic aneurysmectomy. Management with total parenteral hyperalimentation. Ann Surg 1979; 190:631–633.
7. Press OW, Press NO, Kaufman SD. Evaluation and management of chylous ascites. Ann Intern Med 1982; 96:358–364.
8. Huang Q, Jiang ZW, Jiang J, Li N, Li JS. Chylous ascites: treated with total parenteral nutrition and somatostatin. World J Gastroenterol 2004; 10:2588–2591.
9. Leibovitch I, Mor Y, Golomb J, Ramon J. Chylous ascites after radical nephrectomy and inferior vena cava thrombectomy. Successful conservative management with somatostatin analogue. Eur Urol 2002; 41:220–222.
10. Shapiro AM, Bain VG, Sigalet DL, Kneteman NM. Rapid resolution of chylous ascites after liver transplantation using somatostatin analog and total parenteral nutrition. Transplantation 1996; 61: 1410–1411.
11. Collard JM, Laterre PF, Boemer F, Reynaert M, Ponlot R. Conservative treatment of postsurgical lymphatic leaks with somatostatin-14. Chest 2000; 117:902–905.
12. Fernandez Balaguer P, Suarez Miguelez JM, Galeano Diaz F, et al. Use of somatostatin in the conservative treatment of external pancreatic fistula. Rev Esp Enferm Apar Dig 1989; 76:222–228.
13. Ulibarri JI, Sanz Y, Fuentes C, Mancha A, Aramendia M, Sanchez S. Reduction of lymphorrhagia from ruptured thoracic duct by somatostatin. Lancet 1990; 336:258.
14. LeVeen HH, Wapnick S, Grosberg S, Kinney MJ. Further experience with peritoneo-venous shunt for ascites. Ann Surg 1976; 184:574–581.

15. Ablan CJ, Littooy FN, Freeark RJ. Postoperative chylous ascites: diagnosis and treatment. A series report and literature review. Arch Surg 1990; 125:270–273.
16. Bihrle R, Foster RS, Donohue JP. Complications of post chemotherapy retroperitoneal lymph node dissection. Urol Clin North Am 1988; 15:237–242.
17. McKiernan JM, Motzer RJ, Bajorin DF, Bacik J, Bosl GJ, Sheinfeld J. Reoperative retroperitoneal surgery for nonseminomatous germ cell tumor: clinical presentation, patterns of recurrence, and outcome. Urology 2003; 62:732–736.
18. Heidenreich A, Albers P, Hartmann M, et al. Complications of primary nerve sparing retroperitoneal lymph node dissection for clinical stage I nonseminomatous germ cell tumors of the testis: experience of the German Testicular Cancer Study Group. J Urol 2003; 169:1710–1714.
19. Dommisse GF. The blood supply of the spinal cord. A critical vascular zone in spinal surgery. J Bone Joint Surg Br 1974; 56:225–235.
20. Szilagyi DE, Hageman JH, Smith RF, Elliott JP. Spinal cord damage in surgery of the abdominal aorta. Surgery 1978; 83:38–56.
21. Dunki Jacobs PB, Dicke HW. Ischemic damage to the spinal cord following surgery of the abdominal aorta. Neth J Surg 1984; 36:1–5.
22. Ross RT. Spinal cord infarction in disease and surgery of the aorta. Can J Neurol Sci 1985; 12:289–295.
23. Sandson TA, Friedman JH. Spinal cord infarction. Report of 8 cases and review of the literature. Medicine (Baltimore) 1989; 68:282–292.
24. Leibovitch I, Nash PA, Little JS Jr, Foster RS, Donohue JP. Spinal cord ischemia after post-chemotherapy retroperitoneal lymph node dissection for nonseminomatous germ cell cancer. J Urol 1996; 155:947–951.
25. Petersen PM, Skakkebaek NE, Vistisen K, Rorth M, Giwercman A. Semen quality and reproductive hormones before orchiectomy in men with testicular cancer. J Clin Oncol 1999; 17:941–947.
26. Foster RS, McNulty A, Rubin LR, et al. The fertility of patients with clinical stage I testis cancer managed by nerve sparing retroperitoneal lymph node dissection. J Urol 1994; 152:1139–1142; discussion 42–43.
27. Jewett MA, Kong YS, Goldberg SD, et al. Retroperitoneal lymphadenectomy for testis tumor with nerve sparing for ejaculation. J Urol 1988; 139:1220–1224.
28. Donohue JP, Foster RS, Rowland RG, Bihrle R, Jones J, Geier G. Nerve-sparing retroperitoneal lymphadenectomy with preservation of ejaculation. J Urol 1990; 144(2 Pt 1):287–291; discussion 91–92.
29. Wahle GR, Foster RS, Bihrle R, Rowland RG, Bennett RM, Donohue JP. Nerve sparing retroperitoneal lymphadenectomy after primary chemotherapy for metastatic testicular carcinoma. J Urol 1994; 152(2 Pt 1):428–430.
30. Coogan CL, Hejase MJ, Wahle GR, et al. Nerve sparing post-chemotherapy retroperitoneal lymph node dissection for advanced testicular cancer. J Urol 1996; 156:1656–1658.
31. Beck SDW, Peterson MD, Foster RS, Bihrle R, Donohue JP. What is the short-term morbidity of primary retroperitoneal lymph node dissection in a contemporary group of patients? Am Urol Assoc 2006 (Abstract).
32. Jaeger N, Weissbach L, Hartlapp JH, Vahlensieck W. Risk/benefit of treating retroperitoneal teratoid bulky tumors. Urology 1989; 34:14–17.
33. Babaian RJ, Bracken RB, Johnson DE. Complications of transabdominal retroperitoneal lymphadenectomy. Urology 1981; 17:126–128.
34. Skinner DG, Melamud A, Lieskovsky G. Complications of thoracoabdominal retroperitoneal lymph node dissection. J Urol 1982; 127:1107–1110.
35. Carter GE, Lieskovsky G, Skinner DG, Daniels JR. Reassessment of the role of adjunctive surgical therapy in the treatment of advanced germ cell tumors. J Urol 1987; 138:1397–1401.
36. Donohue JP, Thornhill JA, Foster RS, Bihrle R. Vascular considerations in postchemotherapy. Retroperitoneal lymph-node dissection: Part II. World J Urol 1994; 12:187–189.
37. Beck SD, Foster RS, Bihrle R, Koch MO, Wahle GR, Donohue JP. Aortic replacement during post-chemotherapy retroperitoneal lymph node dissection. J Urol 2001; 165:1517–1520.
38. Albers P, Melchior D, Muller SC. Surgery in metastatic testicular cancer. Eur Urol 2003; 44:233–244.
39. Beck SD, Lalka SG, Donohue JP. Long-term results after inferior vena caval resection during retroperitoneal lymphadenectomy for metastatic germ cell cancer. J Vasc Surg 1998; 28:808–814.
40. Spitz A, Wilson TG, Kawachi MH, Ahlering TE, Skinner DG. Vena caval resection for bulky metastatic germ cell tumors: an 18-year experience. J Urol 1997; 158:1813–1818.
41. Flechon A, Bompas E, Biron P, Droz JP. Management of post-chemotherapy residual masses in advanced seminoma. J Urol 2002; 168:1975–1979.
42. Friedman EL, Garnick MB, Stomper PC, Mauch PM, Harrington DP, Richie JP. Therapeutic guidelines and results in advanced seminoma. J Clin Oncol 1985; 3:1325–1332.
43. Ravi R, Vasanthan A. Intraoperative irradiation: another option for the treatment of > or = 3 cm residual mass following chemotherapy for advanced testicular seminoma. Urol Int 1995; 55:137–140.

44. Schultz SM, Einhorn LH, Conces DJ Jr, Williams SD, Loehrer PJ. Management of postchemotherapy residual mass in patients with advanced seminoma: Indiana University experience. J Clin Oncol 1989; 7:1497–1503.
45. Mosharafa AA, Foster RS, Leibovich BC, Bihrle R, Johnson C, Donohue JP. Is post-chemotherapy resection of seminomatous elements associated with higher acute morbidity? J Urol 2003; 169:2126–2128.
46. De Santis M, Becherer A, Bokemeyer C, et al. 2-18fluoro-deoxy-D-glucose positron emission tomography is a reliable predictor for viable tumor in postchemotherapy seminoma: an update of the prospective multicentric SEMPET trial. J Clin Oncol 2004; 22:1034–1039.

15 | Complications of Renal Transplantation

Michael J. Malone, Sanjaya Kumar, and Stefan G. Tullius
Division of Transplant Surgery, Brigham and Women's Hospital, Boston, Massachusetts, U.S.A.

INTRODUCTION

Renal transplantation has flourished since the first reports of successful living-related and cadaveric human transplants by Merrill et al. (1) and Landsteiner and Hufnagle (2) decades ago. Advances in immunosuppression and organ preservation have made renal allograft transplantation the most cost-effective treatment of choice for end-stage renal disease (ESRD).

However, the increasing demand for donor organs has exceeded availability with ever increasing patient listings and waiting times for potential recipients. In 1993, there were 24,704 patients listed for deceased donor renal transplant which had increased to 56,621 by 2003 (3,4). Correspondingly, only 7444 and 9532 deceased donor transplants were performed in those years, respectively. This means that the percentage of patients receiving deceased donor renal transplants in those years decreased from 30% to 17%, respectively. The annual mortality rate among patients waiting for renal transplant is now 6% (5).

Live donor renal transplant has now surpassed deceased donor renal transplant annually. The popularity of laparoscopic donor nephrectomy, both standard and hand-assisted, is largely responsible for this. The less invasive surgical procedure with a less protracted postoperative course for the renal donor has increased both living-related donation (LRD) as well as living-unrelated donation (LURD), including nonfamily members.

This chapter is designed to provide the urologic surgeon with a brief history and detailed overview of the medical and surgical aspects of renal transplantation necessary to understand potential complications and their management. This includes an overview of transplantation immunobiology and immunosuppression, the renal donor and renal transplant recipient evaluations and surgical procedures, and the diagnosis and management of resultant complications and acute rejection.

PATIENT SELECTION AND EVALUATION

Disease processes that result in ESRD in the United States include: diabetes, 36%; hypertensive glomerulosclerosis, 30%; chronic glomerulonephritis, 24%; and autosomal dominant polycystic kidney disease, 12% (6). These patients have limited long-term management options, which include hemodialysis, peritoneal dialysis, or renal transplantation. Most patients, regardless of age, who are experiencing satisfactory health prior to ESRD will choose renal transplantation because it is associated with maintenance or considerable improvement in quality of life. Comparison of hemodialysis or peritoneal dialysis with successful renal transplantation is shown to be considerably more cost-effective, even when the expense of immunosuppressive agents, potential rejection episodes, and multiple hospitalizations are considered.

At the Brigham and Womens' Hospital, we offer renal transplantation whenever possible and inquire about potential donors at initial evaluation. Patients for potential renal transplant are evaluated by the transplant team, which consists of the transplant surgeons, nephrologists, social worker, dietician, and the transplant coordinator.

Absolute contraindications to renal transplantation are active infection, including HIV and active malignancy. Medical conditions that render the patient incapable of tolerating a general anesthetic or surgical procedure, nonreconstructable vascular or cardiac disease, and chronic noncompliance to prior medical conditions and dialysis become contraindications by definition. Morbid obesity, defined as a body mass index of greater than 35, is now included in the absolute contraindication category (7).

Active infections must be eradicated prior to renal transplant. This includes dental disease, hemodialysis or peritoneal dialysis access infections, pulmonary infections, and urinary tract infections. Cytomegalovirus (CMV) can be a major cause for morbidity in the immuno-suppressed patient. CMV serology should be ascertained and a CMV+ kidney transplanted into a CMV– recipient requires systemic treatment post-transplant with gancyclovir (8).

Relative contraindications include systemic and metabolic diseases such as viral hepatitis, focal segmental glomerulosclerosis (FSGS) (9), hemolytic-uremic syndrome, and primary hyperoxaluria (10).

C-antibody-positive and hepatitis B antigenicity is associated with a two- to three-fold increase in morbidity and mortality from progressive cirrhosis. Transplantation may be justi-fied in patients with no biochemical evidence of hepatic dysfunction and patients may consent to receiving a kidney from a hepatitis positive donor (11). FSGS has a higher recurrence rate approaching 35% in patients with a rapidly progressing course and in those with mesangial proliferation on native renal biopsy. Patients with a failed renal transplant because of recur-rence have a recurrence rate of 80% in subsequent transplants. Primary hyperoxaluria can recur rapidly in the renal allograft and may be best treated with combined liver/kidney transplant as the liver transplant corrects the underlying metabolic defect.

Lastly, less common causes of ESRD with potential for recurrence in the renal allograft include amyloidosis, vasculitis, Fabry's disease, systemic lupus erythematosis, and cystinosis. Overall, the basic tenet should be that the benefits of transplant exceed the relative risks of subsequent complications from these diseases with a potential for recurrence in the renal allograft.

Candidates for renal transplantation receive an extensive evaluation including: a detailed medical history, psychological profile, physical examination, and routine laboratory studies as outlined in Table 1. Subsequent evaluation is based upon the patient's age, results of studies, and the primary disease process resulting in ESRD.

Older patients, or any patient with diabetes, have a propensity to develop significant coronary artery disease. Patients in this category undergo exercise tolerance testing with a thallium scan. A positive result on a stress-thallium scan or in patients with a long-standing his-tory of diabetes necessitates more invasive studies including coronary arteriography (12). Serious lesions should be successfully treated either with coronary stenting or coronary artery bypass prior to being activated for renal transplant. Patients with peripheral vascular disease are found in this population as well and need to be evaluated and successfully treated prior to transplant. The iliac vessels are utilized for the renal transplant procedure. Any suspicion for

TABLE 1 Routine Laboratory and Radiologic Evaluation of the Potential Renal Allograft Recipient

Laboratory evaluation
  Blood typing
  Human leukocyte antigen typing
  Hepatitis B and C serology
  Human immunodeficiency virus serology
  Viral serology
  Complete blood count
  Electrolytes, BUN, creatinine
  Liver function testing
  Electrocardiogram
  Serum cholesterol and triglycerides
Radiologic evaluation
  Chest X-ray
  Abdominal ultrasound
  Voiding cystourethrogram
  Upper gastrointestinal series/endoscopy
  Colonoscopy
  Exercise tolerance testing with thallium scan
  Coronary arteriography
  Peripheral noninvasive studies/MRA

Abbreviations: BUN, blood urea nitrogen; MRA, magnetic resonance arteriography.

significant disease in these vessels can be evaluated with magnetic resonance arteriography or venography.

A history of significant gastrointestinal disease, because of association with increased peri- and postoperative complications, demands extensive evaluation. All adults undergo abdominal ultrasonography. Symptomatic gallstones necessitate pretransplant cholecystectomy. A history of peptic ulcer disease necessitates upper gastrointestinal endoscopy and all active lesions need to be treated. Asymptomatic diverticulosis requires observation only, whereas recurrent diverticulitis indicates the need for prophylactic segmental colectomy prior to transplant.

Patients with no evidence of recurrent malignant disease with ESRD are candidates for renal transplantation provided that there has been adequate follow-up and an appropriate disease-free interval from the time of removal of the original malignant tumor. Specific risks have been determined using data derived from the 1993 Transplant Tumor Registry (13). The optimum waiting period for transplantation after removal of the malignant tumor depends upon the grade and stage of the tumor as well as risk for subsequent metastatic potential. One to two years is adequate for tumors with low metastatic potential and five to six years for patients with high-grade tumors. The majority of recurrences post-transplant occur within two years.

The genitourinary tract evaluation of the transplant candidate is designed to identify vesicoureteral reflux, obstructive uropathy, urinary tract infections, and neurogenic entities. A positive result prompts further investigation including cystoscopy, voiding cystourethrography, or retrograde urethrography. If a significant postvoid residual exists, an urodynamic profile is necessary to rule out a neurogenic or hypotonic bladder or urethral obstruction from stricture. Patients with greater than grade 3 reflux may need bilateral nephrectomies prior to transplant while those with a lesser severity may require antibiotic suppression only. When a small, noncompliant bladder is found, cycling the bladder may increase capacity; if not, the patient may need a bladder augmentation prior to transplant. The patient with a nonusable bladder may need supravesical urinary diversion with either an ileal conduit or a continent reservoir (14).

In the older, male, transplant patient we are now seeing lower urinary tract symptoms of bladder outlet obstruction, which need pretransplant prostatic evaluation with flexible cystourethroscopy and uroflow measurement. The patient may need an alpha-blocker or even a transurethral resection of the prostate. Lastly, urethral strictures, when found, can be corrected post-transplantation with the patient being maintained on clean intermittent catheterization or suprapubic tube drainage prior to surgical correction.

Bilateral native nephrectomies, once standard practice, are seldom required prior to renal transplantation. The most common indications include recurrent pyelonephritis; malignant disease; medically uncontrolled hypertension; symptomatic polycystic kidney disease, especially larger kidneys extending below the iliac crest; high-grade vesicoureteral reflux; persistent nephrolithiasis that can not be cleared by minimally invasive modalities including lithotripsy; and immunologically active disease. Most native nephrectomies are bilateral and will be performed through a midline or transverse "chevron" abdominal incision.

For patients undergoing retransplantation after a failed, asymptomatic, chronically rejected renal allograft, transplant nephrectomy is usually unnecessary. Indications for allograft nephrectomy include ongoing rejection with fever, graft tenderness, and malaise; recurrent hematuria; and uncontrolled hypertension. The safest approach for allograft nephrectomy is usually via a subcapsular fashion as this will lessen the potential for iliac vessel injury. Blood loss with resultant transfusion and surgical complication rates are higher in late, failed allograft nephrectomies (15).

DONOR SELECTION
Living-Related Donation

The potential renal donor must have no conditions that could increase the risk of postoperative complication, diminish the function of their remaining solitary kidney, or change their quality

TABLE 2   Evaluation of a Potential Live-Donor Renal Donor

Laboratory evaluation
  Blood typing
  Human leukocyte antigen typing
  Complete blood count
  Serum electrolytes, BUN, creatinine
  Liver function tests
  Coagulation studies
  HIV
  Cytomegalovirus titers
  Urine analysis and culture
  24-Hour urine for creatinine clearance—two determinations
  EKG
Radiologic evaluation
  Renal ultrasound
  Chest X-ray
  CT angiography and urography

Abbreviations: BUN, blood urea nitrogen; CT, computed tomography; EKG, electrocardiogram.

of life. The potential donor must be free of infection, transmissible malignancy, and renal disease. The standard evaluation is outlined in Table 2.

Once the potential donor is medically cleared, three-dimensional computed tomography (CT) angiography (16) with and without intravenous contrast is utilized to evaluate donor renal vascular and urinary collecting system anatomy. This has replaced conventional transfemoral angiography with less morbidity and cost.

Current renal allograft half-life is greater for live donor than for deceased donor renal transplants being 13.4 years versus 8.2 years, respectively (17). When strict protocols are utilized to ensure that only medically suitable donors are selected, long-term follow-up of these patients, as long as 45 years, have consistently demonstrated that renal donation can be performed with acceptable perioperative morbidity, negligible mortality, and no long-term compromise of renal function for the remaining solitary kidney (18,19). Thus, LRD continues to be a valuable and important source of renal allografts both because of superior outcomes and in lessening the impact of the growing shortage of deceased donor organs.

Living-Unrelated Donation

With the growing shortage of deceased donor organs, there has been an increasing utilization of LURD. This also includes the increasing role of the "good samaritan" donor. The entire screening process remains the same as well as radiologic evaluation. Initial results at one year show renal allograft survival in recipients to be from 83% to 93% with a four-year survival comparable to LRD (20). Most recently, these numbers have been substantiated (21) as this mode of organ donation has increased in popularity. It is important to remember that the strict criteria utilized to select appropriate renal donors must be maintained in order to continue LURD, especially from the truly altruistic donor.

Deceased Donor Donation

Although the criteria for appropriate deceased donor donation have been expanded to include the use of nonheart-beating donation, now known as donation after cardiac death (DCD), and expanded deceased donor donation (EDD), potential donors still should have no generalized disease process that could adversely affect renal allograft vascular integrity or function. This includes the absence of severe chronic hypertension, diabetes, malignant disease with significant metastatic potential, or untreatable systemic infection. Using these criteria, the one year allograft and patient survival was 86% and 90%, respectively (22). The 10 year allograft and patient survival now is recorded as 36.4% and 57.9%, respectively (23). This decline is due to chronic allograft dysfunction, which is probably secondary to progressive tissue damage with considerable vasculopathy from the necessity for chronic immunosuppression (24,25). Despite these declining long-term results, deceased donor donation remains a necessity.

The expanded deceased donor criteria has allowed the use of previously discarded kidneys. All EDD and DCD kidneys undergo a renal biopsy prior to allocation. A biopsy finding of significant glomerulosclerosis (>10–20%), intimal hyperplasia, interstitial fibrosis, tubular atrophy, or evidence of disseminated intravascular coagulopathy renders the donor suboptimal to unacceptable. All EDD and DCD kidneys undergo preservation on the pulsatile perfusion machine, which allows assessment of ultimate viability by measurement of perfusion pressures (26).

Procedures for Donors

The most difficult time of management for the potential deceased donor is that during the aggressive neurologic management prior to being declared as an irreversible, brain-dead patient. Fluids may be restricted to prevent cerebral edema and patients with isolated central nervous system pathology may develop diabetes insipidis. This can lead to systemic hypotension and subsequent renal shutdown. Once the donor status is established, aggressive fluid management that promotes systemic hydration and renal perfusion is undertaken. This may even necessitate the use of certain vasopressors to support systemic and renal perfusion.

The next phase of organ procurement is that of matching the potential deceased donor with appropriate recipients from the same blood-type list. This match run, including human leukocyte antigen (HLA) typing, is the same as performed for the live-donor renal transplant once compatible blood type is ascertained. The potential donor's serum or, in the case of deceased donor donation, lymph node tissue is cross-matched with the recipient's serum. The lymph node tissue can be obtained from the deceased donor via groin dissection prior to organ procurement. This will lessen cold-ischemia time as the cross-match process can be performed while the organ procurement is taking place as opposed to postprocurement. Once the negative cross-match is ascertained, the kidney can be offered to the potential recipient.

There is a strong positive correlation between histocompatibility matching for the HLA-A, -B, and -DR locus antigens and allograft survival for LRD renal allografts. First-degree relatives, such as siblings, parents and offspring, have a consistent inherited homogeneity to these histocompatibility complexes found on the sixth chromosome. This implies that matching these loci in closely related individuals means matching for most of the whole chromosome, or haplotype.

HLA matching is more difficult in LURD and deceased donor donation as there is greater heterogeneity in these groups compared to LRD. Clinical effects on renal allograft survival continue to be controversial. Favorable (27,28) and insignificant (29,30) influences on HLA (ABDR) matching have been published. The only generally accepted tenet is that zero-mismatched renal allografts have superior results when compared with other, less well-matched renal allografts. The united network for organ sharing (UNOS) zero-mismatched program reports an 87% one-year allograft survival and a 13-year half-life when compared with a 79% one-year allograft survival and seven-year half-life in other less-matched controls. There are also fewer rejection episodes noted in this population. The conclusion from this is that it is still worthwhile to export zero-mismatched renal allografts from a long distance away whereas the survival advantage is not there for less well-matched allografts, which should remain locally with a shorter cold ischemia time.

Extracorporeal Renal Preservation

Effective ex vivo preservation of deceased donor kidneys for 24 to 36 hours is necessary to provide time for crossmatching and histocompatibility testing and to permit efficient dissemination of allografts throughout the UNOS. The two methods commonly employed are simple cold storage and continuous hypothermic pulsatile perfusion.

Cold (hypothermic) storage is the most commonly used method of preservation. Once the kidneys are removed from the donor, they are flushed out immediately with cold preservation solution. For most LRD kidneys, an extracellular solution such as iced Ringer's lactate is used as the cold ischemia time is minimal, usually less than one to three hours. Longer cold ischemia times are seen with deceased donor renal allografts and require an intracellular solution to prevent cell swelling with acidosis, expansion of the interstitial space, and production of oxygen free radicals. High osmotic solutions are used, the most common of which is University of Wisconsin solution (31).

Pulsatile perfusion is most commonly used for renal allografts of questionable viability and most recently for all EDD allografts (26). Region 1 of the UNOS has used this method of preservation since the inception of its EDD protocols. The quality of perfusion is correlated directly with viability at implantation of the renal allograft.

Donor Nephrectomy

Multiple surgical techniques for live donor nephrectomy have been described. The most common is the extraperitoneal flank approach via an 11th or 12th rib incision. Based upon pre-operative CT angiogram, multiple vessels are usually avoided with greater than 60% of donors having a single artery on one side. Multiple renal arteries can be reconstructed on the "back table" after hypothermic perfusion by the recipient transplant surgeon. This facilitates the arterial anastamosis into the allograft recipient. Multiple arteries that are far apart can be anastamosed to both the external and internal iliac arteries. Smaller upper pole arteries less than 2 cm in size can be sacrificed while lower pole arteries must be preserved.

The introduction of laparoscopic donor nephrectomy has increased the live donor pool (32). The operative techniques and results for laparoscopic and hand-assisted laparoscopic donor nephrectomy have been compared and contrasted in multiple publications (33–35). The utilization of the left kidney is preferred due to the longer length of renal vein obtainable. However, most transplant centers are becoming more comfortable with utilizing right-sided laparoscopic donor nephrectomy where the left side is not indicated that is approaching a similar rate of utilization as with open donor nephrectomy. Results show that the donor has less pain, a shorter hospitalization, and a more rapid return to normal activities, all of which potentially lead to more donors in the future. Hand-assisted transperitoneal laparoscopy versus pure laparoscopy will have a shorter warm ischemia time of 1.6 versus 3.9 minutes, respectively (33). Ultimately, both, techniques will have the same allograft survival and serum creatinine levels when compared with standard open donor nephrectomy.

At the Brigham and Womens' Hospital, we prefer the use of a retroperitoneal hand-assisted laparoscopic technique and have utilized this approach in over 100 renal donors with no conversions to an open donor nephrectomy (S. Kumar, M.J. Malone and S. Tullius, Department of Transplant Surgery, Brigham and Women's Hospital, Boston, Massachusetts, U.S.A.). We utilize a 7 to 8 cm iliac fossa incision and develop the retroperitoneal space for the hand port and insufflation. The ureter and ipsilateral gonadal vein are isolated and tagged with an umbilical tape. Once insufflation has occurred, standard 12 and 5 mm ports are used and the standard hand-assisted laparoscopic technique is utilized in the retroperitoneal space for procurement. Demonstrates the anatomy encountered with a right-sided donor, while shows the anatomic variant of a retroaortic left renal vein encountered with a left-sided donor. We believe that this technique lessens the chance of intra-abdominal organ injury while more closely paralleling the technique of standard open donor nephrectomy.

Recipient Operation

A standard modified Gibson incision is utilized with the renal allograft implanted into the contralateral iliac fossa (36). The transplant renal artery anastamosis is performed first, usually into the recipient external iliac artery in end-to-side fashion using a running 6-0 prolene. A man undergoing repeat renal transplant who has had a prior renal allograft anastamosis to the internal iliac artery should not have the contralateral internal iliac artery utilized as this could lead to impotence.

The transplant renal vein is anastamosed to the recipient external iliac vein in end-to-side fashion using a running 6-0 prolene suture. Furosemide and mannitol, along with the preselected immunosuppressive agents are given prior to vessel cross-clamp removal.

In order to re-establish the continuity of the urinary tract, an extra-vesical, Gregoir-Lich (37) ureteral reimplant is used. A small incision is made on the dome of the bladder. The detrusor muscle is incised and the mucosa is allowed to prolapse. The mucosa is then opened and the transplant ureter is anastamosed using a running 5-0 polyglycolic acid suture (PDS). The overlying muscle can then be reapproximated to create a tunnel to prevent vesicoureteral reflux.

A 6 × 12 double J ureteral stent is used to protect the ureteroneocystostomy from urinary leakage. A 10 F Jackson Pratt drain is used to drain the peritransplant space and the incision is closed in standard fashion.

Occasionally, the renal allograft ureter will have to be reimplanted into an augmented bladder or into a supravesical urinary diversion, which includes an ileal conduit (38) or continent urinary diversion (14). This may require implantation of the renal allograft transperitoneally as opposed to the iliac fossa in order to facilitate establishing urinary tract continuity. Any reconstruction of the bladder or creation of a supravesical urinary diversion should be performed at least three months prior to renal allograft implantation. Patients should be instructed on how to perform clean intermittent catheterization if a bladder augmentation is to be utilized. Poor bladder emptying from augmentation may result in renal allograft dysfunction (39).

A baseline transplant renal ultrasound is obtained within 24 hours of the renal allograft transplant procedure. The information obtained by ultrasound includes vascular patency and flow characteristics, presence of ureteral obstruction or hydronephrosis, lymphocoele formation, and indirect evidence of renal allograft rejection by measurement of resistive index. Acute rejection can be suspected by ultrasound findings of allograft swelling, increased resistive index (>0.7), pelvi-infundibular thickening, reduced sinus fat, and prominent medullary pyramids. If no flow is found on ultrasound, a 99mTc-MAG3 (Tc-99m mercaptoacetylglycerine) renal scan is obtained or magnetic resonance arteriography (MRA) can be utilized to supplant the use of conventional arteriography for diagnosis of vascular thrombosis.

IMMUNOSUPPRESSION

Immunosuppressive agents are utilized to prevent allograft rejection. They can be used as an induction agent immediately after allograft implantation, as maintenance immunotherapy once serum creatinine has normalized, or as treatment of acute rejection.

Early immunosuppressive protocols included the use of azathioprine and corticosteroids. Azathioprine incorporates into DNA and inhibits cell mitosis and proliferation. Its major side effect is bone marrow suppression resulting in leukopenia. It is useful in induction and maintenance immunotherapy but not in acute rejection. Corticosteroids induce inhibition of interleukin (IL)-1 release for antigen-presenting cells. Long-term usage has major side effects and newer immunosuppressive regimens lower the necessity for them. Corticosteroids are useful in induction, maintenance, and for the treatment of acute rejection.

Cyclosporin A (CyA) has a lymphocyte-specific immunosuppressive effect. Its use has helped to reduce the therapeutic steroid dose requirement. CyA inhibits gene transcription for IL-2 production and other genes required for proliferation (calcineurin inhibition) and differentiation of the T-lymphocyte. CyA is used for maintenance immunosuppression but has no role in acute rejection and with resultant decreased renal allograft blood flow is not used for induction therapy. CyA increased one-year cadaveric allograft survival from 50% to nearly 90% after its introduction (40).

Antilymphocyte/antithymocyte globulin (ALG/ATG) are xenoantibodies produced by immunized laboratory animals with human lymphocytes or thymocytes. Resultant ALGs or ATGs have been used successfully to reverse initial acute rejection with an approximate 80% success rate (41). They are now used for induction therapy in higher risk renal allografts such as the expanded donor allografts or for patients retransplanted for the second or third time. They can also be used to reverse acute allograft rejection but are not used as maintenance immunotherapy due to significant side effects.

A monoclonal antibody, OKT3, was developed by injection a mouse with human T-lymphocytes producing a hybridoma of the mouse's spleen and murine myeloma cells. The hybridoma was screened and cloned to produce a pure antibody against the CD3 protein of the antigen recognition complex found on all mature T-cells. When OKT3 binds to the CD3 protien, the antigen recognition complex is altered and the T-cells are rendered blind to the renal allograft antigen. Experience with OKT3 monoclonal antibody in the therapy of primary acute rejection has an effectiveness in excess of 95% (43) and is effective in reversing steroid-resistant rejection. OKT3 is not used for induction or maintenance immunotherapy due to serious side effects. Repeated use for subsequent acute rejection episodes is limited in the recipient who produces OKT3 antibodies.

Newer DNA technology has been used to help lessen some of the clinical problems associated with both OKT3 and ALG/ATG. Chimeric (Basiliximab: Simulect; Novartis, Basel, Switzerland) and humanized (Daclizumab: Xenapac; Roche, Basel, Switzerland) monoclonal antibodies have been generated against specific T-cell CD3 surface protein receptors. A reduction in xenogenic epitomes results in a decrease in development of antixenogenic antibodies resulting in less toxicity.

FK506 (Tacrolimus: Prograft; Astrella Pharmaceuticals Inc., Tokyo, Japan) is similar to CyA in terms of mode of action. It also suppresses IL-2 production from the CD4+ cells. It is now used as maintenance therapy and also may rescue renal allografts undergoing rejection when substituted for CyA (43).

Rapamycin (Sirolimus; Rapamune) also blocks IL-2. Unlike FK506 and CyA, rapamycin does not seem to be nephrotoxic. Rapamycin can be combined with CyA and may be synergistic. Rapamycin can be continued with CyA withdrawal and a steroid taper in newer protocols (44).

Mycophenolate mofetil (Cellcept; Roche) is an antimetabolite drug that inhibits the synthesis of purines. Its effect is more lymphocyte-specific than azathioprine. Initial results are favorable for its use in induction and maintenance immunotherapy with an associated decrease in acute rejection of almost 50% first year post-transplantation (45).

In summary, most institutions in the United States, including the Brigham and Womens' Hospital, use a combination of prednisone, an antimetabolite, with or without anti-CD3 or CD25 antibodies for induction immunosuppression. This avoids the nephrotoxicity of induction CyA or FK506 on early allograft function. Deceased donor and some live donor renal allograft recipients with expected acute tubular necrosis (ATN) or delayed allograft function or with high immunologic risk [prior transplant or panel reactive antigens (PRA) 15%] can be given either ALG/ATG or Sirolimus preoperatively and continued until serum creatinine normalizes to <2.5 mg/dL (46). CyA or FK506 can then be started and antibody preparations discontinued once adequate serum CyA or FK506 levels are achieved. Steroids can be pulsed for acute rejection. Steroid-resistant rejections can be treated with OKT3.

Rejection
Diagnosis of Rejection
In order to diagnose renal allograft rejection, the transplant surgeon needs to understand the basics of the alloimmune response responsible for it. The renal allograft is rejected because the recipient immune system recognizes it as foreign and mounts both a cellular and humoral response. Careful preoperative tissue typing can limit the dissimilarity between the donor allograft and the recipient host and to modify the recipient host's immune response to the renal allograft. The role of the various immunosuppressive agents now available is to alter the immunogenic cascade that occurs when antigenic stimuli are introduced to the allograft recipient.

Many antigen groups can evoke an immune response. The most crucial are those found on the short arm of chromosome 6, known as the major histocompatibility complex or the HLA complex. The HLA complex is further divided into class 1 (A, B, C) and class 2 (DR, DP, DQ) loci. Class 1 antigens are present in all nucleated cells and class 2 antigens are limited to B-lymphocytes, a subpopulation of macrophages, and activated T-cells. The class 1 antigens specifically bind to the antigen receptor complex on cytotoxic T-lymphocytes. Class 2 antigens are involved in the stimulation of helper T-lymphocytes.

The tissue typing process involves the determination of compatibility between class 1 A and B antigens and class 2 DR antigens. Identification of these three antigens on lymphocytes is accomplished using typed monospecific antisera in a complement-mediated cytotoxicity test. The ideal result is to find donors with similar HLA antigenic specificities as the recipient. Some now debate whether this is necessary with newer immunosuppressive agents that inhibit this recognition process leading to rejection.

Helper T-lymphocytes in the presence of class 2 [human leukocyte antigen-DR locus (HLA-DR)] antigen become sensitized and release macrophage stimulating factor. The cascade continues because the now stimulated macrophages make monokine IL-1, which in turn promotes differentiation and proliferation of the helper T-cell line. The helper T-cells produce a variety of proteins, including T-cell growth factor (IL-2), B-cell growth factor (IL-4), and gamma interferon.

IL-2 promotes the activation and proliferation of lymphoid cell lines, including cytotoxic T-cells. The class 1 antigens sensitize these cells in the IL-2 environment to become effector cells capable of allograft destruction. B-lymphocytes in the presence of IL-4 become plasma cells that produce donor-specific antibodies.

Direct cellular allograft destruction is mediated through attack on donor tissue target cells by macrophages, cytotoxic T-cells, and helper T-cells. Donor-specific antibodies synthesized by plasma cells cause damage through both complement-mediated cell lysis and antibody-dependent cell-mediated cytotoxicity. Allograft rejection is thus a result of both activated cellular and humoral responses to an antigenic challenge.

Hyperacute Rejection

Hyperacute rejection is a devastating and irreversible form of rejection that occurs within minutes to a few hours of allograft implantation. It develops in recipients with circulating class 1 HLA antibodies against donor cells, specifically vascular endothelium. Most patients have been sensitized by prior blood transfusions, multiple pregnancies, or a previously rejected allograft. On the microscopic level, the antigen-antibody interaction leads to complement deposition, platelet aggregation, and capillary thrombosis formation. This results in cortical infarction and acellular glomeruli. Macroscopically, the allograft becomes edematous and tense and is dark blue to purple in color.

Diagnosis is usually ascertained on the operating table, which necessitates immediate allograft nephrectomy. If the recipient is a few hours out from surgery, the presentation will be anuria with fever, chills, and severe allograft tenderness. The MAG-3 renal scan will show no uptake of isotope. MRA will differentiate between this and acute renal arterial thrombosis by confirming transplant renal artery patency. Immediate allograft nephrectomy is necessary as the recipient will be toxic secondary to severe rejection. Careful routine cross-matching, especially for highly-sensitized patients, has made the incidence of this type of rejection extremely low.

Acute Rejection

Humoral rejection often occurs within the first week after transplantation. It involves an antibody-mediated allograft damage and progresses on an accelerated basis. Vascular compromise secondary to arteriolar thrombosis results in allograft ischemia. Although acute humoral rejection and hyperacute rejection may appear clinically and pathologically similar, the latter develops immediately after transplantation and demonstrates donor-specific antibodies at the time of implantation. In acute humoral rejection, the recipient has previously been sensitized to class 1 HLA antigens through blood transfusion or prior transplantation. Re-challenge with a large antigenic stimulus produces recall of donor-specific antibodies resulting in accelerated acute rejection with allograft destruction. Most accelerated acute rejections can be successfully treated with the protocols mentioned earlier.

Acute cellular rejection, the most common form of rejection, usually occurs 7 to 10 days after transplantation. It is mediated by the infiltration of T- and B-lymphocytes and macrophages clinically. The recipient presents with manifestations ranging from micro-allograft impairment to oliguric renal failure requiring dialysis as well as hypertension and pulmonary edema.

The recipient will complain of flu-like symptoms including malaise, arthralgias, anorexia, low-grade fever, hypertension or hypotension, and decreased urinary output. The allograft is usually swollen, tender, and painful. Laboratory evaluation includes a rising serum creatinine and white blood cell count. Transplant renal ultrasound may show a high resistive index with allograft swelling.

The differential diagnosis of all types of rejection include renal artery thrombosis and ATN. Also included in the differential are urinary leakage and/or obstruction which will be fully discussed later in the chapter. Transplant renal ultrasound will show characteristics of arterial flow as well as whether flow is present or absent. Ultrasound will also show collections around the allograft suggestive of urinary leakage or, if hydronephrosis is present, an expanding lymphocoele or hematoma. A MAG-3 renal scan can also help to ascertain ATN or urinary leakage if the isotope is present extrarenally.

ATN can be seen in 5% to 40% of renal allografts from deceased donors (47). This injury is usually attributed to prolonged cold ischemia or prolonged anastamotic times. The use of expanded or older donors along with those who are unstable going to the operating room increases the incidence of ATN. Treatment is expectant and may take several weeks to resolve. Immunosuppressive strategies during ATN include sequential use of ALG/ATG or anti-CD25 monoclonal antibodies followed by careful monitoring of IL-2 inhibitor (CyA or tacrolimus) levels.

Once nonrejection diagnoses are excluded, percutaneous renal allograft biopsy under ultrasound guidance will be necessary to diagnose rejection. Light microscopy will be able to differentiate ATN from acute rejection. Acute rejection will show dense interstitial allograft infiltrate consisting of lymphocytes, macrophages, and plasma cells. Complications of renal allograft biopsy include hematoma and gross hematuria. We are very aggressive in utilizing renal allograft biopsy post-transplant as this facilitates early treatment of acute rejection and will diagnose ATN, which requires no change in immunosuppressive treatment.

RESULTS OF RENAL TRANSPLANTATION AND CHRONIC ALLOGRAFT REJECTION

Significant improvements in one-year patient and graft survival have been made in the last two to three decades. One-year patient survival has increased from 50% to 92% (48,49). Similarly, one-year graft survival is currently at 80% to 85% for deceased donor and greater than 90% for live donor renal transplants (47,48).

However, newer data (5,23) show that while rejection rates are at their lowest, the long-term risk of renal allograft loss has not improved. Thus, 10-year patient and graft survival are 57.9% and 36.4%, respectively, for deceased donor renal allografts and 77.4% and 55.2%, respectively, for live donor renal allografts.

Chronic renal allograft rejection is the next problem to be solved and is the most common cause of renal allograft loss after the first year post-transplantation (25). Even in the case of renal allografts with good function and no rejection in the early years post-transplantation, progressive tissue damage and slowly decreasing function may develop. In addition, long-term immunosupression with calcineurin inhibitors can cause fibrosis, which contributes to chronic renal allograft injury and dysfunction (50), which is independent of antigenicity to the renal allograft. Thus, targeting of these factors that are dependent and independent of alloantigens early in the post-transplant course is necessary to improve renal allograft survival.

COMPLICATIONS OF RENAL TRANSPLANTATION
Nonsurgical Complications
Infection

More than 80% of patients undergoing renal transplantation have at least one episode of infection in the first postoperative year. Infection also remains the leading cause of death at all points in the postrenal allograft transplant course. Important factors in the course and intensity of infection are the status of the donor and recipient before renal allograft implantation; the type, intensity and duration of immunosuppressive therapy; and the pathogens the recipient is exposed to while taking immunosuppressive agents.

Bacterial pathogens can lead to urinary, wound, and pulmonary infections in the first postoperative month. These are usually acute and are easily treated once diagnosed. Opportunistic infections predominate throughout the next two to six months. Renal allograft recipients are most susceptible to viruses and intracellular infectious agents because immunosuppressive agents inhibit the cellular component of the immune response. The infectious agents that best exemplify this include CMV, hepatitis B and C (HBV and HCV), and HIV. Pneumocystis carinii infection has been less prevalent by four-fold because of the use of trimethoprim-sulfamethoxazole in the first six months post-transplant.

Cytomegalovirus

Cytomegalovirus is the major viral pathogen during the first two to six month post-transplant period, causing symptomatic disease in 35% and death in 2% of renal allograft recipients (51).

Seronegative recipients of CMV+ donor kidneys are the highest risk of having symptomatic disease. Reactivation disease is also possible when latent infection in CMV+ recipients reactivates after allograft transplantation. Initial symptoms include fever, malaise, fatigue, anorexia, myalgias, and arthralgias. Leukopenia, thrombocytopenia, atypical lymphocytosis, and elevation of serum transaminase levels are common laboratory findings. Respiratory and gastrointestinal tracts are most commonly affected. CMV pneumonitis presents with a dry cough, dyspnea, hypoxia, and an abnormal chest X ray. Diagnosis is made on sputum cytology or lung biopsy. CMV in the gastrointestinal tract may cause ulceration, bleeding, or intestinal perforation, with the stomach, small bowel, and cecum most commonly affected (52). The shell-vial culture technique, which uses monoclonal antibody against an early viral antigen to detect CMV presence, is now commonly used with results available in 24 hours.

Immunosuppressive therapy needs to be reduced along with vigorous rehydration, antipyretics, and the administration of the antiviral agent, gancyclovir (53). Monoclonal and polyclonal antibodies can reactivate CMV while CyA, prednisone, rapamycin, and tacrolimus have no ability for reactivation. However, with initiation of viral replication, CyA will amplify CMV infection with an incidence of 10% to 20%. Addition of ALG or OKT3 will increase the amplification to an incidence of 60%. If gancyclovir is given preemptively and continued for six months, the high incidence of clinical disease is dramatically lessened (54) by decreasing viral shedding and progression of CMV disease.

Hepatitis B and C Viruses

Hepatitis B viruses and HCV can be acquired at the time of renal allograft transplantation. The risk of acquiring HBV with a renal allograft is less than 0.01% (55) as all patients on dialysis are vaccinated. However, once acquired, HBV can be associated with fulminant hepatic failure in 10% to 15% of allograft recipients. After two years, these recipients do poorly and progress to end-stage liver disease, hepatocellular carcinoma, and cardiovascular disease.

Hepatitis C viruses disease acquired at renal allograft transplantation tends not to be associated with an acute clinical syndrome but causes chronic, subclinical hepatocellular dysfunction until end-stage liver disease occurs. Despite this, selective acceptance of HCV seropositive renal allografts for potential recipients with serious medical conditions or in antibody HCV+ recipients with a low incidence of clinical hepatitis and liver failure is advocated by some centers (56).

Human Immunodeficiency Virus

Renal allograft transplantation from a documented HIV+ donor has the potential viral transmission to the recipient approaching 100%. In 70% of recipients of HIV+ organs, acquired immunodeficiency syndrome (AIDS) will develop 2.5 to 3 years later (57). The risk of transmission has been reduced to less than 1%. Patients in whom AIDS develops after renal allograft transplantation while taking CyA have a clinical course similar to that of the nonimmunosuppressed patient (58).

The appropriate management of the asymptomatic HIV+ patient undergoing dialysis is controversial. Data available show that one-third of recipients having undergone allograft transplantation are dead at six months, one-third are alive and well five years or more post-transplant, and one-third will be alive with overt AIDS three years after transplantation (59). Markers are currently available to screen the prospective, asymptomatic recipient who is HIV+ with regard to which clinical course will ensue.

Cancer

Another potential problem is that the immunosuppression necessary for renal allograft transplantation increases the incidence of cancer. Analysis of malignant disease associated with the advent of CyA immunotherapy shows an increasing incidence of lymphoma and sarcoma (60). Post-transplant lymphoproliferative disorders (PTLD) have an incidence of 2.5% in deceased donor renal allografts (61). The mean time of PTLD with CyA use was about 15 months with 32% occurring within four months of allograft implantation. These lesions can be identified as monoclonal or polyclonal populations of B-lymphocytes with the monoclonal lesions having a worse prognosis. Cessation of immunosuppression may be necessary for regression.

Other common cancers that can develop are skin cancers, carcinomas of the cervix, renal tumors, and carcinomas of the vulva and perineum (62). Bladder cancer is also fairly common with an incidence approaching 8% to 10%. Superficial disease should not be treated with bacille calmette-guerin (BCG) suspension intravesically as transplant allograft recipients have a much higher incidence of systemic infection because of immunosuppression. Thiotepa may augment the myelosuppressive effect of immunosuppression especially with mycophenolate mofetil.

New-Onset Diabetes Mellitus
A small percentage of previously nondiabetic renal allograft recipients will develop new-onset diabetes mellitus. This is mostly seen in immunosuppression protocols that include glucocorticoids and calcineurin inhibitors, such as CyA and tacrolimus. Insulin-dependent diabetes mellitus is also higher in protocols utilizing tacrolimus as opposed to CyA.

Surgical Complications
Urologic Complications
Urinary Obstruction and Anastamotic Stricture
Urologic complications are unusual, with a range of 2% to 5% in most series (63,64). Most complications include anastamotic leaks, ureteral or anastamotic stricture formation, ureteral obstruction, and ureteropelvic disruption. Clinically, the recipient will have a decrease in urine output and allograft dysfunction. Diagnosis can be made by ultrasound or renal scan showing an extravesical fluid collection by ultrasound with isotope uptake on a renal scan differentiating from a lymphocoele.

Most of the complications are technical in nature and can be decreased by careful maintenance of the ureteral blood supply by not dissecting the periureteral connective tissue at the time of procurement. The use of the extravesical technique for ureteral reimplantation has also decreased the incidence of stricture and obstruction (65). The only disadvantage of the extravesical technique is a greater rate of urinary reflux (66) but the creation of a muscular tunnel will decrease this risk.

Urinary leakage or obstruction encountered early in the post-transplant period is usually best managed by open techniques. Urinary leakage from the ureteroneocystostomy is best remedied by repeat ureteroneocystostomy. If there is an ischemic ureteral injury encountered with resultant inadequate ureteral length, the transplant ureter can be reanastamosed to the ipsilateral native ureter. The transplant renal pelvis can also be anastamosed to the ipsilateral native ureter or to the recipient's bladder as alternatives.

Treatment of urinary obstruction from an anastamotic stricture encountered months to years after successful renal allograft transplant is undertaken once antegrade percutaneous nephrostogram the level of obstruction. A percutaneous nephrostomy tube can be placed to decompress the obstructed system. Percutaneous ureteral dilatation followed by stent placement has been reported with good success rates (67,68) especially in anastamotic strictures that are short in length. Failure of treatment is usually apparent within one year of treatment. Repeat transplant ureteroneocystostomy may be necessary if there is inadequate ureteral length. Alternatives include the use of transplant to ipsilateral native ureteroureterostomy, ureteropyelostomy with native renal ureter anastamosed to the transplant renal pelvis, or transplant renal pelvis to recipient bladder as a vesicopyelostomy (69). A short segment of the ileum can be used for an ileal ureter if other options are not available (70).

Urinary Tract Infection
Infection of the urinary tract post-transplant is extremely common. Immunosuppression and an indwelling bladder catheter are major contributors along with diabetes mellitus and pre-existing urinary tract abnormalities. Broad-spectrum antibiotics such as trimethoprim-sulfamethoxazole are used for the first six months post-transplant for pulmonary Pneumocystis carinii and will also help in prophylaxis against urinary tract infection.

Pyelonephritis post-transplant can be caused by urinary obstruction or renal stone. Once these are excluded by ultrasound, conventional antimicrobial therapy is utilized to treat the specific organism causing the urinary tract infection. Candida albicans is common in the diabetic population and may need to be treated with amphotericin bladder irrigations and ketoconazole. Calcineurin inhibitor doses have to be reduced as ketoconazole interferes with their metabolism (71).

Urolithiasis

Urolithiasis after renal allograft transplant can be due to recurrent urinary tract infection, obstruction, decreased fluid intake, and hyperparathyroidism. The recipient may not have typical renal colic as the renal allograft is denervated and may present with severe pyelonephritis or worsening renal function. Percutaneous techniques may be easier for renal or ureteral stones that are not amenable to extracorporeal shock wave lithotripsy (ESWL). When the patient is treated with ESWL, the prone position is utilized as with a distal ureteral stone with good success (72).

Kidney-Pancreas with Bladder Drainage

Urologic complications are common after kidney-pancreas transplantation with pancreatic exocrine drainage into the urinary bladder. While they do not adversely affect renal or pancreatic allograft survival (73), there are significant urinary tract complications, which may necessitate conversion to enteral drainage for the pancreatic exocrine secretions. The major complications include hematuria and clot retention with bleeding originating from the duodenovesical anastamosis, allograft pancreatitis, duodenal leaks, and urethral lesions that may require prolonged catheterization to heal. One interesting complication in this series was the presence of postrenal allograft urinary retention in patients with normal preoperative urodynamic studies. The urologic surgeon will be called upon to assist in the complex decision-making related to correcting these debilitating complications.

Vascular Complications

Historically, the incidence of vascular complications, namely arterial thrombosis, disruption, and hemorrhage, pseudoaneurysm, and mycotic aneurysm, approached 6% (74). The incidence of these complications has decreased dramatically as a result of a lower incidence of perinephric infections and the use of monofilament sutures. The major vascular complications that are still evident include vascular thrombosis, allograft rupture, thrombophlebitis, and transplant renal artery stenosis (TRAS).

Vascular Thrombosis

Transplant renal artery thrombosis, while still the leading cause of acute allograft loss in the first postrenal transplant year, is fortunately very rare and occurs less than 0.1% of the time. This is usually secondary to a technical error during the transplant renal artery anastamosis to the recipient external iliac artery. The recipient will present with acute tenderness over the allograft, with fever and chills. Laboratory findings will include an elevated white blood cell count and may show an elevated lactic dehydrogenase level of >1000/dL. Transplant renal ultrasound and renal scan will differentiate this from acute rejection, ATN, or urinary leak, with resultant oliguria or anuria and MRA will confirm the diagnosis demonstrating no flow into the transplant renal artery. Table 3 illustrates the findings seen with each diagnostic modality used for the differential diagnosis. Even with expediency in making the diagnosis, salvage of the allograft is unlikely and allograft nephrectomy is necessary.

TABLE 3 Diagnostic Modalities and the Differential Diagnosis of Acute Allograft Dysfunction

	Renal artery thrombosis	Acute rejection	Acute tubular necrosis	Urinary leak
Allograft tenderness	+	+	+	+
Oliguria anuria	+	+	+	+
Fever chills	+	+	+	+
Elevated WBC	+	+	+	+
Elevated LDH	>1000	+/–	+/–	–
Transplant ultrasound	No flow	+/– flow	+/– flow	flow
Renal scan	No flow	+/– flow	+/– flow	flow extravasation
MRA arterial	Occluded	Open	Open	Open patency

Abbreviations: LDH, lactic dehydrogenase; MRA, magnetic resonance arteriography; WBC, white bloodcell count.

Transplant renal vein thrombosis, although uncommon, can result from expansion of the renal allograft with acute rejection or fluid accumulation in a tight, retroperitoneal pocket, resulting in compression of the transplant renal vein. Transplant renal ultrasound will show no outflow through the transplant renal vein coupled with a high resistive index in the renal artery or reversal of diastolic flow. Salvage is unlikely unless diagnosis is suspected. Treatment is usually allograft nephrectomy.

Occasionally, a compressed or thrombosed iliac artery secondary to deep venous thrombosis can mimic transplant renal vein thrombosis. Noninvasive testing or magnetic resonance venography (MRV) will help to make the diagnosis. The recipient may present with renal allograft tenderness with ipsilateral lower extremity swelling. Thrombectomy with postoperative anticoagulation will be necessary to re-establish vascular flow. Renal allograft salvage is likely in this clinical scenario. Patients taking CyA may have a higher incidence of thromboembolic events as opposed to other immunosuppressive agents (75).

Renal Allograft Rupture
Renal allograft rupture can occur as a result of allograft swelling secondary to acute rejection. This usually occurs on the convex border of the kidney as a result of cortical ischemia from edema and intense cellular infiltration (76). The recipient may present with acute allograft tenderness that can lead to hypovolemic shock secondary to hemorrhage. The renal allograft can be repaired with large mattress (liver) sutures reapproximating the renal capsule with Avitene (Medchem, Woburn, Massachusetts, U.S.A.) and Surgicel (Johnson and Johnson, New Brunswick, New Jersey, U.S.A.) bolsters. Floseal (Baxter, Deerfield, Illinois, U.S.A.) may also play a role in hemostasis. If hemorrhage cannot be controlled, allograft nephrectomy is indicated.

Transplant Renal Artery Stenosis
TRAS may result from atherosclerotic disease in the recipient iliac artery, technical anastamotic error, renal artery injury during donor nephrectomy, or immunologic injury as seen with chronic allograft rejection. The stenotic area is usually at the transplant renal artery-to-external iliac artery anastamosis or just distal to it. Recipients may present with gradually worsening allograft function, uncontrolled hypertension, or a bruit over the allograft. The differential diagnosis includes acute rejection, CyA toxicity, and chronic allograft dysfunction.

TRAS can occur with an incidence of 1.5% to 8% (77,78). TRAS should be suspected in all recipients whose blood pressure cannot be controlled with traditional antihypertensive agents with no evidence of acute or chronic rejection. The sudden appearance of a bruit over the renal allograft with hypertension late in the post-transplant period suggests TRAS and should be evaluated (79). The diagnosis can be made with transplant renal ultrasound or MRA but definitive renal arteriography may be necessary. A percutaneous renal allograft biopsy under ultrasound guidance should be performed to exclude chronic renal allograft dysfunction when stenosis of the main transplant renal artery is associated with diffuse narrowing of secondary and tertiary renal arterial branches. If present, correction of the main TRAS will not correct hypertension or worsening renal allograft function.

Percutaneous transluminal angioplasty (PTA) or open surgical renal arterial reconstruction can be used to correct TRAS. The nonsurgical PTA approach is ideal and has a reported success rate of 50% to 93% (80–83). Tilney et al. (79) reported the first operative series with a success rate of 67% with renal reconstruction using a saphenous vein graft via a transabdominal approach. This allows the surgeon to approach the transplant renal artery anastamosis to the external iliac artery through a virgin plane and also facilitates exposure of the recipient's more proximal arterial circulation if necessary for revascularization. More recently, Roberts et al. (78) reported a success rate of over 70% with an additional 15% having significant improvement in hypertension. Our practice, as with most transplant centers, is to start with PTA and recipients not amenable to this modality will need open revascularization most likely with a saphenous vein bypass graft.

Lymphocoele
Most incidental fluid collections that are found in the immediate post-transplant period using ultrasound imaging require no further intervention. Once an urinoma resultant from a urine

leak has been excluded, the other diagnostic possibilities include hematoma and lymphocoele both of which will spontaneously resolve.

Symptomatic lymphocoeles, including those that are painful, infected, or causing acute urinary obstruction, can be treated by percutaneous aspiration and sclerosis (84) under ultrasound or computed axial tomography scan guidance. If the lymphocoele reaccumulates, open or laparoscopic techniques can be utilized for drainage and marsupialization into the peritoneal cavity (85). Infected lymphocoeles, those that are associated with wound healing problems, and those that are immediately adjacent to vital vascular structures will require open drainage.

FUTURE CONSIDERATIONS

The demand for renal transplantation can logically be diminished only by elimination of the disease processes that result in ESRD. A decrease in this incidence depends upon control or cure of diabetic and hypertensive nephropathies as well as the other less-prevalent glomerulonephropathies. The ever-present organ shortage and long-term immunosuppression complications, including recurrent ESRD and relisting, remain as the limiting factors for increasing the utilization of renal transplantation. The solution to these problems will match the continued demand for renal allografts for the increasing number of recipients listed, as well as to decrease chronic renal allograft dysfunction, which returns these recipients to the list once their allograft has failed.

The increased utilization of LURDs as well as laparoscopic donor nephrectomy has increased the rate of live donor renal transplant to the point of surpassing cadaveric renal transplant. ECD as well as DCD has increased deceased donor donation and subsequent renal transplant rates but not to the point of matching the increased number of patients being listed. Donor kidney exchange protocols (86), such as the one utilized by the New England Organ Bank, allows for either incompatible donor exchange to their respective recipients within the region or an incompatible donor donating to the list with their previously incompatible recipient receiving the next suitable deceased donor renal allograft available within the region. Moreover, protocols to remove isoagglutinin and HLA antibodies by plasmapheresis and intravenous immune globulin administration have made possible the use of ABO-incompatible renal allografts by negating the positive cross-match between the potential live-donor and recipient (87).

Immunosuppression with corticosteroid-sparing protocols have been utilized with great success. The future goal, as always, is to achieve immune tolerance. Knechtle et al. (88) presented protocols to induce tolerance such as the one utilizing the lymphocyte-depleting monoclonal antibody Campath-1H plus sirolimus monotherapy. This demonstrated a one-year patient and allograft survival of 100% and 97.5%, respectively. This may help to lower the rate of chronic renal allograft dysfunction by lessening the amount of chronic immunosuppression necessary once tolerance is induced.

CONCLUSION

Advances in immunosuppression, renal preservation, surgical donor and recipient techniques, and effective management of post-transplant complications has made renal allograft transplantation the therapeutic option of choice for the properly selected patient with ESRD. Continuous refinements in immunosuppression and protocols for treatment of rejection will need to make the transplant option safer and more durable with an acceptable nonrejection complication rate. The urologic surgeon is and must remain an integral member of the transplant team both at the technical and research levels.

REFERENCES

1. Merrill JP, Murray JE, Harrison JH, et al. Successful homotransplantation of the human kidney between identical twins. JAMA 1956; 160:277–282.
2. Landsteiner K, Hufnagle L. Cited by Goodwin WE, Martin DC. Renal transplantation. In: Campbell MF, Harrison JH, eds. Urology. 3rd ed. Philadelphia, PA: WB Saunders, 1970[a1].

3. Neylan JF, Sayegh MH, Coffman TM, et al. The allocation of cadaveric Kidneys for transplantation in the United States: consensus and controversy. J Am Soc Nephrol 1999; 10:2237–2243.

4. Ojo AO, Heinrichs D, Emond JC, et al. Organ donation and utilization in the USA: Am J Transplant 2004; 350(suppl 9):27–37.

5. Organ Procurement and Transplant Network. Reported deaths and annual Death rates per 1,000 patient years at risk: waiting list, 1993–2002. In: OPTN/SRTR 2003 Annual Report: Summary Tables, Transplant Data 1993–2002. Table 1.7 (Accessed July 28, 2005, at http://www.ustransplant.org).

6. Urban Institute. Medicare ESRD Incidence per Million by Primary Diagnosis. The Urban Institute 1980–1986. Based on HCFA Data. Washington, D.C.: U.S. Government Publication. 1986[a2].

7. Modlin CS, Fletchner SM, Goormastic M, et al. Should obese patients lose weight before receiving a kidney transplant? Transplantation 1997; 64:599–604.

8. Dunn DL, Mayoral JL, Gillingham KJ, et al. Treatment of invasive cytomegalovirus disease in solid organ transplant patients with ganciclovir. Transplantation 1991; 51:98–106.

9. Cameron JS. Recurrent disease in renal allografts. Kidney Int 1993; S91:44–45.

10. Jamieson NV. The results of combined liver/kidney transplantation for primary hyperoxaluria (PH1) 1984–1997: the European PH1 Transplant Registry report. European PH1 Transplantation Study Group. J Nephrol 1998; S36:11–13.

11. Marthurin P, Moquet C, Poynardt T, et al. Impact of hepatitis B and C virus on kidney transplantation outcome. Hepatology 1999; 29:257–261.

12. Steinmuller DR. Evaluation and selection of candidates renal transplantation. Urol Clin North Am 1983; 10:217–230.

13. Penn I. The effect of immunosuppression in pre-existing cancers. Transplantation 1993; 55:742–747.

14. Hatch DA, Belitsky P, Barry JM, et al. Fate of renal allograft transplanted in patients with urinary diversion. Transplantation 1993; 56:838–842.

15. Mazzucchi E, Nahas WC, Antonopoulos IM, et al. Surgical complications of graft nephrectomy in the modern transplant era. J Urol 2003; 170:734–737.

16. Tsuda K, Murakami T, Kim T, et al. Helical CT angiography of living renal donors: comparison with 3D Fournier transformation phase contrast MRA. J Comput Assist Tomogr 1998; 22:186–191.

17. Cecka JM. The UNOS Scientific Renal Transplant Registry. In: Cecka JM, Terasaki PI, eds. Clinical Transplants, 1999. Los Angeles UCLA Immunogenics Center, Los Angeles, California: 2000:11–12[a3].

18. Narkun-Burgess DM, Nolan CR, Norman JE, et al. Forty-five year followup after uninephrectomy. Kidney Int 1993; 43:1110–1115[a4].

19. Goldfarb DA, Matin SF, Braun WE, et al. Renal outcome 25 years after donor nephrectomy. J Urol 2001; 166:2043–2047.

20. Wyner LM, et al. Improved success in living unrelated renal transplantation with cyclosporine immunosuppression. J Urol 1993; 149:706–708.

21. Humar A, Durand B, Gillingham K, et al. Living unrelated donors in kidney transplants: better long-term results than with non-HLA-identical living related donors? Transplantation 2000; 69:1942–1945.

22. Evans RW. Executive Summary: The National Cooperative Transplantation Study BHARC-100-91-020. Seattle, WA: Battelle-Seattle Research Center, 1991.

23. Unadjusted graft and patient survival at 3 months, 1 year, 5 years, and 10 years: standard errors of the survival rates. In: OPTN/SRTR 2003 Annual Report: Summary Tables, Transplant Data 1993–2002. Table 1.14. (Accessed July 28, 2005, at http://www.ustransplant.org).

24. Vella JP, Spadafora-Ferreira M, Murphy B, et al. Indirect allorecognition of major histocompatibility complex allopeptides in human renal transplant recipients with chronic graft dysfunction. Transplantation 1997; 64:795–800.

25. Pascual M, Theruvath T, Kawai T, et al. Strategies to improve long-term outcomes after renal transplantation. N Engl J Med 2002; 346:580–590.

26. Matsuno N, Kozaki K, Degawa H, et al. A useful predictor in machine perfusion preservation for kidney transplantation from non-heart-beating donors. Transplant Proc 2000; 32:173–175 .

27. Gjertson DW. Multifactorial analysis of renal transplants reported to the United Network for Organ Sharing Registry: The 1994 Update. In: Cecka JM, Terasaki PI, eds. Clinical Transplants, 1994. Los Angeles, CA: UCLA Tissue Typing Laboratory, 1995:532–534.

28. Leivastad T, Berger L, Thornsby E. Beneficial effects of DR matching on cadaveric renal transplant survival in Scandian Transplant. Transplant Proc 1992; 24:2447–2448.

29. Matas AJ, Sutherland DE, Najarian JS, et al. The impact of HLA matching on graft survival and on sensitization after a failed transplant. Transplantation 1990; 50:599–607.

30. Hayes MJ, Steinmuller DR, Novick AC, et al. A single center experience with shared 6-antigen matched cadaveric renal transplants. Transplantation 1993; 55:669–672.

31. Belzer FO, Hoffmann RM, Rice MJ, et al. Combination perfusion cold storage for optimum cadaver kidney function and utilization. Transplantation 1985; 39:118–121.

32. Nogueira JM, Canero CB, Fink JC, et al. A comparison of renal transplant outcomes with laparoscopic vs open donor nephrectomy. Transplantation 1999; 67:722–728.

33. Ruiz-Deya G, Cheng S, Palmer E, et al. Open donor, laparoscopic donor, and hand-assisted laparoscopic donor nephrectomy: a comparison of outcomes. J Urol 2001; 166:1270–1274.

34. Jacobs SC, Cho E, Dunkin BJ, et al. Laparoscopic live donor nephrectomy: The University of Maryland 3 year experience. J Urol 2000; 164:1494–1499.
35. Ratner LE, Kavoussi LR, Shulam PG, et al. Comparison of laparoscopic live donor nephrectomy versus the standard open approach. Transplant Proc 1997; 29:138–139.
36. Malone MJ, Bihrle W III, Libertino JA. Renal transplantation. In: Libertino JA, ed. Reconstructive Urologic Surgery. 3rd ed. St. Louis, MO: Mosby Yearbook Inc., 1998:93–100.
37. Lich R Jr, Howerton LW, Davis LA. Recurrent urosepsis in children. J Urol 1961; 86:554–558.
38. Surange RS, Johnson RWG, Tavakoli A, et al. Kidney transplantation into an ileal conduit: a single center experience of 59 cases. J Urol 2003; 170:1727–1730 .
39. Alfrey EJ, Salvatierra O, Tanney DC, et al. Bladder augmentation can be problematic with renal failure and transplantation. Pediatr Nephrol 1997; 11:672–676.
40. Ponticelli C, Tarantino A, Montagnino G, et al. A randomized trial comparing triple-drug and double-drug therapy in renal transplantation. Transplantation 1988; 45:913–918.
41. Shield CF III, Cosimi AB, Tolkoff-Rubin N, et al. Use of antithymocyte globulin for reversal of acute allograft rejection. Transplantation 1979; 28:461–464.
42. Norman DJ, Shield CF III, Barry J, et al. A U. S. clinical study of orthoclone OKT3 in renal transplantation. Transplant Proc 1987; 19(2 suppl. 1):21–27.
43. Meier-Kriesche HU, Kaplan B. Cyclosporine microemulsion and tacrolimus are associated with decreased chronic allograft failure and improved long- term graft survival as compared to sandimmune. Am J Transplant 2002; 2:100–104.
44. Cole E, Landsberg D, Russell D, et al. A pilot study of steroid-free immunosuppression in the prevention of acute rejection in renal allograft recipients. Transplantation 2001; 72:845–850.
45. The tri-continental mycophenolate mofetil renal transplantation study group. A blinded, randomized clinical trial of mycophenolate mofetil for the prevention of acute rejection in cadaveric renal transplantation. Transplantation 1996; 61:1029–1037.
46. Vincenti F, Kirkman R, Light S, et al. Interleukin-2 receptor blockade with daclizumab to prevent acute rejection in renal transplantation. N Engl J Med 1998; 338:161–165.
47. Cecka J, Cho Y, Terasaki P. Analysis of the UNOS scientific renal transplant registry at three years: early events affecting transplant success. Transplantation 1992; 53:59–64.
48. Gray J, Kasiske B. Patient and renal allograft survival in the late post-transplant period. Semin Nephrol 1992; 12:343–348.
49. Harihan S, Johnson CP, Bresnahan BA, et al. Improved graft survival after renal transplantation in the United States, 1988–1996. N Eng J Med 2003; 342:605–612.
50. Nankjvell BJ, Borrows RJ, Fung CL-S, et al. The natural history of chronic allograft nephropathy. N Engl J Med 2003; 349:2326–2333.
51. Davis CL. The prevention of cytomegalovirus disease in renal transplantation. Am J Kidney Dis 1990; 16:175–188.
52. Peterson PK, Balfour HH Jr, Marker SE, et al. Cytomegalovirus disease in renal allograft recipients: a prospective study of the clinical features, risk factors and impact on renal transplantation. Medicine 1980; 59:283–300.
53. Markham A, Faulds D. Gancyclovir: an update of its therapeutic use in cytomegalovirus infection. Drugs 1994; 48:455–461.
54. Rubin RH. Preemptive therapy in immunocompromised hosts. N Engl J Med 1991; 324:1057–1059.
55. Jacobson IM, Jaffers G, Dienstag JL, et al. Immunogenicity of hepatitis B vaccine in renal transplant recipients. Transplantation 1985; 39:393–395.
56. Roth D, Fernandez JA, Babischkin S, et al. Transmission of hepatitis C virus with solid organ transplantation: incidence and clinical significance. Transplant Proc 1993; 25(1 pt 2):1476–1478.
57. Schoenfeld P, Feduska NJ. Acquired immunodeficiency syndrome and renal disease: report of the National Kidney Foundation-National Institute of Health Task Force on AIDS and kidney disease. Am J Kidney Disease 1990; 16:14–25.
58. Zaleski C, Burke G, Nery J, et al. Risk of AIDS (HIV) transmission of 581 renal transplants. Transplant Proc 1993; 25(1 pt 2):1483–1486.
59. Abbot KC, Oliver JD III, Ko CW, et al. Patient and renal allograft survival in patients seropositive for human immunodeficiency virus infection. Transplantation 2000; 69:S217.
60. Penn I. Cancers following cyclosporine therapy. Transplantation 1987; 43:32–35.
61. Cockfield SM, et al. Post-transplant lymphoproliferative disorder in renal allograft recipients. Transplantation 1993; 56:88–96.
62. Penn I. Occurrence of cancers in immunosuppressed organ transplant recipients. In: Terasaki PI, Cecka JM, eds. Clinical Transplants 1994. Los Angeles UCLA Tissue Typing Laboratory. 1995:99–109[a8].
63. Loughlin KR, Tilney NL, Richie JP. Urologic complications in 718 renal transplant patients. Surgery 1984; 95:297–302.
64. Shoskes DA, Hanbury D, Cranston D. Urologic complications in 1000 consecutive renal transplant recipients. J Urol 1995; 153:18–21.
65. Thrasher JB, Temple DR, Spees EK. Extravesical versus Leadbetter-Politano ureteroneocystostomy: a comparison of complications in 320 renal transplants. J Urol 1990; 144:1105–1109.

66. Yadav RM, Johnson W, Morris PJ, et al. Vesico-ureteric reflux following renal transplantation. Br J Surg 1972; 59:33–35.
67. Voegeli DR, Crummy AB, McDermott JC, et al. Percutaneous dilatation of ureteric strictures in renal transplant patients. Radiology 1988; 169:185–188.
68. Streem SB. Endourologic management of urological complications following renal transplantation. Semin Urol 1994; 12:123–127.
69. Kennelly MJ, Konnak JW, Herwig KR. Vesicopyeloplasty in renal transplant patients: a 20-year followup. J Urol 1993; 150:1118–1120.
70. Malone MJ, Khauli RB, Lowell J. Use of small and large bowel in renal transplantation. Urol Clin North Am 1997; 24:837–843.
71. Wise GJ. Fungal and actinomycotic infections of the urinary tract. In: Walsh PC, Retik AB, Vaughan ED, Wein AJ, eds. Campbell's Urology. Vol. 1. 8th ed. Philadelphia, PA: Saunders, 2002:807–808.
72. Wheatley M, Ohld DA, Sonda LP III, et al. Treatment of renal transplant stones by extracorporeal shock-wave lithotripsy in the prone position. Urology 1991; 37:57–60.
73. Gettman MT, Levy JB, Engen DE, et al. Urological complications after kidney-pancreas trnasplantation. J Urol 1998; 159:38–43.
74. Goldman MH, Tilney NL, Vineyard GC, et al. A twenty year survey of arterial complications of renal transplantation. Surg Gynecol Obstet 1975; 141:758–763.
75. Vanrenterghem Y, Roels L, Lerut T, et al. Thromboembolic complications in haemostatic changes in cyclosporine-treated cadaveric kidney allograft recipients. Lancet 1985; 1:999–1002.
76. Gaber LW, Moore LW, Gaber AO, et al. Utility of standardized histological Classification in the management of acute rejection. Transplantation 1998; 65:376–382.
77. Sutherland RS, Spees EK, Jones JW, et al. Renal artery stenosis after renal transplantation. J Urol 1993; 149:980–985.
78. Roberts JP, Ascher NL, Fryd DS, et al. Transplant renal artery stenosis. Transplantation 1989; 48: 580–583.
79. Tilney NL, Rocha A, Strom TB, et al. Renal artery stenosis in transplant patients. Ann Surg 1984; 199:454–460.
80. Mollenkopf F, Matas A, Veith FJ, et al. Percutaneous transluminal angioplasty treatment for transplant renal artery stenosis. Transplant Proc 1983; 15:1089–1091.
81. Grossman RA, Dafoe DC, Schoenfeld RB, et al. Percutaneous transluminal angioplasty treatment of renal transplant artery stenosis. Transplantation 1982; 34:339–343.
82. Greenstein SM, Verstandig A, McLean GK, et al. Percutaneous transluminal angioplasty: procedure of choice in the hypertensive renal allograft recipient with renal artery stenosis. Transplantation 1987; 43:29–32.
83. Nicita G, Villari D, Marzocco M, et al. Endoluminal stent placement after percutaneous transluminal angioplasty in the treatment of post-transplant renal artery stenosis. J Urol 1998; 159:34–37.
84. Rivera M, Marcen R, Burgos J, et al. Treatment of post-transplant lymphocoele with povidone-iodine sclerosis: long-term followup. Nephron 1996; 74:324–326.
85. Gill IS, Hodge EE, Munch EC, et al. Transperitoneal marsupialization of lymphocoeles: a comparison of laparoscopic and open techniques. J Urol 1995; 153:706–711.
86. Delmonico FL, Morrissey PE, Lipkowitz GS, et al. Donor kidney exchanges. Am J Transpl 2004; 4:1–7.
87. Jordan SC, Vo A, Bunnapradist S, et al. Intravenous immune globulin treatment inhibits crossmatch positivity and allows for successful transplantation of incompatible organs in living-donor and cadaveric recipients. Transplantation 2003; 76:631–636.
88. Knechtle SJ, Pirsch JD, Fechner JH, et al. Campath-1H induction plus rapamycin monotherapy for renal transplantation: results of a pilot study. Am J Transplant 2003; 3:722–730.

16 | Complications of Genitourinary Trauma

Sean P. Elliott
Department of Urologic Surgery, University of Minnesota, Minneapolis, Minnesota, U.S.A.

Jack W. McAninch
Department of Urology, University of California at San Francisco, San Francisco General Hospital, San Francisco, California, U.S.A.

INTRODUCTION

Compared to other surgical fields there are relatively few emergencies in urology. For this reason we may become unaccustomed to caring for the trauma patient. Therefore, it is important to keep in mind some guiding principles when confronted with genitourinary trauma. If appropriately cared for, urologic trauma patients can have an excellent recovery with relatively few complications compared to trauma injuries of other organ systems; however, missed genitourinary injuries and improperly managed injuries lead to significant morbidity.

KIDNEY

Renal injury occurs in 1% to 3% of trauma cases (1–3). Isolated renal trauma is rare, occurring in only 5% of cases (4). The type of associated injuries varies but includes liver, colon, small bowel, and major vasculature most commonly. The majority of renal injuries are the result of blunt trauma. The degree of injury is minor in most cases. As such, morbidity and mortality are accounted for primarily by associated injuries. Urologic complications are unusual and include urinoma, perinephric abscess, hypertension, Page kidney, vascular complications, renal loss and, rarely, death.

Urinary Extravasation

Urinary extravasation occurs in 10% to 30% of penetrating renal trauma and 2% to 18% of blunt renal trauma (4,5). It is considered a characteristic of renal injury rather than a complication of renal injury. Only 13% to 26% of cases persist longer than a few days (6,7). So, in most patients, urinary extravasation can be managed expectantly. Occasionally, urine leak will persist and may develop into urinoma or perinephric abscess. Level 3 evidence suggests that risk factors for infection include devitalized renal fragments, coexisting pancreatic or intestinal injuries, prolonged central venous catheters, and large areas of soft-tissue loss requiring debridement (2,7,8). Signs and symptoms range from nonspecific to flank pain and tenderness with fever and palpable mass. Imaging by ultrasound demonstrates a low-density fluid collection that may develop a thick capsule or fluid echogenicity in the case of an infected urinoma or abscess. Computed tomography with delayed pyelography (CT-IVP) is the imaging procedure of choice as it shows not only the anatomy of the collection but can also demonstrate communication with the collecting system.

Prolonged urinary extravasation is well treated with retrograde stenting or percutaneous nephrostomy (9,10). If there is a loculated fluid collection without communication to the collecting system then percutaneous drainage of the urinoma or abscess is indicated and avoids open exploration in nearly all cases (10,11).

Vascular Complications

Vascular complications of renal trauma are rare and include delayed bleeding, pseudoaneurysm, and arteriovenous fistula. Pseudoaneurysm and arteriovenous fistula more commonly occur after elective renal surgery or renal biopsy, respectively. In the setting of trauma these complications occur most commonly after renal stab wounds, with a frequency of 6% (12) and 0% to 7%, (4,13,14) respectively. Signs and symptoms of pseudoaneurysm can include hematuria, hypertension, abdominal bruit, flank mass, or pain and abdominal bruit (15). Signs and symptoms of arteriovenous fistula are similar with the occasional additional finding of diastolic hypertension and congestive heart failure (16).

Delayed bleeding can occur due to a pseudoaneurysm, arteriovenous fistula or due to a segmental renal artery injury that may have tamponaded initially due to surrounding hematoma—after the hematoma reabsorbs the artery can rebleed. If a vascular complication is suspected then imaging is done with Doppler ultrasound or CT scan with intravenous contrast. If a lesion is confirmed then angiography can be both confirmatory and therapeutic with selective angioembolization (17,18). Abdominal exploration is rarely necessary and often results in nephrectomy.

Hypertension

The frequency with which hypertension occurs after renal trauma has been the source of much debate. Reported rates range from 0% to 55% (4,8,19–21). Unfortunately, with the poor follow-up of trauma patients there are few studies that look at this issue. Given the high background prevalence of hypertension, those studies that have been performed are likely underpowered to answer this question. Still, there are several reports of new onset hypertension in young, otherwise healthy patients after renal trauma. One study with four years of follow-up suggests that there is a higher incidence in nonoperatively managed patients; (20) however, others have not been able to reproduce this finding. The etiology of hypertension may include renal artery stenosis after injury (21,22) or extrinsic compression of the kidney either acutely from hematoma or chronically from scar (Page kidney) (23,24). A final possible cause is an arteriovenous fistula, which, like renal artery stenosis and Page kidney, leads to renal underperfusion and consequent hyperreninemia.

URETER

Ureteral injuries represent less than 1% of all genitourinary injuries from violent trauma (25). The most common etiology of ureteral trauma is a gunshot wound, accounting for 81% of such injuries (25). While retrograde pyelogram is the most sensitive diagnostic study it is time consuming and requires anesthesia. Therefore, the diagnostic procedure of choice is a CT-IVP, which can be easily incorporated into the radiographic survey of nongenitourinary injuries. In the unstable patient, the injured side can be drained with a nephrostomy tube, the ureter ligated if the abdomen is open, and the defect reconstructed at a later date. In the stable patient, the ureter is debrided back to healthy tissue and reconstructed. Proximal and mid-ureteral injuries are most commonly repaired with ureteroureterostomy and distal injuries are repaired with ureteroneocystostomy. The incidence of complications related to the repair of ureteral trauma is 25% (25–33).

Prolonged urinary leakage at the anastomosis is the most common acute genitourinary complication. Presentation can include urinoma, abscess, or peritonitis. Placement of a drain in the retroperitoneum at the time of initial repair is a preventive measure in that it allows efflux of urine in case of leakage and it allows one to recognize the leakage earlier. High volume output from the drain should be sent for a creatinine level. Delayed recognition of undrained leakage at the anastomosis is associated with additional morbidity such as sepsis, more complicated reconstruction, and prolonged hospital stay (25,30,34–36). Delayed urologic complications include ureteral stricture and retained ureteral stent leading to stone formation (25). Follow-up is difficult due to the transient nature of the trauma patient population; therefore, a true assessment of the incidence of long-term complications is difficult. Acute nonurologic complications and death from other causes are also common in patients with ureteral injury. This is indicative of the gravity of associated injuries and not due to the ureteral injury itself.

BLADDER

Bladder trauma occurs secondary to blunt or penetrating injury. Sixty of ninety percent of blunt bladder injuries occur secondary to pelvic fracture and 2% to 11% of patients with pelvic fracture sustain a bladder injury (37). Combined urethral and bladder injury is present in 2% to 30% of cases (38,39). Blunt injury is further characterized as intraperitoneal or extraperitoneal because the type of rupture dictates management—all intraperitoneal blunt bladder ruptures should be managed operatively whereas nearly all extraperitoneal blunt bladder ruptures may be managed nonoperatively. Indications for exploration and repair of blunt extraperitoneal bladder injuries include hematuria that is not adequately drained by a urethral catheter, and concomitant bladder neck, rectal, or vaginal injuries. Patients undergoing internal fixation of pelvic fracture should undergo cystorraphy to prevent infection of hardware. In addition, hemodynamically stable patients undergoing exploratory laparotomy for the management of intraperitoneal injuries should have repair of their extraperitoneal bladder injury as doing so may speed recovery. All penetrating trauma injuries to the bladder, whether intraperitoneal or extraperitoneal, should be explored and managed with cystorraphy (37). When these principles are followed, complications of bladder trauma are rare (37); however, deviation from these principles may result in multiple complications and prolonged convalescence.

Delayed presentation can occur after relatively minor blunt trauma in an intoxicated patient with a full bladder. In such cases, the patient may present several days later with acute peritonitis. This is a surgical emergency and delayed presentation or delayed diagnosis can lead to death (40). Missed injury may result from failing to perform a cystogram when indicated or from an improperly performed cystogram. It is important that a stress cystogram be performed—that is, the bladder must be filled to 300 cc through the urethral catheter regardless of whether a plain film cystogram or CT cystogram is being performed. In the case of a CT cystogram it is not adequate to clamp the catheter and allow the bladder to fill with contrast as it is excreted from the kidneys as this leads to inadequate bladder distension and missed injuries (41–43). One should suspect a missed bladder injury if there is evidence of urinoma (fever, leukocytosis, and abdominal pain), high volume output from an abdominal drain, a urethral catheter that does not drain well, or persistent gross hematuria. Reabsorption of urine from the abdominal cavity will lead to serum electrolyte abnormalities mimicking renal failure (hyperkalemia, uremia, and elevated serum creatinine). Fluid from abdominal drains with high volume output should be sent for a creatinine level.

Another pitfall is treating all extraperitoneal bladder ruptures nonoperatively, regardless of etiology or concomitant injuries. Failure to repair penetrating bladder injury results in prolonged healing and can be complicated by vesicocutaneous, vesicovaginal, or vesicorectal fistula even if the concomitant injuries are repaired but the bladder injury is not (44). Likewise, attempts to repair bladder injuries through alternative approaches such as a transperineal approach or through a vaginal laceration are fraught with complications (44). Failure to repair a bladder neck injury in the initial hospitalization can lead to bladder neck stenosis and incontinence.

URETHRA

Complications of urethral injury include urethral stricture and erectile dysfunction. Complications vary with the severity and location of the urethral injury as well as with initial treatment of the injury.

Penetrating Anterior Urethral Injury

Anterior urethral injury can occur after penetrating trauma but this is rare. Most experts advocate primary debridement and repair of penetrating anterior urethral injuries. With early repair rather than urethral catheter realignment, the urethral stricture rate is reduced from 67% to 100% down to about 10% to 20% (45–47). Operative exploration also allows for diagnosis and repair of corporal body injuries. A missed corporal body injury can lead to persistent bleeding and cavernosal-spongiosal fistula. Follow-up is poor in these patients and no studies have used validated instruments to gage sexual function so a true assessment of the rate of erectile dysfunction is impossible. Some have reported penile curvature after repair of patients with extensive penile injuries (45).

Blunt Anterior Urethral Injury

The more common etiology of anterior urethral trauma is a straddle injury with compression of the bulbar urethra against the undersurface of the pubic arch. Patients present with ecchymosis and hematuria, or with blood at the meatus and an inability to void. Perhaps counterintuitively, when compared with suprapubic cystostomy, primary alignment with urethral catheterization has been associated with an increase (although not statistically significant) in urethral stricture rate rather than a decrease (100% vs. 88%, $p = 0.37$) (48). One theory is that the surrounding corpus spongiosal injury makes these injuries behave differently than posterior urethral injuries (see subsequently) (49).

Posterior Urethral Injury

Posterior urethral injury is nearly always the result of pelvic fracture; penetrating injury is rare. These patients can be acutely ill due to bleeding from the bony injury. Options for management include primary realignment or suprapubic diversion with delayed repair. Primary realignment was historically accomplished by vesicotomy and antegrade catheter placement, sometimes with prostatic apex dissection to assist with guiding the catheter. Other methods included the use of interlocking sounds or magnetic sounds. Such techniques are to be avoided due to the massive hemorrhage, urethral misalignment, and erectile dysfunction that can occur. Modern endourologic primary realignment does seem to decrease the rate of urethral stricture formation after posterior urethral injury by about 50% when compared with suprapubic urinary diversion (from a mean of 92% down to a mean of 47%) (50). Impotence and incontinence rates are similar with realignment and diversion (34% vs. 42% and 18% vs. 25%). However, no prospective randomized studies comparing the two methods have been done. Those series reporting lower rates of urethral stricture formation with primary realignment suffer from selection bias in that urethral realignment was attempted in all patients unless they were acutely ill. If realignment was unsuccessful, patients underwent suprapubic diversion. Hence, patients with suprapubic diversion were more acutely ill and had more significant urethral injuries.

EXTERNAL GENITALIA
Penetrating Penile Injury and Penile Amputation

All patients with penetrating penile injury should undergo urethrography and operative penile exploration, debridement, and suture repair of urethral and cavernosal injuries. Failure to do so leads to urethral stricture, hemorrhage from missed corporal injuries, and cavernosal-spongiosal fistula. Experience with the amputated penis is rare; however, prompt replantation with anastomosis of the urethra, tunica albuginea, cavernosal nerves, dorsal arteries and veins can be accomplished with few complications (51–54). Nonmicrosurgical replantation is associated with poorer outcomes (55). Penile engorgement due to poor venous and lymphatic drainage is common after replantation and responds to leech therapy (56).

Penile Fracture

Penile fracture occurs most commonly during intercourse, although self-inflicted injuries do occur (57,58). Concomitant injury to the corpus spongiosum occurs in approximately 20% and urethral injury in 3% to 20% (57–59). Urethrography should be performed if there is blood at the meatus, any degree of hematuria, or obstructive urinary symptoms. Missed urethral injuries may lead to stricture and/or cavernosal-spongiosal fistula. Some relief of symptoms is obtained with an ice pack; however, surgical repair should be carried out as early as possible. Expert opinion is that early evacuation of hematoma and primary closure of the tunical defect with absorbable suture minimizes inflammation, fibrosis, and consequent penile curvature (59). Complications are limited to minimal/moderate penile curvature in 7% of those who undergo exploration (58); however, a later series including the same patients reported no penile plaques so the relationship between penile fracture and Peyronie's disease is unclear (60). In one series with good follow-up on 170 patients who were repaired surgically the prevalence of erectile dysfunction, based on answers to a validated questionnaire, was no different from controls (58).

Genital Skin Loss

External genital skin loss results from avulsion injuries, animal or human bites, and necrotizing skin infections. Avulsion injuries and animal bites present acutely and can usually be closed primarily after empirical antibiotic coverage, debridement, and wound irrigation; complications are rare (61). Human bites to the genitalia often present in a delayed fashion resulting in more advanced infection of surrounding tissues. These wounds should not be closed. With proper debridement, irrigation, and antibiotic administration, complications are few. Fournier's gangrene should receive rapid surgical and antibiotic attention to avoid complications of sepsis, extensive tissue loss, and death. Death occurs on average in 15% (range 3–45%) and the rate varies with what is defined as Fournier's gangrene (62). Patients with genitourinary pathology as the underlying cause of their infection had a better chance of survival than patients with underlying recto-anal pathology (63). Other risk factors for death included chronic renal failure and >6% body surface area involvement. While diabetes was commonly present it was not predictive of death.

Testis

Testicular trauma is due to blunt injury in 85% of cases. While testis trauma was at one time managed nonoperatively, this approach has been abandoned as many series have shown improved testicular salvage rates with exploration with 72 hours (64–66). Rapid diagnosis is essential and ultrasound is the imaging procedure of choice in cases where physical examination is nondiagnostic (66). Delayed diagnosis can lead to pain, hematoma that is slow to reabsorb, infection, and perhaps infertility. There is no negative impact on fertility with early operative intervention (67).

CONCLUSION

Genitourinary trauma is rarely life threatening; however, this should not lead to apathy on the part of the consulting urologist. Rapid diagnosis and appropriate intervention can yield excellent results whereas an inappropriate delay in diagnosis or intervention can lead to increased complications.

REFERENCES

1. Wessells H, Suh D, Porter JR, et al. Renal injury and operative management in the United States: results of a population-based study. J Trauma 2003; 54:423–430.
2. Santucci RA, Wessells H, Bartsch G, et al. Evaluation and management of renal injuries: consensus statement of the renal trauma subcommittee. BJU Int 2004; 93:937–954.
3. Krieger JN, Algood CB, Mason JT, Copass MK, Ansell JS. Urological trauma in the Pacific Northwest: etiology, distribution, management and outcome. J Urol 1984; 132:70–73.
4. Kansas BT, Eddy MJ, Mydlo JH, Uzzo RG. Incidence and management of penetrating renal trauma in patients with multiorgan injury: extended experience at an inner city trauma center. J Urol 2004; 172(4 Pt 1):1355–1360.
5. Brandes SB, McAninch JW. Complications of renal trauma. In: Teneja SS, Smith RB, Ehrlich RM, eds. Complications of Urology. 3rd ed. Philadelphia, PA: W.B. Saunders, 2001:205–225.
6. Matthews LA, Smith EM, Spirnak JP. Nonoperative treatment of major blunt renal lacerations with urinary extravasation. J Urol 1997; 157:2056–2058.
7. Moudouni SM, Patard JJ, Manunta A, Guiraud P, Guille F, Lobel B. A conservative approach to major blunt renal lacerations with urinary extravasation and devitalized renal segments. BJU Int 2001; 87:290–294.
8. Husmann DA, Gilling PJ, Perry MO, Morris JS, Boone TB. Major renal lacerations with a devitalized fragment following blunt abdominal trauma: a comparison between nonoperative (expectant) versus surgical management. J Urol 1993; 150:1774–1777.

9. Philpott JM, Nance ML, Carr MC, Canning DA, Stafford PW. Ureteral stenting in the management of urinoma after severe blunt renal trauma in children. J Pediatr Surg 2003; 38:1096–1098.

10. Titton RL, Gervais DA, Hahn PF, Harisinghani MG, Arellano RS, Mueller PR. Urine leaks and urinomas: diagnosis and imaging-guided intervention. Radiographics 2003; 23:1133–1147.

11. Meng MV, Mario LA, McAninch JW. Current treatment and outcomes of perinephric abscesses. J Urol 2002; 168(4 Pt 1):1337–1340.

12. Heyns CF, Van Vollenhoven P. Selective surgical management of renal stab wounds. Br J Urol 1992; 69:351–357.

13. Armenakas NA, Duckett CP, McAninch JW. Indications for nonoperative management of renal stab wounds. J Urol 1999; 161:768–771.

14. Bernath AS, Schutte H, Fernandez RR, Addonizio JC. Stab wounds of the kidney: conservative management in flank penetration. J Urol 1983; 129:468–470.

15. Lee RS, Porter JR. Traumatic renal artery pseudoaneurysm: diagnosis and management techniques. J Trauma 2003; 55:972–978.

16. Morin RP, Dunn EJ, Wright CB. Renal arteriovenous fistulas: a review of etiology, diagnosis, and management. Surgery 1986; 99:114–118.

17. Beaujeux R, Saussine C, al-Fakir A, et al. Superselective endo-vascular treatment of renal vascular lesions. J Urol 1995; 153:14–17.

18. Pinto IT, Chimeno PC. Treatment of a urinoma and a post-traumatic pseudoaneurysm using selective arterial embolization. Cardiovasc Intervent Radiol 1998; 21:506–508.

19. McAninch JW, Carroll PR, Armenakas NA, Lee P. Renal gunshot wounds: methods of salvage and reconstruction. J Trauma 1993; 35:279–283; discussion 83–84.

20. Cass AS, Luxenberg M, Gleich P, Smith C. Long-term results of conservative and surgical management of blunt renal lacerations. Br J Urol 1987; 59:17–20.

21. Haas CA, Dinchman KH, Nasrallah PF, Spirnak JP. Traumatic renal artery occlusion: a 15-year review. J Trauma 1998; 45:557–561.

22. Meyrier A, Rainfray M, Lacombe M. Delayed hypertension after blunt renal trauma. Am J Nephrol 1988; 8:108–111.

23. Haydar A, Bakri RS, Prime M, Goldsmith DJ. Page kidney—a review of the literature. J Nephrol 2003; 16:329–333.

24. Engel WJ, Page IH. Hypertension due to renal compression resulting from subcapsular hematoma. J Urol 1955; 73:735–739.

25. Elliott SP, McAninch JW. Ureteral injuries from external violence: the 25-year experience at San Francisco General Hospital. J Urol 2003; 170(4 Pt 1):1213–1216.

26. Azimuddin K, Milanesa D, Ivatury R, Porter J, Ehrenpreis M, Allman DB. Penetrating ureteric injuries. Injury 1998; 29:363–367.

27. Brandes SB, Chelsky MJ, Buckman RF, Hanno PM. Ureteral injuries from penetrating trauma. J Trauma 1994; 36:766–769.

28. Perez-Brayfield MR, Keane TE, Krishnan A, Lafontaine P, Feliciano DV, Clarke HS. Gunshot wounds to the ureter: a 40-year experience at Grady Memorial Hospital. J Urol 2001; 166:119–121.

29. Carlton CE Jr, Scott R Jr, Guthrie AG. The initial management of ureteral injuries: a report of 78 cases. J Urol 1971; 105:335–340.

30. Campbell EW Jr, Filderman PS, Jacobs SC. Ureteral injury due to blunt and penetrating trauma. Urology 1992; 40:216–220.

31. Rober PE, Smith JB, Pierce JM Jr. Gunshot injuries of the ureter. J Trauma 1990; 30:83–86.

32. Ghali AM, El Malik EM, Ibrahim AI, Ismail G, Rashid M. Ureteric injuries: diagnosis, management, and outcome. J Trauma 1999; 46:150–158.

33. Velmahos GC, Degiannis E. The management of urinary tract injuries after gunshot wounds of the anterior and posterior abdomen. Injury 1997; 28:535–538.

34. Holden S, Hicks CC, O'Brien DP, Stone HH, Walker JA, Walton KN. Gunshot wounds of the ureter: a 15-year review of 63 consecutive cases. J Urol 1976; 116:562–564.

35. Walker JA. Injuries of the ureter due to external violence. J Urol 1969; 102:410–413.

36. Medina D, Lavery R, Ross SE, Livingston DH. Ureteral trauma: preoperative studies neither predict injury nor prevent missed injury. J Am Coll Surg 1998; 186:641–644.

37. Gomez RG, Ceballos L, Coburn M, et al. Consensus statement on bladder injuries. BJU Int 2004; 94:27–32.

38. Cass AS, Gleich P, Smith C. Simultaneous bladder and prostatomembranous urethral rupture from external trauma. J Urol 1984; 132:907–908.

39. Palmer JK, Benson GS, Corriere JN Jr. Diagnosis and initial management of urological injuries associated with 200 consecutive pelvic fractures. J Urol 1983; 130:712–714.

40. Lunetta P, Penttila A, Sajantila A. Fatal isolated ruptures of bladder following minor blunt trauma. Int J Legal Med 2002; 116:282–285.

41. Doyle SM, Master VA, McAninch JW. Appropriate use of CT in the diagnosis of bladder rupture. J Am Coll Surg 2005; 200:973.

42. Horstman WG, McClennan BL, Heiken JP. Comparison of computed tomography and conventional cystography for detection of traumatic bladder rupture. Urol Radiol 1991; 12:188–193.
43. Mee SL, McAninch JW, Federle MP. Computerized tomography in bladder rupture: diagnostic limitations. J Urol 1987; 137:207–209.
44. Elliott SP, McAninch J. Extraperitoneal bladder trauma: mismanagement leads to prolonged convalescence. J Trauma.
45. Hall SJ, Wagner JR, Edelstein RA, Carpinito GA. Management of gunshot injuries to the penis and anterior urethra. J Trauma 1995; 38:439–443.
46. Husmann DA, Boone TB, Wilson WT. Management of low velocity gunshot wounds to the anterior urethra: the role of primary repair versus urinary diversion alone. J Urol 1993; 150:70–72.
47. Gomez RG, Castanheira AC, McAninch JW. Gunshot wounds to the male external genitalia. J Urol 1993; 150:1147–1149.
48. Park S, McAninch JW. Straddle injuries to the bulbar urethra: management and outcomes in 78 patients. J Urol 2004; 171(2 Pt 1):722–725.
49. Santucci RA. Straddle injuries to the bulbar urethra: management and outcomes in 78 patients. Int Braz J Urol 2004; 30:345–346.
50. Mouraviev VB, Coburn M, Santucci RA. The treatment of posterior urethral disruption associated with pelvic fractures: comparative experience of early realignment versus delayed urethroplasty. J Urol 2005; 173:873–876.
51. Shaw MB, Sadove AM, Rink RC. Reconstruction after total penile amputation and emasculation. Ann Plast Surg 2003; 50:321–324; discussion 4.
52. Ishida O, Ikuta Y, Shirane T, Nakahara M. Penile replantation after self-inflicted complete amputation: case report. J Reconstr Microsurg 1996; 12:23–26.
53. Sanger JR, Matloub HS, Yousif NJ, Begun FP. Penile replantation after selfinflicted amputation. Ann Plast Surg 1992; 29:579–584.
54. Jezior JR, Brady JD, Schlossberg SM. Management of penile amputation injuries. World J Surg 2001; 25:1602–1609.
55. Bhanganada K, Chayavatana T, Pongnumkul C, et al. Surgical management of an epidemic of penile amputations in Siam. Am J Surg 1983; 146:376–382.
56. Mineo M, Jolley T, Rodriguez G. Leech therapy in penile replantation: a case of recurrent penile self-amputation. Urology 2004; 63:981–983.
57. Beysel M, Tekin A, Gurdal M, Yucebas E, Sengor F. Evaluation and treatment of penile fractures: accuracy of clinical diagnosis and the value of corpus cavernosography. Urology 2002; 60:492–496.
58. Zargooshi J. Penile fracture in Kermanshah, Iran: the long-term results of surgical treatment. BJU Int 2002; 89:890–894.
59. Miller KS, McAninch JW. Penile fracture and soft tissue injury. In: McAninch JW, ed. Traumatic and Reconstructive Urology. 1st ed. Philadelphia, PA: W.B. Saunders Co., 1996:693–698.
60. Zargooshi J. Trauma as the cause of Peyronie's disease: penile fracture as a model of trauma. J Urol 2004; 172:186–188.
61. Morey AF, Metro MJ, Carney KJ, Miller KS, McAninch JW. Consensus on genitourinary trauma: external genitalia. BJU Int 2004; 94:507–515.
62. Eke N. Fournier's gangrene: a review of 1726 cases. Br J Surg 2000; 87:718–728.
63. Jeong HJ, Park SC, Seo IY, Rim JS. Prognostic factors in Fournier gangrene. Int J Urol 2005; 12:1041–1044.
64. Gross M. Rupture of the testicle: the importance of early surgical treatment. J Urol 1969; 101:196–197.
65. Lupetin AR, King W III, Rich PJ, Lederman RB. The traumatized scrotum. Ultrasound evaluation. Radiology 1983; 148:203–207.
66. Buckley JC, McAninch JW. Use of ultrasonography for the diagnosis of testicular injuries in blunt scrotal trauma. J Urol 2006; 175:175–178.
67. Kukadia AN, Ercole CJ, Gleich P, Hensleigh H, Pryor JL. Testicular trauma: potential impact on reproductive function. J Urol 1996; 156:1643–1646.

17 | Management of the Surgical Complications of Penile Carcinoma

Kevin R. Loughlin
Harvard Medical School and Division of Urology, Brigham and Women's Hospital, Boston, Massachusetts, U.S.A.

Penile carcinoma is relatively common in many underdeveloped countries, but rare in the United States and Europe. Penile carcinoma occurs almost exclusively in uncircumcised men and is associated with poor hygiene and papilloma virus infection. In the United States and Europe the yearly incidence of penile cancer is 0.5 to 1.0 per 100,000 men (1), whereas in less developed areas, penile cancer may account for 10% to 20% of all male malignancies (2).

Because of the rarity of penile carcinoma in the United States, many U.S. surgeons perform the surgery associated with penile cancer, rarely, if it all. Therefore, it is worthwhile to review the surgical techniques involved in treating both the primary penile lesion and the regional lymph nodes with specific attention to the complications that can be associated with each surgical procedure.

PRIMARY LESION

All patients with a penile lesion that is suspicious for malignancy should first have a biopsy performed to confirm the diagnosis. After the histologic diagnosis has been confirmed, the next surgical decision is to determine whether a partial or total penectomy is the appropriate treatment. The major considerations of which option is desirable are the size of the local lesion and the length of the phallus.

Prior to surgery, a magnetic resonance imaging (MRI) or penile ultrasound can be helpful in determining the proximal extent of the penile lesion. The traditional teaching has been that a 2-cm proximal margin in required. However, my own experience has been that a clear surgical margin of any diameter is likely to provide good local control (3). The surgeon must decide if a partial penectomy is to be performed, whether the patient will be left with a phallus that will enable him to stand to void and permit sexual arousal.

Technique of Partial Penectomy

After adequate spinal or general anesthesia has been achieved, the patient is placed in the supine position and his genitalia are prepared and draped in a sterile manner. A tourniquet is positioned around the base of the phallus and the incision is outlined using a surgical pen. A condom or surgical glove can be placed over the penile lesion, depending on the surgeon's preference (Fig. 1A). The circumferential incision is carried down through the skin and subcutaneous tissue and the neurovascular bundle is identified, mobilized, and divided (Fig. 1B). Attention is then turned to the corpora spongiosum and the urethra is isolated and divided (Fig. 1C).

The corpora caverosa are then divided (Fig. 2A) and the corpora are closed with a running absorbable suture (Fig. 2B). It is important to mobilize the urethra in such a manner so that the distal urethra extends beyond the closed, transected corpora cavernosa by 1 to 2 cm (Fig. 2C).

The penile skin is then brought over as a hood on the distal penis and a small opening is made in the reapproximated penile skin to accommodate the urethra. The urethral neomeatus is then "matured" much as one would do with an ileal conduit stoma (4). The dorsal aspect of the distal urethra is incised (Fig. 3A) and is folded back and sewn to the penile skin (Fig. 3B and C). When the neomeatus is completed, a Foley catheter is left indwelling for 24 to 48 hours and a drain is left along the penile shaft to prevent postoperative hematomas (Fig. 3D).

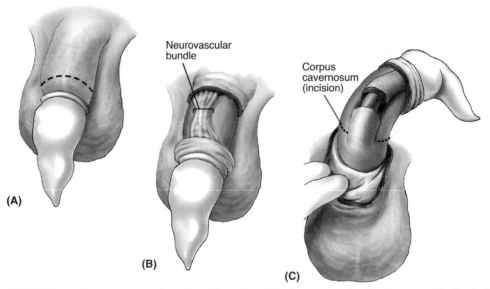

FIGURE 1 Partial penectomy: a circumferential penile incision is made proximal to the lesion (**A**). The incision is carried down through the subcutaneous tissue and the neurovascular bundle is isolated and divided (**B**). The urethra is mobilized and divided (**C**).

Technique of Total Penectomy

A total penectomy is the procedure of choice in cases of large lesions or with a small phallus where a partial penectomy would leave a penis inadequate to stand to void or provide sexual stimulation. A circumferential incision is made at the base of the penis and is carried down to the base of the corpora. The proximal urethra is mobilized and an infant feeding tube is sutured within the urethral lumen. Then a site for the perineal urethrostomy is chosen and a right angle clamp is passed upward through the site and the infant feeding tube is grasped and brought down through the perineal urethrostomy site (Fig. 4A). The perineal urethrostomy is matured in the same fashion as described in the partial penectomy (Fig. 4B).

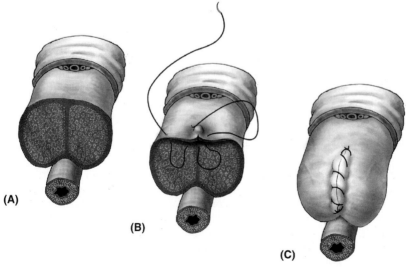

FIGURE 2 Partial penectomy: after the corpora are divided (**A**) they are closed with an absorbable suture (**B**). It is important to mobilize the distal urethra sufficiently to achieve a urethra that extends 1–2 cm beyond the corpora cavernosa (**C**).

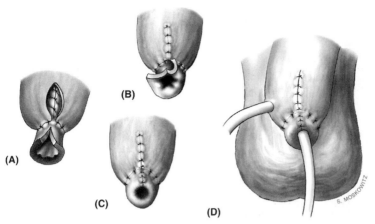

FIGURE 3 Creation of the neomeatus: the penile skin is closed (**A**) and the dorsal aspect of the urethra is incised (**B**) and then matured (**C,D**) much as would be done with an ileal loop stoma.

Technique of Ilioinguinal Lymphadenectomy

An ilioinguinal lymphadenectomy is generally performed in patients with penile cancer who have either palpable inguinal nodes or in those with nonpalpable nodes, but with a high-grade primary penile lesion with invasion into the corpora. Various incisions have been advocated for the ilioinguinal node dissection, but my own preference has been for three parallel incisions (Fig. 5).

The procedure starts with a bilateral pelvic lymphadenectomy, as is done for prostate cancer. After the pelvic nodes have been removed, vertical incisions are made over the femoral triangles up to the inguinal creases. A Scott ring retractor with disposable skin hooks facilitates exposure and minimizes the handling of the skin edges (5). The saphenous vein is utilized as a landmark and is dissected down to the femoral vein. In cases of bulky nodes, the saphenous vein almost always needs to be divided, whereas in cases of nonpalpable nodes, the saphenous vein can often be spared. Many surgeons feel that sparing the saphenous vein may minimize the risk of postoperative lymphedema.

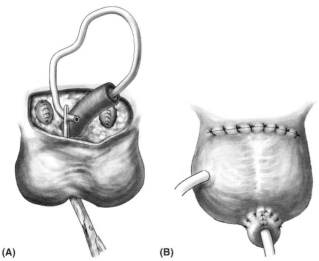

FIGURE 4 Total penectomy: a feeding tube placed in the urethra facilitates the passage of the urethra to the perineal urethrostomy site with a right-angle clamp (**A**). The perineal urethrostomy is then matured in the same fashion as is performed after a partial penectomy (**B**).

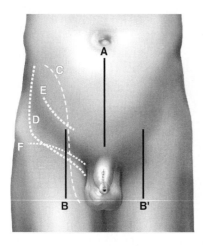

FIGURE 5 Choice of incisions for ilioinguinal lymphadenectomy: several incisions have been advocated for ilioinguinal lymphadenctomies.

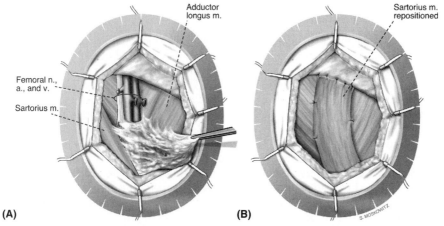

Adductor longus m.

Sartorius m. repositioned

Femoral n., a., and v.

Sartorius m.

(A)   **(B)**

S. MOSKOWITZ

FIGURE 6 Inguinal node dissection: the limits of the dissection are the apex of the femoral triangle inferiorly, the inguinal ligament superiorly, the adductor longus muscle medially, and the sartorius muscle laterally (**A**). The sartorius muscle can be detached from the anterior iliac spine and reattached to the inguinal ligament to provide coverage to the femoral vessels (**B**). *Abbreviations*: a., artery; n., nerve; v., vein.

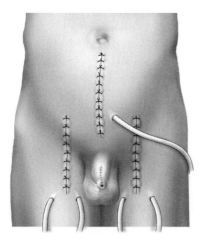

FIGURE 7 Closure of ilioinguinal incisions: the three incisions are closed and surgical drains are left in place.

The dissection proceeds as the femoral nerve, artery and vein are exposed, and the nodal packet is mobilized (Fig. 6A). The limits of the dissection are the apex of the femoral triangle inferiorly, the inguinal ligament superiorly, the adductor longus muscle medially and the sartorius muscle laterally.

After the inguinal node, dissection has been completed, the sartorius muscle can be mobilized to provide additional coverage over the femoral vessels. The superior aspect of the sartorius muscle is detached from the anterior iliac spine and is reattached to the inguinal ligament (Fig. 6B). The transfer of the sartorius muscle provides additional coverage to the femoral vessels in the event of a superficial wound infection.

The incisions are closed in the usual manner and drains are brought out through the skin (Fig. 7). Considerable lymphatic drainage can occur from the inguinal node dissections in some cases and the drains are left in place until the drainage is less than 50 cc per 24 hours from each surgical area.

REFERENCES

1. Gloeckler-Ries LA, Hankey BF, Edwards BK, eds. Cancer Statistics and Review 1973–1987. Bethesda, MD: US Dept of Health and Human Services, Public Health Service, National Institutes of Health, NIH Publications 1990; 789.
2. Narayana AS, Olney LE, Loening SA, et al. Carcinoma of the penis— analysis of 219 cases. Cancer 1982; 49:2185.
3. Hoffman MA, Renshaw AA, Loughlin KR. Squamous cell carcinoma of the penis and microscopic pathologic margins: how much margin is needed for local cure? Cancer 1999; 85:1565–1568.
4. Loughlin KR. The rosebud technique for creation of a neomeatus after partial or total penectomy. Br J Urol 1995; 76:123–124.
5. Loughlin KR. Use of the Scott ring surgical retractor for ilioinguinal node dissection. Br J Urol 1988; 61:267.

18 | Complications of Benign Adult Penile and Scrotal Surgery

Jeffrey C. La Rochelle and Laurence A. Levine
Department of Urology, Rush University Medical Center, Chicago, Illinois, U.S.A.

INTRODUCTION

Surgeries of the penis and scrotum for non-neoplastic reasons are seldom, if ever, life-threatening affairs. They are typically performed for reasons involving sexual function, fertility, or esthetics. Therefore, great attention must be paid to the delicate structures present in this region of the body. The nerves and arteries supplying the various tissues are of a small caliber and must be handled with care. Caution must be exercised when using electrocautery, particularly on the penis, and bipolar devices should be considered. Optical magnification is also often helpful when working in areas where neurovascular injury is a possibility. Hemostasis, particularly in the scrotum, is critical in preventing edema and hematoma formation in this rather dependent portion of the body. Mildly compressive dressings and activity limitation following surgery are recommended for most procedures performed in this area, and skin closures should be made with absorbable sutures to avoid the need for later removal. Techniques for the prevention and management of complications specific to individual surgeries of the penis and scrotum are described in the following sections.

COMPLICATIONS OF PENILE PROSTHESES

Placement of a penile prosthesis is a routine procedure in most cases with a high rate of patient satisfaction. On occasion, complications arise intra- or postoperatively, and surgeons who place penile prostheses need to be prepared to manage them. The risk of complications such as infection or device failure can be minimized but not eliminated with proper technique and attention to detail, but eventually most prostheses will fail. This is the inevitable consequence of placing a complex foreign device into the body. However, the majority of patients will have the use of their prosthesis for 10 years or longer without significant side effects or complications.

Intraoperative Complications
Crural Crossover
Crural crossover occurs during proximal corporal dilation when a dilating instrument perforates the intracorporal septum and crosses into the proximal portion of the contralateral corpus cavernosum. A urethral injury, though not likely in this situation, must be ruled out when the crossover is identified. A careful inspection looking for damage to the corpus spongiosum or blood at the meatus is necessary before proceeding because an unrecognized urethral injury could easily lead to device infection or fistula formation. A crural crossover should be suspected if the dilating instrument deviates from the expected path. Crossover may not be recognized until later when there is difficulty placing the cylinders or when an abnormality or asymmetry is seen when both cylinders are in place.

  If a urethral injury is discovered, a decision to proceed or abort must be made, and this will be discussed in the next section. If no urethral injury is present, dilation of the proximal portion of the corpus cavernosum on the side of the injury still needs to be performed because the dilating instrument has not yet been properly passed into that space. There may be some difficulty getting the dilators to follow the correct path because they continue to preferentially cross over through the perforation. To avoid this, the contralateral corpus should be dilated if it has not yet been done. Once it has been dilated, a 13-mm dilator should remain in the corpus on that side while dilation is resumed on the side of the crossover. The dilator on the opposite side should prevent the instrument from passing back through the septal perforation. Once both corpora have been adequately dilated, the first prosthesis cylinder is placed on the side of the perforation while the dilator is still in place on the contralateral side. After the first cylinder is well seated, the dilator can be removed and the second cylinder can be placed.

Distal Crossover
Distal crossover during corporal dilation is handled similar to crural crossover except that suspicion for urethral injury should be higher. Dilute methylene blue may be infused into the intracorporal space with a bulb syringe to better evaluate the integrity of the urethra. As will be discussed later, the procedure must be aborted in cases of distal urethral injury due to elevated risk of infection.

Crural Perforation
The best method to manage crural perforation during dilation is to prevent it with careful technique. It may occur in spite of proper precautions, however. To avoid perforation, dilation should begin with a 9-mm or larger dilating instrument because they are blunter than smaller instruments and therefore less likely to pierce the tunica (1). When the dilator is advanced into the proximal corpora, it should be directed laterally which is more in line with the angle of the crura. This also directs the main force of the dilator toward the portion of the crus that is supported by the inferior pubic ramus.

Proximal crural perforation is recognized when there is a sudden loss of resistance to the passage of the dilator. When the full length of the proximal corpus cavernosum is dilated properly, the dilator should be felt making contact with a hard surface which is the proximal tip of the corpus cavernosum against the inferior pubic ramus. When a dilator has perforated, it will pass into the perineal space without coming into contact with the inferior ramus. (Fig. 1) In uncertain situations, using measurements from the contralateral crus will help to determine whether the dilator has passed outside of the corpus. If the dilator has perforated the crus on

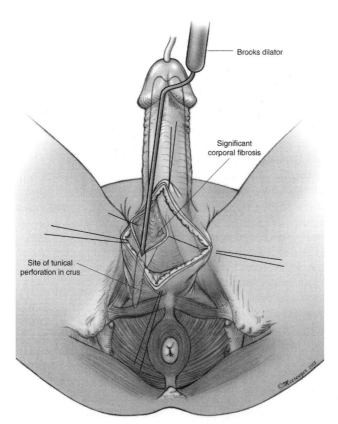

Brooks dilator

Significant
corporal fibrosis

Site of tunical
perforation in crus

FIGURE 1 A corporal perforation in the typical ventromedial direction. *Source*: From Ref. 1.

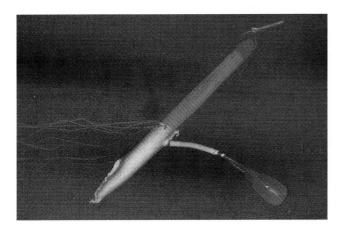

FIGURE 2 A windsock fashioned from polytetrafluroethylene for proximal corporal perforation. Note the tacking sutures placed prior to insertion into the perforated corpus cavernosum.

the dorsomedial aspect away from the proximal corporal tip, it is sometimes possible to reestablish the proper plane of dilation by redirecting the dilator in a more ventrolateral direction. If the perforation is too large or is at the tip of the corpus cavernosum, it requires repair because of the risk of proximal migration of the prosthesis cylinder.

There are several methods of repair. In the past, surgeons would sometimes reposition and redrape the patient to allow for a perineal approach to repair a crural injury. This increases the risk of infection and adds considerable time to the procedure. Instead, two simpler methods are commonly used in the case of proximal perforation: the windsock method and the plug and patch method. The windsock repair involves fashioning a cone-shaped "windsock" out of either polytetrafluroethylene (PTFE), Dacron, or nonsynthetic material, such as processed pericardium (Tutoplast™, Tutogen Medical, Alachua, Florida, U.S.A.) or 4-ply porcine intestinal submucosa (Surgisis™, Cook Biotech, West Lafayette, Indiana, U.S.A.) (Fig. 2). The length of the windsock is determined by measuring the length of the proximal corporal tip to the inferior aspect of the corporotomy of the unperforated crus. The windsock is fitted over the proximal portion of the cylinder, and the cylinder and windsock are then placed inside the corpus cavernosum. The edge of the windsock adjacent to the corporotomy is sutured to the inside of the tunica, securing it in place and preventing proximal migration. Nonsynthetic materials have the advantage of not requiring removal should the prosthesis become infected. The modified windsock repair uses a rear-tip extender from the prosthesis as the windsock by suturing it directly to the tunica. This technique may be difficult if the proximal corporal segment is long, and it has the disadvantage of a difficult removal should infection occur.

The plug-and-patch repair, first described by Szostak et al. (2), is preferred by the authors. This method uses a 5×7 cm polyglycolic acid absorbable mesh or processed pericardium (Tutoplast™), which is the material we prefer. It is incised parallel to the long axis of the piece 1 cm from the edge. This incision is carried along three-fourths of the length of the patch (Fig. 3). The bulk of the material is wadded to form a plug which is passed into the corporal perforation with a dilator. The 1 cm wide tail of the patch which was not wadded should extend back out of the corporotomy. It is sutured to the inside of the tunica after the corpus cavernosum is redilated with the plug in place and then trimmed if necessary.

After either method of repair, additional protection against proximal migration of the device can be obtained by using the PTFE sleeve that covers the tubing where it emerges from the cylinders in American Medical System (Minnetonka, Minnesota, U.S.A.) devices. The sleeve is carefully opened lengthwise with scissors and then sutured to the outside of the tunica near where the tubing exits the corporotomy, taking care to avoid damaging the cylinder inside.

Distal Corporal Perforation

Distal corporal perforation may result from overly vigorous dilation, particularly when using a cavernotome in cases of corporal fibrosis. Urethral injury must be ruled out, as will be discussed in the section on urethral injury. If the perforation is at the distal tip of the corpus cavernosum, it can be repaired by elevating the glans off the corporal body through a dorsolateral

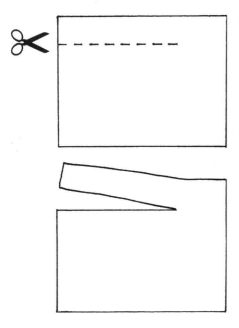

FIGURE 3   Diagram of the incision made in a mesh patch for use in proximal corporal perforation.

semi-circumferential incision. Once the tunical defect is visualized, it is closed with a 2-0 synthetic absorbable suture. If the perforation is on the lateral aspect of the corporal body, a repair can be made through a semi-circumferential incision directly over the perforation without mobilizing the glans. If the tunical tissue has been attenuated and the edges of the perforation are not sufficiently strong to hold the repair, a patch can be sewn over the repair for additional strength to prevent later extrusion. The patch may be made of absorbable or nonabsorbable material, but absorbable materials make potential future revisions for infection much less complex.

Urethral Perforation

Proximal urethral injury can occur early in the procedure during the initial dissection, particularly in revision cases where scarring from the initial prosthesis placement is present. Placement of a Foley catheter at the outset of the case helps in identifying and avoiding the urethra. If a urethral injury occurs before the corpora have been entered, the urethra should be repaired in multiple layers in a transverse direction to avoid luminal narrowing. The repair should be checked for water tightness by instilling methylene blue through the meatus. A Foley catheter should be placed and the prosthesis placement should be delayed eight weeks.

If the proximal urethral injury occurs during corporal dilation, the decision of whether to continue is more complicated. Once the corpora have been opened, not placing the device can potentially lead to corporal fibrosis and loss of penile length. This must be balanced against the increased risk of infection if the device is placed. The following suggestions must be adapted to patient circumstances and surgeon preference and experience. If the patient is at higher risk of infection (diabetes, chronic intermittent or indwelling catheterization, spinal cord injury, immunosuppression) the urethra should be repaired and placement of the device should be delayed. In a non–high-risk patient where the urethral injury is proximal and can be adequately repaired, placement of both cylinders with a Foley left in for five to seven days is a reasonable option. If the injury is in the pendulous urethra, one cylinder can be left in the corpus cavernosum contralateral to the injury after the urethra is repaired and a Foley catheter is placed. This will help prevent penile shortening that would have occurred if no cylinder was in place. In both situations, copious irrigation with antibiotic solutions as described by Mulcahy (3) should be performed prior to the insertion of the cylinders. A suprapubic catheter should also be placed and left in for 10 to 14 days to allow removal of the urethral Foley after five to seven days.

Distal urethral perforation with the dilator protruding through the meatus during distal dilation is the most common urethral injury. To avoid this complication, the dilator should be advanced carefully, and it should be angled dorsolaterally away from the urethra. The free hand should also be used to guide the tip of the dilator in the proper direction. Should perforation occur in spite of precautions, no attempt at cylinder placement is recommended. Instead, a Foley catheter should be placed. Urethral repair or suprapubic diversion is not necessary. Injuries to this portion of the urethra are difficult to repair and will heal with catheter placement alone. Prosthesis placement should be delayed for at least eight weeks and until after a retrograde urethrogram demonstrates complete urethral healing.

Residual Curvature

Penile prostheses are sometimes placed in men with Peyronie's disease to achieve a straight, rigid erection. Occasionally, a residual curve is present after the cylinders are in place. A curve of less than 30° will not interfere with sexual functioning and will also typically straighten with time. However, a curve of greater than 30° may make sexual activity difficult. In these cases, techniques are necessary to further straighten the penis. Wilson and Delk described the technique of manual molding over a prosthesis (4). The prosthesis is maximally inflated, the tubes to the pump are gently clamped to protect the pump mechanism, and the penis is forcibly bent in a direction away from the residual curvature while putting pressure over the corporotomies with the fingers to prevent herniation through these potentially weak areas. The penis is held in this position for 90 seconds and reinspected. A second attempt may be made if sufficient straightening has not been achieved. Urethral injury occurs in 4% of cases of manual molding, usually adjacent to the meatus (5). If this occurs, the cylinder that extruded into the meatus should be removed, and it may be replaced one to two months later. Manual molding may also rupture the plaque, leaving the device exposed. (Fig. 4) A defect in the tunica albuginea less than

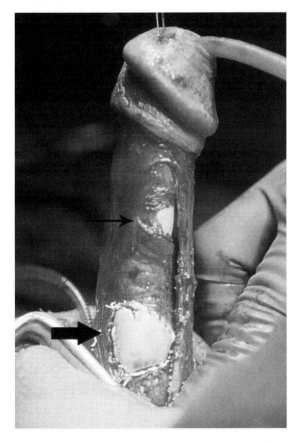

FIGURE 4 Corporal defects resulting from manual molding over a penile prosthesis. The wide arrow shows a patched defect while the thin arrow shows a defect small enough to heal without patching.

2 cm does not require repair, while a graft of PTFE or processed pericardium should be placed for repair of larger defects to prevent device herniation or recurvature from cicatrix contraction. If manual molding is insufficient to straighten the penis, plication sutures may be placed opposite the curve. Alternatively, the tunica may be opened opposite the curve and a graft placed. Care must be taken to not pierce the cylinder while placing the sutures during these repairs.

Postoperative Complications
Infection
Risks and Prevention

Infection of a penile prosthesis is problematic not only because of the necessity of removing the device or the rare occurrence of penile necrosis, but because the consequences of prosthesis infection can be long-lasting. The inflammation resulting from infection leads to corporal fibrosis which shortens the penis after prosthesis removal and makes subsequent reimplantation significantly more difficult. Salvage protocols, which will be discussed later, have been developed for appropriate patients in order to allow immediate reimplantation and preservation of penile length and girth. Prevention of device infection remains key, and minimizing the risk should be foremost in the mind of the implanting surgeon.

Certain subsets of patients with severe erectile dysfunction (ED) are at higher risk for infectious complications. Patients with spinal cord injuries (SCI) and immunocompromised patients, such as transplant patients or those requiring chronic steroid use, have higher rates of infection than patients without these conditions (6,7). Prior to surgery, SCI patients with neurogenic bladders should have sterile urine. Avoiding semi-rigid prostheses in SCI patients also appears to lower their risk toward that of the general population (7,8). Earlier series found that diabetics have a higher risk of infection, but more recent studies have not come to the same conclusion (6,9,10). Wilson et al. did not find elevated serum hemoglobin A_{1C} levels to be correlated with increased infection rates, though a trend toward higher infection rates in diabetics compared to non-diabetics was seen (11). Based on their findings they argued against a strict hgb A_{1C} cutoff that would disqualify candidates for penile prosthesis placement.

Several steps should be taken to minimize bacterial seeding of the prosthesis at the time of operation, which is when the majority of contamination occurs (12). There is not universal agreement as to which preoperative antibiotic(s) should be given, but it should cover both gram-positive and gram-negative organisms and be given prior to incision. The patient should be shaved thoroughly in an atraumatic fashion and scrubbed for 10 minutes. All operative personnel should scrub for 10 minutes, as well. As an extra precaution, we use an Ioban™ incise drape (3M, Rochester, Minnesota, U.S.A.) with the penis and scrotum brought through a small hole that stretches to fit the contour of the genitalia. This diminishes the chance of surgical site contamination from the perineum.

We use a penoscrotal incision, though operative approach has not been shown to influence infection rates (13,14). Copious antibiotic irrigation is used liberally throughout the operation, and the prosthesis is soaked in the antibiotic irrigation before placement. We use rifampin, which has been shown to be the single most active agent against biofilm-forming *Staphylococcus epidermidis* (15), and kanamycin. If the patient is diabetic or immunocompromised, amphotericin B or fluconazole irrigation is added. The incision is closed in several layers. We do not leave drains, though some surgeons prefer their use to prevent hematomas. Postoperatively, we prescribe a 14-day course of cephalexin, or a fluoroquinolone if the patient is penicillin allergic. Many surgeons do not routinely continue antibiotics beyond the perioperative period, which is a reasonable approach.

Recent series have reported an infection rate of approximately 2% to 3% for first-time prosthesis placements (6,9,16,17). Patients who undergo revision surgery for noninfectious causes have higher infection rates, with most series reporting rates of 10% to 20% (6,9,11,18,19). One reason for this may be "reactivation" of bacteria that have colonized the original device without causing signs or symptoms of infection. Licht et al. found that 40% of clinically uninfected devices tested at the time of revision surgery were culture positive (20), while Henry et al. found 70% to be positive under similar circumstances (21). Researchers have speculated that somehow the removal and replacement of an uninfected but colonized prosthesis activates the bacteria left behind in the biofilm and causes more aggressive behavior when the new device is in place (22). Another possible cause of elevated infection rates for revision surgery is diminished antibiotic penetration into the dense, relatively avascular surgical capsule that forms around the original device (18,23). The elevated risk prompted Henry et al. to conduct a prospective study that investigated the use of a modified Mulcahy salvage protocol using an antibiotic irrigation washout during revision surgery for noninfectious causes (24). They found a marked reduction (2.8% vs. 11.6%, $P = 0.034$) for the group that underwent the salvage protocol. Interestingly, the group that did not undergo the washout had antibiotic-eluting prostheses implanted while the salvage protocol group did not. This suggests that the washout with antibiotic irrigation assisted in mechanically removing residual biofilm left from the old device, in addition to introducing high local concentrations of antibiotics. The results of this study strongly suggest that an antibiotic irrigation washout should be used during revision surgery even when the reason for reoperation is not infection-related.

As mentioned above, manufacturers have developed medication-eluting devices that deliver antibiotics to the surrounding tissues for a brief time after implantation. American Medical Systems (Minnetonka, Minnesota, U.S.A.) markets devices impregnated with rifampin and minocycline under the name InhibiZone™ (Minnetonka, Minnesota, U.S.A.). Carson retrospectively reviewed 2261 men who received devices with the InhibiZone™ coating and 1944 men who received noneluting devices (25). All were primary implants, and after 180 days the group that received the InhibiZone™ devices had a lower rate of infection than the group that received conventional devices (0.68% vs. 1.61%, $P = 0.0047$). Coloplast Corporation (Santa Barbara, California, U.S.A.), previously Mentor Corporation, has designed devices with a hydrophilic coating that absorbs antibiotic irrigation when soaked. Wolter and Hellstrom retrospectively reviewed 2357 men receiving hydrophilic-coated devices and 482 men with uncoated Mentor devices (26). Both primary and revision placements were included, and after one year the coated device infection rate was lower than the rate for uncoated devices (1.06% vs. 2.07%, $P = 0.033$). The results from these studies suggest that antibiotic-eluting devices can improve already low infection rates for penile prostheses.

Diagnosis and Management

Recognition of prosthesis infection in the postoperative period can be difficult because the typical symptoms of erythema, induration, and edema are often absent, and the serum leukocyte count is usually normal. These subclinical infections are more common than overt device infection (27). The most frequent complaint when infection is present is persistent penile pain. Pain is expected in the first month after surgery but subsides with time. Pain that persists beyond the first four to six weeks should raise the suspicion of infection, though other causes of prolonged pain, such as placement of an oversized device, do exist. New onset of pain over a device component is particularly suspicious, as is fixation of the device to adjacent tissues. The majority of device infections occur within the first seven months following placement (27). Infections do occur outside of this time period, and cases of hematogenous seeding of penile prostheses have been described (28). Erosion of prosthesis components is also associated with device infection (12).

Management of penile prostheses infections is primarily surgical. Conservative management of subclinical infections with prolonged oral antibiotics, which can be diagnostic if pain resolves on therapy, has been described but is not reliable in resolving the infection (12). Removal is the more definitive method of clearing the infection. *Staphylococcus epidermidis* is the organism most commonly found in infected prostheses (18,21,29,30). Other coagulase-negative *Staphylococcus* species, *Staphylococcus aureus*, *Pseudomonas*, *Enterococcus*, *Candida*, and various gram-negative organisms have also been isolated from infected devices. Adequate coverage of both gram-positive and gram-negative organisms should be initiated once device infection is suspected. When removing the infected device, it is essential that no portion of the device or other foreign material, such as a PTFE graft used as a windsock or corporal patch, is left behind. Rear tip extenders (RTE) can easily be left in the proximal crura, so a thorough search must be performed (31). Use of a rigid cystoscope to retrieve a retained RTE has been described, as has the combination of a nasal speculum and a long, curved clamp (32,33). Palpation and use of a forceps or hemostat should usually suffice. Even small fragments can serve as a nidus for recurrent infections, so care should be taken to avoid fracturing the device during removal (34). The reservoir of three-piece devices should also be removed when infection is present. It can be difficult to remove the reservoir via a penoscrotal incision, so a counter-incision over the external inguinal ring is sometimes necessary. All spaces should be thoroughly irrigated with antibiotic irrigation. A pressure-irrigating device will assist with the removal of bacterial biofilm that is present inside the corpora. If a new device is not being placed at the same operation suction drains should be placed inside the corpora and scrotum, and the wound can be closed. Antibiotic irrigation is instilled through the drains three times a day for 72 hours, after which time the drains are removed (23). The antibiotic irrigation and IV antibiotic regimen should be adjusted depending on the culture results, and appropriate oral antibiotics should be given for 10 to 14 days once the patient is discharged. A new device may be placed two to six months later.

Delaying replacement of the device to allow healing and resolution of infection has important drawbacks. A second operation is required which adds considerable expense. More importantly, without a new device in place the corpora become fibrotic and contracted with penile length commonly losing up to 2 inches (30). Placement of a new prosthesis into a fibrotic, foreshortened penis can be extremely difficult and occasionally impossible (6). In these patients, a device with narrower cylinders may be implanted if a larger device cannot, with the option of placing a larger device 6–12 months later.

For appropriate patients a salvage procedure, first described by Furlow and Goldwasser (35) and since refined by Mulcahy (3), is an effective alternative to removal and delayed replacement of a penile prosthesis. The Mulcahy protocol is the most commonly used technique for prosthesis salvage. Candidates for salvage are men that have infected prostheses without the following relative contraindications: sepsis, necrotic tissue, pus in the presence of diabetes, a rapidly developing infection after device placement (less than two weeks), or an eroded device (3). The protocol uses four antibacterial irrigations starting with a solution of kanamycin 80 mg/L and bacitracin 1 gm/L in saline, followed by half-strength hydrogen peroxide, then half-strength povidone-iodine, and then pressure irrigation with 5 L of saline containing vancomycin 1 gm and gentamicin 80 mg. The wound is then reirrigated with iodine solution, peroxide solution, and finally kanamycin/ bacitracin solution. After irrigation the surgical drapes are removed, the surgeons re-gown and glove, the patient is redraped, and new instruments are used for insertion of the new prosthesis. Mulcahy's long-term success in 65 patients was 82% (30). The majority of reinfections were apparent within one month, which is earlier than infections in primary implants. Other investigators have had similar success rates (29,36). Due to the difficulties of delayed replacement of a penile prosthesis, salvage therapy is a very acceptable treatment for infected penile prostheses provided the patient is fully informed.

Mechanical Complications
Mechanical Failure
Mechanical failure of penile prostheses is a function of time and, to a certain extent, the type of device implanted. Semi-rigid prostheses are less likely to fail over time (19,37), because they do not rely on fluid transfer within the device. Inflatable prostheses have high reliability, particularly within the first five years after implantation.

The integrity of the device can be compromised at the time of surgery by accidental puncture with a suture needle when closing the corporotomy over each cylinder. Injury to the device can also occur if the back of the needle is dragged across the cylinder as the needle is passed through the tunica, so care must be taken at all times during corporotomy closure. To avoid the need for passing a suture near the cylinders, some surgeons place horizontal mattress stay sutures on both sides of the incision along the length of the corporotomy before cylinder placement. These sutures are then tied together over the incision for closure. We use this technique when placing larger two-piece inflatable devices that fill the intracorporeal space because they do not deflate to the same extent that a three-piece device will. However, whenever possible we close the corporotomies with a running 2-0 PDS suture for a tighter closure and better hemostasis. Damage to the device can also occur from traction on the tubing where it enters the cylinders. This is a point of potential leakage so tubing should be handled carefully (38).

Long-term mechanical failure rates are somewhat difficult to predict precisely because design modifications have periodically been made that affect durability. Commonly used inflatable penile prostheses have a 5- and 10-year mechanical failure-free survival rate of 85% to 95% and 60% to 70%, respectively (12,16,39–41). The most common cause of mechanical failure has been fluid loss. Fluid loss becomes apparent when there is diminishing or asymmetric rigidity that progresses to complete flaccidity. There is no way to add fluid to the system, so device replacement is required. At the time of removal and replacement an obvious location for the leak may not found, and the entire device needs to be replaced. The most common site for fluid leakage is the cylinders due to the high pressures they are subjected to during use (12). Individual cylinders are best not replaced as most inflatable prostheses come with the cylinders preconnected to the pumps, so an entirely new device should be inserted. Malleable devices are less likely to fail mechanically, but cases of prosthesis fracture have been reported (42). It has been suggested that larger corporotomies should be used when placing semi-rigid or malleable prostheses in order to avoid the need for excessive bending of the device during insertion which may lead to later fracturing (43).

Whether to replace the reservoir of three-piece devices when other inflatable prosthesis components fail is the subject of some controversy. The reservoir is unlikely to be the cause of mechanical failure, but the surgical capsule surrounding it will often contract as the entire system loses fluid. Simply reconnecting the reservoir to a new device will increase the likelihood of cylinder autoinflation, a complication that will be discussed later. Attempting to stretch the capsule around the reservoir by slowly refilling under pressure is recommended, but injury to the bladder may occur because of adhesions to adjacent structures and loss of compliance in the area from scarring (44). Postoperative hematuria after reservoir re-expansion suggests the possibility of reservoir-associated bladder injury. Investigators have come to differing conclusions regarding the need for replacement of the reservoir when replacing a malfunctioning device due to the relative rarity of subsequent infection or erosion. Rajpurkar et al. found no instances of infection or erosion in 85 patients when reusing the reservoir for a new device (45), but several case reports have demonstrated that in rare instances the reservoir has herniated into the bladder, as well as large and small bowel (34,46–49).

At a minimum, the capacity of the reservoir should be checked carefully to ensure that significant back pressure does not develop when filling to the appropriate volume. This should be done by infusing saline to the recommended capacity and removing pressure from the plunger of the syringe while still cannulating the tubing. Fluid will begin to refill the syringe if under pressure. Gentle but firm pressure may be used to expand the capsule. If significant force is necessary to expand the reservoir to the correct capacity, consideration should be given to removing the reservoir and manually disrupting the capsule, or placing a new one on the opposite side. Replacing the malfunctioning prosthesis soon after fluid loss becomes apparent may help minimize problems of capsule contracture (47). If debris is found inside the reservoir, it should be replaced due to the risk of subsequent clogging of the pump and tubing.

In patients with previous pelvic surgery and a malfunctioning three-piece prosthesis, the placement of a two-piece prosthesis should be considered, which would avoid reservoir-associated problems (49). In situations when a three-piece prosthesis is replaced with a two-piece device or when a three-piece device is being removed without being replaced, it seems reasonable that reservoir removal should be attempted because of the slight risk of later complications if it is left behind. If extensive dissection would be necessary to free the reservoir, it is reasonable to deflate and cap the reservoir and leave it behind if no infection is present.

Autoinflation
Autoinflation occurs in patients with three-piece devices when fluid flows from the reservoir to the cylinders without activation of the pump, resulting in unwanted prosthesis rigidity. Autoinflation has been reported to occur in 0.7% to 11% of patients with three-piece devices, and 1% to 2% will need surgical correction for it (16,19,40,50,51). The cause of autoinflation is pressure on the reservoir, and intraoperative measures should be taken to avoid its occurrence. An adequate pocket must be created wherever the reservoir will be placed. In most implants, the reservoir is placed in the retropubic space anterolateral to the bladder. The transversalis fascia at the floor of the external inguinal ring is pierced medial to the spermatic cord with a Metzenbaum scissors or other sharp instrument. The retropubic space is then bluntly developed with a finger. It is important to ensure that the space being created is deep to the transversalis fascia which can be confirmed by feeling the posterior surface of the superior pubic ramus. Otherwise the reservoir will be placed in a space where higher pressures will develop, causing autoinflation. Once the reservoir has been placed, which can be facilitated with the use of a nasal speculum, it should be filled with saline to the recommended capacity with a large syringe

and needle specifically designed for this purpose. The syringe should then be allowed to passively refill by removing pressure from the plunger. If there is no pressure on the reservoir from surrounding tissue, there will be no refilling. Up to 10 cc of saline can be removed to ensure zero pressure in the reservoir (37). If there is still pressure after the removal of 10 cc, the space should be redilated or a new location for the reservoir should be found. After surgery the cylinders should be left flaccid, which allows the reservoir to remain full. The capsule that forms around the reservoir will therefore be more capacious and less likely to cause autoinflation. Once he begins to use the prosthesis, the patient must be reminded to completely deflate the cylinders when not using it in order to prevent the capsule from tightening around the reservoir. Our particular method of preventing postoperative development of autoinflation is a program of prosthesis cycling whereby the device is completely inflated and deflated twice per day for four weeks. We have the patients start this process four to six weeks postoperatively when pain will not interfere with pump activation.

If autoinflation does develop, most cases can be managed conservatively by actively deflating the cylinders two to three times a day for three to four weeks (12). If autoinflation is present after six months, surgical correction may be necessary (50). A repair can be made by disrupting the capsule by distending the reservoir to the appropriate capacity with firm pressure as described in the previous section. If unsuccessful in creating a pressure-free space in this manner, the capsule may be manually disrupted or a new location for the reservoir may be found.

Wilson et al. reported their experience with a lock-out valve developed by Mentor (50). They reported no occurrences of autoinflation requiring correction in a series of 160 patients with the new device, including eight patients with reservoirs placed in locations where higher pressures were expected. Most patients will not require the added protection of a device with a lock-out valve, but those with previous retroperitoneal surgery or need for ectopic reservoir placement may benefit from the use of one.

Other Postoperative Complications
Pain
Several series have reported the incidence of significant pain following prosthesis placement to be 0.26% to 11% (19,40,51,52), It is unclear whether these numbers reflect patients who had severe pain at anytime following device placement or those who had pain beyond the expected recovery period. Patients commonly report significant pain in the first two to four weeks following prosthesis placement. Diabetics have a tendency to experience pain for a longer period of up to three to four months, perhaps because of increased stress on the tunica albuginea (12). Pain should resolve with time, and if it persists, infection or device malposition should be suspected.

Prosthesis infection, which was discussed in a previous section, often presents with persistent pain. If infection is present, pain should improve with the initiation of antibiotics. If symptoms improve on therapy, antibiotics should be continued for 10 to 12 weeks to attempt a cure of the infection, with expected success in 60% of cases (12). If symptoms recur after the antibiotics are stopped, removal and replacement is necessary using a salvage protocol. If antibiotics do not improve the pain, an infection may be present that is not susceptible to the antibiotics already used or device malposition is responsible for the symptoms. In either case, surgical correction is necessary. At the time of surgery, pus or biofilm may be present that indicates the presence of infection and that a salvage protocol should be initiated. If the prosthesis is found to be buckled or kinked, the cylinders may be too long or the corpora have not been adequately dilated to allow the device to be well positioned. The device should be removed to allow for remeasurement and/or redilation of the space. Antibiotic irrigation should be used liberally to counter the higher infection rates of revision surgery. The original device can be used if removal of an RTE extender or redilation has created enough space for it. A 3–0 suture to be used with the inserting device can be passed through the hole at the tip where the original thread was located. If redilation has not enlarged the intracorporal space, a smaller device should be substituted.

Moncada investigated the use of imaging in determining the cause of pain in 14 patients without signs of device infection (53). With magnetic resonance imaging (MRI), they found buckling of the device in the flaccid state in 12 of 14 (85%) patients. In only a minority of the patients was the buckling apparent on physical examination. They reported resolution of pain in all patients after corporal redilation, removal of RTE, or replacement with a smaller device.

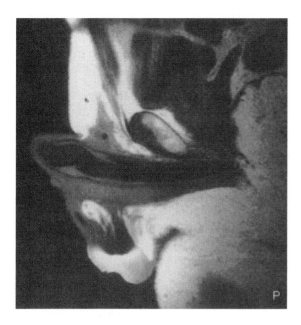

FIGURE 5 An MRI showing a buckled cylinder during prosthesis inflation due to an oversized device, which resulted in persistent pain. *Source*: From Ref. 53.

It appears reasonable that MRI may be used to help define the cause of persistent pain after prosthesis placement, particularly in patients who are reluctant to undergo reoperation without a more definite diagnosis ahead of time (Fig. 5).

Corporoglanular (Supersonic Transport) Deformity

After placement of a penile prosthesis, the glans may tilt in a ventral or lateral direction resulting in the "supersonic transport" (SST) deformity, so called because of its similarity in appearance to the Concorde aircraft. (Fig. 6) The deformity results from poor support of the glans by

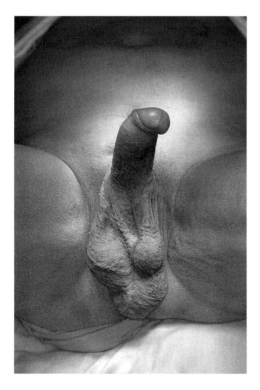

FIGURE 6 A corporoglanular (supersonic transport) deformity.

the distal tips of the corpora. This can occur because of the placement of cylinders that were undersized due to inadequate distal dilation of the corporal bodies, or proximal migration of a cylinder from erosion or unrecognized proximal perforation at the time of surgery. Some patients may have preexisting hypermobility of the glans that has become more apparent after placement of the prosthesis because of diminished glanular engorgement from progressive (ED) (54). The likelihood of the SST deformity after prosthesis placement has been reported to be 0.2% to 0.9% (19,40,51). Patients may complain of the deformity because of its appearance or because it causes discomfort to the patient or his partner due to the loss of cushioning that the glans provides. At the original surgery, placing the largest device that will fit in the intracorporal space without buckling will help avoid the problem postoperatively. Similarly, staying vigilant for crural perforation during the dilation can lessen the risk of subsequent proximal migration and resulting deformity.

If the SST deformity develops postoperatively, physical examination or imaging with MRI will reveal whether there has been proximal migration of a prosthesis cylinder (55), which requires repair if found. If an undersized device is responsible, replacement with a larger device after corporal redilation will correct the deformity. If the cause of the deformity is glans hypermobility, fixation of the glans (glanulopexy) can be done through a dorsal semi-circumferential incision through the skin and dartos fascia. Loupe magnification will facilitate elevating Buck's fascia and the neurovascular bundle. Mulhall and Kim described placing bilateral nonabsorbable vertical mattress sutures through the distal tunica albuginea and fascial undersurface of the glans lateral to the neurovascular bundle in order to pull the glans dorsally into better position over the tips of the corpora cavernosum (Fig. 7) (54). They reported no failure in 10 patients. We performed a similar procedure with absorbable sutures and have also had excellent results (56). When placing the sutures, the cylinders should be pinched back away from the tips of the corpora to avoid puncturing them.

Cylinder Erosion/Extrusion

The cylinders of all penile prosthesis types occasionally erode through the tunica albuginea and more rarely extrude through the skin. Extrusion through the urethra is also seen. Semi-rigid devices are at higher risk for erosion and extrusion due to the constant pressure they exert on surrounding tissues (37), though not all investigators have found them to have higher rates of this complication (57). Reported rates of erosion and extrusion are 1.2% to 8% (16,54,57). Distal erosion becomes apparent when one or more of the cylinder tips is not seated under the glans, but rather protrudes in a lateral, dorsal, or ventral direction. If a cylinder erodes medially, the patient will more likely have dysuria and hematuria or will see the device protruding through the meatus (Fig. 8). Proximal erosion of a cylinder will result in asymmetry or a corporoglanular (SST) deformity when the device is inflated.

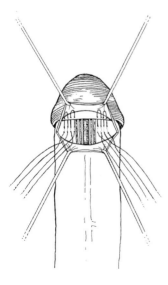

FIGURE 7 Suture placement for glanulopexy for an SST deformity. *Source*: From Ref. 54.

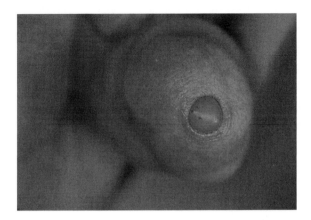

FIGURE 8   A penile prosthesis cylinder extruding through the meatus.

Repair is required when a cylinder erodes through the tunica, and infection must be ruled out at the time of surgery because it is a recognized cause of erosion and extrusion. If the prosthesis has extruded through the skin or urethra, device superinfection should be expected. Distal erosion can be repaired in several ways. Mulcahy described a method of rerouting the tip of the cylinder into the proper subglanular position without the need for a graft with universal success in 14 patients followed for at least two years (58). Through a hemi-circumcising incision, a 4-cm longitudinal corporotomy is made over the protruding cylinder. The cylinder is then retracted out of the capsule that has formed around it. About 3 cm proximal to the glans, a transverse incision is made in the back wall of the capsule, and through that incision a new plane of dissection behind the capsule is carried up toward the glans using a Metzenbaum scissors. The new space is then dilated to the appropriate size for the device. The cylinder is reseated with an inserting device, and the wall that formerly comprised the medial aspect of the capsule around the cylinder now forms the lateral wall. The corporotomy made at the outset is closed with a synthetic absorbable suture to give additional support to the cylinder. A second method involves fashioning a windsock similar to the method used to repair intraoperative crural perforation (see section on intraoperative complications). Carson and Noh compared the outcomes of the two methods and found the "rerouting" technique to be faster and to have lower rates of recurrence, pain, and infection compared to a Goretex windsock repair (59). Nevertheless, if corporal tissue is inadequate to allow the rerouting method, repairing the eroded corpus cavernosum with a windsock fashioned from a synthetic or nonsynthetic material is a reasonable option. We prefer to use non-synthetic materials because of the lower risk of infection and a more natural feel.

Urethral erosion has been successfully managed with a salvage procedure involving removal of the device, irrigation with antibiotic solutions, and replacement of one cylinder in the corpus cavernosum contralateral to the urethral erosion when gross infection is not present (30). Similarly, Wilson and Delk reported an 83% success rate when removing only the cylinder on the side of the erosion, which was replaced six to eight weeks later (6).

Penile Shortening and Hypoesthesia
To avoid unrealistic expectations, patients should be counseled preoperatively that the erections achieved with a penile prosthesis will not replicate those achieved prior to the onset of ED. The rigid penis after device placement will typically be shorter than what they experienced before, and the glans will often not engorge. Wang et al. found the average erect length following implantation to be 0.9 cm less than the erection achieved with the injection of a vasoactive agent before surgery (60). Additionally, Montorsi et al. reported that 30% of men receiving a penile prosthesis complained about shortening or the appearance of the penis (52). It is uncertain if they were counseled preoperatively about expectations regarding penile appearance.

Hypoesthesia of the penis is rare, with a reported rate of 0.2% to 2.5% (16,51,52). The infrapubic approach is more likely to result in dorsal nerve injury, particularly during revision surgery where scarring can distort anatomy (61). Changes in sensation are usually transient and should improve with time.

Hematoma and Superficial Wound Infection
Rates of hematoma formation following prosthesis placement are reported to be 0.2% to 2% (16,39,51,52,57). Hematomas result from inadequate hemostasis and great care should be taken to cauterize all bleeders, particularly in the scrotal dartos fascia. The corporotomy closure should also be inspected before closing the skin incision. We use a running suture to close the corporotomies to ensure adequate hemostasis. Superficial wound infections occur in 2% to 6% of cases, and if treated promptly should not compromise prosthesis survival (16,52,57).

COMPLICATIONS OF SURGERY FOR PEYRONIE'S DISEASE

Several methods are commonly used today to straighten the penis of men with severe curvature from Peyronie's disease (PD). The Peyronie's plaque creates unequal expansion of the corpora cavernosum leading to deformity in which the plaque forms the concave aspect of a penile curvature. Surgery is typically reserved for men with disease that significantly affects their ability to engage in sexual activity. The various techniques are classified into lengthening and shortening procedures. Lengthening procedures involve the incision or partial excision of the plaque with the placement of a graft into the defect left in the tunica albuginea. The release of the plaque eliminates the tethering on the concave side of the penis, thereby allowing it to straighten. Shortening procedures straighten the penis by shortening the convex side to the same degree that the plaque has shortened the concave side, essentially creating symmetric tethering on the penis. Examples of shortening techniques are the Nesbit procedure which involves excising an ellipse of tunica albuginea from the convex side of the penis, and the tunica albuginea plication technique which achieves a similar effect as the Nesbit operation without excising tissue. While the techniques used for each type of straightening surgery are different, the complications that result are similar.

Prior to performing a straightening procedure, the conformation and degree of curvature is assessed. It is sometimes difficult to accurately assess the patient's curvature preoperatively due to an insufficient erection in the office. An injection of alprostadil or similar medication can help achieve a fuller erection which will help determine the appropriate operation for the patient. An assessment of the patient's preoperative erectile function is also advised to guide appropriate therapy and counsel the patient regarding postoperative expectations. Based on the patient's deformity and erectile function, we determine the preferred surgery for the patient, but we counsel patients that intraoperative findings will also affect which procedure we ultimately pursue. We also inform men who are uncircumcised that we perform a circumcision as part of all straightening procedures unless they have a strong objection. Studies have shown that 40% to 50% of uncircumcised men undergoing surgery for PD will later require a circumcision for phimosis or paraphimosis if they are not circumcised at the time of surgery (62,63).

Lengthening Procedures

Lengthening procedures are so called because the goal of the operation is to release the tethering caused by the Peyronie's plaque. At operation, an artificial erection is induced with an infusion of a vasoactive agent and saline. The deformity is assessed with particular attention to points of narrowing and hinging. To access the plaque, the penis is degloved, Buck's fascia is opened longitudinally, and the dorsal neurovascular bundle is elevated under loupe magnification. Incisional techniques involve semi-circumferential incisions through the plaque which widen as the penis straightens. The defects in the tunica are grafted, most often with autologous dermis, vein, temporalis fascia, or off-the-shelf grafts composed of processed pericardium or porcine small intestinal submucosa.

Residual/Recurrent Curvature

Both incisional and excisional techniques are effective in straightening the penis. Reported rates of residual or recurrent curvature for incision and grafting procedures are 5% to 20% (62,64–67). The majority of these are less than 30°, which is unlikely to affect sexual functioning, but up to 6% are greater than 30° (64,66). Excisional procedures have postoperative curvature rates of 2% to 20% (68,69). Penile curvature following grafting procedures can result from insufficient correction, graft contracture, and progressive disease. At the conclusion of any grafting procedure, another artificial erection should be induced to ensure adequate straightening. Residual curvature can be corrected with plication sutures opposite the curve. To avoid the problems with graft shrinkage, it is recommended that the graft be up to 10% larger than the defect that is being covered (65). To prevent postoperative progression of PD resulting in new curvature, surgical correction should not be performed until the deformity has not changed in at least six months (66).

Penile Shortening

Lengthening procedures are often chosen when a patient's penile length has been significantly affected by PD. However, a significant portion of patients lose a small degree of length from the procedure. The penis should be measured on stretch at the start of the operation and documented. It should then be remeasured when the procedure is finished. Incision and grafting techniques usually result in no change or slight lengthening, but complaints of shortening occur in 0% to 50% of cases (62,64–67,70). Patient complaints do not always correlate with objective findings. Yurkanin et al. reported 50% of patients complaining of shortening when objective measurements showed no loss (70). Most subjective and objective measurements show that a loss of penile length of 1 to 2 cm occurs in 25% and a loss of greater than 2 cm in approximately 15% (62,64,65). With partial excisional techniques, we have found that two-thirds of patients complain of shortening but objective measurement show only one-third have lost length of an average of 0.7 cm (68). In spite of the common complaint of penile shortening, few men report that their perceived loss of length has negatively affected sexual functioning (62,64).

There are no simple techniques to avoid shortening. To avoid patient dissatisfaction with the result of a lengthening procedure, preoperative counseling is very important. Patients may have overly optimistic expectations about the postoperative result. They may expect to return to their predisease state which is not realistic.

Erectile Dysfunction

New-onset ED after a lengthening procedure is rare, but worsening of preexisting ED is not uncommon (70). Likewise, patients with ED preoperatively should not expect an improvement in erectile function beyond correction of the deformity. Rates of ED following incision and grafting procedures are 5% to 46%, with most recent series reporting rates of 10% to 15% (62,64–67). The degree to which the operation causes ED is difficult to determine because of the high rate of coexisting ED in this patient population (64). Most men with ED following incision and grafting are able to achieve intercourse with the use of oral phosphodiesterase (PDE-5) inhibitor therapy, intracavernous injections, or vacuum constriction devices (62,65,70). In a series of patients undergoing partial plaque excision and grafting at our institution, we found a rate of ED of 30%, but only 5% were unable to achieve intercourse (68). Graft size did not predict which patients were more likely to experience postoperative ED, but ventral curvature repair with partial excision and grafting resulted in a 50% rate of significant ED. This procedure should not be used to correct ventral curvature without patient consent.

Evidence suggests that veno-occlusive dysfunction is responsible for some ED following plaque incision or excision, though it can also be the cause of ED in Peyronie's patients before surgical correction (71). The grafting techniques involve replacing a portion of the less compliant tunica albuginea with a more compliant graft. This may prevent effective venous trapping of blood in the subtunical venous plexus. Constricting rings and vacuum devices are often effective when treating ED in these men. When determining the best surgical approach for men with a penile deformity and marked ED from vascular insufficiency, a penile prosthesis rather than a plaque incision or excision may be a better choice because of the likelihood of severe ED in these men following grafting procedures. For men refusing prosthesis placement, a Nesbit or plication procedure may be preferred because of a lower rate of postoperative ED. However, in general, men with ED unresponsive to oral erectogenic medications should not be offered straightening procedures without a prosthesis.

Penile Hypoesthesia

To access the plaque during plaque incision and excision procedures, the neurovascular bundle is elevated under loupe magnification. Good visualization helps prevent damage to the nerves, but 2% to 15% of patients report diminished glans sensation following these procedures (64–68,70). Penile sensation normalizes in most men with this complaint. However, El-Sakka et al. and Kadioglu et al. each reported that 10% of men in their series had diminished sensation lasting more than three to six months, though they did not describe the extent to which the hypoesthesia affected sexual function (64,67).

Hematoma, Infection, and Graft Site Complications

Hematomas occur in 2% to 15% of grafting procedures, often forming under the graft (62,66,68,70). The hematoma can easily be drained by aspiration with a needle passed through the graft if the hematoma is causing pain or deformity. This is rarely necessary as the hematoma typically resolves spontaneously with time. Carefully closing Buck's fascia after placing the graft provides a layer of protection against extravasation of blood from the corpora. In addition, we loosely wrap the penis in an elastic Coban™ (3M Health Care, St. Paul, Minnesota, U.S.A.) dressing which provides compression without strangulation.

Infection occurs in 0% to 2% of cases (66,67). El-Sakka reported on graft site complications from harvesting saphenous vein (64). Leg wound infection occurred in 3%, lymphatic drainage from the femoral incision occurred in 2%, and a lymphocele occurred in 1%.

Shortening Procedures

Shortening procedures are not designed to intentionally shorten the penis. Rather, the intention is to limit the expansion of the tunica opposite the plaque to the same degree that the plaque is limiting expansion, resulting in a symmetric, straight erection. The first shortening technique, which is still often used, is the Nesbit procedure which involves removing one or more small, transversely-oriented elliptical pieces of tunica from the convex side of the penile curvature and closing the resulting defect. A modification of this technique involves making short longitudinal incisions on the convex side of the penis and closing them in a horizontal, Heineke-Mikulicz fashion, thereby shortening the tunica. Another modification involves plicating the tunica on the convex side without removing a full thickness piece of the tunica, which is the method we prefer. The Nesbit procedure and its modifications appear to have similar results regarding success and complications (72). The benefits of Nesbit-type procedures when compared with plaque incision or excision are their relative simplicity, less frequent need for neurovascular bundle mobilization, and lower incidence of ED (72). Drawbacks include the greater chance of penile shortening and the inability to correct penile narrowing or hinging caused by the plaque. The best candidates for plication-type procedures are men with well-preserved penile length and curvature less than 60° without severe narrowing or hinge effect (73).

Residual/Recurrent Curvature

The Nesbit procedure and its modifications are very effective at straightening penile deformities. As with other straightening procedures, an artificial erection is induced intraoperatively with a vasodilating agent and saline infusion in order to assess the deformity and plan the location of tunica excision or plication. Buck's fascia is opened longitudinally over the convex side of the curvature. By grasping the tunica longitudinally with an Allis clamp, the surgeon is able to simulate the degree of straightening that sutures would achieve when placed in the same position. When the desired degree of straightening is achieved with clamps, they are removed and the indentations left by the clamps serve as markers for the position of tunica excision or plicating suture placement. An artificial erection is again induced once all sutures have been placed to ensure adequate straightening. Some of the sutures that are placed should be non-absorbable to prevent subsequent release of the closure and recurrence of angulation.

Andrews et al. analyzed patients with recurrent deformity after a Nesbit procedure and concluded that the use of absorbable suture contributed to 25% of the failures with disease progression accounting for the rest (74). As with grafting procedures, correction should not be attempted until the disease process has stabilized for 6 to 12 months.

Penile Shortening

Some degree of shortening is common after penile straightening using the Nesbit technique or other related procedures, with 17% to 78% of men experiencing some shortening (72,75–77). However, the percentage of men reporting sexual difficulties or dissatisfaction as a result of shortening are much lower and has been reported at 0% to 12% (75,77). The average loss of length is 0.34 cm (78), though up to 5% of men will lose more than 2 cm (79). The degree of shortening is affected by the preoperative severity and position of the curvature, with greater curvature and ventral direction often leading to greater loss of length after correction (78). Preoperative counseling regarding the possible loss of length is necessary, and men with significant shortening from the disease process with good erectile function may be better candidates for plaque incision or partial excision procedures.

Penile Hypoesthesia, Palpable Sutures, Hematoma, and Infection

A decrease in penile sensation after straightening by plication or Nesbit has been reported in 2% to 21% of patients (72,75,79). The neurovascular bundle seldom requires mobilization as part of the procedure, and the sensory changes are typically mild and transient. Patients will sometimes complain of the ability to feel sutures under the penile skin. To avoid this we use a 3-0 PDS to bury the knots of the nonabsorbable sutures used to plicate the tunica albuginea. Hematomas and infection are relatively rare with rates of 0% to 5% and 0% to 2%, respectively (75,77,79).

COMPLICATIONS OF OTHER BENIGN ADULT PENILE AND SCROTAL SURGERIES

Hydrocelectomy

Many surgical techniques exist for the treatment of hydrocele, but most are variations on three primary approaches: excision, eversion, and window procedures (internal drainage). Hydrocele excision involves dissection of the hydrocele sac from the overlying dartos fascia followed by excision of the parietal tunica vaginalis up to its reflection with the visceral layer overlying the epididymis and testis. Eversion techniques avoid excising the tunica vaginalis and instead evert the sac to put it in direct apposition to the dartos fascia. Window procedures involve making an aperture in the hydrocele sac to allow excessive fluid to be absorbed by the overlying dartos. The technique chosen to treat a hydrocele affects the likelihood of complications, the most common of which are edema, hematoma, infection, and recurrence.

Edema

Edema is the most common complication and is defined as any swelling that distorts the rugae of the scrotum. Techniques that use extensive dissection to mobilize the hydrocele sac are more likely to cause edema. Rodriguez et al. compared complication rates of various techniques and found hydrocele excision to be followed by marked edema in 76% of cases and the Jaboulay procedure, an eversion technique with extensive mobilization of the sac, to have a rate of 91% (80). In contrast, the Lord procedure, an eversion technique with no dissection of the hydrocele sac from the dartos layer, (Fig. 9A, B) had a 10% rate of postoperative edema. Ku et al. also found a similar divergence in rates of edema between excision and the Lord procedure (74% vs. 8%, P < 0.001) (81).

Hematoma

Hematoma formation after hydrocelectomy is associated with prolonged scrotal swelling and discomfort with an increased risk of infection. The inability of the scrotum to tamponade bleeding combined with its dependent position can lead to very large hematomas in spite of reasonable attempts at intraoperative hemostasis. The various procedures have different rates of hematoma which also appears to be affected by the amount of dissection when mobilizing the hydrocele sac. Rodriguez et al. reported a 20% rate of hematoma after excision and 22%

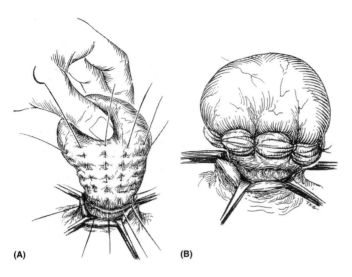

FIGURE 9 The Lord procedure. (**A**) Placement of the plication sutures through the dartos and everted tunica vaginalis. (**B**) After the sutures are tied. *Source*: From Ref. 141.

after the Jaboulay procedure whereas the Lord procedure resulted in no hematomas (80). Lord specifically limited dissection to avoid bleeding and reported no hematomas in 22 patients when first describing the procedure (82). When excising the hydrocele sac, the cut edge should be carefully oversewn with a locking stitch to minimize bleeding. Regardless of the technique used, advising the patient to avoid strenuous physical activity for a week after surgery is necessary to reduce the risk of late bleeding.

Infection, Recurrence, and Other Complications
Infection rates are similar across all techniques. Authors have reported infections in 5% to 14% without significant differences amongst the various procedures (80,81). Recurrence rates are similar with the notable exception of the window technique, which is much higher. Excision and eversion procedures have a 0% to 4% risk of recurrence while window procedures result in recurrence in 85% to 91% of cases (81,83). The reason appears to be gradual closure of the hole made in the hydrocele sac (84,85). For this reason, window procedures have largely been abandoned in spite of their low rates of edema and hematoma formation.

A rare and possibly under-recognized risk of hydrocelectomy is epididymal injury. Ross and Flom reported three cases of azoospermia following hydrocele repair in men with documented presence of sperm preoperatively (86). In the three cases surgical exploration revealed scarred and kinked epididymes where the cut edges of the hydrocele sac had been sewn behind the epididymes in a bottleneck fashion. It therefore seems prudent that great care should be taken to avoid injury to the epididymis and vas deferens if excising the hydrocele sac and especially if sewing the cut edges behind the testis.

Vasectomy
Failure
The most common method of vasectomy in the 1960s and 1970s was division and removal of a short segment of the vas with suture ligation of each end, but this method had a failure rate of 1.2% to 3.3% (87,88). Interposition of fascia between the cut ends decreased the failure rate to below 1% (88). Schmidt and Free reported reducing their failure rate to zero by omitting ligation and instead combining fascial interposition and electrocautery of the lumen of each end of the vas (87). Others have disputed the efficacy of placing the cut ends in different fascial planes (89). When clipping or tying the cut ends of the vas, excessive force that crushes or cuts the vas should not be used because this may allow leakage of sperm proximal to the clip or suture. Methods that allow formation of sperm granulomas to form at the cut end of the vas may have higher recanalization rates (89–91).

Men must be counseled to continue alternate methods of contraception until two consecutive semen analyses at least four weeks apart are azoospermic which usually requires at least

10 to 15 ejaculations. Esho et al. reported 94% of men achieving azoospermia by 16 weeks, 97% by 26 weeks, and over 99% by 48 weeks (92). Rare cases of late recanalization do occur at a rate of 1 in 2000 to 7000 cases, and patients must be counseled that this very unusual event is possible though unlikely (88,93). They may elect to have yearly semen analysis if they are particularly concerned about this possibility.

Pain

One of the more troublesome adverse effects following vasectomy is chronic pain. Pain is a common complaint after vasectomy with 27% of men responding to a follow-up questionnaire reporting pain at anytime following vasectomy, but only 5% had pain lasting longer than three months (94). Other patient surveys have found complaints of chronic testicular pain after vasectomy in 19% to 33%, with 2% to 15% reporting the pain as troublesome (95,96). In the majority of men with the complaint of chronic postvasectomy pain, the onset was one to six months postoperatively (94).

Chronic pain after vasectomy, also called postvasectomy pain syndrome (PVPS), can be unilateral or bilateral and is often described as a dull ache or sharp pain that worsens with ejaculation or physical exertion. The cause of the pain is not known precisely, but many researchers suspect congestive changes in the epididymis to be the source (90,97–99). Sperm granulomas from leakage of spermatozoa from the vas or epididymis have also been blamed for the symptoms (100), but pain from these lesions appears to be the exception rather than the rule (90,99,101). In fact, a sperm granuloma resulting from leakage from the epididymis (epididymal blow-out) may be protective for PVPS because pressure in the epididymis has been vented, thereby alleviating congestion that might otherwise cause chronic pain (90,99). Moss advocated the use of open-ended vasectomies where the abdominal end is closed and the testicular end of the vas is left open to prevent congestion of the epididymis (101). In a series of over 6000 patients, he found congestive epididymitis in 6% of men with closed-end vasectomies and 2% of those with the open-end technique. Shapiro and Silber also compared open- and closed-end vasectomies in 800 patients (90). Sperm granulomas formed in 97% of men with the open-end method, and none of them were painful. They found a 4% recanalization rate with the open-end technique when the abdominal end was only cauterized, and the failure rate fell to 0.4% when the abdominal end was clipped.

The initial treatment for PVPS should be conservative with recommendations for non-steroidal anti-inflammatory drugs (NSAIDs), scrotal supports, warm compresses, and spermatic cord nerve blocks. Many patients will not achieve lasting results from these measures, and more aggressive treatment is necessary. Two methods, microsurgical vasovasostomy and microsurgical spermatic cord denervation, offer reasonable probabilities of relief from symptoms. Microsurgical vasovasostomy has been reported to be 84% to 100% effective in resolving or significantly improving PVPS (90,102,103). The drawback, of course, is the reestablishment of fertility. Spermatic cord denervation offers an alternative and is the method we prefer. A subinguinal approach is used, and the contents of the spermatic cord are divided with the exception of the internal spermatic arteries and one or two lymphatics. The vas is also divided again. Rates of complete and significant improvement have been reported at 77% to 100% (94,104,105). In the series at our institution, a 2% rate of testicular atrophy was seen. Caddedu et al. reported a laparoscopic approach for denervation by dividing the vessels proximal to the internal inguinal ring (106). They reported a 77% success rate and no cases of testicular atrophy in nine patients, a result they felt was due to reconstituted blood flow distal to the point of arterial division. A spermatic cord nerve block using 20 cc of 0.5% bupivicaine should be performed prior to a denervation procedure to ascertain whether surgical denervation will alleviate symptoms. A good response to nerve block correlates with surgical success (107). Epididymectomy has also been used to treat PVPS when the pain is strictly in the congested epididymis, while orchiectomy is more radical and has lower success rates as initial therapy (98,108,109). If physical examination reveals localized tenderness of a nodule over the epididymis or vasectomy site, a painful sperm granuloma may be present. Excision of these lesions may alleviate the pain (90). The mechanism by which sperm granulomas cause pain may be impingement of nerve bundles traveling in close proximity to the wall of the lesion (100).

Hematoma, Infection, and Testicular Atrophy

As with most scrotal surgeries, hematoma is a risk after vasectomy with rates reported to be 0.9% to 2.3% and an additional 3% experiencing scrotal echymosis (92,93). The majority of the hematomas do not require intervention and can be managed with scrotal elevation. Patients should be advised to avoid strenuous activity for several days following the procedure. Superficial wound infection occurs in 1.3% to 4.5% (92,93,95). In addition to antibiotics, sitz baths and scrotal support should be recommended. Testicular atrophy is a very unlikely event following vasectomy under normal circumstances, and it has not been regularly reported as a complication in large series. However, patients with a history of varicocelectomy or inguinal surgery may be at risk (110). Prior surgery can partially devascularize the testis, and the artery of the vas may be its only blood supply. Great care should be taken to separate the vessels accompanying the vas before dividing it.

Varicocelectomy

Palpable varicoceles are usually treated to improve fertility and sometimes to alleviate discomfort. Several approaches have been described, and historically the most commonly used were inguinal varicocelectomy (Ivanissevich) (111) and retroperitoneal high ligation (Palomo) (112). More recently, microsurgical techniques have become popular because of lower rates of the most common complications which are recurrence and hydrocele. Laparoscopic approaches have also grown in popularity, particularly in cases of bilateral varicoceles. Efficacy, as measured by pregnancy rates and semen parameters, is comparable amongst the various techniques. Hematoma and infection are both less than 1% after varicocelectomy (113–115), though epigastric arterial injury does occasionally occur during laparoscopy (116,117).

Recurrence

Recurrence rates following varicocelectomy vary by technique. Retroperitoneal high ligation has recurrence rates of 7% to 18% (114,118–120). In contrast, microsurgical inguinal and subinguinal approaches have recurrences in 0% to 2% of cases (114,118,119). Goldstein et al. demonstrated the benefits of optical magnification in preventing recurrence in a series of 640 varicocelectomies (113). They reported a 9% recurrence when not using magnification, 8% using 2.5× loupes, and 0.6% using an operative microscope. Laparoscopic approaches have recurrence rates of 0% to 14% (116,121,122).

The explanations for differences in recurrence rates are controversial. Microsurgical subinguinal techniques allow the visualization of minute venous channels that may later dilate if not identified intraoperatively. Higher approaches ligate the spermatic vein(s) at a point where fewer small branches exist, making it less likely that a branch will be missed, but radiographic studies have shown that high ligation procedures will miss internal spermatic vein (ISV) collaterals that bypass the point of division (123–126) (Fig. 10). The role of dilated external spermatic (ES) veins originating from the common iliac vein is also controversial. Dilated ES veins larger than 2 mm are present in 93% of varicoceles (127), and ES veins larger than 4 mm are present in 50% (128). Retroperitoneal high ligation and laparoscopic approaches cannot treat these ES veins, yet the large majority of failures from those methods are from persistent dilated internal, not external, spermatic veins (124–126). Authors dubious of ES vein involvement in varicocele pathogenesis point out that a much higher percentage of failures would be attributable to persistent ES veins if they were an important factor (116). Nevertheless, cases have been reported of improved reproductive function when persistent ES veins were ligated after failure of the primary treatment (129). Dilated ES veins can often be demonstrated by venography (130,131), and it seems reasonable to recommend that when a patient has a recurrence after a high or laparoscopic approach, a subinguinal or interventional radiologic approach should be used that can identify and treat possible lower avenues of collateral flow. Deferential veins, which drain to the hypogastric vein, are rarely, if ever, responsible for recurrence and do not generally require ligation during primary treatment (110,132).

Hydrocele

Hydroceles form after varicocelectomy because of disruption of lymphatic channels along the spermatic cord that drain the tunica vaginalis and other intrascrotal tissues. Szabo and

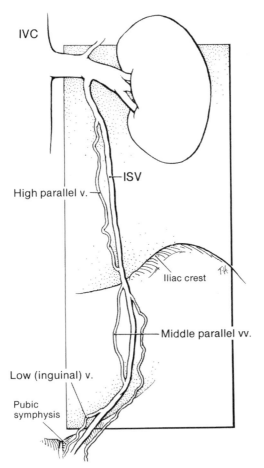

FIGURE 10 Parallel collateral channels of the left internal spermatic vein (ISV). *Source*: From Ref. 123.

Kessler reported a 7.2% rate of postoperative hydrocele when using the retroperitoneal approach, and other authors have found comparable rates of 6% to 9% using the same technique (114,119,133). Nonmagnified inguinal approaches have had similar hydrocele rates of 7.3% to 9% (113,115,128). Microsurgical procedures, which use an inguinal or subinguinal approach, allow the visualization and sparing of lymphatic channels and have lower rates of hydrocele formation (127). Goldstein et al. reported a 9% rate of hydrocele using a subinguinal approach without magnification which then fell to zero after the implementation of the use of loupes or an operating microscope (113). Several other series have also found fewer postoperative hydroceles using microsurgical techniques (114,119,121), and our own experience using an operating microscope has had the same result. Hydrocele rates after laparoscopic varicocelectomy have been reported at 0% to 8.5% (116,121,122).

Hydroceles following varicocelectomy usually appear after several months, with an average onset of 18.2 months postprocedure (133). They may be triggered by trauma well after the initial postoperative period (110). Many hydroceles after varicocelectomy will resolve with conservative measures such as scrotal elevation, but a significant number will persist and require surgical correction (115,133,134). Their effect on fertility is uncertain, as several men have fathered children in spite of hydrocele formation (133).

Testicular Atrophy

The three sources of blood flow to the testis are the testicular, cremasteric, and deferential arteries. When not branched, the testicular artery has an average diameter of 1 mm, and in more than half of men the testicular artery is larger than the cremasteric and deferential arteries combined (135) (Fig. 11). At the inguinal level the testicular artery is surrounded by densely adherent veins in 30% of cases, and this increases to 90% in the subinguinal portion of the cord

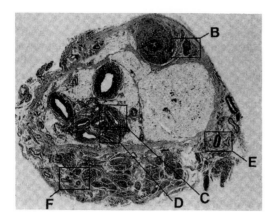

FIGURE 11 Transverse section through the spermatic cord showing comparative size of the arteries. **B**, deferential artery. **C** and **D**, internal spermatic arteries. **E**, possible external spermatic arteries. **F**, cremasteric arteries. *Source:* From Ref. 142.

(127). In spite of this, arterial injury during microsurgical subinguinal surgery is rare. Chan et al. reported 19 (0.9%) instances of accidental arterial ligation in 2102 varicocelectomies (136). Only one of the 15 patients followed clinically after arterial injury developed any testicular atrophy, which in this case was a loss of 20% of volume. Jarow et al. and Ralph et al. both reported an approximately 20% rate of arterial injury during laparoscopic varicocelectomy, though Jarow et al. reported significant improvement with experience (116,122). They both reported no cases of testicular atrophy. Palomo, who intentionally divided the testicular artery during high retroperitoneal ligation, reported no instances of atrophy in 40 cases (112). He attributed this result to flow from the more distally located cremasteric and deferential arteries.

The majority of patients in the series reported by Chan et al. (136) who suffered arterial injury still had improved semen parameters, though not to the same degree as the general population undergoing varicocelectomy. The authors pointed out that the patients with arterial injury had on average smaller testes at baseline than the majority of men with varicoceles which could potentially account for their smaller improvement. It is also likely that in this series the artery that was injured was often not the only branch of the testicular artery, given that 43% of men have multiple branches in the subinguinal region (127). Silber encountered a case of prior bilateral ligation of the testicular arteries during varicocelectomy being done for poor sperm motility but normal sperm concentration (137). The patient subsequently became azoospermic in spite of maintaining normal testicular volume. Though injury to a portion of the arterial supply of the testis does not seem overly deleterious to testicular function in most cases, it is best to make every effort to avoid ligating an arterial branch through the use of optical magnification and intraoperative Doppler ultrasonography (138).

Circumcision

Circumcision in the adult population is relatively rare and is usually carried out for phimosis or neoplastic conditions, although some patients will request a circumcision for esthetic reasons. There are very little data on complication rates of adult circumcisions. Neonatal circumcisions, which are far more common, are typically performed with techniques that differ from the methods used for adults. It is therefore problematic to predict the nature and frequency of complications for adult circumcision based on those of children. Nevertheless, certain complications, such as bleeding and excessive penile skin removal, do occasionally follow adult circumcision, and techniques to avoid and manage these unusual results should be known to practitioners.

Excessive Penile Skin Removal

The removal of an excessive amount of penile skin should be avoided to prevent the appearance of a loss of penile length. When determining the location of the proximal circumferential incision, an erection should be simulated by stretching the penis while applying pressure to the abdominal skin over the pubis at the base of the penis. This prevents migration of abdominal skin onto the penile shaft, and allows the surgeon to identify the position of the penile shaft skin during erection along with the proximal extent of the redundant foreskin. The incision should be made immediately proximal to where the redundant skin extends over the corona of the glans.

Should it become evident that an excessive amount of penile skin has been removed, a full thickness skin graft should be placed over the distal penile shaft (Fig. 12A–D). We have typically harvested skin from the anterior thigh. The thickness of the graft should be 0.018–0.020 inches and the dimensions are determined by the deficit of distal shaft skin. The distal aspect of the native skin should be secured to the underlying dartos fascia with 4–0 chromic suture. The graft should then be placed over the exposed dartos or Buck's fascia. When placed on the penis the graft forms a cylinder, and the seam where the edges of the graft meet should be on the ventral aspect of the penis to provide a better cosmetic result. Once in place, the edges of the graft should be sutured to the native penile skin with 4-0 chromic suture. Small (3–4 mm) incisions are then made throughout the graft (pie-crusting) to prevent fluid accumulation beneath the graft which could compromise graft take. It should then be covered with a bulky cotton gauze that has been saturated with mineral oil and squeezed to remove the excess. The gauze is secured in place with 2-0 silk sutures that are placed in the native penile skin proximal and distal to the graft. The proximal sutures are tied to the distal sutures over the top of the gauze,

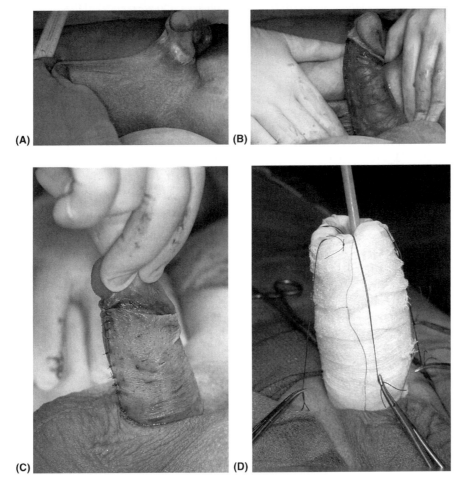

(A)　　　　(B)

(C)　　　　(D)

FIGURE 12 Repair of excessive skin removal during circumcision. (**A**) Tethered penis from excessive skin removal. (**B**) Degloved penis showing normal-sized corporal bodies. (**C**) After the skin graft has been placed. Note the position of the seam on the ventral aspect of the penis. (**D**) Placement of the bulky, mineral-oil soaked dressing.

cinching the dressing down against the graft to improve graft-bed apposition. It should not be so tight as to strangulate the underlying tissue. The dressing can be removed after seven days.

Bleeding/Hematoma

Good hemostasis is crucial to prevent postoperative bleeding or hematoma. Bipolar cautery forceps are a convenient tool to coagulate bleeding while avoiding possible injury to the underlying dorsal neurovascular bundle. If using monopolar electrocautery, it is better to first pick up bleeding sites with a forceps to better isolate it from sensitive nerve fibers in adjacent tissue. Postoperatively, we apply a mildly compressive dressing over the incision that does not extend the full length of the penis.

The paucity of reports on large series of adult circumcisions makes rates of bleeding and hematomas uncertain. However, one report described a 1% rate of postoperative bleeding requiring intervention and 1.6% rate of hematoma requiring evacuation (139). Whether these numbers are generally applicable is unknown.

Sexual Effects

Fink et al. conducted a novel study of the sexual effects of circumcision in light of anecdotal reports of beneficial and harmful effects on sexual functioning resulting from circumcision (140). A survey was sent retrospectively to patients who had undergone circumcision as adults for a variety of causes. The response rate was relatively low at 44%, but several interesting results were seen amongst the responders. A slight decline in erectile function was reported that reached statistical significance. Trends were also seen toward decreased penile sensitivity and sexual activity. However, sexual satisfaction increased after circumcision to a modest, but statistically significant, degree. The role that an underlying disease process, such as balanitis, or other reason for circumcision played in the results is uncertain and could conceivably affect the results.

REFERENCES

1. Mulcahy JJ. Crural perforation during penile prosthetic surgery. J Sex Med 2006; 3:177–180.
2. Szostak MJ, DelPizzo JJ, Sklar GN. The plug and patch: a new technique for repair of corporal perforation during placement of penile prosthesis. J Urol 2000; 163:1203–1205.
3. Brant MD, Ludlow JK, Mulcahy JJ. The prosthesis salvage operation: immediate replacement of the infected penile prosthesis. J Urol 1996; 155:155–157.
4. Wilson SK, Delk JR. A new treatment for Peyronie's disease: modeling the penis over an inflatable penile prosthesis. J Urol 1994; 152:1121–1123.
5. Wilson SK, Cleves MA, Delk JR. Long-term followup of treatment for Peyronie's disease: modeling the penis over an inflatable penile prosthesis. J Urol 2001; 165:825–829.
6. Wilson SK, Delk JR. Inflatable penile implant infection: predisposing factors and treatment suggestions. J Urol 1995; 153:659–661.
7. Gross AJ, Sauerwein DH, Kutzenberger J, Ringert RH. Penile prostheses in paraplegic men. Br J Urol 1996; 78:262–264.
8. Zermann DH, Kutzenberger J, Sauerwein D, Schubert J, Loeffler U. Penile prosthetic surgery in neurologically impaired patients: long-term followup. J Urol 2006; 175:1041–1044.
9. Jarow JP. Risk factors for penile prosthetic infection. J Urol 1996; 156:402–404.
10. Montague DK, Angermeier KW, Lakin MM. Penile prosthesis infections. Int J Impot Res 2001; 13: 326–328.
11. Wilson Sk, Carson CC, Cleves MA, Delk JR. Quantifying risk of penile prosthesis infection with elevated glycosylated hemoglobin. J Urol 1998; 159:1537–1540.
12. Carson CC. Postoperative complications of penile prosthesis implantation. Atlas Urol Clin 2002; 10:203–216.
13. Garber B, Marcus SM. Does surgical approach affect the incidence of inflatable penile prosthesis infection? Urology 1998; 52:291–293.
14. Montague DK. Periprosthetic infection. J Urol 1987; 138:68–69.
15. Peck KR, Kim SW, Jung SI, et al. Antimicrobials as potential adjunctive agents in the treatment of biofilm infection with Staphylococcus epidermidis. Chemotherapy 2003; 49:189–193.
16. Carson CC, Mulcahy JJ, Govier FE. Efficacy, safety and patient satisfaction outcomes of the AMS 700CX inflatable penile prosthesis: results of a long-term multicenter study. J Urol 2000; 164:376–380.
17. Govier FE, Gibbons RP, Correa RJ, Pritchett TR, Kramer-Levien D. Mechanical reliability, surgical complications, and patient and partner satisfaction of the modern three-piece inflatable penile prosthesis. Urology 1998; 52:282–286.

18. Thomalla JV, Thompson ST, Rowland RG, Mulcahy JJ. Infectious complications of penile prosthetic implants. J Urol 1987; 138:65–67.
19. Lotan Y, Roehrborn CG, McConnell JD, Hendin BN. Factors influencing the outcome of penile prosthesis at a teaching institution. Urology 2003; 62:918–921.
20. Licht MR, Montague DK, Angermeier KW, Lakin MM. Cultures from genitourinary prostheses at reoperation: questioning the role of Staphylococcus epidermidis in periprosthetic infection. J Urol 1995; 154:387–390.
21. Henry GD, Wilson SK, Delk JR, et al. Penile prosthesis cultures during revision surgery: a multicenter study. J Urol 2004; 172:153–156.
22. Silverstein A, Donatucci CF. Bacterial biofilms and implantable prosthetic devices. Int J Impot Res 2003; 15(Suppl. 5):S150–S154.
23. Mulcahy JJ. Treatment alternatives for the infected penile implant. Int J Impot Research 2003; 15(Suppl. 5):S147–149.
24. Henry GD, Wilson SK, Delk JR, et al. Revision washout decreases penile prosthesis infection in revision surgery: a multicenter study. J Urol 2005; 173:89–92.
25. Carson CC. Efficacy of antibiotic impregnation of inflatable penile prosthesis in decreasing infection in original implants. J Urol 2004; 171:1611–1614.
26. Wolter CE, Hellstrom WJG. The hydrophilic-coated inflatable penile prosthesis: 1-year experience. J Sex Med 2004; 1:221–224.
27. Carson CC.Diagnosis, treatment and prevention of penile prosthesis infection. Int J Impot Research 2003; 15(Suppl. 5):S139–S146.
28. Carson CC, Robertson CN. Late hematogenous infection of penile prostheses. J Urol 1988; 139: 50–52.
29. Knoll LD. Penile prosthetic infection: management by delayed and immediate salvage techniques. Urology 1998; 52:287–290.
30. Mulcahy JJ. Long-term experience with salvage of infected penile implants. J Urol 2000; 163: 481–482.
31. Ilbeigi P, Sadeghi-Nejad H, Kim MK. Retained rear-tip extenders in redo penile prosthesis surgery: a case for heightened suspicion and thorough physical examination. J Sex Med 2005; 2:149–150.
32. Schaber JD, Paquette EL, Peppas DS, Preston DM, Zorn B. Endoscopic retrieval of a proximal corpus cavernosum polytetrafluoroethylene sleeve during explantation of an infected penile prosthesis. J Urol 1999; 162:1691.
33. Hellstrom WJG. Three-piece inflatable penile prosthesis components (surgical pearls on reservoirs, pumps, and rear-tip extenders). Int J Impot Res 2003; 15(Suppl. 5):S136–S138.
34. User H, Hoff F, McVary KT. Occult retained penile prosthetic fragments in persistent urogenital infections. J Urol 2001; 165:531–533.
35. Furlow WL, Goldwasser B. Salvage of the eroded inflatable penile prosthesis: a new concept. J Urol 1987; 138:312–314.
36. Kaufman JM, Kaufman JL, Borges FD. Immediate salvage procedure for infected penile prosthesis. J Urol 1998; 159:816–818.
37. Montague DK, Angermeir KW. Penile prosthesis implantation. Urol Clin North Am 2001; 28:355–361.
38. Kim SC, Seo KK, Yoon SH. Fracture at the input tube-cylinder junction of AMS 700 inflatable penile prostheses as a complication of a modified implantation technique in a series of 99 patients. Urology 1999; 54:148–151.
39. Levine LA, Estrada CR, Morgentaler A. Mechanical reliability and safety of, and patient satisfaction with the Ambicor inflatable penile prosthesis: results of a 2 center study. J Urol 2001; 166:932–937.
40. Dubocq F, Tefilli MV, Gheiler EL, Li H, Dhabuwala CB. Long-term mechanical reliability of multi-component inflatable penile prosthesis: comparison of device survival. Urology 1998; 52:277–281.
41. Wilson SK, Cleves MA, Delk JR. Comparison of mechanical reliability of original and enhanced Mentor Alpha 1 penile prosthesis. J Urol 1999; 162:715–718.
42. Lee WH, Xin ZC, Choi HK. Spontaneous breakage of malleable prosthesis. Int J Impot Res 1998; 10:255–256.
43. Lockyer R, Gingell C. Spontaneous breakages of malleable prosthesis. Int J Impot Res 1999; 11:237–8 (letter).
44. Fitch WP, Roddy T. Erosion of inflatable penile prosthesis reservoir into bladder. J Urol 1986; 136:1080.
45. Rajpurkar A, Bianco FF, Al-Omar O, Terlecki R, Dhabuwala C. Fate of the retained reservoir after replacement of 3-piece penile prosthesis. J Urol 2004; 172:664–666.
46. Munoz JJ, Ellsworth PI. The retained penile prosthesis reservoir: a risk. Urology 2000; 55: 949viii–949ix.
47. Leach GE, Shapiro CE, Hadley R, Raz S. Erosion of inflatable penile prosthesis reservoir into bladder. J Urol 1984; 131:1177–1178.
48. Park JK, Jang SW, Lee SW, Cui Y. Rare complication of multiple revision surgeries of penile prosthesis. J Sex Med 2005; 2:735–736.

49. Singh I, Godec CJ. Asynchronous erosion of inflatable penile prosthesis into small and large bowel. J Urol 1992; 147:709–710.

50. Wilson SK, Henry GD, Delk JR, Cleves MA. The Mentor Alpha 1 penile prosthesis with reservoir lock-out: effective prevention of auto-inflation with improved capability for ectopic reservoir placement. J Urol 2002; 168:1475–1478.

51. Goldstein I, Newman L, Baum N, et al. Safety and efficacy outcome of Mentor Alpha-1 inflatable penile prosthesis implantation for impotence treatment. J Urol 1997; 157:833–839.

52. Montorsi F, Rigatti P, Carmignani G, et al. AMS three-piece inflatable implants for erectile dysfunction: a long-term multi-institutional study in 200 consecutive patients. Eur Urol 2000; 37:50–55.

53. Moncada I, Hernandez C, Jara J, et al. Buckling of cylinders may cause prolonged pain after prosthesis implantation: a case control study using magnetic resonance imaging of the penis. J Urol 1998; 160:67–71.

54. Mulhall JP, Kim FJ. Reconstructing penile supersonic transporter (SST) deformity using glanulopexy (glans fixation). Urology 2001; 57:1160–1162.

55. Thiel DD, Broderick GA, Bridges M. Utility of magnetic resonance imaging in evaluating inflatable penile prosthesis malfunction and complaints. Int J Impot Research 2003; 14(Suppl. 5):S155–S161.

56. Levine LA, Latchamsetty KC. Management of intraoperative complications, perforation, hypermobile glans, crural crossover, and penile curvature. Atlas Urol Clin 2002; 10:189–201.

57. Minervini A, Ralph DJ, Pryor JP. Outcome of penile prosthesis implantation for treating erectile dysfunction: experience with 504 procedures. BJU Int 2005; 97:129–133.

58. Mulcahy JJ. Distal corporoplasty for lateral extrusion of penile prosthesis cylinders. J Urol 1999; 161:193–195.

59. Carson CC, Noh CH. Distal penile extrusion: treatment with distal corporoplasty or Goretex windsock reinforcement. Int J Impot Res 2002; 14:81–84.

60. Wang R, Chaves JM, Jacobsohn KM. Comparison of erect penile length induced by intracavernosal injection to that obtained with inflatable penile prosthesis. J Sex Med, 2006; 3(Suppl. 1):63 (abstract).

61. Montague DK, Angermeir KW. Surgical approaches for penile prosthesis implantation: penoscrotal vs infrapubic. Int J Impot Res 2003; 15(Suppl. 5):S134–S135.

62. Adeniyi AA, Goorney SR, Pryor JP, Ralph DJ. The Lue procedure: an analysis of the outcome in Peyronie's disease. BJU Int 2002; 89:404–408.

63. Nooter RI, Bosch JLHR, Schroder FH. Peyronie's disease and congenital penile curvature: long-term results of operative treatment with the plication procedure. Br J Urol 1994; 74:497–500.

64. El-Sakka AI, Rashwan HM, Lue TF. Venous patch graft for Peyronie's disease. Part II: outcome analysis. J Urol 1998; 160:2050–2053.

65. Backhaus BO, Muller SC, Albers P. Corporoplasty for advanced Peyronie's disease using venous and/or dermis patch grafting: new surgical technique and long-term patient satisfaction. J Urol 2003; 169:981–984.

66. Montorsi F, Salonia A, Maga T, et al. Evidence based assessment of long-term results of plaque incision and vein grafting for Peyronie's disease. J Urol 2000; 163:1704–1708.

67. Kadioglu A, Tefekli A, Demirel S, Tellaloglu S. Surgical treatment of Peyronie's disease with incision and venous patch technique. Int J Impot Res 1999; 11:75–81.

68. Levine LA, Estrada CR. Human cadaveric pericardial graft for the surgical correction of Peyronie's disease. J Urol 2003; 170:2359–2362.

69. Leungwattanakij S, Bivalacqua TJ, Reddy S, Hellstrom WJG. Long-term follow-up on use of pericardial graft in the surgical management of Peyronie's disease. Int J Impot Research 2001; 13: 183–186.

70. Yurkanin JP, Dean R, Wessells H. Effect of incision and saphenous vein grafting for Peyronie's disease on penile length and sexual satisfaction. J Urol 2001; 166:1769–1773.

71. Dalkin BL, Carter MF. Venogenic impotence following dermal graft repair for Peyronie's disease. J Urol 1991; 146:849–851.

72. Licht MR, Lewis RW. Modified Nesbit procedure for the treatment of Peyronie's disease: a comparative outcome analysis. J Urol 1997; 158:460–463.

73. Levine LA, Lenting EL. A surgical algorithm for the treatment of Peyronie's disease. J Urol 1997; 158:2149–2152.

74. Andrews HO, Al-Akraa M, Pryor JP, Ralph DJ. The Nesbit operation for Peyronie's disease: an analysis of the failures. BJU Int 2001; 87:658–660.

75. Syed AH, Abbasi Z, Hargreave TB. Nesbit procedure for disabling Peyronie's curvature: a median follow-up of 84 months. Urology 2003; 61:999–1003.

76. Richter S, Shalev M, Nissenkorn I. Correction of congenital or acquired penile curvature through simple corporoplication technique. Int J Impot Res 1996; 8:255–258.

77. Rolle L, Tamagnone A, Timpano M, et al. The Nesbit operation for penile curvature: an easy and effective technical modification. J Urol 2005; 173:171–174.

78. Greenfield JM, Lucas S, Levine LA. Factors affecting the loss of length associated with tunica albuginea placation for correction of penile curvature. J Urol 2006; 175:38–41.

79. Ralph DJ, Al-Akraa M, Pryor JP. The Nesbit operation for Peyronie's disease: 16-year experience. J Urol 1995; 154:1362–1363.

80. Rodriguez WC, Rodriguez DD, Fortuno RF. The operative treatment of hydrocele: a comparison of 4 basic techniques. J Urol 1981; 125:804–805.

81. Ku JH, Kim ME, Lee NK, Park YH. The excisional, placation, and internal drainage techniques: a comparison of the results for idiopathic hydrocele. BJU Int 2001; 87:82–84.

82. Lord PH. A bloodless operation for the radical cure of idiopathic hydrocele. Bri J Surg 1964; 51: 914–916.

83. Yachia D. Window technique for hydrocele. Urology 1986; 27:576 (letter).

84. Jahnson S, Johansson JE. Results of window operation for primary hydrocele. Urology 1993; 41: 27–28.

85. Greene WR. "Window operation" for hydrocele. Urology 1987; 30:513 (letter).

86. Ross LS, Flom LS. Azoospermia: a complication of hydrocele repair in a fertile population. J Urol 1991; 146:852–853.

87. Schmidt SS, Free MJ. The bipolar needle for vasectomy: experience with the first 1000 cases. Fertil Steril 1978; 29:676–680.

88. Esho JO, Cass AS. Recanalization rate following methods of vasectomy using interposition of fascial sheath of vas deferens. J Urol 1978; 120:178–179.

89. Rhodes DB, Mumford SD, Free MJ. Vasectomy: efficacy of placing the cut vas in different fascial planes. Fertil Steril 1980; 33:433–438.

90. Shapiro EI, Silber SJ. Open-ended vasectomy, sperm granuloma, and postvasectomy orchalgia. Fertil Steril 1979; 32:546–550.

91. Schmidt SS. Technics and complications of elective vasectomy: the role of spermatic granuloma in spontaneous recanalization. Fertil Steril 1966; 17:467–482.

92. Esho JO, Cass AS, Ireland GW. Morbidity associated with vasectomy. J Urol 1973; 110:413–415.

93. Philp T, Guillebaud J, Budd D. Complication of vasectomy: review of 16,000 patients. Br J Urol 1984; 56:745–748.

94. Ahmed I, Rasheed S, White C, Shaikh NA. The incidence of post-vasectomy chronic testicular pain and the role of nerve stripping (denervation) of the spermatic cord in its management. BJU Int 1997; 79:269–270.

95. Choe JM, Kirkemo AK. Questionnaire-based outcomes study of nononcological post-vasectomy complications. J Urol 1996; 155:1284–1286.

96. McMahon AJ, Buckley J, Taylor A, Lloyd SN, Deane RF, Kirk D. Chronic testicular pain following vasectomy. Br J Urol 1992; 69:188–191.

97. Selikowitz SM, Schned AR. A late post-vasectomy syndrome. J Urol 1985; 134:494–497.

98. Chen TF, Ball RY. Epididymectomy for post-vasectomy pain: histological review. Br J Urol 1991; 68: 407–413.

99. Christiansen CG, Sandlow JI. Testicular pain following vasectomy: a review of postvasectomy pain syndrome. J Androl 2003; 24:293–298.

100. Schmidt SS. Spermatic granuloma: an often painful lesion. Fertil Steril 1979; 31:178–181.

101. Moss WM. A comparison of open-end versus closed-end vasectomies: a report on 6220 cases. Contraception 1992; 46:521–525.

102. Nangia AK, Myles JL, Thomas AJ. Vasectomy reversal for the post-vasectomy pain syndrome: a clinical and histological evaluation. J Urol 2000; 164:1939–1942.

103. Myers SA, Mershon CE, Fuchs EF. Vasectomy reversal for the treatment of the post-vasectomy pain syndrome. J Urol 1997; 157:518–520.

104. Levine LA, Matkov TG. Microsurgical denervation of the spermatic cord as primary surgical treatment of chronic orchalgia. J Urol 2001; 165:1927–1929.

105. Choa RG, Swami KS. Testicular denervation: a new surgical procedure for intractable pain. Br J Urol 1992; 70:417–419.

106. Caddedu JA, Bishoff JT, Chan DY, Moore RG, Kavoussi LR, Jarrett TW. Laparoscopic testicular denervation for chronic orchalgia. J Urol 1999; 162:733–736.

107. Levine LA, Matkov TG, Lubenow TR. Microsurgical denervation of the spermatic cord: a surgical alternative in the treatment of chronic orchalgia. J Urol 1996; 155:1005–1007.

108. Costabile RA, Hahn M, McLeod DG. Chronic orchalgia in the pain prone patient: the clinical perspective. J Urol 1991; 146:1571–1574.

109. Davis BE, Noble MJ, Weigel JW, Foret JD, Mebust WK. Analysis and management of chronic testicular pain. J Urol 1990; 143:936–939.

110. Amelar RD. Early and late complications of inguinal varicocelectomy. J Urol 2003; 170:366–369.

111. Ivanissevich O. Left varicocele due to reflux: experience with 4470 operative cases in forty-two years. J Int Coll Surg 1960; 34:742–755.

112. Palomo A. Radical cure of varicocele by a new technique: preliminary report. J Urol 1949; 61: 604–607.

113. Goldstein M, Gilbert BR, Dicker AP, Dwosh J, Gnecco C. Microsurgical inguinal varicocelectomy with delivery of the testis: an artery and lymphatic sparing technique. J Urol 1992; 148:1808–1811.

114. Ghanem H, Anis T, El-Nashar A, Shamloul R. Subinguinal microvaricocelectmoy versus retroperitoneal varicocelectomy: comparative study of complications and surgical outcome. Urology 2004; 64:1005–1009.

115. Ross LS, Ruppman N. Varicocele vein ligation in 565 patients under local anesthesia: a long-term review of technique, results and complications in light of proposed management by laparoscopy. J Urol 1993; 149:1361–1363.

116. Jarow JP, Assimos DG, Pattaway DE. Effectiveness of laparoscopic varicocelectomy. Urology 1993; 42:544–547.

117. Enquist E, Stein BS, SIgman M. Laparoscopic versus subinguinal varicocelectomy: a comparative study. Fertil Steril 1994; 61:1092–1096.

118. Barbalias GA, Liatsikos EN, Nikifordis G, Siablis D. Treatment of varicocele for male infertility: a comparative study evaluating currently used approaches. Eur Urol 1998; 34:393–398.

119. Cayan S, Kadioglu T, Tefekli A, Kadioglu A, Tellaloglu S. Comparison of results and complications of high ligation surgery and microsurgical high inguinal varicocelectomy in the treatment of varicocele. Urology 2000; 55:750–754.

120. Sayfan J, Soffer Y, Orda R. Varicocele treatment: prospective randomized trial of 3 methods. J Urol 1992; 148:1447–1449.

121. McManus MC, Barqawi A, Meacham RB, Furness PD, Koyle MA. Laparoscopic varicocele ligation: are there advantages with the microscopic subinguinal approach? Urology 2004; 64:357–361.

122. Ralph DJ, Timoney AG, Parker C, Pryor JP. Laparoscopic varicocele ligation. Br J Urol 1993; 72: 230–233.

123. Murray RR, Mitchell SE, Kadir S, et al. Comparison of recurrent varicocele anatomy following surgery and percutaneous balloon occlusion. J Urol 1986; 135:286–289.

124. Kaufman SL, Kadir S, Barth KH, Smyth JW, Walsh PC, White RI. Mechanisms of recurrent varicocele after balloon occlusion or surgical ligation of the internal spermatic vein. Radiology, 1983; 147: 435–440.

125. Punekar SV, Prem AR, Ridhorkar VR, Deshmukh HL, Kelkar AR. Post-surgical recurrent varicocele: efficacy of internal spermatic vemography and steel-coil embolization. Br J Urol 1996; 77:124–128.

126. Feneley MR, Pal MK, Nockler IB, Hendry WF. Retrograde embolization and causes of failure in the primary treatment of varicocele. Br J Urol 1997; 80:642–646.

127. Hopps CV, Lemer ML, Schlegel PN, Goldstein M. Intraoperative varicocele anatomy: a microscopic study of the inguinal versus subinguinal approach. J Urol 2003; 170:2366–2370.

128. Chehval MJ, Purcell MH. Varicocelectomy: incidence of external vein involvement in the clinical varicocele. Urology 1992; 39:573–575.

129. Sayfan J, Adam YG, Soffer Y. A new entity in varicocele subfertility: the "cremasteric reflux". Fertil Steril 1980; 33:88–90.

130. Sayfan J, Adam YG. Intraoperative internal spermatic vein phlebography in the subfertile male with varicocele. Fertil Steril 1978; 29:669–675.

131. Coolsaet BLRA. The varicocele syndrome: venography determining the optimal level for surgical management. J Urol 1980; 124:833–839.

132. Marmar J, Benoff S. Editorial: new scientific information related to varicoceles. J Urol 2003; 170: 2371–2373.

133. Szabo R, Kessler R. Hydrocele following internal spermatic vein ligation: a retrospective study and review of the literature. J Urol 1984; 132:924–925.

134. Dubin L, Amelar RD. Varicocelectomy: 986 cases in a twelve-year study. Urology 1977; 10:446–449.

135. Raman JD, Goldstein M. Intraoperative characterization of arterial vasculature in spermatic cord. Urology 2004; 64:561–564.

136. Chan PK, Wright J, Goldstein M. Incidence and postoperative outcomes of accidental ligation of the testicular artery during microsurgical varicocelectomy. J Urol 2005; 173:482–484.

137. Silber SJ. Microsurgical aspects of varicocele. Fertil Steril 1979; 31:230–232.

138. Wosnitzer M, Roth JA. Optical magnification and Doppler ultrasound probe for varicocelectomy. Urology 1983; 22:24–26.

139. Tucker SC, Cerqueiro J, Bracka A. Circumcision: a refined technique and 5 year review. Ann R Coll Surg Engl 2001; 83:121–125.

140. Fink KS, Carson CC, DeVellis RF. Adult circumcision outcomes study: effect on erectile function, penile sensitivity, sexual activity and satisfaction. J Urol 2002; 167:2113–2116.

141. Dahl DS, Singh M, O'Connor VJ. Lord's operation for hydrocele compared with conventional techniques. Arch Surg 1972; 104:40–41.

142. Jarow J, Ogle A, Kaspar J. Testicular artery ramification within the inguinal canal. J Urol 1992; 147:1290–1292.

19 | Complications of Female Incontinence Surgery

Craig V. Comiter
Department of Surgery, Section of Urology, University of Arizona Health Sciences Center, Tucson, Arizona, U.S.A.

INTRODUCTION

Over the past two decades, there has been an increased interest in female incontinence surgery in urologic practice. As with any form of surgery, adverse events occur, and both patient and surgeon should be aware of the common complications that may accompany female incontinence surgery, and how they and their sequelae are best managed. This chapter will focus on the complications associated with the most common surgeries for urinary incontinence, as well as those related to anterior vaginal wall prolapse surgery, which is often performed in the setting of incontinence surgery.

When evaluating a woman with urinary incontinence, it is necessary to determine whether the leakage is due to bladder or outlet causes. One must consider the patient's symptoms, the urologist's findings, and the actual diagnosis. Symptoms are determined by the urologic history, and usually consist of stress incontinence, urgency incontinence, and/or leakage without sensation. The urologist must base his findings on the physical examination (with demonstration of leakage if possible), basic laboratory testing (urinalysis and culture if indicated) measurement of postvoid residual urine, and appropriate diagnostic studies (urodynamics and/or cystoscopy) if indicated. Determination must be made whether the incontinence is due to bladder causes—such as detrusor overactivity, diminished vesical compliance, or overflow incontinence; or due to outlet causes—such as urethral hypermobility or intrinsic sphincteric incompetence. Pelvic organ prolapse should also be identified in the incontinent patient, as prolapse and incontinence often coexist.

A trial of conservative management is usually indicated prior to surgical treatment. If surgery is indicated, it is vital that the patient fully understand the surgical plan. Informed consent goes beyond a mere signature—there must be a dialogue in which the patient is informed of the risks of the surgical procedure itself, the risk of foregoing surgery, any reasonable alternatives to the planned surgery, appropriate expectations of success, and the length of surgery, the hospital stay, and expected convalescence. The discussion of surgical risks should include those complications that are most common, those that are less common, but still reported, as well as the general treatment of such complications.

ABDOMINAL APPROACH FOR STRESS INCONTINENCE SURGERY

Although the majority of stress incontinence surgeries are now performed transvaginally, (1) the abdominal urethropexy is still offered, especially in the setting of concomitant abdominal surgery. The Marshall-Marchetti-Kranz (MMK) urethropexy and the Burch colposuspension (often combined with a paravaginal repair) are the most common stress urinary incontinence (SUI) surgeries performed abdominally. The MMK involves placing sutures in the periurethral tissue and the pubic symphysis, while the Burch involves placing sutures in the paravaginal tissue and Cooper's ligament. Complications of transabdominal urethropexy include: osteitis pubis (OP) in approximately 2.5% undergoing MMK, but is rare with Burch colposuspension; significant bleeding requiring transfusion in 1% to 2% (2); bladder or urethral injury in 1.6% with resultant fistula formation in 0.3%; prolonged urinary retention 3% to 7%; de novo voiding dysfunction 11% to 12%; wound infection 5%, urinary tract infection 4% (3,4). With a lateral defect cystocele, a paravaginal repair can be performed at the time of urethropexy. The complications associated with paravaginal repair are similar to that of urethropexy.

Osteitis pubis is a self-limiting nonbacterial inflammation of the periosteum overlying the symphysis pubis that is associated with, but not unique to, incontinence surgery. This condition has also been associated with pelvic trauma, childbirth, and prolonged running (5). While OP tends to be self-limiting, it can be quite distressing and incapacitating for up several months following surgery. The patient usually complains of pubic pain in the immediate postoperative period, exacerbated by walking, climbing steps, and standing, and demonstrates pubic bony tenderness, adductor spasm, and a wide-based gait (6). Laboratory evaluation usually demonstrates leukocytosis and an elevated erythrocyte sedimentation rate, and pelvic reontgenography may show a "moth-eaten" lytic lesion that evolves over several weeks. Treatment includes rest, anti-inflammatory medication, and physical therapy. Steroid injections into the pubic symphysis may also be helpful (7).

It is important, but often difficult to rule out osteomyelitis—a true infection of the bone. Osteomyelitis tends to present three to six weeks postoperatively, with signs and symptoms similar to OP, but which are usually more progressive. Diagnosis is best determined by culture, and treatment involves long-term intravenous antibiotics, and occasionally pubic bone resection (8).

VAGINAL APPROACH FOR STRESS INCONTINENCE SURGERY

Over the past five years, transvaginal surgery has replaced transabdominal surgery as the most common surgical treatment for SUI (1). Vaginal surgery is performed with the patient in dorsal lithotomy position.

Nerve damage may complicate anti-incontinence and prolapse surgery, and may result from either malpositioning of the patient (9) or from actual intraoperative ligation/division/ injury to a nerve. The lithotomy (especially exaggerated lithotomy) position may put the sciatic nerve under stress during hip flexion, resulting in weakness of knee flexion; or it may result in femoral nerve compression during hip flexion, resulting in weakness of the quadriceps muscle. Less commonly, the saphenous nerve may be stretched during hip flexion, resulting in pain in the medial calf (10). The common peroneal nerve is at risk for compression against stirrups, and injury may result in ipsilateral foot drop. Such adverse events may be prevented by careful attention to positioning, padding of the legs, and avoidance of excessive abduction and flexion of the thighs.

Ileoinguinal nerve injury is more likely to result from entrapment during passage of the urethral suspension sutures (11,12). Postoperative complaints usually include groin, labial or medial thigh pain, or numbness. Obturator nerve entrapment may result from inappropriate lateral passage of urethral suspension sutures. Treatment usually involves removal of the offending suture, but this does not universally reverse the symptoms. This complication can be avoided if fixation to the pubic bone is used (13).

SLING SURGERY

Suburethral synthetic sling surgery has replaced the Burch colposuspension as the most frequently performed procedure for the treatment of female SUI (1). The most common complication related to operative technique is bladder perforation during needle passage, with an incidence of 1% to 15% (14–17), with an average rate of 5% in most large series. It usually occurs on the side opposite the surgeon's dominant hand, and occurs with greater frequency in patients after previous incontinence surgery, and in those undergoing concomitant vaginal surgery (18). Management includes recognition of the injury on cystourethroscopy, withdrawal and repositioning of the needle laterally, and catheter drainage for 72 hours postoperatively.

Bladder injury may occur during dissection of the vaginal wall off the pubocervical fascia or during perforation of the endopelvic fascia into the retropubic space (which may be necessary for transvaginal paravaginal repair and for placement of certain bone anchors). Transvaginal repair should be performed if possible, with a two-layer closure using absorbable sutures. If exposure is sub-optimal, it may be necessary to approach the bladder transabdominally. Catheter drainage is recommended for one week.

Injury of the urethra or bladder during vaginal dissection is best avoided by placing a urethral catheter, infiltrating the anterior vaginal wall with 1:100,000 epinephrine solution, and using sharp dissection rather than blunt, and staying superficial to the pubocervical fascia. Cystotomy during perforation of the endopelvic fascia is best avoided by emptying the bladder, staying superficial (lateral) to the perivesical fascia. Bladder perforation during needle passage is best avoided by emptying the bladder, and providing finger guidance during needle passage through the retropubic space (not routine with tension-free vaginal tape (TVT) and similar procedures). Early reports of the transobturator sling report a lower rate of bladder and urethral injury by needle passage (19).

Bleeding may occur during vaginal dissection, during perforation of the retropubic space, or during needle passage. Bleeding upon entry into the retropubic space can be difficult to manage, as exposure of the perivesical venous plexus is difficult. An attempt at suture ligation is indicated, followed by packing with a laparotomy pad, or a sponge-wrapped catheter with a 30-cc balloon (20). If bleeding persists, but is not excessive, the sling should be placed, and tying of the sling sutures or bone anchor sutures should tamponade the bleeding. The vaginal wall should be closed and the vagina packed with gauze. Ultimately, persistent heavy bleeding may require abdominal incision and an open retropubic repair. Major bleeding during needle passage may signify external iliac or femoral vessel injury, which is usually caused by exaggerated flexion of the thigh and excessively lateral passage of the needle. Symptomatic retropubic hematoma and vaginal or labial hematoma occurs with a frequency of 1% to 5% (21,22). Management is usually with rest and observation.

Sling-related complications vary with the material composition of the sling. While surgery with prepackaged synthetic slings are associated with a quicker recovery, shorter operative time, shorter hospital stay, and lower rate of urinary retention compared to autologous rectus fascial slings, synthetic slings are associated with a 10 times higher rate of vaginal extrusion and urethral erosion compared to organic slings (23). Urethral erosion likely results from placement of the sling deep to the periurethral fascia (24), too close to the urethral spongy tissue or mucosa, or due to excessive tension causing ischemic necrosis (25). Intraoperative cystourethroscopy is always indicated to rule out urethral or bladder perforation.

With monofilament woven polypropylene slings, vaginal extrusion or urethral erosion occurs at a rate of approximately 1.1% (26) in most contemporary series. Other synthetics, such as polytetrafluoroethylene (PTFE), polyester, or silicone have a higher erosion/extrusion rates, ranging from 4% to 30% (27,28).

Solid and excessively woven materials have a higher complication rate than do meshed slings (29,30). Furthermore, attaching the sling to a mobile structure such as the rectus sheath (as opposed to the fixed pubic bone) may also inhibit tissue ingrowth by permitting sling movement, leading to sinus formation and erosion (29). Similarly, a stiff graft may not conform to the surrounding host tissue, further interfering with tissue ingrowth. The lower rate of urethral erosion and vaginal extrusion with monofilament woven polyester are likely due to the favorable characteristics of the loosely woven polypropylene tape. A loose fiber weave with pores >80 microns theoretically permits the passage of macrophages and tissue ingrowth, thereby allowing integration of the graft into the surrounding tissues (24). This favorable property makes observation a feasible option in the case of vaginal extrusion of a monofilament polypropylene graft (24).

Management of urethral erosion depends on the sling material. With synthetic sling erosion, complete removal of the sling and any permanent suture material is necessary, but bone anchor removal is not necessary unless osteomyelitis is present. The urethral defect should be closed over a catheter, and similar to a urethral diverticulectomy, the periurethral fascia should be reapproximated, with placement of a labial fat graft if the repair is tenuous. Care should be taken to inspect for bladder erosion (which often demonstrates encrustation, Fig. 1), which may necessitate partial cystectomy. The urethral catheter should remain for two weeks. The likelihood of postoperative incontinence ranges from 44% to 83% (31,32). While success rates for synchronous anti-incontinence surgery as high as 87% have been reported, caution is advised—as the risk of surgery is potentially high in the setting of urethral erosion and repair. While erosion with organic material is 15 times less likely than with synthetics, such complications do occur. In cases or nonsynthetic sling erosion, incision or partial excision of the sling and multi-layer urethral closure usually suffices (31,33).

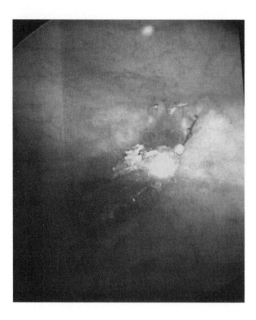

FIGURE 1 Erosion of synthetic sling into the bladder. Note encrustation.

Sling fixation with transvaginal bone anchors enjoyed popularity in the late 1990s. While the placement of permanent urethral suspension sutures through the periosteum of the pubic bone or pericondrium of the pubic symphysis during MMK is clearly associated with a higher risk of OP (1–10%), it is not clear if the use of bone anchors during transvaginal surgery is associated with an elevated risk. The group from Cedars Sinai reports an incidence of OP of 0.45% and no cases of osteomyelitis with the use of transvaginal bone anchors in 440 patients (34). Other reports from centers of excellence include the Northwestern University group, with an incidence of OP of 0.4% and an incidence of osteomyelitis of 1.3% (35), and the group from Cleveland clinic reports osteomyelitis and OP occurrence at rates of significantly less than 1% (36).

TRANSVAGINAL CYSTOCELE REPAIR

Coexisting anterior vaginal wall prolapse should be repaired at the time of incontinence surgery. Often the patient will complain of a symptomatic vaginal bulge, with a feeling of fullness in the vagina. In the incontinent patient with an asymptomatic moderate to severe cystocele, repair is also indicated, because providing urethral support and ignoring a cystocele may result in bladder outlet obstruction. With a transvaginal approach to a large cystocele, both a central defect repair and lateral defect repair are indicated. The anterior vagina is incised from the midurethra to the vaginal cuff, and the vaginal wall is dissected off the pubocervical fascia. The margins of dissection are the mid urethra anteriorly, the cardinal ligaments posteriorly, and the obturator internus fascia laterally.

Injury to the bladder during dissection should be managed via transvaginal repair with a two-layer closure using absorbable sutures. If exposure is sub-optimal, it may be necessary to approach the bladder transabdominally. Catheter drainage is recommended for one week. Cystotomy is best avoided by infiltrating the anterior vaginal wall with 1:100,000 epinephrine solution, using sharp dissection superficial to the pubocervical fascia, and keeping the bladder empty. Bleeding during vaginal dissection should be managed with temporary packing or with suture ligation rather than electrocautery, in order to minimize the risk of vesicovaginal fistula formation.

Ureteral ligation is another potential complication of transvaginal cystocele repair, but this complication should always be recognized and remedied intraoperatively. Cystourethroscopy is absolutely indicated, and visualization of urine efflux should be observed from both ureteral orifices. Difficulty visualizing efflux may be overcome by administration of intravenous indigo carmine, and fluid challenge. Lack of visualization should be further investigated

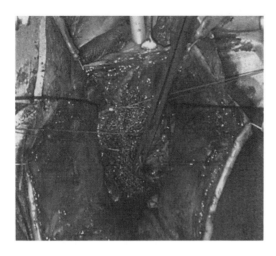

FIGURE 2 Absorbable mesh is used to reduce the cystocele, protect the ureters from suture ligation, and reinforce the central defect repair.

with attempted passage (and then removal) of a ureteral stent. Inability to pass a stent implies ureteral ligation, and requires removal of the offending suture, which usually involves the cardinal ligament or posterior pubocervical fascial suture(s). Subsequent confirmation of urine reflux should suffice, without the need for further evaluation or treatment.

With significant prolapse, the trigone may be displaced inferiorly and anteriorly, increasing the risk of ureteral occlusion during the central defect repair. Reduction of the cystocele with a biodegradable mesh (Fig. 2) reduces the risk of ureteral injury as well as reducing the risk of recurrent prolapse (37). The use of permanent or organic material to bolster the central repair and provide lateral support has increased in popularity over the past several years. The complications of such material are similar to those discussed with sling surgery. In addition, the complications of urinary tract infection, vaginal infection, bleeding, dyspareunia, and de novo voiding dysfunction are similar to those of sling surgery.

URETHRAL DIVERTICULECTOMY

A urethral diverticulum results from infection of the periurethral glands (38) of the distal two-thirds of the urethra, and usually opens into the mid or distal urethra (39). Dilated glands beneath the periurethral fascia expand posterior to the urethra (anterior vaginal wall mass, Fig. 3), and rupture into the urethral lumen, ultimately establishing a communication between the diverticulum and the urethra. Indications for surgery include dyspareunia, postvoid dribbling, recurrent urinary tract infections, pain, and lower urinary tract symptoms. Rarely, patients present with urinary retention.

The principles governing repair of a urethral diverticulum include: (*i*) water-tight and tension-free closure of the urethra; (*ii*) reapproximation of the periurethral fascia with nonoverlapping suture lines; (*iii*) use of vascularized tissue flaps to re-enforce the repair if necessary. The periurethral fascia is a distinct layer surrounding the urethral diverticulum. Preservation of this fascia provides a second layer of vascularized tissue.

In the setting of a large periurethral abscess, drainage of the abscess is recommended first, with a staged urethral diverticulectomy to follow several weeks later (40). Occasionally, a stone may form in the diverticulum, and must be removed at the time of diverticulectomy (Fig. 4). It is helpful to have preoperative assessment of the extent of the diverticulum (i.e., proximal extension, circumferentiality, etc.). This is best done with magnetic resonance imaging (MRI), which has become the modality of choice for imaging a urethral diverticulum (41). If the diverticulum has significant proximal extension, care must be taken to avoid injuring the striated sphincter, bladder neck, trigone, and ureters. Ureteral integrity is verified by observation of urinary efflux, and bladder integrity may be demonstrated cystoscopically or by intravesical instillation of methylene blue.

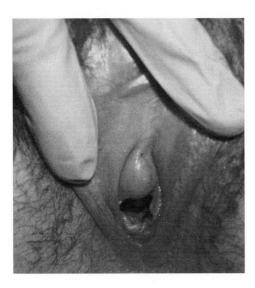

FIGURE 3 Urethral diverticulum. Patient presented with dribbling, dyspareunia, and dysuria.

De novo SUI occurs with a rate of 2% to 16% (40–43). The risk is increased if the diverticulum lies near the midurethral complex. Injury of the sphincteric mechanism may cause intrinsic sphincter deficiency (ISD), or removal of an obstructing diverticulum may unmask SUI. Placement of a suburethral sling should be considered at the time of surgery if there is pre-existing SUI (42), or if the surgeon suspects a high likelihood of postoperative SUI. However, synthetic material is contra-indicated due to a high risk of infection and erosion. Postoperative ISD may be managed with sling surgery or periurethral injection after healing is complete.

Urethral stricture occurs in 0% to 5% of cases, but is unusual if the urethra can be reconstructed around a 12 F Foley catheter. Urinary tract infection occurs 3% to 13% of the time, but recurrent infections may indicate recurrent diverticulum (43). Diverticular recurrence occurs in 1% to 30% of instances. The likelihood of recurrence may be minimized by complete excision of the diverticular sac, and adequate reapproximation of the urethral mucosa, urethral spongy tissue, and periurethral fascia.

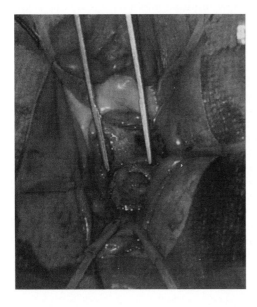

FIGURE 4 Stone in urethral diverticulum.

Urethrovaginal fistulization has been reported postoperatively at a rate of incidence of 1% to 8% (40–43), or may even present preoperatively if the diverticulum ruptures through the vaginal wall. Fistulae involving the proximal urethra or bladder neck present with continuous incontinence; midurethral fistulae often present with SUI. Distal fistulae often have urinary spraying, split stream, vaginal voiding, or may even be asymptomatic.

Keys to Preventing Formation of a Urethro-Vaginal Fistula

Fistula formation is usually related to an error in surgical technique. During dissection of the vaginal wall, care should be taken to remain superficial to be periurethral fascia and perivesical fascia. Dissection is best performed sharply, without the use of electrocautery. Entry into the correct plane between the vaginal wall and pubocervical fascia usually leads to a relatively bloodless dissection. Hemostasis may be achieved via temporary vaginal packing or accurate suture placement with a 4-0 self-absorbing suture (SAS). The differential diagnosis includes vaginal discharge, severe SUI, and vesicovaginal fistula. Work-up should include history, physical examination, cystoscopy, vaginoscopy, and voiding cystourethrography. Surgical repair of an urethrovaginal fistula is similar to the technique described for urethral diverticulectomy. Interposition of a labial fat graft is often recommended.

FISTULAE

While hysterectomy is not indicated for the treatment of urinary incontinence, it is, however, indicated with symptomatic uterine prolapse in the setting of incontinence surgery, and therefore the incontinence surgeon should be aware of the urologic complications associated with hysterectomy (44). Injury to the urinary tract may occur during transabdominal or transvaginal hysterectomy, resulting in formation of a vesico-vaginal fistula (VVF) or an uretero-vaginal fistula (UVF), both of which present with urinary incontinence.

Keys to Preventing Formation of Vesico-Vaginal Fistula

A VVF results from simultaneous injury to the bladder and vagina. The surgery most commonly associated with VVF is a transabdominal hysterectomy, followed by transvaginal hysterectomy. The risk increases with a history of steroid use (45), pelvic radiation, prior uterine surgery, endometriosis, previous cervical conization, or distorted anatomy secondary to fibroids or adnexal mass (46). Therefore, elective hysterectomy in a high-risk patient should be performed by an experienced surgeon with the availability of urologic assistance if necessary (47). The vulnerability of the bladder arises from its proximity to the cervix and anterior vaginal wall. The most common site of bladder injury is supratrigonal, and may occur from overt laceration, electrocautery, or when the vaginal cuff closure inadvertently incorporates the bladder (Fig. 5).

Preventive measures include continuous bladder drainage and sharp dissection rather than electrocautery to separate the bladder off the uterus (48). Specific hemostatic suturing is preferable to excessive cauterization. Prior to ligation of the uterosacral ligaments, the inferior and lateral aspect of the bladder must be adequately mobilized, and the ligaments should be taken close to the uterus (49). With extensive pelvic and perivesical fibrosis, intentional anterior cystotomy may be performed in order to prevent accidental injury to the bladder base (50).

If cystotomy is suspected, the bladder should be filled with colored fluid to visualize any leakage. Repair should be attempted only after adequate tissue mobilization (51). Given the 10% incidence of concomitant ureteral injury, the surgeon must always demonstrate the integrity of the ureters. Intentional extension of the cystotomy anteriorly provides trigonal exposure, and inspection for other injuries and for visualization of urinary efflux from the ureteral orifices is easily accomplished, often helped by intravenous indigo carmine. If efflux is not demonstrated, or if high suspicion remains, retrograde ureteral stents should be passed over a floppy-tipped wire, with fluoroscopic guidance. The patient should be transferred to a fluoroscopy-ready table prior to attempting passage of a guide-wire, ureteral stent, or ureteroscope, thereby minimizing the risk of additional iatrogenic ureteral injury.

The cystotomy should be closed with SAS in two layers. If the closure is tenuous, interposition of adjacent vascularized tissue between the cystotomy repair and the vagina is

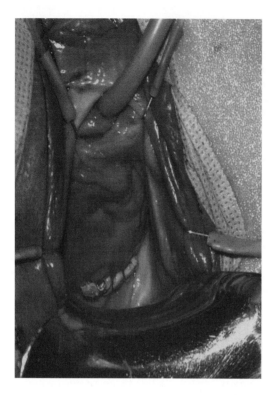

FIGURE 5 Vaginal stones formed from multiple small fistulae secondary to incorporation of the bladder in vaginal cuff staple line during hysterectomy.

recommended. The bladder should be drained continuously for two weeks, with catheter removal only after cystographic confirmation of complete healing.

Keys to Preventing Ureteral Injury

The ureter is vulnerable during pelvic surgery because it lies close to the rectum and female reproductive organs within the pelvis. During laparoscopic hysterectomy, the distal ureters may be injured during ligation of the uterine arteries (52), or when the cardinal ligaments are dissected and divided below the uterine vessels (53). Ureteral injury occurs in 0.5% to 1% of all pelvic surgeries (54) and in 1.4% to 2% of patients undergoing radical hysterectomy (55,56).

It is incumbent upon the surgeon to identify both ureters. While familiarity with normal anatomy is vital, it is the cases with abnormal anatomy that likely pose the highest risk. Intravenous urography (IVU) may be considered if a pre-existing abnormality is suspected. In two contemporary series of patients with pelvic organ prolapse and no known malignancy, the prevalence of hydronephrosis on routine preoperative IVU was 7%, with only 1% of patients rated as severe dilation (57). The incidence of hydroureteronephrosis did increase, however, with worsening pelvic prolapse. While ureteral injuries during hysterectomy occur in up to 2.5% of cases (58), routine preoperative IVU has not been shown to reduce the incidence of ureteral injury (57). Furthermore, approximately 3% of patients will have a significant adverse reaction to the contrast agent.

Identification of urethral, bladder, or ureteral injury is crucial, because the best time for repair is at the time of injury. The tissues are in their best condition, all options for repair are still present, and the morbidity of a second trip to the operating room may be avoided.

Repair of Vesico-Vaginal Fistula

Patients typically present with continuous daytime and nighttime leakage per vagina, following pelvic surgery. Depending on the size of the fistula, the amount of urine voided versus the amount lost per vagina varies. Pelvic examination often identifies the fistulous opening at the vaginal cuff. Filling the bladder with a blue solution can be helpful. The vagina may then be inspected for leakage, or packed with a tampon and re-examined after ambulation.

Both lower and upper tract evaluation are indicated. Voiding cystourethrography may demonstrate the fistula, as well as any concomitant prolapse. Cystoscopy is necessary to evaluate bladder capacity, and the size and location of the fistula relative to the ureteral orifices. Biopsy is recommended if there is a history of genitourinary malignancy. Upper tract evaluation is useful to rule out UVF or ureteral obstruction.

A trial of conservative management should be offered for small fistulae. Continuous catheter drainage plus oral antimuscarinics and antibiotics have been associated with a 2% to 10% closure rate (59,60). There are anecdotal reports of success for de-epithelialization using silver nitrate, mechanical curettage (61), or electrocautery (62). Success has also been reported using fibrin glue (63–65) or Nd-YAG laser welding (66) in fistulae <3 mm.

For large VVFs, and for those that fail conservative management, surgery is required. Urine should be sterilized, and preoperative estrogen replacement is recommended in postmenopausal women (67). As many series document excellent success rates with early fistula repair (68–72), immediate surgical intervention for uncomplicated VVF caused by iatrogenic injury is now recommended, thus avoiding the discomfort associated with urinary leakage (odor, skin excoriation, urinary tract infection) as well as the adverse psychological and medicolegal impact of prolonged urinary leakage.

The principles of surgical repair are adequate exposure of the fistulous tract, and a tension-free, watertight, multi-layered repair with nonoverlapping suture lines. Whether the approach is vaginal or abdominal, the initial attempt at repair has the highest success rate. The approach should be individualized, based on the patient's anatomy, location of the fistula, and reconstructive considerations.

Compared to abdominal surgery, the transvaginal approach has less morbidity and a shorter hospitalization (73). Abdominal repair is recommended, however, when: (*i*) the fistulous opening cannot be adequately exposed vaginally; (*ii*) simultaneous bladder augmentation is planned; (*iii*) simultaneous ureteral surgery/ureteroneocystostomy is planned. Through a Pfannenstiel or lower abdominal midline incision, an intraperitoneal, extraperitoneal, or transvesical approach (74,75) to the bladder may be utilized. The bladder and vagina are each closed in two layers using SAS (76,77). Interposition of perivesical or extraperitoneal fibrofatty tissue, or greater omentum (78) between the bladder and vaginal closures should be considered. A suprapubic tube is placed in addition to the urethral catheter, to allow maximal bladder drainage. A Penrose drain should be brought out through a separate stab wound.

The transvaginal approach is far less burdensome for patients than is an abdominal approach (79,80). Contraindications include severe vaginal stenosis and an inability to tolerate the dorsal lithotomy position. If the fistula encroaches upon the ureteral orifices, transurethral placement of ureteral stents is indicated. The fistulous tract should be dilated with lacrimal duct probes and pediatric urethral sounds until an 8Fr Foley catheter can be inserted into the bladder (useful for traction). Instillation of saline into the vaginal wall is recommended to aid dissection, and the fistula is circumscribed sharply.

Vaginal wall flaps are raised anteriorly, posteriorly, and laterally. Excision of the tract is not necessary, and might increase the risk of bleeding. Furthermore, the fibrous ring of the fistula provides a strong anchor for suture placement. The intrafistula catheter is removed, and the tract is closed transversely with interrupted 2-0 SAS. The perivesical fascia and detrusor muscle are then imbricated perpendicular to the first layer, 5 mm from the previous closure. Integrity of the closure is tested by bladder filling. The proximal vaginal wall flap is advanced anteriorly beyond the fistula, covering the repair with healthy tissue. In cases of recurrent fistula or tenuous repair, a labial fat graft can be tunneled under the labia minora to the site of repair (81,82). Alternatively, a peritoneal flap may be harvested, by dissecting posteriorly toward the cul-de-sac, and mobilizing the preperitoneal fat and peritoneum caudally. The peritoneal flap can then be advanced over the repair with interrupted 3-0 SAS. Other sources of tissue include the sartorius, gluteus, rectus, and gracilis muscles (83–87).

Postoperatively, the vagina is packed with an antibiotic-impregnated gauze for several hours. Urethral and suprapubic catheter drainage is recommended until the urine is clear of blood. The urethral catheter may then be removed to minimize mucosal irritation at the site of repair. Oral antibiotics should minimize the risk of infection. Bladder spasms have been postulated to compromise healing of the repair (88), and should be treated. Oral or topical estrogen has been demonstrated to promote healing (89). Cystography is performed at two weeks to document complete healing of the fistula, followed by catheter removal.

Early complications include vaginal bleeding, bladder spasms, and urinary or vaginal infection. Intraoperative bleeding should be controlled with suture ligation. Postoperative bleeding is usually controlled by vaginal packing and bed rest. Late complications include vaginal stenosis, unrecognized ureteral injury, and fistula recurrence. Vaginal stenosis usually results from over-aggressive resection of vaginal tissue. Delayed recognition of a ureteral injury is best managed by percutaneous drainage, with definitive surgical repair only after several months, so as not to jeopardize the VVF repair. Recurrent fistula mandates reoperation, but should be delayed until the inflammation associated with the original surgery has completely subsided. Labial fat graft or peritoneal flap interposition is recommended for repair of recurrent VVF.

Repair of Uretero-Vaginal Fistula

The most common cause of UVF is total abdominal hysterectomy for either benign or malignant disease (90). Fistulization occurs when a ureteral leak persists and the urine makes its way to the vaginal cuff. Any unexplained abdominal or flank pain or costovertebral angle tenderness should alert the surgeon to the possibility of a ureteral injury, yet often there are no symptoms before urinary incontinence occurs. The typical presentation is one of sudden onset leakage from the vagina one to four weeks postoperatively. The patient additionally voids per urethra as the contralateral ureter fills the bladder.

In a female with vaginal leakage after pelvic surgery, a double dye test may differentiate between VVF and UVF (91). The vagina is packed and methylene blue is given intravenously, while red carmine is instilled intravesically. The vaginal pack will stain red if a VVF is present, and blue if a UVF is present. An IVU may demonstrate varying degrees of hydronephrosis, or even a silent kidney (92). If IVU is not revealing, a retrograde ureterogram should demonstrate the location and magnitude of the fistula.

Treatment options include internal drainage via ureteral stent, external drainage via percutaneous nephrostomy, open surgical repair, or even nephrectomy. Controversy exists regarding timing of repair, with some surgeons performing immediate, while others advocate early upper tract drainage followed by delayed ureteral repair (93–98).

Retrograde ureteropyelography is recommended may be diagnostic and therapeutic. If a ureteral catheter cannot be passed, the diagnosis of a distal obstruction is confirmed. If distal ureteral obstruction remains, spontaneous healing is unlikely. Should a stent be placed to bypass the fistula, spontaneous healing is likely without further intervention (99,100). If retrograde ureteral stenting is unsuccessful, antegrade percutaneous nephrostomy is recommended. Obstruction is relieved, and access for antegrade ureteral stenting is made available. If spontaneous healing does not occur, an attempt at antegrade stenting is recommended. Once a stent is placed, there is a 50% to 70% chance that the UVF will heal without the need for open surgical intervention (99,100). Because of the chance of ureteral stricturing, close follow-up is needed.

If neither antegrade nor retrograde ureteral access is successful, open surgical repair is indicated. Early surgical repair may be undertaken if there is not significant urosepsis and renal function is relatively well preserved. End-to-end uretero-ureterostomy may be performed, but frequently, ureteroneocystostomy is the favored repair. Ureteroneocystostomy bypasses the site of injury, eliminating the difficult dissection of the distal ureter (101). Success rates are close to 100% with ureteral reimplantation (101–103) and the risk of ureteral obstruction is minimized by avoiding an antirefluxing anastamosis.

The location of the injury and the degree of ureteral and bladder mobility will dictate the method of implantation. An ureteroneocystostomy may be aided by a psoas bladder hitch to minimize anastomotic tension (103). A Boari flap replacement of the distal ureter is indicated when the obstructive segment lies proximally (104,105). With high or long ureteral strictures, a more complex reconstruction such as transureteroureterostomy, renal decensus, renal autotransplantation, or ileouretero-cystoplasty may be necessary. Nephrectomy should only be undertaken as a last resort (104,105).

ARTIFICIAL URINARY SPHINCTER

Sphincteric incompetence in women is most commonly treated with suburethral sling surgery or with periurethral bulking agents. The familiarity, safety, and efficacy of these procedures have relegated artificial urinary sphincter (AUS) surgery as a "procedure of last resort." However, AUS placement surgery can be performed via a transvaginal (106,107) or transabdominal approach (108,109), and in the properly selected patients has been associated with excellent outcome. Appell (106) and Hadley (107) report >90% success without revision in >90% of patients status post-transvaginal AUS placement.

However, the transvaginal approach is relatively contraindicated in patients after previous incontinence surgery or radiation, due to the difficult dissection between the vaginal wall and the urethra/bladder neck, and the increased risk of vaginal cuff extrusion. The transabdominal approach allows better exposure, with relatively straightforward placement of the cuff around the bladder neck between the periurethral fascia and the vagina (107,109–111). In instances of difficult dissection, intentional cystotomy (cephalad to the cuff placement) can be helpful, to better allow discernment of the plan between the vagina and periurethral fascia, and prevent accidental bladder or urethral injury.

Success rates generally range from 76% to 89% (108,109,111), with lower success rates and a higher revision rate in patients with neurogenic bladder dysfunction. Infection, erosion, or extrusion of any single component requires explantation of the entire device. With urethral erosion, urethral reconstruction is necessary, often with labial fat graft interposition, followed by at least one week of urethral catheterization. Attempt at replacement should wait at least six weeks.

PERIURETHRAL BULKING AGENTS

Stress urinary incontinence resulting from ISD may be treated via periurethral bulking. Success rates with transurethral injection of gluteraldehyde cross-linked collagen, the most commonly used injectable agent, success rates are generally greater than 65% at one year (112), but decline significantly thereafter (113–115). One of the limitations of collagen is its susceptibility to bioabsorption over time. More "permanent" materials, including carbon coated zirconium beads, and polydimethylsiloxane (silicone rubber) solid particles suspended in a nonsilicone carrier gel are available. However, long-term data is not available for these newer agents (116,117).

Complications associated with periurethral injection include: transient urinary retention, hematuria, irritative symptoms, urinary tract infection, particle migration, delayed hypersensitivity reaction, and periurethral abscess formation. Temporary retention ranges from 1% to 21% (118–123). The highest rates of urinary retention are associated with PTFE, an older injectable agent, which is not, FDA-approved (124). Large-bore catheterization should be avoided, as this may mold the soft injectable in an open position, thereby "undoing" the coaptive injection. Treatment for retention should be intermittent catheterization with a 12 or 14 F catheter. When self- catheterization is not feasible, a 10 or 12 F Foley catheter should be placed for 12 to 24 hours. Retention beyond 48 hours is very rare.

Transient minor hematuria occurs in 2% to 16% (118,121) of instances. Temporary irritative symptoms are not uncommon, occurring at a rate of 8% to 10% (125,126), and should be managed expectantly. Urinary tract infection occurs at a rate of 0% to 12% (121,125,127), but may be reduced with the administration of perioperative antibiotics. New-onset urgency is another well-known complication of periurethral injection, occuring at a rate of 1% to 25%. Stothers et al. recently reported a series with de novo urgency occurring in 13% of patients, 21% of whom did not improve with anticholinergics (128).

Particle migration has been demonstrated with carbon coated (local and distant lymph nodes), but the clinical effect of bead migration is yet uncertain (129). Particle migration is also associated with PTFE (130), with reports of migration to pelvic nodes, brain, kidneys, and lungs (131), with an instance of alveolitis (54) reported from the inflammatory response (132). Silicone microimplants with particle size >100 microns do not migrate. However, concerns remain about the migration of smaller silicone particles (133). Autologous fat injection has been associated with fat embolism, as well as donor site hematoma and infection (134). Delayed hypersensitivity reaction (135) associated with collagen injection is uncommon (2%), but can be associated with arthralgias. Periurethral abscess formation is a rare complication (136) (Fig. 6) and may result in urethral diverticulum or urethrovaginal fistulization.

URINARY RETENTION

Urinary retention is a well-known complication of incontinence surgery, but the incidence depends on the definition of "retention." Frank retention requiring catheterization beyond one week typically occurs in about 4% to 8% of patients following sling surgery, and in 3% to 7% following abdominal urethropexy (3,137–139). The risk of retention increases with age and parity, as well as with concomitant vaginal surgery. Additionally, the risk is increased in those of increased age, those who are post hysterectomy, and in those with adverse urodynamics characteristics—that is, low flow and/or low voiding pressures (140,141). Physical examination is necessary to identify any hypersuspension of the urethra, vertical axis of the urethra, or hyper-support of the mid-urethra with an obstructing cystocele posteriorly.

Urinary retention is best avoided by adhering to the principles of incontinence surgery: to provide urethral support from above to prevent descent, or to provide a backboard from below to prevent descent. Urodynamic investigation has demonstrated that a properly placed suburethral sling does not produce obstruction as long as the position of the sling material is carefully determined from bladder neck to mid-urethra and excessive tension is avoided (142,143).

With abdominal urethropexy, care should be taken to avoid overly medial suture placement, which may result in urethral kinking or periurethral scarring. With sling surgery, the sling should not be placed too distally, especially with a poorly supported bladder neck. Many techniques have been described to avoid overtightening of a suburethral sling, and usually involve placing an instrument between the sling and periurethral fascia during tensioning. With ISD, tighter sling tension may be required in order to close the incompetent outlet.

Treatment of urinary retention can begin conservatively, with alpha blockers and clean intermittent catheterization (at least four times per day) as long as the patient is satisfied, and does not suffer from irritative symptoms or recurrent infections. The majority of patients will, however, require reoperation. Urodynamic demonstration of bladder outlet obstruction is not necessary in the face of retention, because sling incision/urethrolysis should be offered regardless of the

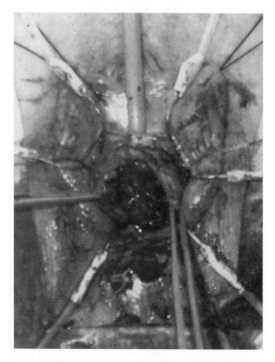

FIGURE 6 Periurethral abscess was drained previously. Urethral diverticulum repair—note preservation of the periurethral fascia, which will be closed over the urethra.

presence or absence of adequate detrusor contractility. While urethral dilation and transurethral urethrotomy have been described (144), a more appropriate treatment for early retention after sling surgery (i.e., less than 8 weeks postoperatively) is sling incision (145–147) in the midline. If relaxation of the urethral support is not obvious, then unilateral or bilateral incision of the sling as it enters the endopelvic fashion is recommended (148). Early relief of obstruction may be associated with less permanent voiding dysfunction than is delayed treatment (149).

In cases of long-standing urinary retention, a formal urethrolysis is indicated—either transvaginally or transabdominally (150,151). With the former, consideration should be given to omental flap interposition between the urethra and pubis, and with the latter, use of a labial fat graft should be considered, especially in the setting of failed previous urethrolysis or sling incision. Success rates are generally high, with 65% to 93% of patients voiding well, resolution of urgency incontinence in 67%, and a recurrent SUI rate of less than 10%. Recurrent SUI is uncommon, in less than 10% of patients (152,153). Complications of urethrolysis are similar to those of sling surgery—namely bleeding, infection, urethral or bladder injury, and voiding dysfunction.

VOIDING DYSFUNCTION

Voiding dysfunction is the most common complication following incontinence surgery. Although the incidence reported varies with the definition of voiding dysfunction, up to 20% of patients will have new urinary complaints postoperatively, most commonly de novo urgency. Unfortunately, obstructive and irritative symptoms do not necessarily correspond to urethral or bladder dysfunction, respectively. Behavioral management with fluid restriction, caffeine restriction, timed voiding, and double voiding is often helpful, and empiric pharmacotherapy is often utilized—with alpha blockers for retentive symptoms and antimuscarinics for irritative symptoms. Persistent voiding dysfunction is an indication for urodynamics evaluation. However, failure to demonstrate unstable bladder contractions does not rule out detrusor overactivity, and there is no standard definition of bladder outlet obstruction. While some investigators suggest a voiding pressure >20 cm water and peak urinary flowrate <15 mL/s signifies obstruction, in many instances there is no bladder contraction during urodynamics studies (154,155). Bladder outlet obstruction may therefore be difficult to diagnose. At the University of Arizona, video urodynamics has proven useful, where narrowing or cutoff of radiocontrast at the level of the sling may suggest surgical obstruction (Fig. 7).

If the voiding dysfunction is due to bladder outlet obstruction, and conservative management fails, then urethrolysis is recommended (156). If detrusor overactivity is the diagnosis, and pharmacotherapy is unsuccessful, consideration should be given to sacral neuromodulation or augmentation cystoplasty.

RECURRENT PELVIC ORGAN PROLAPSE

Postoperative pelvic organ prolapse may be due to a true recurrence, or on the other hand secondary to an anatomic defect that was not properly repaired with the original surgery. Factors

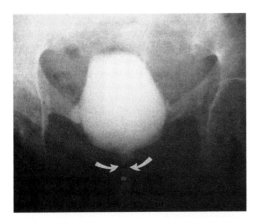

FIGURE 7 Bladder outlet obstruction, clearly visible on fluoroscopy, following sling. Patient had significant voiding dysfunction postoperatively.

that increase the risk of recurrent prolapse include advanced age, menopausal status, obesity, steroid use, and malnutrition. Failure to identify an anatomic defect preoperatively may result from competition among prolapsing organs filling a finite introital space, thereby obscuring concomitant prolapse. The incontinence surgeon must identify all prolapse preoperatively, because repairing only anterior vaginal prolapse may exacerbate prolapse of the middle and posterior compartments. Initial procedure may disturb the balance of the structural parts and thus predispose to a second defect occurring or cause an already present defect to increase after the initial procedure (157,158). In the case of pelvic floor relaxation, often seen in multiparous women, widening of the levator hiatus leads to a diminution in the pubococcygeal response to straining. This in turn results in insufficient vaginal angulation, with the proximal vagina becoming more vertically oriented. Similarly, surgery to augment urethral support without proper repair of concomitant pelvic floor relaxation results in anterior displacement of the vagina. The cul-de-sac is left unprotected and exposed to increases in intraabdominal pressure, thereby predisposing to enterocele formation. With inadequate support of the vaginal cuff following hysterectomy, separation of the sacrouterine and cardinal ligaments may then predispose to peritoneal herniation through the vaginal apex. For example, the risk of enterocele formation following Burch colposuspension is generally 8% to 14% at one to two years, with approximately two-thirds of those requiring reoperation (159,160).

Dynamic MRI has evolved as the procedure of choice for evaluating patients with complex vaginal prolapse (161). MRI is more accurate than physical examination in identifying cystocele, enterocele (Fig. 8), vault prolapse, and pelvic organ pathology such as uterine fibroids, urethral diverticula, ovarian cysts, and Bartholin's gland cysts (162). Accurate diagnosis of complex pelvic organ prolapse with dynamic MRI has been shown to alter surgical planning in more than 30% of cases, most often because of occult enterocele not appreciated on physical examination (163).

SUMMARY

Female incontinence and pelvic organ prolapse surgery has become a routine part of urologic care. The incontinence surgeon must be aware of these complications and inform the patient of the appropriate risks. Preoperative evaluation, astute knowledge of surgical anatomy, and intraoperative vigilance are necessary to minimize the risk of complications. The best management results from intraoperative recognition and immediate repair. Postoperative

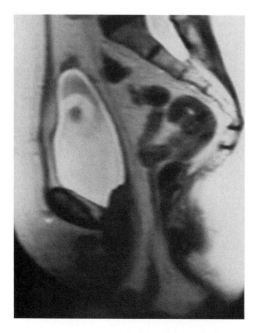

FIGURE 8 Magnetic resonance imaging of complex vaginal prolapse. Large enterocele is demonstrated.

complications do, however, occur, and management of these adverse events should follow a stepwise approach, with appropriate diagnostic studies, conservative management if possible, and surgical management if necessary.

REFERENCES

1. Bhargava S, Chapple CR. Rising awareness of the complications of synthetic slings. Curr Opin Urol 2004; 14:317–321.
2. Wiskind AD, Stanton SL. The Burch colposuspension for genuine stress incontinence. In: Thompson JD, Rock JA, eds. TeLinde's Operative Gynecology Updates. Philadelphia, PA: J.B. Lippincott, 1993:1–13.
3. Mainprize TC, Drutz HP. The Marshall-Marchetti-Kranz procedure: a critical review. Obstet Gynecol Surv 1988; 43:724–729.
4. Walters MD. Retropubic operations for genuine stress incontinence. In: Walters MD, Karram MM, eds. Urogynecology and Reconstructive Pelvic Surgery. St. Louis, MO: Mosby, 2003:159–170.
5. Gamble JG, Simmons SC, Freedman M. The symphysis pubis: anatomic and pathologic considerations. Clin Orthop 1986; 203:261–272.
6. Winters JC, Scarpero HM, Appell RA. Use of bone anchors in female urology. Urology 2000; 4:15–22.
7. Lentz SS. Osteitis pubis: a review. Obstet Gynecol Surv 1995; 50:310–315.
8. Ross JJ, Hu LT. Septic arthritis of thepubic symphysis: review of 100 cases. Medicine (Baltimore) 2003; 82:340–345.
9. Phillips TH, Zeidman KJ, Thompson IM, et al. Complications following needle bladder-neck suspension. Int Urogynecol J 1992; 3:38–42.
10. Karram MM. Transvaginal needle suspension. In: Hurt GW, ed. Urogynecologic Surgery. Gaithersburg, MD: Aspen Publishers, 1992:61–72.
11. Miyazaki F, Shook G. Ilioinguinal nerve entrapment during needle suspension for stress incontinence. Obstet Gynecol 1992; 80:246–248.
12. Monga M, Ghoniem GM. Ilioinguinal nerve entrapment following needle bladder suspension procedures. Urology 1994; 44:447–450.
13. Kelly MJ, Zimmern PE, Leach GE. Complications of bladder neck suspension procedures. Urol Clin North Am 1991; 18:339–348.
14. Nilsson CG, Kuuva N, Falconer C, et al. Long term results of the tension-free vaginal tape (TVT) procedure for surgical treatment of female stress urinary incontinence. Int Urogynecol J 2001; 12:S5–S8.
15. Kuuva N, Nilsson CG. A nationwide analysis of complications associated with the tension-free vagnal tape (TVT) procedure. Acta Obstet Gynecol Scand 2002; 81:72–77.
16. Lebret T, Lugagne PM, Herve JM, et al. Evaluation of tension-free vaginal tape procedure. Eur Urol 2001; 40:543–547.
17. Meschia M, Pifarotti P, Bernasconi F, et al. Tension-free vaginal tape: analysis of outcomes and complications in 404 stress incontinent women. Int. Urogynecol J 2001; 12:S24–S27.
18. Meltomaa S, Backman T, Haarala M. Concomitant vaginal surgery did not affect outcome of tension-free vaginal tape operation duringa a prospective 3-year follow-up study. J Urol 2004; 172:222–226.
19. de Leval J. Novel surgical technique for the treatment of female stress urinary incontinence: Transobturator vaginal tape inside out. Eur Urol 2003; 44:724–730.
20. Katske FA, Raz S. Use of Foley catheter to obtain transvaginal tamponade. Urol Urotechnol 1987; 8:18.
21. Dwyer NT, Kreder KJ. An update on slings. Curr Opin Urol 2005; 15:244–249.
22. Flock F, Reich A, Muche R, et al. Hemmorhagic complications associated with tension-free vaginal tape procedure. Obstet Gynecol 2004; 104:989–994.
23. Leach GE, Dmochowski RR, Appell RA, et al. Female Stress Urinary Incontinence Clinical Guidelines Panel summary report on surgical management of female stress urinary incontinence. J Urol 1997; 158:875–880.
24. Kobashi KC, Govier FE. Management of vaginal erosion of polypropylene mesh slings. J Urol 2003; 169:2242–2243.
25. Wai CY, Atnip SD, Williams KN, et al. Urethral erosion of tension-free vagnal tape presenting as recurrent stress urinary incontinence. Int Urogynecol J 2004; 15:353–355.
26. Cody J, Wyness L, Wallace S, et al. Systemic review of the clinical effectiveness of tension-free vaginal tape for treatment of urinary stress inctontinence. Health Technol Assessment 2003; 7:21–31.
27. Morgan JE. A sling operation using marlex polypropylene mesh for treatment of recurrent stress incontinence. Am J Obstet Gynecol 1970; 106:369–377.
28. Comiter CV, Colegrove PM. High rate of vaginal exgtrusion of silicone-coated polyester sling. Urology 2004; 63:1066–1070.

29. Giberti C, Rovida S. Transvaginal bone-anchored synthetic sling for the treatment of stress urinary incontinence: an outcomes analysis. Urology 2000; 56:956–961.

30. Duckett JR, Constantine G. Complications of silicone sling insertion for stress urinary incontinence. J Urol 2000; 163:1835–1837.

31. Blaivas JG, Sandhu J. Urethral reconstruction after erosion of slings in women. Curr Opin Urol 2004; 14:335–338.

32. Clemens JQ, De Lancey JO, Faerber GJ, et al. Urinary tract erosions after synthetic pubovaginal slings: diagnosis and management strategy. Urology 2000; 56:589–594.

33. Amundsen CL, Flynn BJ, Webster GD. Urethral erosion after synthetic and nonsythetic pubovaginal slings: differences in management and continence outcome. J Urol 2003; 170:134–137.

34. Frederick RW, Carey JM, Leach GE. Osseous complications after transvaginal bone anchor fixation in female pelvic reconstructive surgery: report from single largest prospective series and literature review. Urology 2004; 64:669–674.

35. Goldberg RP, Tchetgen MB, Sand PK, et al. Incidence of pubic osteomyelitis after bladder neck suspension using bone anchors. Urology 2004; 63:704–708.

36. Rackley RR, Abdelmalak JB, Madjar S, et al. Bone anchor infections in female pelvic reconstructive procedures: a literature review of series and case reports. J Urol 2001; 165:1975–1978.

37. Sand PK, Koduri S, Lobel RW, et al. Prospective randomized trial of polyglactin 920 mesh to prevent recurrence of cystoceles and rectoceles. Am J Obstet Gynecol 2001; 184:1357–1362.

38. Bennett SJ. Urethral diverticula. Eur J Obstet Gynecol Reprod Biol 2000; 89:135–139.

39. Rufford J, Cardozo L. Urethral diverticula: a diagnostic dilemma. BJU Int 2004; 94:1044–1047.

40. Leach GE, Schmidbauer CP, Hadley HR, et al. Surgical treatment of female urethral diverticulum. Semin Urol 1986; 4:33–42.

41. Dmochowski R. Urethral diverticula: evolving diagnostics and improved surgical management. Curr Urol Rep 2001; 2:373–378.

42. Leach GE, Bavendam TG. Female urethral diverticula. Urology 1987; 30:407–415.

43. Peters W III, Vaughan ED Jr. Urethral diverticulum in the female. Etiologic factors and postoperative results. Obstet Gynecol 1976; 47:549–552.

44. Langer R, Ron-El R, Neuman M, et al. The value of simultaneous hysterectomy during Burch colposuspension for urinary stress incontinence. Obstet Gynecol 1988; 72:866–869.

45. Rackley RR, Appell RA. Vesicovaginal Fistula: Current Approach. AUA Update Series. Lesson 21. 1998; 17(21):162–167.

46. Smith GL, Williams G. Vesicovaginal fistula. BJU Int 1999; 83:564–569.

47. Neale G. Clinical analysis of 100 medico-legal cases. Br Med J 1993; 307:1483–1494.

48. Schleicher DJ, Ojengbede OHA, Elkins TE. Urologic evaluation after closure of vesico-vaginal fistulae. Urogynaecol J 1993; 4:262–267.

49. Chassar-Moir J. Vesico-vaginal fistulae as seen in Britain. J Obstet Gynaecol Br Com 1983; 80: 598–604.

50. Symmonds RE. Incontinence: vesical and urethral fistulas. Clinical Obstet Gynecol 1984; 27: 499–505.

51. Stothers L, Chopra A, Raz S. Vesicovaginal fistula. In: Raz S, ed. Female Urology. 2nd ed. Philadelphia, PA: W.B. Saunders Co., 1996:492–506.

52. Nouira Y, Oueslati H, Reziga H, et al. Ureterovaginal fistulas complicating laparoscopic hysterectomy: a report of two cases. Eur J Obstet Gynecol Reprod Bio 2001; 96:132–134.

53. Tamussino K, Lang P, Breinl E. Ureteral complications with operative gynecologic laparoscopy. Am J Obstet Gynecol 1998; 178:967–971.

54. Mattingly RF, Borkowf HI. Acute operative injury to the lower urinary tract. Clin Obst Gynaec 1978; 5:123–125.

55. Brown RB. Surgical and external ureteric trauma. Aust N Z J Surg 1977; 47:4741–4747.

56. Baltzer J, Kaufmann C, Ober KG, et al. Complications in 1,092 radical abdominal hysterectomies with pelvic lymphadenectomies. Geburtshilfe Frauenkeild 1980; 40:1–9.

57. Piscitelli JT, Simel DL, Addison A. Who should have intravenous pyelograms before hysterectomy for benign disease? Obstet Gynecol 1987; 69:541–545.

58. Solomons E, Levin EJ, Bauman J. A pyelographic study of ureteric injuries sustained during hysterectomy for benign conditions. Surg Gynecol Obstet 1960; 111:41–46.

59. O'Conor VJ. Nonsurgical closure of vesicovaginal fistulae. Trans Am Assoc Genito Urin Surg 1938; 31:255–257.

60. Davits RJAM, Miranda SI. Conservative treatment of vesicovaginal fistulas by bladder drainage alone. Br J Urol 1991; 68:155–156.

61. Aycinea JF. Small vesicovaginal fistula. Urology 1977; 9:543–545.

62. Stovsky MD, Ignatoff JM, Blum MD, et al. Use of eletrocoagulation in the treatment of vesicovaginal fistulas. J Urol 1994; 152:1443–1444.

63. Hedelin H, Nilson AE, Teger-Nilsson AC, et al. Fibrin occlusion of fistulas postoperatively. Surg Gynecol Obstet 1982; 154:366–367.

64. Petersson S, Hedelin H, Jansson I, et al. Fibrin occlusion of a vesicovaginal fistula. Lancet 1979; 1:933.
65. Kanaoka Y, Hirai K, Ishiko O, et al. Vesicovaginal fistula treated with fibrin glue. Int J Gyneacol Obstet 2001; 73:147–149.
66. Dogra PN, Nabi G. Laser welding of vesicovaginal fistula. Int Urogeynecol J Pelvic Floor Dysfunct 2001; 12:69–70.
67. Thacker HL. Current issues in menopausal hormone replacement therapy. Cleveland Clinic J Med 1996; 63:344–353.
68. Wang Y, Hadley HR. Nondelayed transvaginal repair of high lying vesicovaginal fistula. J Urol 1990; 144:34–36.
69. Robertson JR. Vesicovaginal fistulas. In: Slate WG, ed. Disorders of the Female Urethra and Urinary Incontinence. Baltimore, MD: Williams and Wilkins, 1982:242–249.
70. Persky L, Herman G, Guerrier K. Non delay in vesicovaginal fustula repair. Urology 1979; 13:273–277.
71. Raz S, Little NA, Juma S. Female Urology. In: Walsh PC, Retik AB, Stamey TA, eds. 6th ed. Campbell's Urology. Philadelphia, PA: W.B. Saunders, 1992:2782–2828.
72. Carbone JM, Kaveler E, Raz S. Transvaginal repair of vesicovaginal fistula: success with the use of a peritoneal flap. J Urol 2000; 163:167–171.
73. Raz S, Bregg KJ, Nitti VW, et al. Transvaginal repair of vesicovaginal fistula using a peritoneal flap. J Urol 1993; 150:56–60.
74. Cetin S, Tazicioglu A, Ozgur S, et al. Vesicovaginal fistula repair: a simple suprapubic transvesical approach. Int Urol Nephrol 1988; 20:265–268.
75. Gelabert A, Arango OJ, Borau A, et al. Rectangular vesical flap. Exptraperitoneal suprapubic approach to close vesicovaginal fistulae. Acta Urol Belg 1988; 56:64–68.
76. O'Conor VJ, Sokol JK. Vesicovaginal fistula from the standpoint of the urologists. J Urol 1951; 66:367–370.
77. O'Conor VJ, Sokol JK, Bulkley GJ, et al. Suprapubic closure of vesicovaginal fistula. J Urol 1973; 109:51–53.
78. Wein AJ, Malloy TR, Greenberg SH, et al. Omental transposition as an aid in genitourinary reconstructive procedures. J Trauma 1980; 20:473–475.
79. Barnes R, Hadley H, Johnston O. Transvaginal repair of vesicovaginal fistulas. Urology 1977; 10:258–261.
80. Little NA, Juma S, Raz S. Vesicovaginal fistulae. Sem Urol 1989; 7:78–82.
81. Martius H. Die operative wiedeherstellung der volkommen fehlenden harnorohre und des schiessmuskels derselben. Zentralbl Gynakol 1928; 52:480–482.
82. Margolis T, Elkins TE, Seffah J, et al. Full-thickness Martius grafts to preserve vaginal depth as an adjunct in the repair of large obstetric fistulas. Obstet Gynecol 1994; 84:148–151.
83. Byron RL Jr, Ostergard DR. Sartorius muscle interposition for the treatment of the radiation-induced vaginal fistula. Am J Obstet Gynecol 1969; 104:104–106.
84. Stirnemann H. Treatment of recurrent recto-vaginal fistula by interposition of a gluteus maximus muscle flap. Am J Proctol 1969; 20:52–54.
85. Menchaca A, Akhyat M, Gleicher N, et al. The rectus abdominis muscle flap in a combined abdominovaginal repair of difficult vesicovaginal fistulae. A report of three cases. J Reprod Med 1990; 35:565–569.
86. Tancer ML. A report of thirty-four instances of urethrovaginal and bladder neck fistulas. Surg Gynecol Obstet 1993; 177:77–81.
87. Patil U, Waterhouse K, Laungani G. Management of 18 difficult vesicovaginal and urethrovaginal fistulas with modified Ingelman-Sundberg and Martius operations. J Urol 1980; 123:653–655.
88. Carr LK, Webster G. Abdominal repair of vesicovaginal fistula. Urology 1996; 48:10–13.
89. Jonas U, Petro E. Genito-urinary fistulas. In: Stanton SL, ed. Clinical Gynecologic Urology. St. Louis, MO: C.V. Mosby Co. 1984:238–255.
90. Symmonds RE. Ureteral injuries associated with gynecologic surgery: prevention and management. Clin Obstet Gynecol 1976; 19:623–627.
91. Raghavaiah NV. Double-dye test to diagnose various types of vaginal fistulas. J Urol 1975; 112:811–812.
92. Benchekroun A, Lachkar A, Soumana A, et al. Ureterovaginal fistulas.45 cases. Ann Urol 1988; 32:295–298.
93. El Ouakdi J, Jlif H, Boujnah B, et al. Uretero-vaginal Fistula. Apropos of 30 Cases. J Gynecol Obstet Biol Reprod 1989; 18:891–895.
94. Badenoch DF, Tiptaft RC, Thakar DR, et al. Early repair of accidental injury to the ureter or bladder following gynaecological surgery. Br J Urol 1987; 59:516–518.
95. Beland G. Early treatment of ureteral injuries found after gynecological surgery. J Urol 1977; 118:25–28.
96. Witeska A, Kossakowski J, Sadowski A. Early and delayed repair of gynecological ureteral injuries. Wiad Lek 1989; 42:305–307.

97. Meirow D, Moriel EZ, Zilberman M, et al. Evaluation and treatment of iatrogenic ureteral injuries during obstetric and gynecologic operations for non-malignant conditions. J Am Coll Surg 1994; 178:144–147.

98. Onoura VC, al-Mohalhal S, Youssef AM, et al. Iatrogenic urogenital fistulae. Br J Urol 1993; 71:144–146.

99. Peterson DD, Lucey DT, Fried FA. Nonsurgical management of ureterovaginal fistula. Urology 1974; 4:677–679.

100. Patel A, Werthman PE, Fuchs GJ, et al. Endoscopic and percutaneous management of ureteral injuries, fistulas, obstruction, and strictures. In: Raz S, ed. Female Urology. Baltimore, MD: Williams and Wilkins, 1996:521–538.

101. Kihl B, Nilson AE, Pettersson S. Ureteroneocystotomy in the treatment of postoperative ureterovaginal fistula. Acta Obstet Gynecol Scand 1982; 61:341–343.

102. Selzman A, Spirnak J, Kursh ED. The changing management of ureterovaginal fistulas. J Urol 1995; 153:626–629.

103. Bennani S, Joual A, El Mrini M, et al. Ureterovaginal fistulas. A report of 17 cases. J Gynecol Obstet Biol Reprod 1996; 25:56–59.

104. Falandry L. Uretero-vaginal fistulas: diagnosis and operative tactics. Apropos of 19 personal cases. J Chir 1992; 129:2093–3013.

105. Server G, Alonso M, Ruiz JL, et al. Surgical treatment of uretero-vaginal fistulae caused by gynecologic surgery. Actas Urol Esp 1992; 16:1–4.

106. Appell RA. Techniques and results in the implantation of the artificial urinary sphincter in women with type III stress urinary incontinence by a vaginal approach. Neurourol Urodyn 1988; 7:613–619.

107. Hadley RH. The artificial sphincter in the female. Probl Urol 1991; 5:123–133.

108. Heitz M, Olianas R, Schreiter F. Therapy of female urinary incontinence with the AMS 800 artificial sphincter. Indications, outcome, complication as and risk factors. Urologe A 1997; 36:426–431.

109. Costa P, Mottet N. Rabut B, et al. The use of an artificial urinary sphincter in women with type III incontinence and a negative Marshall test. J Urol 2001; 165:1172–1176.

110. Sanz Mayayo E, Gomez Garcia I, Fernandez Fernandez E, et al. AMS-800 artificial sphincter. Our experience in the last 20 years. Arch Esp Urol 2003; 56:989–997.

111. Webster GD, Perez LM, Khoury JM, et al. Management of type III stress urinary incontinence using artificial urinary sphincter. Urology 1992; 39:499–503.

112. Meschia M, Pifarotti P, Gattei U, et al. Injections therapy for the treatment of stress urinary incontinence in women. Gynecol Obstet Invest 2002; 54:67–72.

113. Monga DK, Robinson D, Stanton SL. Periurethral collagen injections for genuine stress incontinence: a 2-year follow-up. Br J Urol 1995; 76:156–160.

114. Gorton E, Stanton S, Monga A. Periurethral collagen injection: a long-term follow-up study. BJU Int 1999; 84:966–971.

115. Chrouser KL, Fick F, Goel A, et al. Carbon coated zirconium beads in beta-glucan gel and bovine glutaraldehyde corss-linked collagen injections for intrinsic sphincter deficiency: continence and satisfaction after extended followup. J Urol 2004; 171:1152–1155.

116. Tamanini JT, D'Ancona CA, Netto NR Jr. Treatment of intrinsic sphincter deficiency using the Macroplastique Implantation System: two-year follow-up. J Endourol 2004; 18:906–911.

117. Madjar S, Covington-Nichols C, Secrest CL. New periurethral bulking agent for stress urinary incontinence: modified technique and early results. J Urol 2003; 170:2327–2329.

118. Faerber GJ. Endoscopic collagten injection for elderly women with type I stress incontinence. J Urol 1996; 155:512–514.

119. Goldenberg SL, Warkentin MJ. Periurethral collagen injections for patients with stress urinary incontinence. J Urol 1994; 151:479A.

120. Herschorn S, Steele DJ, Radomski S. Followup of intraurethral collagen for female stress urinary incontinence. J Urol 1996; 156:1345–1347.

121. O'Connell HE, McGuire EJ, Aboseif S, et al. Transurethral collagen therapy in women. J Urol 1995; 153:433A.

122. Stricker P, Haylen B. Injectable collogen for type 3 female stress incontinence: the first 50 Australian patients. Med J Aust 1993; 158:89–91.

123. Herschorn S. Current status of injectable agents for remale stress urinary incontinence. Can J Urol 2001; 8:1281–1289.

124. Berg S. Polytef augmentation urethroplasty. Correction of surgically incurable urinary incontinence by injection technique. Arch Surg 1973; 107:379–381.

125. Schulz JA, Nager CW, Stanton SL, et al. Bulking agents for stress urinary incontinence: short-term results and complications in a randomized comparison of periurethral and transurethral injections. Int Urogynecol J Pelvic Floor Dysfunct 2004; 15:261–265.

126. Haab F, Zimmern PE, Leach GE. Urinary stress incontinence due to intrinsic sphincter deficiency: experience with fat and collagen periurethral injections. J Urol 1997; 157:1283–1285.

127. Santarosa RP, Blaivas JG. Periurethral injection of autologous fat for the treatment of sphincter incompetence. J Urol 1994; 151:607–608.

128. Stothers L, Goldenberg SL, Leone EF. Complications of periurethral collagen injection for stress urinary incontinence. J Urol 1998; 159:806–807.

129. Pannek J, Brands FH, Senge T. Particle migration after transurethral injection of carbon coated beads for stress urinary incontinence. J Urol 2001; 166:1350–1353.

130. Dewan PA, Fraundorfer M. Skin migration following periurethral polytetrafluorethylene injection for urinary incontinence. Aust N Z J Surg 1996; 66:57–59.

131. Malizia AA Jr, Reiman HM, Myers RP, et al. Migration and granulomatous reaction after periurethral injection of polytef (Teflon). JAMA 1984; 251:3277–3281.

132. Claes H, Stroobants D, Van Meerbeek J, et al. Pulmonary migration following periurethral polytetrafluoroethylene injection for urinary incontinence. J Urol 1989; 142:821–822.

133. Henly DR, Barrett DM, Weiland TL, et al. Particulate silicone for use in periurethral injections: local tissue effects and search for migration. J Urol 1995; 153:2039–2043.

134. Sweat SD, Lightner DJ. Complications of sterile abscess formation and pulmonary embolism following periurethral bulking agents. J Urol 1999; 161:93–96.

135. Stothers L, Goldenberg SL. Delayed hypersensitivity and systemic arthralgia following transurethral collagen injection for stress urinary incontinence. J Urol 1998; 159:1507–1509.

136. McLennan MT, Bent AE. Suburethral abscess: a complication of periurethral collagen injection therapy. Obstet Gynecol 1998; 92:650–652.

137. Levin I, Groutz A, Gold R, et al. Surgical complications and medium-term outcome results of tension-free vaginal tape: a prospe ctive study of 313 consecutive patients. Neurourol Urodyn 2004; 23:7–9.

138. Abousassaly R, Steinberg JR, Lemieux M, et al. Complications of tension-free vaginal tape surgery: a multi-institutional review. BJU Int 2004; 94:110–113.

139. Klutke C, Siegel S, Carlin B, et al. Urinary retention after tension free vaginal tape procedure: incidence and treatment. Urology 2001; 58:697–701.

140. McLennan MT, Melick CF, Bent AE. Clinical and urodynamic predictors of delayed voiding after fascia lata suburethral sling. Obstet Gynecol 1998; 92:608–612.

141. Miller EA, Amundsen CL, Toh KL, et al. Preoperative urodynamic evaluation may predict voiding dysfunction in women undergoing pubovaginal sling. J Urol 2003; 169:2234–2237.

142. Kuo HC. Comparison of video urodynamics results after the pubovaginal sling procedure using rectus fascia and polypropylene mesh for stress urinary incontinence. J Urol 2001; 165:163–168.

143. Yoshimura Y, Hashimoto T, Honda K, et al. The voiding after the suburethral sling operation, obstructive or non-obstructive? Hinyokika Kiyo 2001; 47:83–88.

144. Sokol AI, Jelovsek JE, Walters MD, et al. Incidence and predictors of prolonged urinary retention after TVT with and without concurrent prolapse surgery. Am J Obstet Gynecol 2005; 192:1537–1543.

145. Thiel DD, Gettit PD, McClellan WT, et al. Long-term urinary continence rates after simple sling incision for relief of urinary retention following fascia lata pubovaginal slings. J Urol 2005; 174:1878–1881.

146. Goldman HB. Simple sling incision for the treatment of iatrogenic urethral obstruction. Urology 2003; 62:714–748.

147. Nitti VW, Carlson KV, Blaivas JG, et al. Early results of pubovaginal sling lysis by midline sling incision. Urology 2002; 59:47–51.

148. Long CY, Lo TS, Liu CM, et al. Lateral excision of tension-free vaginal tape for the treatment of iatrogenic urethral obstruction. Obstet Gynecol 2004; 104:1270–1274.

149. Leng WW, Davies BJ, Tarin T, et al. Delayed treatment of bladder outlet obstruction after sling surgery: association with irreversible bladder dysfunction. J Urol 2004; 172:1379–1381.

150. Carr LK, Webster GD. Voiding dysfunction following incontinence surgery: diagnosis and treatment with retropubic or vaginal urethrolysis. J Urol 1997; 157:821–823.

151. Margulis V, Defreitas G, Zimmern PE. Urinary retention after tension-free vaginal tape procedure: from incision to excision to complete urethrolysis. Urology 2004; 64:590.

152. Scarpero HM, Nitti VW. Management of urinary retention and obstruction following surgery for stress urinary incontinence. Curr Urol Rep 2002; 3:354–359.

153. Petrou SP, Young PR. Rate of recurrent stress urinary incontinence after retropubic urethrolysis. J Urol 2002; 167:613–615.

154. Rosenblum N, Nitti VW. Post-urethral suspension obstruction. Curr Opin Urol 2001; 11:411–416.

155. Nitti VW, Tu LM, Gitlin J. Diagnosing bladder outlet obstruction in women. J Urol 1999; 161:1535–1540.

156. Nitti VW, Raz S. Obstruction following anti-incontinence procedures: diagnosis and treatment with transvaginal urethrolysis. J Urol 1994; 152:93–96.

157. DeLancey JO. Anatomy and biomechanics of genital prolapse. Clin Obstet Gynecol 1993; 36:897–909.

158. DeLancey JO. The anatomy of the pelvic floor. Curr Opin Obstet Gynecol 1994; 6:313–316.

159. Langer R, Lipshitz Y, Halperin R, et al. Prevention of genital prolapse following Burch colposuspension: comparison between two surgical procedures. Urogynecol J Pelvic Floor Dysfunct 2003; 14:13–16.

160. Burch JC. Cooper's ligament urethrovesical suspension for stress incontinence. Nine years' experience—results, complications, techniques. 1968. Am J Obstet Gynecol 2002; 187:512–516.

161. Comiter CV, Vasavada SP, Barbaric ZL, et al. Grading pelvic prolapse and pelvic floor relaxation using dynamic magnetic resonance imaging. Urology 1999; 54:454–457.

162. Comiter CV. Radiographic Evaluation of Pelvic Organ Prolapse. In: Vasavada S, Appell RA, Sand P, Raz S, eds. Female Urology. Philadelphia, PA: Williams and Wilkins, 2005:507–524.

163. Comiter CV, Vasavada S, Raz S. Abstracts of Papers, 29th Annual Meeting of the International Continence Society, Denver, CO, August 1999. Denver, CO: International Continence Society, 1999.

20 | Complications of Orchiopexy

Sutchin R. Patel and Anthony A. Caldamone
Division of Pediatric Urology, Hasbro Children's Hospital, Brown Medical School, Providence, Rhode Island, U.S.A.

INTRODUCTION

The study of cryptorchidism began with the anatomic descriptions of fetal testes in the abdominal position first described by Baron Albrecht von Haller and John Hunter in the 18th century. Von Haller in his work *Opuscula Pathologica*, published in 1755, accurately described the abdominal position of the fetal testis and stimulated Hunter to identify the neurovascular supply, cremaster muscles, and gubernaculum of the abdominally positioned fetal testes. From observations on post-mortem dissections, Hunter observed that the testes descend around the eighth month and determined that the descent of the testes was guided by the gubernaculum. Hunter went on to further state that failure of testicular descent may be intrinsic to the testis itself and that after a period of observation, undescended testes should be treated (1).

Thomas B. Curling in 1840 defended John Hunter's original observations in the *Lancet* and in 1866 summarized what was known regarding undescended testes at the time in his work *A Practical Treatise on the Disease of the Testis* (2). Besides describing the gubernaculum, Curling reaffirmed the presence of the cremasteric muscle fibers. During this time surgical intervention was rarely attempted except for instances of unbearable pain or signs of infection when an orchiectomy was performed. James Adams, a London surgeon, published the first account of correction of an undescended testis in an infant in 1871 (3). Adams' rationale for correcting the undescended testis was that he believed the scrotum would not develop on the empty side. Adams performed the first orchiopexy with Curling, but the postoperative course was complicated by a wound infection which led to fatal peritonitis. The importance of identifying and ligating a patent processus vaginalis during orchiopexy was not recognized during this time. In 1877, Thomas Annandale, a surgeon in Edinburgh, Scotland, performed the first successful orchiopexy (4). Annandale credited Curling with the idea of affixing the testicle to the bottom of the scrotum and benefited from Lister's antiseptic technique as his patient's wound healed satisfactorily. The history of the management of undescended testes illustrates many key concepts that are used in the orchiopexy operations of today.

Cryptorchidism is one of the most common congenital male anomalies, affecting 3% to 5% at birth and 0.8% to 1.6% by the first year of life. Treatment for undescended testes is hormonal or surgical. Because the overall efficacy of hormonal treatment is less than 20% and is dependent on pretreatment location, surgery remains the gold standard in the management of cryptorchidism. The primary goal of surgical treatment is to achieve a viable scrotally positioned testis. The success rates for orchiopexy are dependent on the preoperative testicular position and the technique utilized. A meta-analysis by Docimo determined the success rates based on the preoperative anatomical position of the testis as 74% for abdominal, 82% for peeping, 87% for canalicular, and 92% for those distal to the external ring. The success rate of various operative techniques was 89% for standard inguinal, 67% for Fowler–Stephens, 77% for staged Fowler–Stephens, 81% for transabdominal, 73% for two-stage, and 84% for microvascular orchiopexy (5). The data demonstrate that higher testes have a lower chance of successful repositioning in the scrotum.

The management of undescended testes requires proper identification of the anatomy, position and viability of the undescended testis (Table 1). The technical principles aiding in successful orchiopexy have long been established and include adequate mobilization of the

TABLE 1   Surgical Principles for Successful Orchiopexy

Knowledge of anatomy
Loupe magnification
Complete inguinal dissection
Extensive retroperitoneal dissection
Tension-free placement of testis in scrotum
   Division of cremasteric fibers
   High ligation of processus vaginalis
   Division of lateral and medial spermatic fascia
   Prentiss maneuver
Secure scrotal fixation

cord structures, repair of the accompanying indirect inguinal hernia, and fixation of the mobilized testis in a low intrascrotal postion. Several complications may occur including testicular retraction, testicular atrophy or infarction, hematoma formation, ilioinguinal nerve injury, postoperative torsion, and damage to the vas deferens (Table 2).

TESTICULAR ATROPHY

Atrophy of the testis is the most devastating complication but is seldom seen with the standard orchiopexy. Testicular atrophy is cause by disruption of the blood supply to the testis and may result from any one of the following:

1. Direct injury to the spermatic vessels can result from aggressive skeletonization of the cord or overzealous use of electrocautery.
2. Inadvertent torsion of the spermatic vessels can result during passage of the testis into the scrotum.
3. The purposeful ligation and division of the spermatic vessels as in a Fowler–Stephens orchiopexy can result in atrophy when there is poor collateral blood supply. Fowler and Stephens in 1959 studied the vascular anatomy of the testis and described a technique for the high undescended testis, preserving its blood supply via collateral circulation from a long looping vas deferens (6). The testis has three sources of arterial blood supply: the testicular artery, the deferential artery of the vas deferens, and the cremasteric artery. Thus, when the spermatic vessels are divided, the collateral circulation from the deferential artery and the cremasteric arteries become, responsible for supplying blood to the testis. However, the cremasteric muscles and their blood supply are not likely to contribute to testicular blood flow for the high undescended testis and for the canalicular testis so these are usually stripped away. A wide strip of peritoneum should be left attached between the vas and distal spermatic vessels to preserve the collateral vessels. A bleeding test can also be performed to assure adequacy of the vasal artery. This is carried out by incising the tunica albuginea after the testicular artery has been occluded with a vascular clamp. A brisk arterial bleed verifies the adequate circulation.
4. Excessive axial tension on the spermatic vessels, because of a very high testis or inadequate proximal dissection of the cord, or arterial spasm can compromise testicular blood flow. The Prentiss maneuver may be employed to shorten the course of the spermatic vessels by positioning the spermatic vessels medially to the naturally positioned internal ring (7). This

TABLE 2   Incidence of Complications of Standard Orchiopexy

Complication	Incidence	References
Testicular atrophy	Not reported	–
Testicular retraction	0.2–10%	(8,9)
Ilioinguinal nerve injury	7–11%	(17[a], 18[a])
Damage to vas deferens	0.3–7.2%	(22[a], 23[a])
Postoperative torsion	Isolated cases reported	(24)

[a]Based on open herniorrhaphy studies

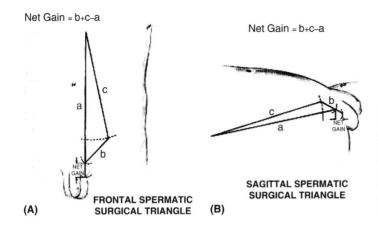

Net Gain = b+c–a

Net Gain = b+c–a

(A) FRONTAL SPERMATIC SURGICAL TRIANGLE

(B) SAGITTAL SPERMATIC SURGICAL TRIANGLE

FIGURE 1 (**A**) Left frontal spermatic triangle superimposed on course of spermatic vessels. Conversion of b and c to a demonstrates relative length gain. (**B**) Specimen in supine position. Diagram of sagittal triangle. Conversion of b and c to a demonstrates relative length gain. *Source*: From Ref. 7.

creates a more direct route to the scrotum by creating a more medially reconstructed internal ring (Fig. 1). When adequate length cannot be obtained, a staged procedure should be performed rather than attempting to place the testis into the scrotum with excess tension on the cord. If, however, the Fowler–Stephens approach is used as a salvage procedure after the spermatic cord has been skeletonized, adequate residual collateral flow would be extremely limited.

TESTICULAR RETRACTION

Recurrence of an undescended testis is most often due to an inadequate operation or utilization of an inadequate technique. The testis must be brought down into the scrotum with adequate mobilization of the spermatic vessels so that it is not under tension and should be secured in the scrotum using a dartos pouch (Fig. 2). Thus, inadequate mobilization of the cord, incomplete transection of cremaster muscle fibers or improper fixation of testis in the subdartos pouch may

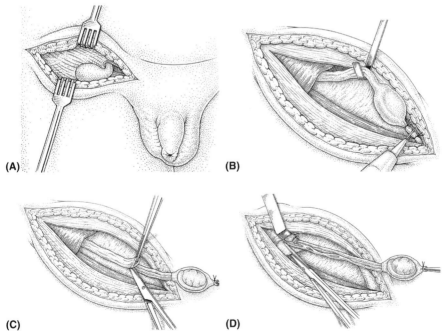

FIGURE 2 (**A**) Transverse inguinal incision. (**B**) Division of gubernacular attachments. (**C**) Dissection of processus vaginalis. (**D**) Division of lateral spermatic fascia. *Source*: From Ref. 42.

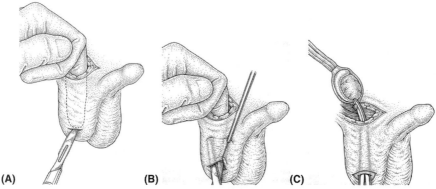

FIGURE 3 Creation of sub-dartos pouch. (**A**) A transverse incision is made in the scrotum over a finger placed from the inguinal incision. (**B**) Blunt dissection of the sub-dartos space. (**C**) A hemostat is passed retrograde to the inguinal incision to grasp the gubernaculum. *Source*: From Ref. 42.

all lead to testicular retraction. The rate of recurrence following orchidopexy is variable ranging from 0.2% to 10% and is directly related to the preoperative position of the testis (8,9).

Failure of adequate proximal dissection of cord structures through the internal inguinal ring resulting in inadequate mobilization of the cord is the main reported cause for surgical failure (9). It was the cause of 10/10 of failed primary orchiopexies in the observations of reoperations reported by Noseworthy (10). Failure to perform high ligation of the patent processus vaginalis can also contribute to testicular retraction. This was thought to be the cause in 6 of 34 (17.6%) cases of reoperative orchiopexy reported by Pesce et al. (8). An unrepaired hernia or inadequate dissection/ligation of the processus vaginalis was the cause of surgical failure in 20 of 32 (62.5%) cases of reoperative orchiopexy in the report by Ziylan et al. (11). Another factor may be the failure to reposition the testis in a low intrascrotal position. This may be primary or secondary to an inadequate proximal dissection of the spermatic cord. Similarly, excessive tension and inadequate scrotal fixation, though often cited as causes of failed primary orchiopexy, are secondary causes resulting from inadequate mobilization of the cord structures. Fixation using the subdartos pouch technique is widely accepted as the standard for the undescended testis (Fig. 3).

NEURALGIAS

The ilioinguinal, iliohypogastric, and genital branch of the genitofemoral nerve are the nerves of concern during orchiopexy. Both the ilioinguinal nerve and the iliohypogastric nerves arise from T12 and L1, and are responsible for sensation to the upper and medial aspects of the thigh and the skin of the base of the penis as well as the anterior portion of the thigh. The ilioinguinal nerve is typically found on the lateral aspect of the spermatic cord. It passes through the superficial inguinal ring to reach the subcutaneous tissues and the skin. The iliohypogastric nerve lies on the internal oblique abdominal muscle and penetrates the aponeurosis of the external oblique muscle near the rectus muscle to reach the subcutaneous tissue and the skin. The genital nerve has both motor and sensory components and innervates the cremaster muscle and the skin of the side of the scrotum. In the inguinal canal it lies on the iliopubic tract and is accompanied by the cremasteric vessels to form a neurovascular bundle that passes through the superficial inguinal ring.

Ilioinguinal nerve injury is an infrequent complication in orchiopexy. Injury can occur from traction, electrocautery, transection, or entrapment. Transient neuralgias can occur and are usually self-limited and resolve within a few weeks of the operation (12). Persistent neuralgic inguinodynia is characterized by hyperesthesia along the corresponding dermatome and exquisite pain at the site of a neuroma or trapped nerve with the patient describing painful exacerbations similar to electric shocks (13). The chronic pain results from repeated activation of pain fibers by compression of the nerve by scar or suture. The symptoms can sometimes be reproduced by palpation over the area of the entrapment. Transection of a sensory nerve usually results in an area of numbness corresponding to the distribution of the involved nerve (12). Various approaches to the management of residual neuralgias have been described and include analgesics, local anesthetic nerve blocks, and various medications. Patients with symptoms of nerve entrapment are usually best treated by repeat exploration with neurectomy (14–16).

The most common neural injury during orchiopexy is injury to the ilioinguinal nerve, which is most likely to occur during opening of the inguinal canal. The nerve should be isolated during the procedure to ascertain its location and integrity. Transection of the nerve, when it occurs, results in loss of sensation in the skin of the inner upper thigh, upper scrotum, and the base of the penis. Ilioinguinal nerve entrapment, on the other hand, is more likely to occur when closing the aponeurosis of the external oblique at the external ring. It should be noted that even careful operative protection of the ilioinguinal nerve does not completely prevent the development of inguinodynia (14).

There are no current reports regarding the incidence of ilioinguinal nerve injury following orchiopexy in the pediatric or adult population. However, the incidence of nerve injury should be relatively similar to that for inguinal hernia repair. The incidence of chronic groin pain (inguinodynia) in adults after nonmesh inguinal hernia repair has been shown to be as high as 7% to 11% (17,18). Amid reported a six-year experience of 49 patients referred with posthernior-rhaphy pain (19). Neuromas (12%) and nerve entrapment (20%) were identified in only a third of the cases, but 96% of the patients in the study were satisfied with their outcome. The most common histologic finding in these patients was some degree of perineural fibrosis.

DAMAGE TO THE VAS DEFERENS

Injury to, or division of, the vas deferens is uncommon but is most likely to occur during dissection of the hernia sac from the spermatic cord. Histologic changes in the vas even with minor degrees of manipulation have been shown in animal studies and inadvertent temporary clamping of the vas with a hemostat is equivalent to complete transaction (20). Resection of the vasal nerves has been shown to cause subfertility proportional to the extent of mobilization. Denervation of the vas deferens results in a loss of vas mobility or contraction leading to a functional obstruction, which may have a detrimental effect on semen transport (21).

During orchiopexy, therefore, extensive mobilization of the vas deferens, including vascular and neural structures can lead to functional obstruction of the vas. If transaction of the vas occurs and is recognized intraoperatively, repair may be accomplished via microsurgery (22). The repair is technically difficult, particularly in the young child and is best performed by a surgeon experienced in microsurgical techniques. Results of microsurgical repair of iatrogenic injury to the vas deferens are somewhat lower than for patients with obstructive azoospermia caused by vasectomy. This is because iatrogenic injuries are associated with longer vasal defects, impaired blood supply, and longer obstructive intervals resulting in secondary epididymal obstruction.

Thus the vas must be identified and handled gently during the operation. The use of loupe magnification and visualization of the vas along with precise cautery point for hemostasis to avoid thermal injury to the vas deferens should decrease the risk for inadvertent vasal injury. Discovery of an injury to the vas deferens may be delayed until later in the patient's life if the patient presents with azoospermia.

Pediatric inguinal hernia repair has been shown to be the most common cause of iatrogenic injury to the vas deferens. Some studies have suggested that the incidence of vasal injury ranges from 0.3% to 7.2%, however, the true incidence of damage to the vas deferens during orchiopexy or open herniorrhaphy is unknown and likely to be underreported for several reasons (22,23). Some vasal injuries may be identified intraoperatively, but in many cases delayed obstruction of the vas deferens due to extrinsic compression or vascular compromise may remain unrecognized. Furthermore a patient would require either bilateral obstruction or unilateral obstruction with a poorly functioning contralateral testis for a patient to present with azoospermia. Because invasive diagnostic studies such as a vasogram would be needed to determine the actual frequency of injuries, the incidence of vasal injury following orchiopexies will remain difficult to ascertain.

POSTOPERATIVE TORSION

Testicular torsion is another possible cause of vascular insufficiency with subsequent atrophy of the testis resulting from ischemia. The injury is usually iatrogenic and occurs when the testis is passed into the scrotum. When the testis is delivered into the dartos pouch, care must be taken to ensure the correct relationship between the testis, epididymis, and the vas deferens and vessels. The spermatic cord should be carefully examined to make certain that it is not twisted. The testis should appear pink and viable in the dartos pouch. If it looks ischemic, the cord orientation in the inguinal canal should be inspected, the dartos hiatus through which the cord passed widened and the integrity of the cord inspected for avulsion injury.

Although rare, there are reports of testicular torsion occurring in patients after orchiopexy. At least 50 cases of spermatic cord torsion in previously fixed testes have been reported by 30 different authors since 1970 (24). In the reported cases, fixation had been attempted by: (*i*) sutures, (*ii*) adhesions between the testis and the scrotal wall, (*iii*) the dartos pouch technique, and (*iv*) sutures combined with the other procedures. The findings at reoperation in which the operative findings were described included 26 cases where the testis was found to be lying freely in the tunica vaginalis cavity without any remnants of the previous fixation, one case where the testis rotated around a previous suture and nine cases where the testis was anchored by a stretched out adhesion, which acted like an axis on which the testis could rotate to favor torsion.

The cause of most postoperative torsions due to failed orchiopexies is the lack of scar tissue formation and adhesion. The evolution of adhesions include a two-fold mechanism that includes the normal healing of a serosa and the process of absorption of the scar tissue. The regeneration is accomplished by (*i*) metaplasia of fibroblasts migrating from the underlying connective tissue toward the surface, (*ii*) implants of mesothelial cells from the intact serosa that attach as free grafts on the facing raw surface, and (*iii*) eccentric growth of its borders. The expansion of one border will continue until it unites with its counterpart and completely reconstructs the cavity of the tunica vaginalis.

Thus the strength of the dartos pouch technique is that placement of the testis within a dartos pouch results in complete circumferential adherence of the tunica albuginea to the scrotal skin.

SCROTAL SWELLING/HEMATOMA/WOUND INFECTION/RARE COMPLICATIONS

Scrotal swelling after an orchiopexy may be caused by a number of processes. Scrotal edema is most marked after the Fowler–Stephens procedure due to compromised venous return. As in any surgery there may be hematoma formation after the procedure. Small hematomas may be inconsequential but larger ones may require surgical drainage. Blind needle aspiration of scrotal masses after orchiopexy should be avoided. Rarely, scrotal swelling following orchiopexy may be due to a recurrent hernia or development of a hydrocele. The occurrence of a hydrocele weeks or months after the procedure may be avoided by removing excess processus vaginalis at the time of the operation. Wound infections after orchiopexies are rare and their treatment is the same as for any other wound infection, mainly drainage if a collection is identified, local wound care, and appropriate antibiotics.

Some of the rarer complications of orchiopexy include bowel, bladder or ureteral injury. Though there are very few cases of these injuries reported in the literature one would expect the incidence of these complications to mirror those for open herniorrhaphy.

The rare instances of injury to the bladder have occurred at the time of repairing indirect inguinal hernias, especially the sliding variety (25). A case of vasal traction following a Fowler–Stephens orchiopexy causing obstruction of the ipsilateral ureter has been reported (26).

COMPLICATIONS OF LAPAROSCOPIC ORCHIOPEXY

One of the most problematic aspects of undescended testis is the diagnosis and treatment of the nonpalpable testis. Nonpalpable testes have been reported to comprise 20% of undescended testes, and, if present, the testis may be located anywhere between the kidney and upper scrotum. Laparoscopy has been established as a safe and effective method in diagnosing and

TABLE 3   Incidence of Complications of Laparoscopic Orchiopexy

Complication	Incidence (%)	References
Testicular atrophy	4–6.1	(30,31)
Testicular retraction	0–7.2	(5,30,38–40)
Vas deferens injury	0.3	(30)
Bladder injury	0.2–0.7	(27,30,34)
Spermatic vessel injury	0.4–1.2	(27,30,41)
Bowel injury	0.2–0.3	(37,30)

managing the nonpalpable testis. The complications unique to laparoscopy include: (*i*) trocar injuries, most of which occur during initial insertion, (*ii*) prolonged carbon dioxide insufflation time leading to hypercapnia, and (*iii*) injury to abdominal viscera either during trocar insertion or during intraperitoneal dissection (Table 3). Significant predictors of complications include the experience of the operator and the access technique utilized (27–29).

The most commonly reported complications in the literature regarding laparoscopic orchiopexy are testicular atrophy and testicular retraction (or improperly positioned testis). A large multi-institutional analysis of laparoscopic orchidopexy by Baker et al. showed an overall success rate of 93% with an atrophy rate of 6% (30). Overall success was defined as a proper scrotal position and the absence of atrophy during follow-up. In the 299 laparoscopic procedures, there was a major complication rate of 3% and a minor complication rate of 2%. Major complications included cecal volvulus (one), bladder perforation (two), ileus (two), torn spermatic vessels leading to a one-stage Fowler–Stephens orchiopexy (two), small laceration of the vas deferens (one), and Veress needle puncture into the sigmoid colon (one). Minor complications included preperitoneal insufflation (two), desaturation with an intrabdominal pressure >10 mmHg (one), wound separation (one), hydrocele (one) and wound infection (one). This series also found that single-stage Fowler–Stephens orchiopexy had a higher failure rate than the two-stage repair (26% vs. 12%, though not statistically significant) and that the combined laparoscopic orchiopexy groups had a higher success rate than the previously reported success rate for the same open procedures (one-stage 74% vs. 67%; two-stage 88% vs. 73%).

A summary of a smaller series on laparoscopic orchiopexy by Lindgren et al. showed a similar incidence of testicular atrophy in 3 of 83 patients (4%) when compared with the multi-institutional study by Baker et al. (30,31). The complication rates for testicular atrophy following a primary laparoscopic orchiopexy are much lower than when compared with a Fowler–Stephens orchiopexy. In the series reported by Samadi et al. 4 of 58 testes underwent testicular atrophy following a laparoscopic Fowler–Stephens orchiopexy (two of which required extensive mobilization because of dense adhesions to the adjacent peritoneum) (32). This is compared to no cases of atrophy in 139 direct laparoscopic orchiopexies. Radmayr et al. had 2 of 29 cases of testicular atrophy for two-stage Fowler–Stephens orchiopexy compared to 0 of 28 for direct laparoscopic orchiopexy (33). Samadi et al. further showed a 3% (6/203) reoperation rate due to unsatisfactory positioning of the testis during laparoscopic orchiopexy (32). Esposito et al. reported one complication of opening of the bladder during Fowler–Stephens orchiopexy in 250 cases of laparoscopic orchiopexy (34). It should also be noted that during laparoscopic orchiopexy the inner spermatic vessels may become very fragile after isolation from the posterior peritoneum and can disrupt easily if excessive traction is placed (34). In terms of nerve injury, during laparoscopic orchiopexy, the lateral femoral cutaneous and the genitofemoral nerves are most commonly affected in contrast to standard orchiopexy.

TECHNICAL ASPECTS OF REDO-ORCHIOPEXY

The basic principles that apply to primary orchiopexy also apply to orchiopexy for recurrent undescended testis. Knowledge of the anatomy and application of loupe magnification for visualization are of paramount importance, especially given the fact that one will encounter altered anatomy and scarred tissue on reoperation. The timing for reoperation is generally no earlier than six months after primary orchiopexy unless there is a perioperative complication (35). The incision is made through the original inguinal incision unless it was poorly placed and

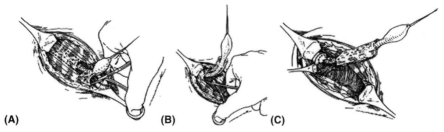

FIGURE 4   En Bloc Spermatic Cord Mobilization. (**A**) Initial dissection is begun at the inferior pole of testis. Dotted lines mark two incisions up the external oblique fascia, one medial and one lateral to the spermatic cord. (**B**) Plane posterior to the spermatic cord incisions may be made safely in external oblique aponeurosis on each side of the cord. (**C**) Above internal inguinal ring two external oblique fascial incisions are connected leaving a rectangle of fascia adherent to the spermatic cord. *Source*: From Ref. 36.

is slightly extended both medially and laterally to allow entry into unscarred tissue. This also allows better visualization and safer mobilization of the spermatic cord in the proximal aspect near the internal inguinal ring (10). Two techniques for reoperative dissection are an approach through the cremasteric fascia and an en bloc cord mobilization (35,36). The maximum area of scar tissue formation is generally between the spermatic cord and the posterior surface of the external oblique aponeurosis, the site of the original incision in the external oblique fascia. Mobilization of the testis and cord structures by dividing the surrounding scar tissue is the next step allowing one to elevate the cord from the floor of the inguinal canal and avoid cord injury. Initial dissection is begun at the inferior pole of the testis and development of a posterior plane allows for controlled incision of the external oblique aponeurosis away from spermatic cord structures (Fig. 4). If the canalicular portion of the cord has dense adhesions and is difficult to mobilize, an "en bloc" dissection to include the external oblique fascia can be used for safe and full cord mobilization (36). The dissection of the cord should be carried upward to the internal ring. Many times fresh tissue planes may be found at this level reflecting inadequate proximal mobilization of the cord, one of the causes of primary orchiopexy failure. A patent processus vaginalis should always be examined for and ligated to achieve adequate cord mobilization. If after extensive dissection and religation of the processus vaginalis there is doubt regarding adequate cord length, then the Prentiss maneuver should be employed (7). The inguinal floor is incised, the inferior epigastric vessels are ligated and divided, and the testis and cord structures should be transposed medially. The floor of the inguinal canal is closed lateral to the transposed cord structures. Anchoring of the remobilized testis is the final step and is generally accomplished using the subdartos pouch technique.

Results after reoperative orchiopexy include "satisfactory outcomes" in 38% to 95% of cases (9,37). No clear definition of "satisfactory outcome" for reoperative orchiopexy has been defined, however. A successful outcome has been described as a testis of reasonable size (i.e., not atrophied), good palpable consistency, and located in a scrotal position. No prospective studies have been performed with objective criteria. Pesce et al. assessed the success of reoperative orchiopexy on the basis of fertility and performed semen analysis on 20 of 34 boys after reoperation (8). They reported that even though the reoperative testes were significantly smaller than the controls, decreased fertility was noted in only three (19%) patients. This suggests that that a proper reorchiopexy does not necessarily translate into a higher rate of fertility.

REFERENCES

1. Hunter J. A description of the situation of the testis in the foetus, with its descent into the scrotum. In: Observations on Certain Parts of the Animal Oeconomy. Chapter 1. With notes by Owen, R. Philadelphia, PA: Haswell, Barrington and Haswell, 1840:5–57.
2. Curling JB. Observations on the structure of the gubernaculum and on the descent of the testis in the foetus. Lancet 1840; 2:70–74.
3. Adams JE. Remarks on a case of transition of the testicle into the perineum. Lancet 1871; 1:710–711.

4. Fischer MC, Milen MT, Bloom DA. Thomas Annandale and the first report of successful orchiopexy. J Urol 2005; 174:37–39.
5. Docimo SG. The results of surgical therapy for cryptorchidism: A literature review and analysis. J Urol 1995; 154:1148–1152.
6. Fowler R, Stephens FD. The role of testicular vascular anatomy in the salvage of high undescended testes. Aust N Zeal J Surg 1959; 29:92–106.
7. Prentiss RJ, Weickgenant CJ, Moses JJ, et al. Undescended testis. Surgical anatomy of spermatic vessels, spermatic surgical triangles and lateral spermatic ligament. J Urol 1960; 83:686–692.
8. Pesce C, d'Agostino S, Costa L, et al. Reoperative orchiopexy: surgical aspects and functional outcome. Pediatr Surg Int 2001; 17:62–64.
9. Maizels M, Gomez F, Firlit CF. Surgical correction of the failed orchiopexy. J Urol 1983; 130:955–957.
10. Noseworthy J. Recurrent undescended testes. Semin Pediatr Surg 2003; 12:90–93.
11. Ziylan O, Oktar T, Korgali E, et al. Failed orchiopexy, leading causes and surgical management. Urol Int 2004; 73:313–315.
12. Stephenson BM. Complications of open groin hernia repairs. Surg Clin North Am 2003; 83:1255–1278.
13. Woolf CJ, Mannion RJ. Neuropathic pain: aetiology, symptoms, mechanisms and management. Lancet 1999; 353:1959–1964.
14. Bendavid R. Complications of groin hernia surgery. Surg Clin North Am 1998; 78:1089–1103.
15. Wantz GE. Testicular atrophy and chronic residual neuralgia as risks of inguinal hernioplasty. Surg Clin North Am 1993; 73:571–581.
16. Aasvang E, Kehlet H. Surgical management of chronic pain after inguinal hernia repair. Br J Surg 2005; 92:795–801.
17. Hay JM, Boudet MJ, Fingerhut A, et al. Shouldice inguinal hernia repair in the male adult: the gold standard? A multicenter controlled trial in 1578 patients. Ann Surg 1995; 222:719–727.
18. Cunningham J, Temple WJ, Mitchell P, et al. Cooperative hernia study. Pain in the postrepair patient. Ann Surg 1996; 224:598–602.
19. Amid PK. A 1-stage surgical treatment for postherniorrhaphy neuropathic pain. Arch Surg 2002; 137:100–104.
20. Smith EM, Dahms BB, Elder JS. Influence of vas deferens mobilization on rat fertility: implications regarding orchiopexy. J Urol 1993; 150:663–666.
21. Lekili M, Gumus B, Kandiloglu AR, et al. The effects of extensive vas mobilization on testicular histology during orchiopexy. Int Urol Nephrol 1998; 30:165–170.
22. Sheynkin YR, Hendin BN, Schlegel PN, et al. Microsurgical repair of iatrogenic injury to the vas deferens. J Urol 1998; 159:139–141.
23. Pollak R, Nyhus LM. Complications of groin hernia repair. Surg Clin North Am 1983; 63:1363–1371.
24. Gesino A, Bachman De Santos ME. Spermatic cord torsion after testicular fixation. A different surgical approach and a revision of current techniques. Eur J Pediatr Surg 2001; 11:404–410.
25. Nguyen DH, Mitchell ME. Ureteral obstruction due to compression by the vas deferens following fowler-stephens orchiopexy. J Urol 1993; 149:94–95.
26. Colodny AH. Bladder injury during herniorrhaphy. Manifested by ascites and azotemia. Urology 1974; 3:89–90.
27. Peters CA. Complications in pediatric urological laparoscopy: results of a survey. J Urol 1996; 155:1070–1073.
28. Kaouk JH, Gill IS. Laparoscopic reconstructive urology. J Urol 2003; 170:1070–1078.
29. El-Ghoneimi A. Paediatric laparoscopic surgery. Curr Opin Urol 2003; 13:329–335.
30. Baker LA, Docimo SG, Surer I, et al. A multi-institutional analysis of laparoscopic orchidopexy. BJU Int 2001; 87:484–489.
31. Lindgren BW, Franco I, Blick S, et al. Laparoscopic Fowler–Stephens orchiopexy for the high abdominal testis. J Urol 1999; 162:990–994.
32. Samadi AA, Palmer LS, Franco I. Laparoscopic orchiopexy: report of 203 cases with review of diagnosis, operative technique, and lessons learned. J Endourol 2003; 17:365–368.
33. Radmayr C, Oswald J, Schwentner C, et al. Long-term outcome of laparoscopically managed nonpalpable testes. J Urol 2003; 170:2409–2411.
34. Esposito C, Lima M, Mattidi G, et al. Complications of pediatric urological laparoscopy: mistakes and risks. J Urol 2003; 169:1490–1492.
35. Redman JF. Inguinal reoperation for undescended testis and hernia: approach to the spermatic cord through the cremaster fascia. J Urol 2000; 164:1705–1707.
36. Cartwright PC, Velagapudi S, Snyder HM, et al. A surgical approach to reoperative orchiopexy. J Urol 1993; 149:817–818.
37. Palacio MM, Sferco A, Garcia Fernanndez AE, et al. Inguinal cordopexy: a Simple and effective new technique for securing the testis in reoperative orchiopexy. J Pediatr Surg 1999; 34:424–425.
38. Lindgren BW, Darby EC, Faiella L, et al. Laparoscopic orchiopexy: Procedure of choice for nonpalpable testis? J Urol 1998; 159:2132–2135.

39. Poppas DP, Lemack GE, Mininberg DT. Laparoscopic orchiopexy: clinical experience and description of technique. J Urol 1996; 155:708–711.
40. Jordan GH, Winslow BH. Laparoscopic single stage and staged orchiopexy. J Urol 1994; 152:1249–1252.
41. Esposito C, Damiano R, Sabin MA, et al. Laparoscopy-assisted orchidopexy: an ideal treatment for children with intra-abdominal testes. J Endourol 2002; 16:659–662.
42. Carr M. Standard inguinal orchiopexy. Dialogues Pediatr Urol 2005;26:4–6.

21 | Complications of Hypospadias Surgery

Joseph G. Borer and Alan B. Retik
Department of Urology, Children's Hospital and Harvard Medical School, Boston, Massachusetts, U.S.A.

INTRODUCTION

In the male, hypospadias is defined as a urethral meatus abnormally located anywhere from the ventral aspect of the glans penis to the scrotum or perineum, often with associated ventral curvature of the penis (chordee), and abnormal distribution of foreskin with a "hood" present dorsally and deficient foreskin ventrally (1). Hypospadias is typically diagnosed at newborn physical examination, although some may escape diagnosis until the foreskin is fully retracted or circumcision is performed. It is a relatively common congenital defect of the male external genitalia with hypospadias occurring in approximately one of every 250 live births (2). Many a successful technique is available to the surgeon faced with reconstruction for hypospadias. This chapter provides a detailed account of complications encountered as a result of the surgical care of the individual with hypospadias, and their management.

COMPLICATIONS

Complications of hypospadias repair include bleeding/hematoma, meatal stenosis, urethrocutaneous fistula, urethral stricture, urethral diverticulum, wound infection, impaired healing, and breakdown of the repair (3–6). When reoperation is indicated, complications such as meatal stenosis, urethrocutaneous fistula, and urethral stricture can be repaired rather expeditiously, with appropriate timing. However, more serious complications involving either partial or complete breakdown of the hypospadias repair may require a major reconstructive effort. At times, this involves the task of performing a complete repair in the face of less than optimal tissues and conditions.

Diagnosis
Bleeding/Hematoma
Bleeding is the most common complication of hypospadias repair. Typically diagnosed as an oozing of blood from the repair site, the source may be a capillary or arteriolar vessel at the skin level or from a vascularized subcutaneous (dartos) tissue flap used as a second layer of coverage for the neourethra. Glans or corpus spongiosum may also be sources of persistent bleeding. Bleeding from the corpus spongiosum may be especially troublesome in repair of severe, proximal defects. A rare source is the corpus cavernosa following incision of these structures and placement of an interposition graft during treatment of severe penile curvature.

Meatal Stenosis
Diagnosis of meatal stenosis is often made at follow-up examination by the surgeon. However, stenosis may be of such a severe grade that obstructive symptoms such as straining at urination, dribbling, or decreased force of urinary stream may present. The complication of meatal stenosis is typically due to technical issues at the time of repair such as fashioning of the urethral meatus with too narrow a lumen or performance of glanuloplasty too tightly leaving little room for the passage of the distal urethra and urethral meatus.

Urethrocutaneous Fistula
The suspicion of a urethrocutaneous fistula is often reported by a parent or caregiver. The fistula is often noted as the presence of two streams during voiding or dripping of urine from a second opening other than the distal meatus, anywhere along the ventral aspect of the hypospadias

repair site. This can be confirmed on physical examination with or without voiding, and documented on either voiding cystourethrogram (Fig. 1) or with retrograde injection of dye such as methylene blue either alone or with glycerin intraoperatively (3,5). Fistula may result from, or be associated with, distal stricture or meatal stenosis.

Infection
Infection at the hypospadias repair site may be suspected secondary to pain beyond that expected in the immediate postoperative period. New onset of pain following resolution of immediate postoperative pain should also raise the index of suspicion for infection. Erythema, edema, and warmth at the repair site or anywhere along the penile glans, shaft and/or base may also be present with an infection. When infection at the hypospadias repair site is suspected, culture of the urine and any repair site exudates should be performed immediately.

Urethral Diverticulum
Although infrequent, urethral diverticulum formation may follow hypospadias repair. Similar to urethrocutaneous fistula, urethral diverticula may be associated with distal stricture or meatal stenosis. A diverticulum may be described as a "bulge" or "lump" anywhere along the course of the urethra following hypospadias repair. This finding reported by the patient or caregiver may be particularly apparent during micturition. Physician observation of voiding may be helpful in confirming this report. Diagnosis is usually confirmed by either retrograde or antegrade urethrogram (Fig. 2), or at cystoscopy.

Balanitis Xerotica Obliterans
Balanitis xerotica obliterans (BXO) is a chronic inflammatory process of unknown etiology. Skin at or near the repair site that is thickened and discolored may be the first evidence of BXO. BXO can arise spontaneously, follow minor trauma or it may complicate hypospadias repair (7). Kumar and Harris reported eight patients with histologically proven BXO (8). Seven of the patients presented with difficult micturition, and meatal stenosis or neourethral stricture, at varying periods from one to eight years following primary hypospadias repair. Recurrent meatal stenosis may also be a sign of a hypospadias repair site that is affected with BXO.

Recurrent Penile Curvature
Recurrent penile curvature may be described by the patient as an exaggerated, shortened aspect of the penile shaft, often appreciated only during an erection. There may be associated pain,

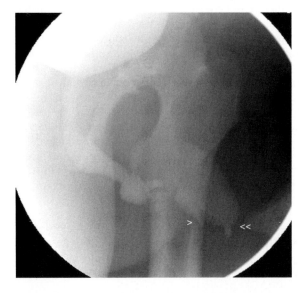

FIGURE 1 Urethrocutaneous fistula (*single arrow*) documented on voiding cystourethrogram (via suprapubic cystostomy tube) following hypospadias repair. Note small proximal urethral diverticulum and drop of contrast material at the urethral meatus (*double arrow*).

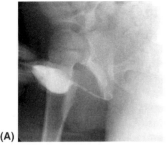 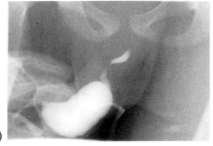

(A) **(B)**

FIGURE 2 Appearance of a large urethral diverticulum following hypospadias repair on (**A**) retrograde and (**B**) antegrade urethrogram.

particularly during erection in severe cases. An examiner may be suspicious of this entity upon palpation of dense fibrous scar tissue on the ventral aspect of the penis in the absence of an erection. Penile curvature may be documented intraoperatively by artificial erection with injection of normal saline into the corpora directly by insertion of a needle through the lateral aspect of one or the other corpora cavernosa. Alternatively, intracorporeal injection of the arterial vasodilator prostaglandin E1 (PGE1) has been used for pharmacological induction of erection for assessment of penile curvature (9,10).

Late-onset, recurrent curvature has been described as a complication of orthoplasty alone or in conjunction with hypospadias repair. Farkas reported that a second operation (and sometimes more) was required in approximately 50% of cases of hypospadias and initial severe curvature (11). In a more contemporary report, late-onset curvature in 22 patients with initial proximal penile or penoscrotal hypospadias and successful orthoplasty was felt to be due equally to either extensive fibrosis of the reconstructed urethra, corporeal disproportion, or both (12).

Urethral Stricture

Urethral stricture other than meatal stenosis may be a complication of proximal hypospadias repair. Patients may present with obstructive symptoms such as straining at micturition, dribbling, decreased force of stream, or urinary retention. The proximal anastomotic site of a tubularized repair such as the transverse preputial island flap appears to be particularly at risk. Urethral stricture following hypospadias repair may present several years following repair and can also occur following repair of distal defects. Similar to urethrocutaneous fistula, diagnosis of stricture may be confirmed by either retrograde or antegrade urethrogram (Fig. 3), or cystoscopy.

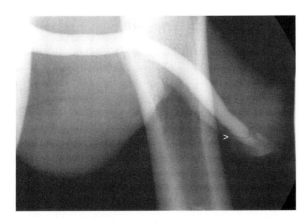

FIGURE 3 Distal urethral stricture (*arrow*) in a 15-year-old boy who presented with decreased force of stream and straining at urination 14 years after Mathieu hypospadias repair.

Intraurethral Hair Growth

Hair growth from tissues incorporated into a hypospadias repair may not be overtly evident. Complaints of irritative or obstructive symptoms may account for the initial presentation of this patient and result from either encrustation of the hair, infection in the urine, or both. Occasionally, if hair-bearing skin was used at the distal extent of the hypospadias repair, hair may be seen emanating from the meatus, the so-called "bearded urethra."

Repair Breakdown

Complete breakdown of a hypospadias repair may yield an appearance of the penis quite similar to that prior to performance of the repair. There may be little or no scar tissue or there may be multiple fistulae with only small skin bridges as evidence of previous attempted repair.

Hypospadias Cripple

Hypospadias cripple is a term used to describe the patient who has undergone several failed attempts at hypospadias repair. For diagnosis of this entity, one need see not only repair breakdown, but also the presence of dense scar tissue over the previous attempted repair site(s).

Prevention
Bleeding/Hematoma

Adequate hemostasis during hypospadias repair may be achieved with one of several methods. Selective use of bipolar electrocautery with fine-point neurologic forceps is one such method (13). Topical application of iced saline-soaked gauze, or dilute epinephrine (epinephrine diluted 1:200,000 with xylocaine) either as an intermittent topical administration with compression or as an injection into glans or corpus spongiosum tissue prior to incision are alternatives. Vasoconstrictive agents that provide temporary hemostasis without permanent tissue devitalization are preferable.

Meatal Stenosis

During closure of the distal extent of the neourethra, care must be taken to leave the meatus of a sufficient caliber. Any distal traction or tension on the penis should be released in order to more accurately assess the caliber of the meatus. Sufficient space for accommodation of the distal urethra between the glans should also be assured by adequate deepening of the glans wing incisions. Awareness of these critical principles during hypospadias repair should significantly decrease the likelihood of meatal stenosis.

Urethrocutaneous Fistula

Fistula may result from, or be associated with, distal stricture or meatal stenosis. Other risk factors include failure to invert all epithelial edges at urethroplasty, devitalization of tissue with excessive use of electrocautery, or failure to add appropriate second-layer urethroplasty coverage. The latter of these, second-layer coverage of the neourethra, has been shown to significantly reduce the fistula rate as reported by several authors (3,14–16).

Infection

The use of intravenous antibiotics in the perioperative period for hypospadias repair is commonly practiced and likely decreases the risk of infection with coverage for the typical epithelial surface bacteria. This practice may also limit the risk for cystitis and thus decrease the risk for repair site infection. With bacterial cystitis, and subsequent passage of infected urine through the urethral (hypospadias) repair site, the repair site may become infected secondarily and therefore, the prevention of bacterial cystitis is particularly important.

Urethral Diverticulum

Limiting the use of preputial skin as this skin dilates and expands easily at the slightest urethral narrowing, increased resistance to urine outflow or turbulent urinary flow should decrease the risk of diverticulum formation. Widely patent anastomotic sites in order to decrease the likelihood of distal narrowing, stricture formation or meatal stenosis development are practices that are also likely to decrease this risk.

Balanitis Xerotica Obliterans

Limit infection, irritation to the repair site. Whenever possible, the use of healthy, well-vascularized skin for the hypospadias repair including skin coverage of the penis is essential for successful repair and decreasing the risk of BXO. Instruction of the patient or caregiver with regard to routine hygiene is also of great importance.

Recurrent Penile Curvature

Although there are many different techniques available for the management of penile curvature, it appears that the dermal graft is the most reliable with the least risk for recurrence in those patients requiring treatment of severe penile curvature at the time of hypospadias repair. Soergel et al. recommended against the use of four-layer small intestinal submucosa because of a high rate of recurrent penile curvature (17).

Urethral Stricture

When it occurs, urethral stricture is usually a complication of the more severe, proximal defects that often require complex repair. During these repairs, special attention needs to be given to anastomoses. Spatulating anastomotic sites where neourethral tubes and native urethra are connected, thus fashioning a widely patent anastomosis is of critical importance in limiting the risk of urethral stricture. Using well-vascularized pedicled flaps in order to decrease the likelihood of ischemia playing a role in stenosis at the distal, peripheral extents of these tissues is also crucial.

Intraurethral Hair Growth

The use of nonhair-bearing skin is the key to prevention of hair growth within the repaired urethra. Avoidance of a scrotal skin component to the neourethra at repair of severe, proximal defects is an important principle. This principle also applies during use of the Mathieu (flip-flap) technique wherein the proximal extent of the ventral penile shaft skin flap should not incorporate scrotal skin.

Repair Breakdown

This unfortunate complication of hypospadias repair is uncommon. It may occur following infection, hematoma formation, or excessive manipulation of the repair site by the patient.

Hypospadias Cripple

Preventing the occurrence or development of a hypospadias cripple is dependent upon adherence to strict principles and goals of any hypospadias repair whether it be a primary or reoperative repair. These include meticulous technique with attention to detail, use of well-vascularized local tissue when possible, and use of extragenital tissue when necessary during the first and desirably only primary repair or reoperation.

Management

In general, unless immediate re-exploration is indicated for bleeding/hematoma, infection or debridement, reoperation for complication(s) should not be performed less than six months following previous repair.

Bleeding/Hematoma

Bleeding following hypospadias repair may require simple addition of a temporary compressive dressing for management. At other times, significant postoperative bleeding may require exploration in order to identify and treat the source. Hematoma may form as a result of persistent bleeding and if large in size may require wound exploration and hematoma evacuation. Consequences of hematoma formation range from simple temporary cosmetic issues to wound or repair breakdown (18). Patients with excessive bleeding and/or hematoma formation, particularly those requiring reoperation, should undergo evaluation for bleeding diathesis or dyscrasia (5).

Meatal Stenosis
Urethral (meatal) dilation or meatotomy may be sufficient for the mildest forms of meatal stenosis. However, a more complex distal urethral stricture also involving the meatus may require a more extensive flap procedure (19). Repeat recurrence of meatal stenosis may be particularly troubling and require the use of extragenital tissues and staged repair for definitive management.

Urethrocutaneous Fistula
Repair of urethrocutaneous fistula is optimized by the same principles as those for initial neourethral closure at hypospadias repair (3,20–26). In addition, assessment for stricture distal to the fistula site prior to fistula repair and excision of devitalized tissue edges at the time of repair are critical components of successful management. At times, larger or multiple fistulae may require incision of the intact skin bridges and repeat hypospadias repair.

Infection
Administration of broad-spectrum antibiotic(s) should begin immediately when infection of the repair is suspected and after urine and wound cultures have been obtained. Incision and drainage, and debridement when indicated, are added to appropriate antibiotic therapy. Treatment should be prompt and aggressive as severe, untreated infection may lead to breakdown of the entire repair. In this setting, an appropriate interval of at least six months prior to entertaining reoperation would be particularly important.

Urethral Diverticulum
Zaontz et al. described repair of urethral diverticulum with circumferential skin incision, penile shaft skin degloving, diverticula excision and urethral closure, followed by "pants over vest" subcutaneous tissue coverage of the repair, with excellent results (27). A similar technique has been described by others (28). For more extensive lesions, Aigen et al. described repair similar to that for megalourethra (29). Repair of a urethral diverticulum is depicted in Figure 4.

Balanitis Xerotica Obliterans
Kumar and Harris reported eight patients with BXO (8). These authors recommended be use of bladder or buccal mucosal-free grafts for repair of such cases, in order to improve upon an alarming 50% complication rate with the use of skin grafts for urethroplasty. Venn and Mundy have described similar techniques for repair in this difficult setting (30).

Recurrent Penile Curvature
The use of a dermal graft appears to be the most reliable means of managing severe ventral penile curvature and has been used extensively for this indication (31–36). After assessing the degree of curvature, the dermal graft is harvested from a nonhair-bearing donor site typically in the groin. The donor site is marked in an elliptical shape at a length slightly longer than the ventral defect to be created by transverse linear corporotomy. The graft is sharply dissected, defatted, and placed in saline. A transverse incision is made at the site of maximal curvature (concavity) and the dermal graft is anastamosed to the edges of the corporal defect with a running simple suture of 6-0 polyglactin.

Urethral Stricture
A thin, film-like urethral stricture of short distance may be successfully treated with less invasive means such as endoscopic cold-knife urethrotomy (37). However, Hsiao et al. reported a success rate of only 50% in 20 patients who underwent direct vision internal urethrotomy for urethral stricture following hypospadias repair (38). The authors suggested that the 50% success rate should not deter the surgeon from a single attempt to treat a stricture with this technique. We would reserve this for a short, film-like stricture. A more extensive stricture may warrant a free graft or preferably, vascularized flap urethroplasty with either of these two techniques achieving greater success when used as an onlay versus a tubularized segment. In a thorough review of anterior urethral stricture repair techniques, Wessells and McAninch reported near-identical overall success rates of approximately 85% for both free graft and pedicled skin flap methods (39). However, these authors noted that many of the reports reviewed did not

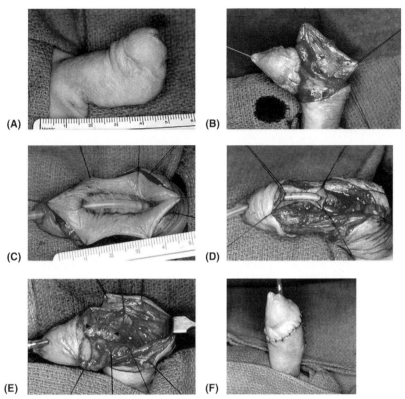

FIGURE 4 Repair of urethral diverticulum depicted in Figure 2 in a five-year-old boy four years following free graft urethroplasty with preputial skin. (**A**) Note protruding ventral aspect of penis (measurement in centimeters). (**B**) A circumferential skin incision has been made proximal and parallel to the corona of the glans. Initial dissection exposes the large diverticulum held here with a silk stay suture placed at the proximal and distal extents. (**C**) View within the opened diverticulum with proposed oval, longitudinally oriented line of incision in order to excise peripheral redundant diverticular tissue. (**D**) Remaining urethral channel following excision of excess tissue demarcated in (**C**). (**E**) Suture line of urethral closure (between *arrows*). Note tissue held by silk stay suture (other than skin) to be used as "pants-over-vest" second- and third-layer coverage of the urethral closure. (**F**) Completed repair with indwelling urethral catheter.

specifically state the site of repair. Others have discussed the usefulness of mucosal grafts for the treatment of urethral stricture disease (40,41). In 1989, Schreiter described a two-stage mesh-graft urethroplasty using split thickness skin, for application in the absence of available pedicled flap tissue or an appropriate graft bed (39,42). The mesh-graft technique would be useful in those instances when all other options have failed.

Intraurethral Hair Growth
Intraurethral hair growth is an uncommon complication of hypospadias repair and occurs when hair-bearing skin is incorporated into the repair either as transferred skin or tubularization of proximal penile or scrotal skin. Crain et al. have described laser hair ablation for management of this complication (43).

Repair Breakdown
Repair breakdown may occur secondary to devascularization of local tissues or flaps used in urethroplasty or other components of hypospadias repair. Breakdown may also result from urethroplasty and/or approximation of the glans (glanuloplasty) under tension. Breakdown of the repair may also result from devitalized tissue due to excessive use of electrocautery, unidentified vascular pedicle injury during repair, or from hematoma formation (18). Regardless of the etiology, repair breakdown may require debridement of devascularized, necrotic tissue prior to repair (5). Options for repeat hypospadias repair are discussed later in this chapter.

Hypospadias Cripple

Horton and Devine (44) used the term "hypospadias cripple" to describe the patient who has undergone multiple, unsuccessful hypospadias repair attempts, with significant resultant penile deformity. These patients represent perhaps the most perplexing of hypospadias repair complications in that they require extensive repair amidst scarred and devitalized tissue (45,46). Options for the repair of the hypospadias cripple are discussed in the following (Reoperative Hypospadias Repair) section.

Reoperative Hypospadias Repair
General Principles

In general, attempts at reoperative hypospadias surgery should not be undertaken less than six months following the previous failure. Certainly, no attempt at repair should be entertained until all edema, infection, and/or inflammation has resolved and healing is complete. Radiographic imaging with retrograde urethrogram and/or voiding cystourethrogram for complete urethral visualization may be necessary in complex reoperative hypospadias cases as an important aspect of preparation for definitive repair. Inspection of available tissue to determine whether adequate local tissue exists, versus the need for an extragenital tissue graft, will significantly impact and dictate repair options. This decision-making process is critical to achieving a successful result.

Immediately Adjacent or Local Tissue Flap

When possible, the use of immediately adjacent or local pedicled, well-vascularized tissue is preferred for reoperative hypospadias surgery. This may be in the form of a simple tubularization procedure or a modification such as the tubularized incised plate (TIP) urethroplasty. The use of TIP urethroplasty in reoperative hypospadias repair was first reported in a multi-center experience (47). Results are similar to that for primary repair when all components of the TIP technique, as described for primary repair, are incorporated (48,49). Several institutions have reported excellent success rates with TIP urethroplasty in reoperative hypospadias (48,50–54). Complications consisted mostly of urethrocutaneous fistulas and complication rates had a narrow range among these institutions with rates ranging from 15% to 28% of patients.

For reoperative hypospadias repair, advantages of the TIP urethroplasty include use of local, usually supple tissue with well-established vascularity for urethroplasty and skin coverage, as well as a cosmetically superior result. The TIP urethroplasty technique is ideal for repair following failed Mathieu, onlay island flap and tubularization procedures as, theoretically, the native vascularity of the urethral plate remains intact. The absence of preputial skin in reoperative cases makes TIP urethroplasty an ideal option as additional skin flaps are typically not necessary either for urethroplasty or for skin coverage of the penis.

In a recent report of reoperative repair using Mathieu and onlay island flap techniques, secondary complications occurred in 24% and 14% of reoperative surgeries performed with these techniques, respectively (55). Emir and Erol reported a 25% complication rate in 55 patients who underwent reoperation with the Mathieu technique (56). With similar concerns regarding skin coverage and a complication rate of 30% in reoperative cases (57), we would not recommend the modified Barcat technique as a viable alternative in such cases. The Duckett tube has been used in reoperative hypospadias with a complication rate of 24% (5 of 21 patients, including distal fistula, proximal diverticula, and stenosis of the meatus and proximal anastomosis (58). Johanssen described a useful two-stage technique for repair of severe urethral stricture following hypospadias repair (59).

Free Graft with Local or Extragenital Tissue

Horton and Devine described the use of a tubularized free skin graft urethroplasty in patients with multiple, previously failed hypospadias repairs (44). This nonhirsute skin graft may be from a genital or extragenital source. Similarly, and perhaps for use in more severe reoperative cases, free graft bladder mucosa (40), buccal mucosa ("dry" or "wet," onaly, or tubularized) (40,41,60,61), or a combination of the above may be used (62,63). It appears that for the skin-deficient hypospadias requiring reoperation, buccal mucosa has become the preferred material for reconstruction (64).

Buccal mucosa as a "dry" onlay (stage 1 of a planned two-stage repair) followed by tubularization at the second stage repair for reoperative hypospadias is becoming an attractive alternative (64,65). Snodgrass and Elmore reported 25 patients who underwent stage 1 of the repair with complete graft take in 22 (88%) cases. Three had focal scarring or graft contracture successfully "patched" prior to tubularization (stage 2) (65). At publication, 20 patients had undergone stage 2 with fistula in 1 of 18 when dartos or tunica vaginalis second-layer coverage was used and partial glans dehiscence in four boys. Fichtner et al. reported a complication rate of 24% (12 of 49 patients) using buccal mucosa strictly as an onlay method (66). In the 49 cases with available follow-up >5 years, 9 of the 12 complications occurred within the first postoperative year including two graft contractures.

Hensle et al. reported the use of buccal mucosa as either a tube graft in 12 patients or as an onlay graft in 35 patients requiring complex urethroplasty (67). The overall complication rate was 32% with rates of 50% for free tube grafts and 20% for onlay grafts. Major complications of graft contracture or slough were seen in six patients, four when buccal mucosa was used as a tube and four in the authors' early experience (first 10 cases) (67). Buccal mucosa has also been used in adult reoperation urethroplasty for multiple indications (68). Free graft of bladder mucosa has also been used for successful repair in complex reoperative cases (69).

Split thickness mesh skin graft as first stage, followed by tubularization at second stage may be a last resort for the hypospadias cripple in whom multiple previous attempts at repair have failed (42). Ehrlich and Alter have described the use of split-thickness skin graft and tunica vaginalis flaps for reoperative hypospadias (70). Using a two-stage procedure, 10 patients with failed hypospadias repair(s) were treated by a varied combination of split-thickness mesh graft urethroplasty and tunica vaginalis flap. A tunica vaginalis flap was placed as a bed for the mesh graft in three patients. Tunica vaginalis flaps were also used as an intermediate layer during stage 2 of the repair. No strictures or fistulas occurred in eight patients. Two patients await second stage of repair after successful placement of the mesh-graft. The combination of split-thickness mesh graft urethroplasty and a tunica vaginalis flap appears to achieve success in the difficult patient with complex hypospadias subsequent to multiple failed repairs.

It is predicted that tissue-engineered constructs for urethral replacement may have a major impact on reoperative hypospadias repair in the future (71). Intestinal free flap urethroplasty has also been described for use in reoperative hypospadias (72).

SUMMARY

Bleeding/persistent oozing from the repair site is the most common complication of hypospadias repair. A well-vascularized second layer of tissue coverage placed over the neourethral suture line is perhaps the single most important step in decreasing the risk of urethrocutaneous fistula. Clinically significant stricture of the neourethra may occur at the meatus (meatal stenosis) or at the proximal anastomotic site of the repair—such as with use of the transverse preputial island flap technique. As a general rule, reoperation for failed hypospadias repair should not be attempted less than six months following failure. Provided sufficient penile tissue of appropriate quality is available, several techniques applicable to primary repair may also be used for reoperation. Multiple previous failures of hypospadias repair in a patient may be best treated with a two-stage technique that, at times, incorporates extragenital skin or buccal mucosa.

CONCLUSIONS

Meticulous technique is the key for successful hypospadias repair. Patience and a thoughtful approach with appreciation for all available options are keys to a successful outcome for management of complications of hypospadias repair.

REFERENCES

1. Mouriquand PD, Persad R, Sharma S. Hypospadias repair: current principles and procedures. Br J Urol 1995; 76(suppl 3):9–22.
2. Paulozzi LJ, Erickson JD, Jackson RJ. Hypospadias trends in two US surveillance systems. Pediatrics 1997; 100:831–834.
3. Retik AB, Keating M, Mandell J. Complications of hypospadias repair. Urol Clin North Am 1988; 15:223–236.

4. Keating MA, Duckett JW. Failed hypospadias repair. In: Cohen MS, Resnick MI, eds. Reoperative Urology. Boston, MA: Little, Brown and Company, 1995:187–204.
5. Horton CE Jr, Horton CE. Complications of hypospadias surgery. Clin Plast Surg 1988; 15:371–379.
6. Duckett JW, Kaplan GW, Woodard Jr, Devine CJ Jr. Panel: complications of hypospadias repair. Urol Clin North Am 1980; 7:443–454.
7. Gargollo PC, Kozakewich HP, Bauer SB, et al. Balanitis xerotica obliterans in boys. J Urol 2005; 174(4 Pt 1):1409–1412.
8. Kumar MV, Harris DL. Balanitis xerotica obliterans complicating hypospadias repair. Br J Plast Surg 1999; 52:69–71.
9. Perovic S, Djordjevic M, Djakovic N. Natural erection induced by prostaglandin-E1 in the diagnosis and treatment of congenital penile anomalies. Br J Urol 1997; 79:43–46.
10. Kogan BA. Intraoperative pharmacological erection as an aid to pediatric hypospadias repair. J Urol 2000; 164:2058–2061.
11. Farkas LG. Hypospadias: some causes of recurrence of ventral curvature of the penis following the straightening procedure. Br J Plast Surg 1967; 20:199–203.
12. Vandersteen DR, Husmann DA. Late onset recurrent penile chordee after successful correction at hypospadias repair. J Urol 1998; 160(3 Pt 2):1131–1133; discussion 1137.
13. Winslow BH, Devine CJ Jr. Principles in repair of hypospadias. Semin Pediatr Surg 1996; 5:41–48.
14. Smith D. A de-epithelialised overlap flap technique in the repair of hypospadias. Br J Plast Surg 1973; 26:106–114.
15. Churchill BM, van Savage JG, Khoury AE, McLorie GA. The dartos flap as an adjunct in preventing urethrocutaneous fistulas in repeat hypospadias surgery. J Urol 1996; 156:2047–2049.
16. Belman AB. De-epithelialized skin flap coverage in hypospadias repair. J Urol 1988; 140(5 Pt 2):1273–1276.
17. Soergel TM, Cain MP, Kaefer M, et al. Complications of small intestinal submucosa for corporal body grafting for proximal hypospadias. J Urol 2003; 170(4 Pt 2):1577–1579.
18. Elbakry A, Shamaa M, Al-Atrash G. An axially vascularized meatal-based flap for the repair of hypospadias [see comments]. Br J Urol 1998; 82:698–703.
19. De Sy WA. Aesthetic repair of meatal stricture. J Urol 1984; 132:678–679.
20. Goldstein HR, Hensle TW. Simplified closure of hypospadias fistulas. Urology 1981; 18:504–505.
21. Davis DM. The pedicle tube-graft in the surgical treatment of hypospadias in the male: with new method of closing small urethral fistulas. Surg Gynecol Obstet 1940; 71:790–796.
22. Cecil AB. Repair of hypospadias and urethral fistula. J Urol 1946; 56:237–242.
23. Waterman BJ, Renschler T, Cartwright PC, Snow BW, DeVries CR. Variables in successful repair of urethrocutaneous fistula after hypospadias surgery. J Urol 2002; 168:726–730; discussion 729–730.
24. Santangelo K, Rushton HG, Belman AB. Outcome analysis of simple and complex urethrocutaneous fistula closure using a de-epithelialized or full thickness skin advancement flap for coverage. J Urol 2003; 170(4 Pt 2):1589–1592; discussion 1592.
25. Richter F, Pinto PA, Stock JA, Hanna MK. Management of recurrent urethral fistulas after hypospadias repair. Urology 2003; 61:448–451.
26. Landau EH, Gofrit ON, Meretyk S, et al. Outcome analysis of tunica vaginalis flap for the correction of recurrent urethrocutaneous fistula in children. J Urol 2003; 170(4 Pt 2):1596–1599; discussion 1599.
27. Zaontz MR, Kaplan WE, Maizels M. Surgical correction of anterior urethral diverticula after hypospadias repair in children. Urology 1989; 33:40–42.
28. Radojicic ZI, Perovic SV, Djordjevic ML, Vukadinovic VM, Djakovic N. "Pseudospongioplasty" in the repair of a urethral diverticulum. BJU Int 2004; 94:126–130.
29. Aigen AB, Khawand N, Skoog SJ, Belman AB. Acquired megalourethra: an uncommon complication of the transverse preputial island flap urethroplasty. J Urol 1987; 137:712–713.
30. Venn SN, Mundy AR. Urethroplasty for balanitis xerotica obliterans. Br J Urol 1998; 81:735–737.
31. Pope JC, Kropp BP, McLaughlin KP, et al. Penile orthoplasty using dermal grafts in the outpatient setting. Urology 1996; 48:124–127.
32. Lindgren BW, Reda EF, Levitt SB, Brock WA, Franco I. Single and multiple dermal grafts for the management of severe penile curvature. J Urol 1998; 160(3 Pt 2):1128–1130.
33. Horton CE Jr, Gearhart JP, Jeffs RD. Dermal grafts for correction of severe chordee associated with hypospadias. J Urol 1993; 150(2 Pt 1):452–455.
34. Hendren WH, Keating MA. Use of dermal graft and free urethral graft in penile reconstruction. J Urol 1988; 140(5 Pt 2):1265–1269.
35. Hendren WH, Caesar RE. Chordee without hypospadias: experience with 33 cases. J Urol 1992; 147:107–109.
36. Devine CJ Jr, Horton CE. Use of dermal graft to correct chordee. J Urol 1975; 113:56–58.
37. Scherz HC, Kaplan GW, Packer MG, Brock WA. Post-hypospadias repair urethral strictures: a review of 30 cases. J Urol 1988; 140(5 Pt 2):1253–1255.
38. Hsiao KC, Baez-Trinidad L, Lendvay T, et al. Direct vision internal urethrotomy for the treatment of pediatric urethral strictures: analysis of 50 patients. J Urol 2003; 170:952–955.

39. Wessells H, McAninch JW. Current controversies in anterior urethral stricture repair: free-graft versus pedicled skin-flap reconstruction. World J Urol 1998; 16:175–180.

40. Baskin LS, Duckett JW. Mucosal grafts in hypospadias and stricture management. AUA Update Series 1994; XIII:270–275.

41. Ahmed S, Gough DC. Buccal mucosal graft for secondary hypospadias repair and urethral replacement. Br J Urol 1997; 80:328–330.

42. Schreiter F, Noll F. Mesh graft urethroplasty using split thickness skin graft or foreskin. J Urol 1989; 142:1223–1226.

43. Crain DS, Miller OF, Smith LJ, Roberts JL, Ross EV. Transcutaneous laser hair ablation for management of intraurethral hair after hypospadias repair: initial experience. J Urol 2003; 170:1948–1949.

44. Horton CE, Devine CJ Jr. A one-stage repair for hypospadias cripples. Plast Reconstr Surg 1970; 45:425–430.

45. Gershbaum MD, Stock JA, Hanna MK. A case for 2-stage repair of perineoscrotal hypospadias with severe chordee. J Urol 2002; 168(4 Pt 2):1727–1728; discussion 1729.

46. Amukele SA, Lee GW, Stock JA, Hanna MK. 20-year experience with iatrogenic penile injury. J Urol 2003; 170(4 Pt 2):1691–1694.

47. Snodgrass W, Koyle M, Manzoni G, Hurwitz R, Caldamone A, Ehrlich R. Tubularized incised plate hypospadias repair: results of a multicenter experience. J Urol 1996; 156(2 Pt 2):839–841.

48. Borer JG, Retik AB. Reoperative surgery for hypospadias with tubularized incised plate urethroplasty. In: Snodgrass W, ed. Dialogues in Pediatric Urology. Pearl River, NJ: William J. Miller Associates, Inc., 2002:2–4.

49. Borer JG, Bauer SB, Diamond DA, et al. Reoperative surgery for hypospadias with the tubularized, incised plate urethroplasty. J Urol 2001; 165(suppl):192.

50. Yang SS, Chen SC, Hsieh CH, Chen YT. Reoperative Snodgrass procedure. J Urol 2001; 166: 2342–2345.

51. Shanberg AM, Sanderson K, Duel B. Re-operative hypospadias repair using the Snodgrass incised plate urethroplasty. BJU Int 2001; 87:544–547.

52. Nguyen MT, Snodgrass WT. Tubularized incised plate hypospadias reoperation. J Urol 2004; 171(6 Pt 1):2404–2406; discussion 2406.

53. Elbakry A. Further experience with the tubularized-incised urethral plate technique for hypospadias repair. BJU Int 2002; 89:291–294.

54. El-Sherbiny MT, Hafez AT, Dawaba MS, Shorrab AA, Bazeed MA. Comprehensive analysis of tubularized incised-plate urethroplasty in primary and re-operative hypospadias. BJU Int 2004; 93: 1057–1061.

55. Simmons GR, Cain MP, Casale AJ, Keating MA, Adams MC, Rink RC. Repair of hypospadias complications using the previously utilized urethral plate. Urology 1999; 54:724–726.

56. Emir L, Erol D. Mathieu urethroplasty as a salvage procedure: 20-year experience. J Urol 2003; 169:2325–2326; author reply 2326–2327.

57. Koff SA, Brinkman J, Ulrich J, Deighton D. Extensive mobilization of the urethral plate and urethra for repair of hypospadias: the modified Barcat technique. J Urol 1994; 151:466–469.

58. Soutis M, Papandreou E, Mavridis G, Keramidas D. Multiple failed urethroplasties: definitive repair with the Duckett island-flap technique. J Pediatr Surg 2003; 38:1633–1636.

59. Johanssen B. Reconstruction of the male urethra in stricture. Acta Chir Scand Suppl 1953; 176:1.

60. Duckett JW, Coplen D, Ewalt D, Baskin LS. Buccal mucosal urethral replacement [see comments]. J Urol 1995; 153:1660–1663.

61. Caldamone AA, Edstrom LE, Koyle MA, Rabinowitz R, Hulbert WC. Buccal mucosal grafts for urethral reconstruction. Urology 1998; 51(suppl 5A):15–19.

62. Retik AB. Proximal hypospadias. In: Marshall FF, ed. Textbook of Operative Urology. 1st ed. Philadelphia, PA: W. B. Saunders Company, 1996:977–984.

63. Ransley PG, Duffy PG, Oesch IL, Van Oyen P, Hoover D. The use of bladder mucosa and combined bladder mucosa/preputial skin grafts for urethral reconstruction. J Urol 1987; 138(4 Pt 2):1096–1098.

64. Bracka A. Two-stage urethroplasty revisited. In: Snodgrass W, ed. Dialogues in Pediatric Urology. Pearl River, NJ: William J. Miller Associates, Inc., 2002:7–8.

65. Snodgrass W, Elmore J. Initial experience with staged buccal graft (Bracka) hypospadias reoperations. J Urol 2004; 172(4 Pt 2):1720–1724; discussion 1724.

66. Fichtner J, Filipas D, Fisch M, Hohenfellner R, Thuroff JW. Long-term followup of buccal mucosa onlay graft for hypospadias repair: analysis of complications. J Urol 2004; 172(5 Pt 1):1970–1972; discussion 1972.

67. Hensle TW, Kearney MC, Bingham JB. Buccal mucosa grafts for hypospadias surgery: long-term results. J Urol 2002; 168(4 Pt 2):1734–1736; discussion 1736–1737.

68. Andrich DE, Mundy AR. Substitution urethroplasty with buccal mucosal-free grafts. J Urol 2001; 165:1131–1133; discussion 1133–1134.

69. Mollard P, Mouriquand P, Bringeon G, Bugmann P. Repair of hypospadias using a bladder mucosal graft in 76 cases. J Urol 1989; 142:1548–1550.

70. Ehrlich RM, Alter G. Split-thickness skin graft urethroplasty and tunica vaginalis flaps for failed hypospadias repairs. J Urol 1996; 155:131–134.
71. Atala A, Guzman L, Retik AB. A novel inert collagen matrix for hypospadias repair. J Urol 1999; 162:1148–1151.
72. Bales GT, Kuznetsov DD, Kim HL, Gottlieb LJ. Urethral substitution using an intestinal free flap: a novel approach. J Urol 2002; 168:182–184.

22 | Complications of Antireflux Surgery

Julian Wan, David Bloom, and John Park

Department of Urology, University of Michigan, Ann Arbor, Michigan, U.S.A.

INTRODUCTION

Vesicoureteral reflux (VUR) was one of the principle disorders, if not the key condition, that defined pediatric urology as a distinct field of surgical practice within the past half century. Although Galen, among others who followed, understood the antireflux nature of the uretero-vesical junction (UVJ), it took modern radiology and the voiding cystourethrogram in the 1950s to make accurate clinical diagnoses of reflux. Only then did VUR become recognized as a common condition in children with serious potential sequellae when combined with urinary tract infection (UTI) (1,2). Chronic pyelonephritis, a common cause of renal failure in children, had previously been thought to be due to blood-borne bacteremia that lodged in the kidney. Experimental studies and clinical practice however showed that VUR of bacteria was the far more usual cause. The sequellae of pyelonephritis, renal scarring, and renal failure spurred interest in the management of reflux. Most reflux resolves. This has become clear in the personal practices of all pediatric urologists and careful large clinical reports (3). Timed voiding, treatment of overactive bladders, bowel management, probiotics, and low-dose antibiotic prophylaxis are the principal strategies to prevent infection and renal injury from reflux during the vulnerable years of early childhood.

A small percentage of refluxers (14% in our experience of nearly 25 years) end up with surgical correction of reflux because of "breakthrough" infections or failure of reflux resolution. Reimplantation of the ureter became an index case for pediatric urology as the new subspecialty emerged and over the past half century many innovative procedures has been deployed. Operative repair usually has excellent results in the hands of experienced pediatric urologists. Nevertheless, a learning curve continues not only individually but also for the entire subspecialty as new techniques accrue in the pediatric urology repertoire. Reimplantation of the ureter and ureteroneocystostomy are well-recognized terms dating from the earliest days of UVJ reconstruction. However, a number of current antireflux procedures defy those descriptions related to traditional detachment and reattachment of the ureter. The extravesical approach has been called "detrussoraphy" wherein the actual UVJ is left intact at the epithelial level, but detrusor is rearranged to create a long intramural tunnel for the ureter. Injection techniques are called implantations, because a synthetic (or homograft) material is injected to improve the coaption of the ureteral orifice. O'Donnell's acronym, *STING* (subureteric injection), put minimally invasive antireflux surgery on the centerstage (4). This chapter focuses on complications of all of these operative treatments of VUR and offers guidance in recognition and management of them. Two categories of complications exist. First is failure of antireflux surgery and this will be a matter of postoperative VUR or obstruction of the distal ureter. The second category includes the assorted complications of bleeding, diverticulum, bladder dysfunction, and neurologic problems. The best approach to complications is that "ounce of prevention," which is worth well more than a pound of cure.

GENERAL COMMENTS ON ANTIREFLUX COMPLICATIONS

The selection of the procedure must match the patient and pathophysiology. Whereas the Ledbetter-Politano and the Ahmed-Cohen cross-trigonal reimplantations gave good service in the formative years of pediatric urology, enough other effective options exist to allow consideration of a UVJ reconstruction that offers a natural course for the ureter so as to allow easy retrograde catheterization, should that ever become necessary. Still, certain anatomic situations may favor a Ledbetter-Politano or a cross-trigonal approach, which will usually provide the longest intramural ureteral course. Each procedure has inherent hazards (Table 1). The old style advancements gave a fair chance of persisting reflux, the Ledbetter-Politano risked intraperitoneal transit and obstruction, and the cross-trigonal method also risked obstruction from angulation. All procedures are susceptible to ureteral devascularization. When tapering wide ureters, by excision or placation, the risks of obstruction or persisting reflux are increased. Newer procedures also have their downsides, some of which we may not yet recognize.

Some technical details are not procedure-specific. For example, we believe open bladder procedures should generally be avoided in infants and very young children. The infant bladder can be easily damaged by degrees of manipulation and retraction that seem "routine" to the surgeon, but may produce transient ischemia or other trauma that sets in motion deleterious tissue remodeling and late fibrosis. We have seen youngsters with VUR and no other underlying pathology who have undergone ureteral reimplantation described as "routine," at very early ages, yet ended up with bladders that we could only describe as hypertonic neuropathic bladders (also known as "hostile bladders"). This is not to deny a careful and effective operative solution for a young child with obstruction or reflux plus breakthrough infections. However, we believe one should tread lightly in these situations proceeding only with very delicate open surgery when clearly necessary. Retraction should be gentle and tissues must be handled with finesse. The distal ureter should be managed by stay sutures, not by repeated forceps squeezes. A vessel loop passed around the ureter and a fine vein retractor are other ways to maneuver the ureter gently. The pediatric ureter is a delicate structure with a precarious blood supply, particularly when the blood supply is surgically interrupted at one end. Even a moment of excessive axial tension may result in late fibrosis and jeopardize the long life expectancy we have for pediatric ureters.

Electrocautery near the ureter surely can have a similar effect and should be used sparingly, if at all. Bipolar electrocautery is preferable to monopolar current when in proximity to the pediatric ureter. Cautery settings should be carefully set to the lowest levels necessary. When monopolar devices are used, a fine shielded tip is necessary and "cut" and coagulation settings are deliberately selected, recognizing that the latter causes more extensive visible and invisible tissue damage and should be used mainly for isolated blood vessels far from the ureter.

When a new intramural tunnel is created for the ureter, the length of the passage should be four to five times the ureteral diameter. The ureter should enter the hiatus of the tunnel in a natural course without kinking, angulation, torsion, or tension. The muscular backing of the intramural tunnel must be sound.

TABLE 1   Concerns with Reimplantation Procedures

Specific advice with certain procedures
   Take care when placing retractor blades intravesically to be sure the desired effect is achieved. The posterior bladder wall is elevated and flattened thereby bringing the trigone and ureteral orifice closer to the surface and into the middle of the operative field.
The Leadbetter-Politano method
   Be sure that the peritoneal lining is bluntly displaced away from the bladder and ureter. When dissecting into a pristine space a fine gauze dissector or cotton-tipped applicator can gently peel away the peritoneum. In boys care must be taken to recognize and avoid the vas deferens which can be drawn into the surgical field and inadvertently injured (20). The placement of the new hiatus should be directly cephalad from the original opening; a laterally placed hiatus may cause obstruction during bladder filling. The backwall must be reconstructed to provide adequate support to the ureter.
Cross trigonal method
   If a patulous opening at the hiatus is encountered, it must be carefully closed to prevent diverticulum formation. If more length is needed, the original hiatus can be incised superiorly and laterally, thereby utilizing a broader area of the posterior bladder wall. If both ureters are being reimplanted, it is preferable to place the more severely refluxing ureter above the ureter with the lesser grade.
Extravesical method
   Caution must be taken in bilateral extravesical repair due to concerns about urinary retention; denervation of the subtrigonal nerve plexus during ureteral dissection and tunnel development (50–52).

EVALUATION OF FAILURES

The two main failures of antireflux procedures are postoperative reflux or obstruction. Ultrasonography and voiding cystourethrography (VCUG) are the fundamental postoperative studies to diagnose or rule out these two adverse outcomes. Yet, some good arguments exist for obviating the routine postoperative VCUG, a test children detest. (The equivalent of the pediatric urology Nobel Prize should go to the team that figures out how to do a catheter-less VCUG with the same or greater accuracy of the standard version.) After extravesical detrussoraphy, the reported success rate of 98% argues for skipping a postoperative VCUG in the absence of clinical problems or the finding of ultrasonography changes (5–7). The cystoscopy evaluation of the ureteral orifice after implantation, as suggested by Edmondson et al., may also substitute for a formal postoperative radiographic study (8). A normal postoperative ultrasonogram or one that shows no significant changes after antireflux procedures is essential in our opinion. Persistent hydronephrosis beyond the postoperative period requires further study to rule out reflux or obstruction. The further study must include an elimination history (the elimination diary is an important tool), a VCUG, and in many instances some study to rule out obstruction such as a diuretic renal scan (9). Doppler resistive indices have not proved very useful for the diagnosis of pediatric obstructive uropathy (10). A pressure–perfusion study may be necessary in extraordinarily equivocal cases (11). When voiding dysfunction is suspected a cystometrogram (CMG) may help define an underlying neuropathic bladder. After treatment of any significant underlying voiding or bowel dysfunction, the postoperative ultrasound and VCUG may normalize. The bottomline when evaluating the failure of antireflux surgery is that detrusor dysfunction or other elimination disorders such as constipation need to be ruled out before declaration of a surgical failure.

POSTOPERATIVE REFLUX

Three types of postoperative VUR exist: persistent, recurrent, and unexpected contralateral VUR. Persistent reflux is reflux that was not solved by the operative procedure due to an inadequate intramural tunnel, insufficient detrusor backing, a wide ureter, a dysfunctional ureter, or a hostile bladder that overwhelms the UVJ. Recurrent reflux occurs after demonstration of postoperative competence. One must always be aware that a single VCUG is imperfect proof of competence of a UVJ. Technical aspects of this study are important and often overlooked. The filling volume must be appropriate for the child (filling volumes per bladder cycle should be recorded) and several cycles are preferable to a single one if a small caliber catheter is left in place. We have seen occasional patients who demonstrated reflux only on a third or fourth VCUG cycle in a single study where each cycle was physiologic. Thus a postoperative VCUG with a single cycle with unmeasured volume and no actual voiding image (because the child could not void on the radiographic table) really cannot be considered proof of a competent UVJ. Recurrent reflux may actually be persistent reflux if a postoperative study does not meet basic technical standards. Instances of bone fide recurrent reflux are likely to be related to detrusor dysfunction such as overactivity or an unrecognized hostile bladder. Bladder and bowel function therefore require careful scrutiny if recurrent VUR is identified. Unexpected contralateral reflux may similarly be related to pre-existing reflux that was simply unobserved preoperatively, or it may be new reflux related to unanticipated detrusor dysfunction. An alternative explanation in some instances may be that deformation of the trigone at the initial antireflux procedure may have rendered a borderline contralateral UVJ incompetent. Another technical point regarding the VCUG is that it not be performed too soon postoperatively or in the face of infection wherein edema of the bladder wall may mask reflux standards for a good VCUG (Table 2). The VCUG, at best, is imperfect proof of the absence of VUR.

Contralateral reflux can develop in patients who had only unilateral reimplantation (12). A history of prior resolved reflux in the contralateral ureter is a significant risk factor. Ross et al. examined instances of postoperative contralateral reflux. They found that contralateral reflux only occurs in up to 10% of ureters, which had no prior history of reflux. Where as, 45% of ureters with prior histories of reflux were at risk of post reimplant reflux (13). Unless two separate VCUGs show resolution of reflux, it was recommended that a contralateral historically

TABLE 2   Voiding Cystourethrogram Criteria

A proper voiding cystourethrography should have
  Physiologic filling volume
  Images that capture the patient voiding on the table
  Appropriate caliber catheter
  No urinary tract infection at the time of the study
  No constipation at the time of the study
  Sufficient time after surgery

refluxing ureter undergo simultaneous reimplantation with the currently refluxing unit. Diamond et al. found that high-grade unilateral reflux may mask a vulnerable contralateral reflux and suggested that this may also be a major risk factor (14). Spontaneous resolution has been reported in 60% to 95% contralateral refluxing ureters (12–14). For this reason, we recommend that a period of observation back on antibiotic prophylaxis should be the preferred approach for patients with contralateral reflux.

BLADDER DYSFUNCTION AND PERSISTENT REFLUX

Vesicoureteral reflux in some patients is a secondary manifestation of another condition. Patients with neurogenic or obstructed bladders can have high intravesical storage pressures or abnormal voiding pressures that produce VUR. Spina bifida, spinal cord injury, and posterior urethral valves are among the common primary conditions that manifest secondary reflux. Management of reflux in these patients requires understanding and treating the primary diagnosis. It would be a mistake, for example, to operate on one of these patients for reflux without documenting normal storage and emptying pressures and no obstruction in the urethra (15).

Some patients who are normal neurologically and anatomically can have bladder dysfunction due to abnormal voiding patterns and habits. Failure to relax and coordinate the pelvic floor during bladder contraction may produce recurrent UTIs, VUR, pyelonephritis, hydronephrosis, dysuria, and incontinence. Concomitant bowel problems such as marked constipation with bowel accidents and poor emptying are common in these patients. The condition is termed "non-neurogenic neurogenic bladder" and is also known as the Hinman syndrome (16). Recognition of this condition is important because operative failure would be likely. A familial form termed urofacial or Ochoa syndrome suggests subtle microstructural anomalies in the brainstem that makes these patients vulnerable to voiding problems (17). Patients with reflux, concomitant bowel problems, voiding problems, and incontinence should suggest Hinman syndrome or other primary lower urinary tract dysfunction.

OBSTRUCTION

Obstruction of the reimplanted ureter occurs in two distinct forms. Early transient obstruction is caused by edema of the ureter and its new surrounding tunnel. This temporary form of obstruction usually subsides after several days to a week. Gentle tissue handling, careful control of hemostasis, and judicious use of electrocautery will minimize postoperative edema. In procedures where the ureter is detached and reconnected, peristalsis and passage of urine are good signs. If the surgical conditions lead to concern about edema and obstruction, a stent can be placed. This can be either a double J indwelling stent or a simple feeding tube passed up the ureter and led out of the bladder and skin. If urine is seen exiting a newly reimplanted orifice a stent is usually not necessary. Early obstruction usually is discovered in the immediate recovery period. Fever, flank pain, and low urinary output are typical findings. A ultrasonogram (USN) of the kidneys and bladder usually will confirm the diagnosis unless substantial preoperative hydroureteronephrosis existed. Early management consists of patience and careful observation in most instances where the obstruction is edematous. Typically the edema subsides after two to four weeks. During this time if the patient has significant discomfort or there is concern about a mechanical obstruction an attempt should be made to pass a retrograde stent or place an antegrade pyelostomy.

If the obstruction does not improve by four to eight weeks after the operation, one must be concerned that something other than edema is causing the problem. Ischemia, torsion, kinking, angulation, or extrinsic compression at the ureteral tunnel hiatus are the usual suspects. Devascularization of the ureter can occur to aggressive handling and dissection that strips away the supporting adventitial vascular plexus. Axial torsion and compression from instruments also harm delicate pediatric ureters. Torsion of the ureter can easily occur when passing the ureter through the tunnel. Observation of the course of the ureter and the placement of a fine stay suture near the orifice of the ureter helps define the proper orientation of the ureter. If a new hiatus is created the ureter may kink if it is placed up on the mobile side wall of the bladder. Intermittent obstruction can occur because the hiatus shifts position leading an acute angulation termed "J" hooking (18).

These problems can occur not just with procedures that detach the ureter such as the Leadbetter-Politano or Ahmed-Cohen but also with extravesical methods. Usually the bladder is mobilized and rolled medially; after mobilization of the ureter, the course of the new ureteral tunnel is guided toward an imaginary line to the contralateral shoulder. By using this landmark, when the bladder is returned to its normal position, the new hiatus follows a more natural course. Extrinsic compression of the ureter can occur because of hematoma formation within the tunnel, ultimately leading to inflammation, fibrosis and obstruction (19). Finally, peritoneal attachment and adhesion, and even intraperitoneal injury can occur when blindly passing the ureter through a new hiatus (20). Management of these problems requires initial drainage by ureteral stent if possible or antegrade nephrostomy. Intravenous pyelogram or antegrade injection may be required to help define the anatomy prior to reoperation.

Management of significant obstruction requires open reoperation after the underlying problem has been identified. Any ischemic or fibrotic segment must be excised. Kinks and severe angulations have to be corrected leaving a smooth gentle course. The hiatus should be repositioned so that it rests on or very near the floor.

LEAKAGE

Urinary extravasation is an uncommon complication of antireflux surgery. Typically this occurs in cases where the bladder is opened and extensive dissection of the ureteral hiatus is necessary. Urine can leak out of either a hole along the anterior bladder suture line or from a gap in the ureteral hiatus. Usually this is discovered by persistent drainage from a Penrose drain. We favor a drain be left whenever the bladder is opened. When leakage is suspected, the first step is to be sure the Foley or suprapubic catheter is not obstructed. Often leaks will resolve spontaneously with good catheter and penrose drainage. Cystography can help differentiate between leakage from these more common sites and rarer ureteral leakage. Treatment is initially drainage and waiting for possible spontaneous closure but if this does not occur after a week, re-exploration may be necessary to seal the leak, particularly if it is coming from the ureteral hiatus.

To prevent leakage, we recommend a two-layer closure of the bladder; the first layer closes the epithelium and the inner half of the musculature, the outer layer closes the outer half of the musculature and the adventitia. The ureteral hiatus should be closed in two layers as well, with care that the ureter is not obstructed.

POSTOPERATIVE URINARY TRACT INFECTION, HEMATURIA, FREQUENCY, AND URGENCY

Transient gross hematuria postoperatively is quite common and usually lasts only one to four days. Typically the urine lightens with each successive day. Microscopic hematuria may persist, however, for weeks to months, afterward. Heavy hematuria with clot formation is more worrisome and can pose significant problems besides blood loss (21,22). Hematomas within the new tunnel, in the bladder, or in the retrovesical space can obstruct the ureter (19). Initial management consists of fluid support and ruling out underlying coagulopathy. Irrigation of the catheter, cystoscopy, and clot evacuation and finally open exploration are other options.

Urgency, urge incontinence, and frequency are common after reimplantation surgery. These are usually short-lived symptoms, which last a few days or until catheters or stents are removed. They are typically caused by irritation and disturbance of the trigone and bladder wall by the newly created ureteral tunnel or from catheter or stent. Anticholinergics (oxybutynin 5 mg po b.i.d.), pyridium, and occasional use of banthine and opium suppositories are usually sufficient to suppress any over-active bladder contractions.

Occasionally nocturnal enuresis can occur after surgery of any sort and not just with genitourinary surgery. This is usually self-limiting and does not require specific therapy. Conservative therapy with fluid restrictions before bedtime and patients usually resolves this form of secondary nocturnal enuresis within six months. Curiously, we have also seen recalcitrant nocturnal enuresis disappear abruptly after antireflux procedures.

The fundamental aim of reimplantation is to halt reflux and thereby prevent the ascension of bacteria to the kidney and the subsequent development of pyelonephritis and renal scarring. The other aims are the prevention of the sequellae of scarring, namely hypertension and renal insufficiency. After successful reimplantation, patients can still develop UTIs. Around 20% of patients may have UTIs even after successful surgery (23). In particular, girls, whose reflux was corrected, will increase their UTI risk with maturation and the onset of sexual activity (24). The effect of UTIs on the miscarriage rates in women who had corrected reflux is not clear; there are many mitigating factors, including the quality of the prenatal care (25). The development of later scarring from subsequent UTIs seems to be greater among patients who already have scars. Because these manifestations may not appear until adulthood, some have advocated lifelong follow-up for patients who have VUR regardless of the success of surgery (24).

URINARY RETENTION

Transient voiding disturbances are normal in the immediate postoperative period. For patients who had an intravesical procedure, the irritation to the trigone and bladder epithelium may produce urgency, frequency, hesitancy, dysuria, and urge incontinence. Disturbances to nocturnal continence are also not unexpected. These are usually self-limiting and improve rapidly as healing progresses, edema resolves, and catheters or stents are removed. Care and caution are needed when using oral anticholinergics and banthine and opium suppositories to control bladder spasms. They may work too well and place the patient in retention either directly due to their pharmacologic effects on bladder contractility and sensation and also indirectly by promoting constipation and bladder overdistention.

The neuroanatomy of the bladder makes urinary retention after reimplantation a natural concern. The detrusor at the bladder base and trigone are well innervated (26). Intravesical procedures do not affect the detrusor innervation at the trigone or bladder base. Likewise, extravesical unilateral reimplantation affects only one side. Fung et al. found that these types of reimplantation procedures did not increase the risk of postoperative urinary retention (27). This observation held true even in cases with high-grade reflux, which required extensive dissection of a larger caliber dilated ureter. When a bilateral detrusorrhaphy was performed, voiding inefficiency as well as urinary retention was noted early on in up to 22% of the patients but it was transient and all but one patient resolved rapidly with further bladder drainage. Neuropraxia of the pelvic plexus has been proposed as a possible mechanism and has been studied in both animals and humans. Extravesical reimplantation may risk injury to the pelvic plexus and its efferent nerves when the dissection proceeds extensively distal to the ureter and dorsal to the trigone (28,29). Electrocautery and the placement of anchor sutures to prevent the ureter from sliding out of position have been theorized as the major risk factors. McArchran and Palmer proposed further that the afferent fibers of the pelvic plexus near the obliterated pelvic plexus maybe equally important. They found that anchoring sutures did not seem to have a critical effect and were able to discharge patients home without a catheter after only a one-day stay in the hospital (29).

MANAGEMENT OF COMPLICATIONS

The initial steps when faced with a complication after antireflux surgery is to first be sure that the patient is stabilized. Antibiotic prophylaxis should be maintained and any obstruction or retention relieved by urinary catheter, stent, or percutaneous nephrostomy tube. Because of the high degree of success expected, when a reimplantation operation fails, after stabilizing the patient, one should not immediately reoperate but perform a thorough evaluation to be sure the situation is well understood and that no other issues have been overlooked (Fig. 1). It can be a stressful time for the surgeon and the family who both may be keen to resolve the situation quickly. A period of time to allow for edema and swelling to subside and a systematic evaluation into why the complication occurred is recommended. Usually a three- to six-month period of time is recommended, longer if it is just persistent, or contralateral reflux which as noted previously can resolve spontaneously with time (30) The only instance where immediate reoperation is worth considering is in the case of large volume leak from the bladder or a gross mechanical obstruction of the distal ureter.

If there is persistent grade I or II VUR after reimplantation it may be worth considering subureteric injection of dextranomer/hyaluronic acid. This method is advantageous because it can be performed endoscopically but also has issues about its long-term consequences (see subsequent section below). A growing body of literature that suggests VUR a select subgroup of patients may tolerate low-grade VUR off antibiotic prophylaxis with little risk of future renal scarring (31–33). For these very select patients, we speculate that it may not be necessary to treat any residual low-grade reflux.

Reimaging with a VCUG, USN, or intravenous pyelogram (IVP) and urodynamics are all prudent actions. If a nephrostomy tube had been placed, an antegrade study can be performed to help visualize the site or region of obstruction. The antegrade image of a long thin atretic line of contrast, for example, is suggestive of an ischemic distal ureter and would be important when planning reoperation. Cystoscopy can be helpful at this juncture. It can help ascertain whether the original tunnel failed because of insufficient length, inadequate muscle backing, or widely patulous orifice. It can also help identify the rare cases of recurrent reflux due to a VUR (34).

Choose an incision that gives sufficient exposure to handle what you may find. While using the old incision it may be necessary to make a new incision. If the original transverse skin incision is utilized we extend it laterally, then open and divide the fascia in a vertical fashion and split the rectus muscles vertically. This approach allows the original skin incision to be used while allowing more lateral exposure with access to the peritoneum.

Various techniques and maneuvers should be considered. If the distal ureter is ischemic and unusable because of extensive scarring and adhesion, consider either a psoas hitch and/or

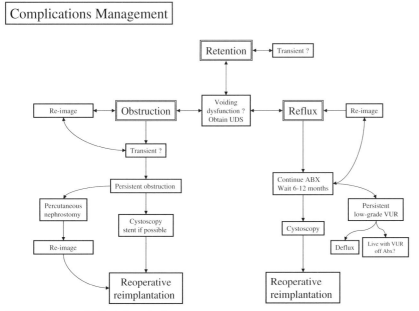

FIGURE 1 Complications flow chart.

Boari flap to allow a new reimplantation with healthier more proximal ureter. If the ureter is in good shape and can be mobilized without jeopardizing its vascular supply mobilize it carefully both intravesically and extravesically. Choose a method of reimplantation, which is comfortable and familiar and which can be performed without tension or torsion to the ureter. Take care to be sure there is adequate muscular backing and sufficient tunnel length. Taper if needed. If the ureter is sufficiently flexible a folding technique may be preferable to the excision technique as it preserves the blood supply. An indwelling stent or feeding tube should be left in instances of reoperation. For cases of a duplicated system, with persistent reflux into one ureter or there is obstruction, consider an ipsilateral ureteroureterostomy draining the troublesome ureter into the unobstructed nonrefluxing one. This option is only possible if there is sufficient flexibility to allow a side-to-side or end-to-side anastomosis. In many cases the ureters are too tightly sheathed together that this is not possible in the distal ureter. In cases where both the left and right ureters have to be reoperated, there may be only sufficient room for one good reimplant. In this case consider a transureteroureterostomy with the recipient ureter being carefully mobilized and reimplanted (35,36).

KIDNEY TRANSPLANT

Patients with VUR and end-stage renal failure requiring renal transplantation pose particular concerns. In general, correction of VUR to the native kidneys before transplantation is desirable. In patients with a history of symptomatic UTI and VUR, the majority (63%) will develop another UTI within three months of the transplantation (37). Evaluation of the adequacy of bladder storage compliance and emptying and the underlying cause of the renal failure should be part of any pre-transplantation evaluation. It is best to correct any lower urinary tract problems before the transplant is performed and the patient is placed on immunosuppression. Pyelonephritis related to VUR has been found to be an important long-term complication, which affects survival of renal allografts (38).

Most renal transplant ureters are anastomosed to the bladder by a dismembered extravesical method. Typically this approach works well and has few complications (leakage, stricture, or obstruction) (39) Only 2.1% in a study of over 800 transplants performed by a small cohort of surgeons had anastomosis-related complications using an unstented extravesical ureteroneocystotomy approach (39). In contrast, Mangus and Haag in a meta-analysis found that stented ureteroneocystotomy in renal transplants had a significant lower complication rate of only 1.5% (40). We usually suggest a stent whenever the procedure is more difficult than usual or when implanting into abnormal bladder (e.g., trabeculated, thick walled, augmented). One option to keep in mind is to connect the transplant kidney to a native nonrefluxing ureter. This approach has been successfully used but is clearly dependent on the availability of a viable native ureter (41).

Complications after renal transplantation are evaluated and managed similar to those of other reimplanted ureters with one major difference. If an obstruction or leakage develops, an attempt to stent the ureter by retrograde cystoscopy is likely to be unsuccessful. Percutaneous placement under ultrasound or computed tomography guidance offers both excellent relief of the obstruction and also allows for later diagnostic and therapeutic procedures (42).

INJECTION THERAPY COMPLICATIONS

The treatment of VUR by the subureteric injection of dextranomer/hyaluronic acid (Dx/HA or Deflux™, Uppsala, Sweden) (43) offers a less invasive alternative method of treating VUR. It has been applied quite successfully to primary reflux grades I and II (44). New contralateral VUR occurs in up to 13% of patients who received unilateral Dx/HA injections (45). This figure is similar in magnitude to that seen with open surgery but its etiology remains unknown. Obstruction of the ureter has been reported in less than 1% of the thousands of ureters treated by injection therapy using polytetrafluouroethylene (46). Snodgrass reported a patient with unilateral hydroureteronephrosis after bilateral Dx/HA injections of only 0.8 mL on each side. The ureters preoperatively were dysmorphic and he speculates that peristalsis in such ureters may be more easily disrupted making them more prone to obstruction (47).

Because of the newness of Dx/HA injection, long-term follow-up will be necessary. Recently Knudson et al. noted that calcifications have been found in the bladder neck of children who had received glutaraldehyde cross-linked collagen injections (48). These were found almost 10 years after the injection. There is already a case report of a symptomatic granuloma found five years after Dx/HA injection (49). For this reason longer follow-up extending 20 to 30 years and through maturity, puberty, aging, and pregnancy will be needed to uncover any other late complications.

CONCLUSIONS

Urology is often described as both an "art and science." The science is beyond dispute. In the past century advances such as the germ theory of disease, antibiotics, modern anesthesia, positive pressure ventilation, clean intermittent catheterization, pressure-based management of neurogenic bladder, fiberoptic endoscopy, extracorporeal shock wave lithotripsy, computed tomography, ultrasonography, and molecular genetics are among the major advances, which have altered how we evaluate and care for patients. The "art" refers to that intangible aspect of medicine where experience and judgment are paramount. Perhaps it is a misnomer to use "art" and we should consider instead the term "craft" as is used by artisans and craftsmen. An artist can have many false starts and have bold experiments which end as glorious failures. An artist can accept failures on the way to creating a masterpiece. We as surgeons cannot accept such an approach. While we do hope to achieve masterpieces, mostly we seek constant improvement of our craft so that our daily work is consistent in its excellence and reliability.

The treatment of VUR reflects this tradition. Careful planning, gentle tissue handling, and proper execution of the appropriate procedure will usually yield an excellent outcome. When complications do occur, the same reasoned approach should be applied. Familiarity with the possible complications, their manifestations, and treatment offers the best chance of resolving the situation satisfactorily.

REFERENCES

1. Arant BS Jr. Vesicoureteric reflux and renal injury. Am J Kidney Dis 1991; 17:491–511.
2. Birmingham reflux study group. Prospective trial of operative versus non-operative treatment of severe vesicoureteric reflux in children: five years' observation. BMJ 1987; 295:237–241.
3. Belman AB, Skoog SJ. Nonsurgical approach to the management of vesicoureteral reflux in children. Pediatr Infect Dis J 1989; 8:556–559.
4. O'Donnell B. Reflections on reflux. J Urol 2004; 172:1635–1636.
5. Bomalaski MD, Ritchey ML, Bloom DA. What imaging studies are necessary to determine outcome after ureteroneocystostomy? J Urol 1997; 158(3 Pt 2):1226–1228.
6. Grossklaus DJ, Pope JC, Adams MC, Brock JW. Is postoperative cystography necessary after ureteral reimplantation? Urology 2001; 58:1041–1045.
7. Bisignani G, Decter RM. Voiding cystourethrography after uncomplicated ureteral reimplantation in children: is it necessary? J Urol 1997; 158:1229–1231.
8. Edmondson JD, Maizels M, Alpert SA, et al. Multi-institutional experience with PIC cystography—incidence of occult vesicoureteral reflux in children with febrile urinary tract infects. Urology 2006; 67:608–611.
9. Bloom DA, Faerber G, Bomalaski MD. Urinary incontinence in girls. Urol Clin N Amer 1995; 22: 521–538.
10. Rawashdeh YF, Djurhuus JC, Mortensen J, Horlyck A, Frokiaer J. The intrarenal resistive index as a pathophysiological marker of obstructive uropathy. J Urol 2001; 165:1397–1404.
11. Tchetgen MB, Bloom DA, Robert H. Whitaker and the Whitaker test: a pressure-flow study of the upper urinary tract. Urology 2003; 61:253–256.
12. Hoenig DM, Diamond DA, Rabinowitz R, Caldamone AA. Contralateral reflux after unilateral ureteral reimplantation. J Urol 1996; 156:196–197.
13. Ross JH, Kay R, Nasrallah P. Contralateral reflux after unilateral ureteral reimplantation in patients with a history of resolved contralateral reflux. J Urol 1995; 154:1171–1172.
14. Diamond DA, Rabinowitz R, Hoenig D, Caldamone AA. The mechanism of new onset contralateral reflux following unilateral ureteroneocystostomy. J Urol 1996; 156(suppl 2S):665–667.
15. Bomalaski MD, Anema JG, Coplen DE, Koo HP, Rozanski T, Bloom DA. Delayed presentation of posterior urethral valves: a not so benign condition. J Urol 1999; 162:2130–2132.
16. Hinman F Jr. Nonneurogenic neurogenic bladder (the Hinman syndrome)—15 years later. J Urol 1986; 136:769–777.

17. Ochoa B. Can a congenital dysfunctional bladder be diagnosed from a smile? The ochoa syndrome updated. Pediatr Nephrol 2004; 19:6–12.

18. Hensle TW, Berdon WE, Baker DH, Goldstein HR. The ureteral "J" sign: radiographic demonstration of iatrogenic distal ureteral obstruction after ureteral reimplantation. J Urol 1982; 127: 766–768.

19. Ellsworth PI, Barraza MA, Stevens PS. Bilateral ureteral obstruction secondary to a retrovesical hematoma following bilateral ureteral reimplantation via the Cohen technique. J Urol 1995; 154: 1498–1499.

20. Kaufman JM, McGuire EJ, Baskin AM. Viscus perforation: unusual complication of ureteroneocystostomy. Urology 1974; 4:728–730.

21. plantation. J Urol 1976; 115:731–735.

22. Garrett RA, Schlueter DP. Complications of antireflux operations: causes and management. J Urol 1973; 109:1002–1004.

23. Willscher MK, Bauer SB, Zammuto PJ, Retik AB. Infection of the urinary tract after anti-reflux surgery. J Pediatr 1976; 89:743–747.

24. Bukowski TP, Betrus GG, Aquilina JW, Perlmutter AD. Urinary tract infections and pregnancy in women who underwent antireflux surgery in childhood. J Urol 1998; 159:1286–1289.

25. Mansfield JT, Snow BW, Cartwright PC, Wadsworth K. Complications of pregnancy in women after childhood reimplantation for vesicoureteral reflux: an update with 25 years of followup. J Urol 1995; 154:787–790.

26. McGuire EJ. The innervation and function of the lower urinary tract. J Neurosurg 1986; 65:278–285.

27. Fung LC, McLorie GA, Jain U, Khoury AE, Churchill BM. Voiding efficiency after ureteral reimplantation: a comparison of extravesical and intravesical techniques. J Urol 1995; 153:1972–1975.

28. Martinez Portillo FJ, Seif C, Braun PM, et al. Risk of detrusor denervation in antireflux surgery demonstrated in a neurophysiological animal model. J Urol 2003; 170(2 Pt 1):570–573; discussion 573–574.

29. McArchran SE, Palmer JS. Bilateral extravesical ureteral reimplantation in toilet trained children: is 1-day hospitalization without urinary retention possible? J Urol 2005; 174:1991–1993.

30. Siegelbaum MH, Rabinovitch HH. Delayed spontaneous resolution of high grade vesicoureteral reflux after reimplantation. J Urol 1987; 138:1205–1206.

31. Grechi G, Selli C, Pecori M, Carini M. Recurrent reflux caused by vesicoureteral fistula. Urology 1981; 17:360–361.

31. Al-Sayyad AJ, Pike JG, Leonard MP. Can prophylactic antibiotics safely be discontinued in children with vesicoureteral reflux? J Urol 2005; 174(4 Pt 2):1587–1589; discussion 1589.

32. Thompson RH, Chen J, Pugach J, Naseer S, Steinhardt GF. Cessation of prophylactic antibiotics for managing persistent vesicoureteral reflux. J Urol 2001; 166:1465–1469.

33. Cooper CS, Chung BI, Kirsch AJ, Canning DA, Snyder HM III. The outcome of stopping prophylactic antibiotics in older children with vesicoureteral reflux. J Urol 2000; 163:269–272; discussion 272–273.

34. Burbige KA, Miller M, Connor JP. Extravesical Ureteral Reimplantation: Results in 128 Patients. J Urol 1996; 155:1721–1722.

35. Hendren WH. Reoperative ureteral reimplantation: management of the difficult case. J Pediatr Surg 1980; 15:770–786.

36. Hendren WH. Reoperation for the failed ureteral reimplantation. J Urol 1974; 111:403–411.

37. Crowe A, Cairns HS, Wood S, Rudge CJ, Woodhouse CR, Neild GH. Renal transplantation following renal failure due to urological disorders. Nephrol Dial Transplant 1998; 13:2065–2069.

38. Ohba K, Matsuo M, Noguchi M, et al. Clinicopathological study of vesicoureteral reflux (VUR)-associated pyelonephritis in renal transplantation. Clin Transplant 2004; 18(suppl 11):34–38.

39. Ohl DA, Konnak JW, Campbell DA, Dafoe DC, Merion RM, Turcotte JG. Extravesical ureteroneocystostomy in renal transplantation. J Urol 1988; 139:499–502.

40. Mangus RS, Haag BW. Stented versus nonstented extravesical ureteroneocystotomy in renal transplantation: a metaanalysis. Am J Transplant 2004; 4:1889–1896.

41. Lapointe SP, Charbit M, Jan D, et al. Urological complications after renal transplantation using ureter-ureteral anastomosis in children. J Urol 2001; 166:1046–1048.

42. Swierzewski SJ III, Konnak JW, Ellis JH. Treatment of renal transplant ureteral complications by percutaneous techniques. J Urol 1993; 149:986–987.

43. Q-Med AB, Seminariegatan 21, 752 28 Uppsala, Sweden.

44. Kirsch AJ, Perez-Brayfield M, Smith EA, Scherz HC. The modified sting procedure to correct vesicoureteral reflux: improved results with submucosal implantation within the intramural ureter. J Urol 2004; 171(6 Pt 1):2413–2416.

45. Elmore JM, Kirsch AJ, Lyles RH, Perez-Brayfield MR, Scherz HC. New contralateral vesicoureteral reflux following dextranomer/hyaluronic acid implantation: incidence and identification of a high risk group. J Urol 2006; 175:1097–1101.

46. Puri P, Granata C. Multicenter survey of endoscopic treatment of vesicoureteral reflux using polytetrafluoroethylene. J Urol 1998; 160(3 Pt 2):1007–1011; discussion 1038.

47. Snodgrass WT. Obstruction of a dysmorphic ureter following dextranomer/hyaluronic acid copolymer. J Urol 2004; 171:395–396.
48. Knudson MJ, Cooper CS, Block CA, Hawtrey CE, Austin JC. Calcification of glutaraldehyde cross-linked collagen in bladder neck injections in children with incontinence: a long-term complication. J Urol 2006; 176:1143–1146.
49. Bedir S, Kilciler M, Ozgok Y, Deveci G, Erduran D. Long-term complication due to dextranomer based implant: granuloma causing urinary obstruction. J Urol 2004; 172:247–248.
50. Leissner J, Allhoff EP, Wolff W, et al. The pelvic plexus and antireflux surgery: topographical findings and clinical consequences. J Urol 2001; 165:1652–1655.
51. David S, Kelly C, Poppas DP. Nerve sparing extravesical repair of bilateral vesicoureteral reflux: description of technique and evaluation of urinary retention. J Urol 2004; 172(4 Pt 2):1617–1620.

23 | Complications of Exstrophy and Epispadias Surgery

Joseph G. Borer and Alan B. Retik
Department of Urology, Children's Hospital and Harvard Medical School, Boston, Massachusetts, U.S.A.

INTRODUCTION

Epispadias is a defect of lower urinary tract development in which there is incomplete closure of the urethra to varying degrees. The urethra is open on the dorsal surface of the corpora cavernosa of the penis, ranging from a glanular to a penopubic junction defect (Fig. 1A). The penopubic variant may also be associated with bladder neck deficiency resulting in urinary incontinence and these patients may also have vesicoureteral reflux (VUR).

Bladder exstrophy is a complex anomaly involving the urinary, genital and intestinal tracts, and the musculoskeletal system. Typically, the diagnosis is made at newborn examination (Fig. 1B) or on fetal ultrasound performed by an experienced observer. Management of bladder exstrophy presents several challenges beginning with initial repair using either the more conventional approach of the modern staged repair of exstrophy (MSRE) or the complete primary repair of exstrophy (CPRE) technique. The MSRE consists of three specific, scheduled components. First, bladder, posterior urethra, and abdominal wall closure with bilateral innominate and vertical iliac osteotomy, when indicated, are performed in the newborn period. Secondly, epispadias repair is then performed at six months to one year of age. Thirdly, bladder neck reconstruction (BNR) and bilateral ureteral reimplantation are performed at age four to five years when adequate bladder capacity for BNR and motivation to participate in a postoperative voiding program are documented (1,2). Grady and Mitchell have described their technique of complete primary exstrophy repair (CPER) for single-stage reconstruction of bladder exstrophy (3,4). The goal of this technique is to combine the goals of staged reconstruction at a single operation; bladder closure and epispadias repair (4) with achievement of urinary continence, if possible, without formal BNR.

Major goals in the management of bladder exstrophy are preservation of normal kidney function, observation for development of adequate bladder function including urinary continence, and provision of acceptable cosmesis and function of the external genitalia. Many of these goals are similar for management of epispadias. This chapter will present a discussion of complications encountered during the care of patients with epispadias, bladder exstrophy, and a brief discussion of complications of cloacal exstrophy management will also be included.

COMPLICATIONS

Complications encountered during the care of patients with epispadias or exstrophy range from minor complications such as urinary tract infection (UTI/cystitis) to major complications that include dehiscence of the repair, obstruction to the outflow of urine (either upper or lower urinary tract) and end-stage renal disease (ESRD).

Intraoperative Complications: Bleeding, External Genitalia Tissue Loss

Significant complications of the total penile disassembly technique for repair of epispadias itself (5), or the epispadias component during complete primary repair of bladder exstrophy have also been reported (6–9). Complications included loss of corpora cavernosa, penile skin, urethral plate and glans tissue either alone or in combination following this technique which is appropriate only for those with adequate experience with exstrophy in general and complete penile disassembly in particular.

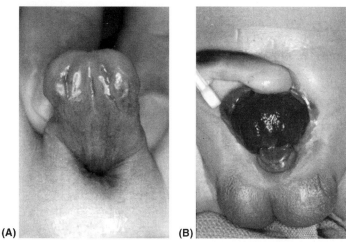

FIGURE 1   Male newborn with (**A**) penopubic epispadias, and (**B**) bladder exstrophy.

Diagnosis

Intraoperative complications such as bleeding or tissue loss are, at times, related. There is often a significant amount of bleeding from the corpus spongiosum during repair of epispadias or exstrophy, particularly in the male. This occurs during dissection of the urethral plate off of the anterior surface of the penis. Risk of tissue loss is increased with some modes of obtaining hemostasis. Injection of dilute epinephrine solution into the penis appears to be particularly risky (6,9). These injuries are often recognized during the progress of the surgical procedure with an appearance of devascularized and/or devitalized tissue.

Prevention

Topical application of iced saline or dilute epinephrine (epinephrine diluted 1:200,000 with xylocaine) as an intermittent topical administration may be adequate for control of bleeding while limiting risk of major complications such as irreversible tissue loss. Judicious use of electrocautery would also be advised. Exquisite care should be exercised when dissecting near the neurovascular bundles that run on the lateral aspect of the corpora cavernosa in exstrophy and epispadias.

Management

Reconstruction of the external genitalia in the face of tissue loss is one of the most challenging surgical exercises faced by the surgeon who care for these complex patients (10). Penile degloving, division of suspensory ligament, and rotational skin flaps are available techniques to achieve penile augmentation and enhancement. Reasonable cosmesis and penile length are attainable goals. In the most severe injuries, microsurgical phalloplasty is a technically feasible and successful option (10).

Immobilization Complications
Diagnosis

Meldrum et al. reviewed various forms of immobilization of patients following exstrophy repair (11). They found that the spica cast and "mummy wrapping" immobilization techniques were less effective and were associated with significant complications when compared with modified Bryant's and modified Buck's traction following repair of exstrophy. Ulcers, friction burns, and skin breakdown are the most common complications from immobilization following repair.

Prevention

Appropriate choice of immobilization method is based upon age of the child, and use of osteotomy at repair. Regardless of the immobilization method chosen, diligent daily observation of the skin areas in contact with any part of the traction mechanism is, perhaps, the most important means by which these complications may be prevented.

Management
Management involves wound care specific to the needs of the patient. Occasionally the assistance of plastic surgery colleagues is indicated.

Dehiscence of Wound or Repair/Bladder Prolapse
Diagnosis
This devastating complication may be evident in the immediate postoperative period following any stage of the MSRE or following CPRE. Dehiscence of the repair may be either partial or complete and is often preceded by a UTI and/or local infection of the site of surgery itself. This may be noticed initially as a small area of wound breakdown that becomes more prominent, involving a larger area over time. The eventual result may be a physical appearance similar to the initial epispadias or bladder exstrophy at presentation. The importance of successful initial bladder closure either in MSRE or CPRE cannot be overstated. In a 10-year review of bladder exstrophy management, Oesterling and Jeffs noted the importance of successful initial bladder closure on eventual outcome of the staged approach in these patients (12). They found that for criteria of bladder capacity at the time of BNR—the third stage of MSRE, interval between initial closure and BNR (time to develop sufficient capacity for BNR) and rate of urinary continence, there was a statistically significant difference favoring those patients with versus those without successful initial bladder closure. As with the MSRE, dehiscence and bladder prolapse have been reported following CPRE (7).

Prevention
One measure of prevention is the use of appropriate antibiotic coverage in the perioperative period in order to decrease the likelihood of an infectious process. Technical aspects include secure closure of the urethra in epispadias repair, the bladder and posterior urethra in MSRE, and the bladder and urethra in CPRE. The closure/approximation of tissues without tension is of critical importance in preventing repair breakdown whether it be epispadias repair alone, or bladder closure with or without epispadias repair in exstrophy patients. Selective use of osteotomy in the newborn (1) or perhaps in all newborns (13), may decrease tension at the point of approximating the pubic bones in the anterior midline at exstrophy closure and in this way decrease the likelihood of dehiscence.

Management
Following repair dehiscence there should be a minimum of six months for full recovery from the previous failed surgical procedure(s). This allows for healing as much as possible and resolution of the inflammatory process prior to performing reoperation or alternative surgical intervention. Dehiscence of the initial repair, particularly in patients with bladder or cloacal exstrophy, has significant negative impact on eventual probability of urinary continence and ability to void spontaneously and effectively (12).

Vesicocutaneous/Urethrocutaneous Fistula
Diagnosis
This complication may be suspected on physical examination and confirmed at the first postoperative cystogram (Fig. 2) following epispadias repair, CPRE, or at latter stages of the MDRE.

Prevention
Limiting use of electrocautery around delicate bladder neck and urethral plate tissues is critical as well as the use of meticulous surgical technique.

Management
Many of these fistulas will heal with continued and at times prolonged bladder decompression and urinary diversion with a suprapubic catheter. For those fistulous tracts that do not heal conservative management is indicated with a waiting period of at least six months prior to

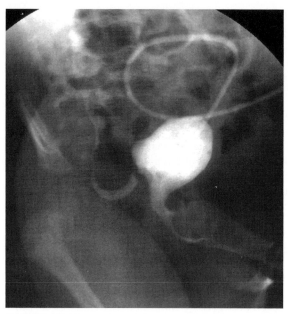

FIGURE 2 Voiding cystogram via suprapubic cystostomy catheter in a three-week-old male following complete primary repair of exstrophy on the second day of life. Note reflux into distal "J" hooking right ureter, urethrocutaneous fistula at funneled bladder neck, and normal appearing penile urethra.

reoperation and fistula repair. Techniques and principles similar to those used in the repair of hypospadias fistulae are often advantageous in this setting as well.

Bladder Outlet Obstruction/Urethral Stricture
Diagnosis
Bladder outlet obstruction or urethral stricture may occur following epispadias or exstrophy repair. Patients may present with obstructive symptoms (14) such as straining with voiding, a dribbling "stream," decreased force of stream, or urinary retention. Urethral stricture following epispadias or exstrophy repair may present in the immediate postoperative period or several months to years following repair. Similar to urethrocutaneous fistula, diagnosis of stricture may be confirmed by either retrograde or antegrade voiding cystourethrogram (VCUG) (Fig. 3A), or cystoscopy. Partial obstruction at the bladder outlet level or in the urethra may result in increased voiding pressures and exacerbation of reflux (Fig. 3B).

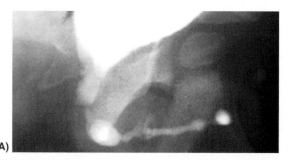
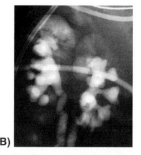

(A)   **(B)**

FIGURE 3 Voiding cystourethrogram showing (**A**) irregular and strictured urethra responsible for high-pressure voiding, exacerbation of vesicoureteral reflux, and eventual urinary retention and bladder calculus formation in a three-year-old male following complete primary repair of exstrophy as a newborn, and (**B**) bilateral high-grade vesicoureteral reflux on the same cystogram. Note the presence of intrarenal reflux that is most prominent in the upper pole, bilaterally.

Prevention

Meticulous technique at closure of the bladder neck region and during any of the intricate surgeries of urethral closure at CPRE or isolated epispadias repair is critical in decreasing the risk of stricture or obstruction. Opinionated use of catheters by many surgeons and on the other hand some surgeons that recommend against routine use of urethral catheters (2) at repair of epispadias and/or exstrophy make recommendations on this issue difficult to defend for either case.

Management

The management of epispadias or exstrophy patients with urethral stricture is complex and may require the use of extragenital tissue sources such as buccal mucosa for reconstruction or repair (14). At times, bladder neck closure and continent urinary diversion are indicated.

Complications of Impaired Bladder Function

Diagnosis

A history of urinary incontinence or more importantly the other end of the spectrum, urinary retention should raise concern regarding deficiency in one or more aspects of bladder functions of storage and emptying. Urodynamic evaluation with noninvasive uroflowmetry coupled with post-void residual urine check by ultrasound (15) with or without invasive cystometrogram have been used to diagnose and objectively treat bladder function abnormality in patients with exstrophy or epispadias (16,17).

Prevention

Conscientious follow-up with a serial history from the caretaker and/or patient coupled with upper and lower urinary tract function assessment are th e best means of identifying trouble with bladder function as early as possible ideally prior to any permanent impairment sets in.

Management

Following unsuccessful or unsatisfactory primary treatment in patients with bladder exstrophy, the options for a surgical solution in order to preserve the upper urinary tract and to achieve continence are limited. After failure of primary treatm ent, the upper urinary tract must be stabilized. Several authors have published results with augmentation and continent diversion following multiple failed exstrophy repair, including those patients who underwent single-stage repair (7,18,19) or MSRE (20). Stein et al. have advocated the use of a rectal reservoir in those patients with a normal or slightly dilated upper urinary tract and intact anal sphincter (21). Alternatively, a gastrointestinal (stomach and ileum) composite urinary reservoir has been shown to provide electrolyte neutrality in a small number of patients with bladder exstrophy (22). Regardless of the surgical approach to repair of patients with failed initial exstrophy closures, proper long-term follow-up and careful monitoring of metabolic parameters must be encouraged (23).

Vesicoureteral Reflux/Pyelonephritis/Renal Scarring

Diagnosis

VR is present in some patients with epispadias and in nearly 100% of patients with exstrophy. Spontaneous resolution of VUR is unlikely in patients with exstrophy secondary to abnormal insertion of the distal ureter into the bladder (ureterovesical junction). The distal ureter is in the shape of a "J" such that it enters the bladder in a perpendicular plane versus obliquely and thus, there is little or no intramural tunnel and no antireflux flap valve mechanism (Fig. 2). UTI/cystitis with infected urine in the bladder may then be carried cephalad directly into the renal collecting system and parenchyma resulting in pyelonephritis and renal scarring if not treated promptly and aggressively. The most sensitive means of diagnosing renal scarring is with technetium[99] dimercapto succinic acid (DMSA) renal scan (Fig. 4). Bolduc et al. recognized the significant risk to the upper urinary tract—24% of patients with renal scarring and/or significant hydronephrosis at a mean follow-up of 4.5 years after the most recent continence procedure (24). A similar rate of renal scarring was reported in a series of exstrophy patients closed initially via CPRE (6). Careful monitoring of this aspect of care in the patient with epispadias or exstrophy cannot be overstressed.

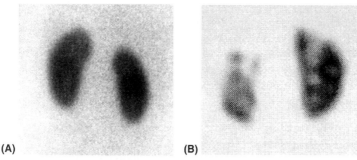

FIGURE 4 Technetium[99] dimercapto succinic acid renal scan from (**A**) a patient with a normal scan, and (**B**) patient shown in Figure 3 with bilateral cortical defects (more pronounced in the left kidney in this posterior view) secondary to recurrent pyelonephritis.

Prevention

Daily antibiotic prophylaxis in patients with VUR should decrease the risk of cystitis and pyelonephritis. Early antireflux surgery, is advocated in those patients with breakthrough pyelonephritis (25).

Management

Careful follow-up with antireflux surgery is advocated in those patients with breakthrough pyelonephritis (25).

End-Stage Renal Disease

This grave complication in epispadias or bladder exstrophy may be seen in patients with persistent VUR with or without associated obstruction in either the upper or lower urinary tract, recurrent pyelonephritis and progressive renal scarring to the point of renal failure. In patients with cloacal exstrophy, there are often abnormalities such as renal agenesis, renal ectopia, and renal dysplasia. Renal dysplasia carried to the extreme and manifested bilaterally or in a solitary kidney may predispose the patient to ESRD early in life.

Diagnosis

Early suspicion of ESRD may be based upon appearance of kidneys with available imaging such as an appearance typical for dysplasia. Plasma creatinine, creatinine clearance, and DMSA renal scan are helpful in making a diagnosis with renal insufficiency or ESRD.

Prevention

Perhaps, the best preventative mechanism against ESRD is aggressive treatment of VUR and prevention of pyelonephritis. Serial evaluations with plasma creatinine, creatinine clearance and DMSA, and involvement of nephrology colleagues in the care of patients with epispadias and bladder exstrophy and particularly in patients with cloacal exstrophy may optimize potential for prevention of ESRD.

Management

Renal replacement therapy is the key form of management in these patients. Bladder function should be assessed to assure that the bladder is an appropriately functioning reservoir to receive urine from a transplanted kidney, particularly if bladder dysfunction was, in part, causative of ESRD.

SUMMARY

The essential goals in the treatment of patients with the bladder exstrophy are preservation of the upper urinary tract, urinary continence, and a functionally as well as cosmetically satisfactory reconstruction of the genitalia. Surgical options include early urinary diversion or reconstruction of the exstrophic bladder in one of either a planned staged or complete primary technique. Although the argument regarding the optimal technique for repair of bladder exstrophy will continue, it should be conceded by all that ultimate success is most dependant upon successful initial reconstruction. Flawless technique carried out by an experienced surgical team is undoubtedly the foundation of a good outcome for patients with epispadias or exstrophy.

CONCLUSIONS

Strict attention to detailed, prospective periodic assessment clear to both physician and caregiver charged as partners with the shared responsibility for lifelong care of the patient with bladder exstrophy. Timely evaluation regarding response of the bladder, upper urinary tracts, and the patient as a whole to surgical intervention in any form—particularly following those procedures that increase bladder outlet resistance—is critical for the realization of a good outcome. Anticipation of VUR and an approach to prevention of upper urinary tract deterioration is most important in the care of these complex patients.

REFERENCES

1. Baker LA, Gearhart JP. The staged approach to bladder exstrophy closure and the role of osteotomies. World J Urol 1998; 16:205–211.
2. Gearhart J. Exstrophy, epispadias, and other bladder anomalies. 8th ed. Philadelphia, PA: WB Saunders, 2002.
3. Grady RW, Mitchell ME. Newborn exstrophy closure and epispadias repair. World J Urol 1998; 16:200–204.
4. Mitchell ME, Bagli DJ. Complete penile disassembly for epispadias repair: the Mitchell technique. J Urol 1996; 155:300–304.
5. Zaontz MR, Steckler RE, Shortliffe LM, Kogan BA, Baskin L, Tekgul S. Multicenter experience with the Mitchell technique for epispadias repair. J Urol 1998; 160:172–176.
6. Borer JG, Gargollo PC, Hendren WH, et al. Early outcome following complete primary repair of bladder exstrophy in the newborn. J Urol 2005; 174(4 Pt 2):1674–1678; discussion 1678–1679.
7. Gearhart JP. Complete repair of bladder exstrophy in the newborn: complications and management. J Urol 2001; 165(6 Pt 2):2431–2433.
8. Hammouda HM, Kotb H. Complete primary repair of bladder exstrophy: initial experience with 33 cases. J Urol 2004; 172(4, Part 1 of 2):1441–1444.
9. Husmann DA, Gearhart JP. Loss of the penile glans and/or corpora following primary repair of bladder exstrophy using the complete penile disassembly technique. J Urol 2004; 172(4 Pt 2): 1696–1701.
10. Amukele SA, Lee GW, Stock JA, Hanna MK. 20-year experience with iatrogenic penile injury. J Urol 2003; 170(4 Pt 2):1691–1694.
11. Meldrum KK, Baird AD, Gearhart JP. Pelvic and extremity immobilization after bladder exstrophy closure: complications and impact on success. Urology 2003; 62:1109–1113.
12. Oesterling JE, Jeffs RD. The importance of a successful initial bladder closure in the surgical management of classical bladder exstrophy: analysis of 144 patients treated at the Johns hopkins Hospital between 1975 and 1985. J Urol 1987; 137:258–262.
13. Halachmi S, Farhat W, Konen O, et al. Pelvic floor magnetic resonance imaging after neonatal single stage reconstruction in male patients with classic bladder exstrophy. J Urol 2003; 170(4 Pt 2): 1505–1509.
14. Baker LA, Jeffs RD, Gearhart JP. Urethral obstruction after primary exstrophy closure: what is the fate of the genitourinary tract? J Urol 1999; 161:618–621.
15. Yerkes EB, Adams MC, Rink RC, Pope JI, Brock JW III. How well do patients with exstrophy actually void? J Urol 2000; 164(3 Pt 2):1044–1047.
16. Borer JG, Gargollo PC, Kinnamon DD, et al. Bladder growth and development after complete primary repair of bladder exstrophy in the newborn with comparison to staged approach. J Urol 2005; 174(4 Pt 2):1553–1557; discussion 1557–8.
17. Diamond DA, Bauer SB, Dinlenc C, et al. Normal urodynamics in patients with bladder exstrophy: are they achievable? J Urol 1999; 162(3 Pt 1):841–844; discussion 844–845.
18. Gearhart JP, Sciortino C, Ben-Chaim J, Peppas DS, Jeffs RD. The Cantwell-Ransley epispadias repair in exstrophy and epispadias: lessons learned. Urology 1995; 46:92–95.
19. Surer I, Ferrer FA, Baker LA, Gearhart JP. Continent urinary diversion and the exstrophy-epispadias complex. J Urol 2003; 169:1102–1105.
20. Shaw MB, Rink RC, Kaefer M, Cain MP, Casale AJ. Continence and classic bladder exstrophy treated with staged repair. J Urol 2004; 172(4, Part 1 of 2):1450–1453.

21. Stein R, Fisch M, Black P, Hohenfellner R. Strategies for reconstruction after unsuccessful or unsatisfactory primary treatment of patients with bladder exstrophy or incontinent epispadias. J Urol 1999; 161:1934–1941.

22. Austin PF, Rink RC, Lockhart JL. The gastrointestinal composite urinary reservoir in patients with myelomeningocele and exstrophy: long-term metabolic followup. J Urol 1999; 162(3 Pt 2):1126–1128.

23. Kalloo NB, Jeffs RD, Gearhart JP. Long-term nutritional consequences of bowel segment use for lower urinary tract reconstruction in pediatric patients. Urology 1997; 50:967–971.

24. Bolduc S, Capolicchio G, Upadhyay J, Bagli DJ, Khoury AE, McLorie GA. The fate of the upper urinary tract in exstrophy. J Urol 2002; 168:2579–2582; discussion 2582.

25. Mathews R, Hubbard JS, Gearhart JP. Ureteral reimplantation before bladder neck plasty in the reconstruction of bladder exstrophy: indications and outcomes. Urology 2003; 61:820–824.

24 | Complications of Shock Wave Lithotripsy

Nicole L. Miller
Department of Endourology and Minimally Invasive Surgery, Clarian Health, Indiana University School of Medicine and International Kidney Stone Institute, Indianapolis, Indiana, U.S.A.

James E. Lingeman
Clarian Health, Indiana University School of Medicine and International Kidney Stone Institute, Indianapolis, Indiana, U.S.A.

INTRODUCTION

The development of shock wave lithotripsy (SWL) began when engineers at Dornier, a German aerospace firm, started researching the effects of shock waves on military hardware. They discovered that shockwaves created by aircraft traveling at supersonic speeds caused damage to the metal exterior of the aircraft. Funded by the German ministry of defense, Dornier expanded their research to study the effects of shock waves on tissue. They were able to demonstrate that shock waves generated in water could be passed through living tissue, except for the lung, without discernible injury. However, brittle materials were subject to fragmentation by the shock waves. Development for human applications continued when Dornier engineers discovered that they could generate low-energy shock waves by an underwater electrical spark discharge in a predictable and reproducible manner. During the 1970s, further investigation of SWL for the treatment of nephrolithiasis proceeded through in vitro and in vivo experiments performed at the University of Munich. This experimental work led to the development of the first lithotriptor, the Dornier HM1. On February 20, 1980, the HM1 was used for the first time clinically in Munich, Germany (1) Further refinement of the lithotriptor led to the Dornier HM2 and HM3. Following promising reports of SWL outcomes by Chaussy and associates (2), clinical trials began in the United States in 1984 using the Dornier HM3 lithotriptor. The lithotriptor received approval by the U.S. Food and Drug Administration in 1984. The report of the United States cooperative study of SWL reaffirmed the effectiveness of this therapy for the treatment of calculi in the upper urinary tract and proximal ureter with stone free rates of 77.4% at three months for patients with single stones (3).

Despite having revolutionized the treatment of nephrolithiasis, SWL is not without treatment-related side effects and complications. These complications may occur as a result of infection, direct injury to the kidney and surrounding tissues, or as a result of stone fragmentation. This chapter will review the acute and chronic effects of SWL.

BASIC PRINCIPLES OF SHOCK WAVE LITHOTRIPSY

During SWL, shock waves are generated by a source external to the patient that propagates through the body before being focused on a kidney stone. The practical application of shock waves for the treatment of nephrolithiasis relies on the ability to focus these nonlinear low-frequency waves on the targeted stone where they can generate enough force to cause fragmentation. Lithotripsy shock waves are generated by one of three mechanisms: (*i*) electrohydraulic spark gap; (*ii*) electromagnetic deflection of a plate; and (*iii*) piezoelectric transduction. Electrohydraulic lithotriptors generate shock waves by vaporization of water at the tip of a spark gap electrode positioned at (F1) of a hemi-ellipsoid reflector. The shock wave is then refocused at the second focal point (F2). Electromagnetic lithotriptors generate shock waves by the application of electric current to an electromagnetic coil. Two conducting cylindrical plates produce a strong magnetic field when electric current is applied. The electromagnetic force results in the creation of a plane or cylindrical shock wave. The shock waves are then focused by an acoustic lens or parabolic reflector. Piezoelectric lithotriptors generate shock waves by application of an electrical current to piezoceramic crystals. The piezoceramic crystals are arranged within a spherical dish to allow convergence of the shock wave front at the desired focal point (F1).

Electrohydraulic lithotriptors typically have larger focal zones than electromagnetic or piezoelectric lithotriptors. The focal zone is the area where the shock wave energy converges. The size of the focal zone determines the ease of stone targeting, and the area of shock wave effect. Therefore, larger focal zones not only improve stone targeting, but also expose a greater area to the effect of shock wave application. Lithotriptors also vary in the size of the shock wave aperture. A wider aperture spreads the acoustic energy over a broader area of skin thus producing less discomfort. Unfortunately, widening the aperture of the shock wave source narrows the focal zone making targeting of the stone more difficult.

Regardless of the mechanism used to generate shock waves, all lithotriptors produce a pressure pulse with the same fundamental waveform (4,5). A typical shock wave consists of an acoustic pulse of short duration (5 μs) with a compressive phase (positive pressure) followed by a tensile tail (negative pressure) (Fig. 1) (6). The amplitudes of the positive and negative phases are dependent on the charging potential of the shock wave source and the mechanism used to focus the pulse. Peak positive pressures range from 15 to 110 MPa and negative pressure range from −5 to −15 MPa depending on the lithotripter and the chosen power (6).

Once generated, the shock wave must be coupled to the patient to allow transmission. The original Dornier HM3 lithotriptor achieves shock wave coupling by submersing a patient in a water bath. In an effort to improve portability, subsequent lithotriptors have been designed using a dry gel coupling system. The shock head is enclosed in a water-filled chamber capped by a latex membrane that can be coupled to the patient's body with ultrasound gel.

Shock waves are thought to result in stone fragmentation by producing mechanical stresses on the stone produced either directly by the incident shock wave or indirectly by the collapse of cavitation bubbles. These events could be occurring simultaneously or separately at the surface of the stone or within the interior of the stone (Fig. 2). Several potential mechanisms for SWL stone breakage have been described: (*i*) spall fracture, (*ii*) squeezing, (*iii*) shear stress, (*iv*) superfocusing, (*v*) acoustic cavitation, and (*vi*) dynamic fatigue.

Spall fracture results in stone comminution because of differences in acoustic impedance. This difference may occur at the distal surface of the stone at the stone–fluid (urine) interface, or at internal sites, such as cavities in the stone and interfaces of crystalline and matrix materials. A compressive wave is created when a shock wave encounters this interface between low and high acoustic impedance. As the compressive wave travels through the stone, it is reflected and inverted in phase to a tensile or negative pressure wave. If the tensile wave exceeds the tensile strength of the stone, there is an induction of nucleation and growth of microcracks, which eventually coalesce resulting in stone fragmentation, termed spallation. Spallation is affected by stone size, shape, and physical properties (7).

The second mechanism for stone breakage, termed squeezing/splitting or circumferential compression, is thought to occur because of a difference in sound speed between the stone and the surrounding fluid (8). The shock wave inside the stone advances faster through the stone

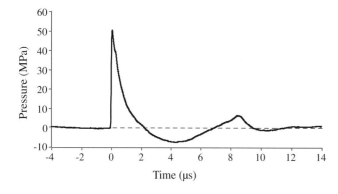

FIGURE 1 Typical shock wave at the focus of the electromagnetic lithotripter Dornier DoLi-50. Note the compressive phase (positive pressure) followed by a tensile tail (negative pressure).

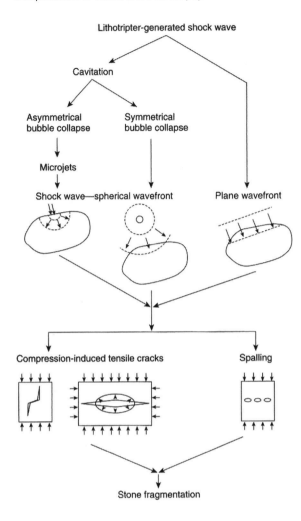

FIGURE 2 Summary of how the various mechanical forces generated by a lithotripsy shockwave might cause a kidney stone to fracture. *Source*: From Ref. 187.

than the shock wave propagating in the fluid outside of the stone. The shock wave that propagates in the fluid outside of the stone thus produces a circumferential force, resulting in a tensile stress at the proximal and distal ends of the stone. The squeezing force splits the stone in a plane parallel to the direction of shock wave propagation.

Shear stress will be generated by shear waves (also termed transverse waves) that develop as the shock wave passes into the stone. The shear waves propagate through the stone and result in regions of high shear stress. Calcium oxalate stones commonly possess alternating layers of mineral and matrix, and the shear stress induced by the transverse wave could cause stone failure. Recent theoretical work by Sapozhnikov et al. (9) suggests that the shear wave mechanism will lead to a tensile strain in cylindrical stones that is 5 to 10 times larger than that induced by spall, initiating cracks in the center of the stone.

Superfocusing is a potential mechanism for stone fragmentation by the amplification of stresses inside a stone. The reflected shock wave at the distal surface of the stone can be focused either by refraction or by diffraction from the corners of the stone. These reflected waves can be focused to regions of high stress in the interior of the stone leading to failure (10,11). The regions of high stress (both tensile and shear) are dependent on the geometry and elastic properties of the stone.

The fifth potential mechanism for stone breakage is cavitation (12–16). Cavitation is defined as the formation and subsequent dynamic behavior of bubbles. The lithotripter-generated pressure field has been found to induce cavitation in both in vitro and in vivo studies. The negative pressure in the trailing part of the pulse causes bubbles to grow at nucleation sites. Bubbles form from these cavitation nuclei, grow rapidly, and ultimately collapse. The violent collapse of these bubbles releases energy primarily by sound radiation in the form of a shock wave. This shock wave can induce all of the fragmentation mechanisms described earlier. However, in the presence of a boundary, a liquid jet, also termed a cavitation microjet, forms inside the bubble during the collapse (13). If the liquid jet is near the surface of a stone, it creates a locally compressive stress field in the stone, which propagates spherically into the stone interior. Recent studies have suggested that cavitation plays a significant role in stone comminution (17,18).

The final mechanism of stone fragmentation is a process known as dynamic fatigue or the growth and coalescence of minute flaws within a stone caused by tensile and/or shear stress that accumulates during SWL (19). Renal calculi have numerous sites of pre-existing flaws (microcracks) due to the presence of both crystalline and noncrystalline material. Repetitive shock waves result in growth of these microcracks until overall stone failure occurs.

MECHANISMS OF SHOCK WAVE INJURY

Although the exact mechanisms for tissue injury related to SWL remain unknown, cavitation and shear stress are thought to play a role. Lithotriptor shock waves have been shown to generate cavitation in vitro (12,20). The hypothesis is that cavitation within blood vessels is responsible for shock wave-induced hemorrhage (21). Crum (13) documented that SWL-induced cavitation microjets are forceful enough to pit or deform metal test foils. Bailey et al. (18) demonstrated lithotriptor-induced cavitation within the renal parenchyma. To further test the hypothesis that cavitation is the primary mechanism of tissue injury, Evan et al. (22) compared the degree of injury induced in the pig kidney following treatment with a clinical dose of shock waves using a standard brass reflector versus a brass reflector fitted with a Styrofoam insert. The insert reverses the normal pressure wave so that the negative tail precedes the positive portion of the wave thereby reducing cavitation (18). The pigs treated with the standard brass reflector developed a hemorrhagic lesion within the renal parenchyma while those treated with the modified reflector had only microscopic damage. These data strongly implicate cavitation in shock wave-induced renal injury.

Another potential mechanism for tissue injury is shear stress. Lokhandwalla and Sturtevant (19) demonstrated, by numerical modeling, that shock waves have the potential to cause cell lysis by inducing unsteady flows (shear waves) in the surrounding media. Subsequent experimental studies using overpressure to eliminate cavitation and a parabolic reflector to refocus the wave field within the sample vial showed that shock waves could damage intracellular organelles by a mechanism other than cavitation validating shear as a potential mechanism of shock wave injury (23).

ACUTE EFFECTS OF SHOCK WAVE LITHOTRIPSY

The acute effects of SWL may be due to direct tissue injury induced by shock wave application or as a result of stone fragmentation.

Acute Renal Injury

The acute tissue effects of SWL have been well studied in animal models. The primary injury appears to be a vascular insult. Histopathologic analysis has revealed regions of hemorrhage at the site of F2 characterized by the rupture of thin-walled veins, small arteries, and glomerular and peritubular capillaries. Venous thrombi have been found in adjacent interlobular and arcuate veins with evidence of endothelial injury. Damage to the endothelium manifests as a form of vasculitis with loss of endothelial cells and activation of platelets and polymorphonuclear cells on the luminal surface. Macroscopically, injury is identified by the presence of hematuria, hemorrhage, and renal enlargement. Bleeding can be found within the renal parenchyma, beneath the capsule or into the perirenal fat. Sites of intraparenchymal hemorrhage generally extend from the papillary tip to the capsule, and appear to be most significant at the corticomedullary junction (24,25). Willis et al. (26) quantified the hemorrhagic lesion as a result of SWL with the unmodified HM3 lithotriptor (2000 shocks at 24 kV) to be about 2% of the functional mass in the adult pig.

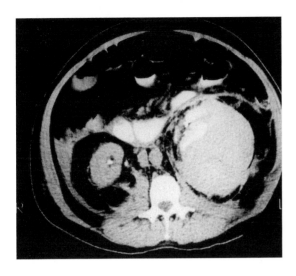

FIGURE 3 Computed tomography scan obtained 48 hours following left shock wave lithotripsy with Dornier HM3 lithotriptor for a 1-cm calculus within the renal pelvis. Note the large hematoma surrounding the left kidney.

The pattern of injury seen in human kidneys as a result of SWL corresponds to that demonstrated in animal studies. The most common clinical sign of renal trauma is gross hematuria (27). Computed tomography (CT) and magnetic resonance imaging (MRI) have demonstrated renal injury, including enlargement of the kidney, loss of corticomedullary junction demarcation, low signal intensity changes in the perirenal fat and hematomas in 63% to 85% of patients treated with SWL (Fig. 3) (28–35). As demonstrated in animal studies, hemorrhage can be intraparenchymal, subcapsular, or perirenal (36). While perirenal collections have been shown to resolve in a few days (37), subcapsular hematomas may take six weeks to six months or longer to resolve (28). Intraparenchymal hemorrhage is preferentially located at the corticomedullary junction which may be more susceptible to injury as a result of differing tissue densities in this location (38). The thin-walled arcuate veins located in the corticomedullary junction are especially vulnerable to shock wave injury.

In addition to the vascular insult, SWL has been shown to produce nephron injury. This injury has been assessed by detecting the spillage of tubular enzymes into the urine immediately after treatment (39–48). These tubular enzymes include: *N*-acetyl-beta-D-glucosaminidase (NAG), alkaline phosphatase, and beta-galactosidase (BGAL) as proximal tubular lysosomal enzymes; gamma-glutamyltransaminase (GGT) and angiotensin-converting enzymes (ACE) for brush border of proximal tubular cells; calbindin-D for distal tubular cells and beta-2-microglobulin as a small circulating protein that is freely filtered but almost completely reabsorbed in the proximal tubule. Karlin et al. (49) noted that elevations in NAG, GGT, ACE, and BGAL occurred immediately following SWL with a piezoelectric lithotripter, but normalized within seven days. Most studies have reported similar results with only a transient elevation in biochemical markers of nephron injury (40,50,51). Significant proteinuria has been reported following SWL (48), however it resolves within three to six months without a change in glomerular filtration rate (GFR) (52).

The acute effects of SWL on renal function have been studied in animals and humans. Jaeger et al. (53) reported a significant decrease in creatinine clearance and an elevation of glucose excretion one-hour post-SWL in dogs treated with 3000 shocks (1500 shocks per pole of kidney). Both values returned to normal by 24 hours post-SWL. Willis et al. have conducted a more recent series of experiments in pigs investigating the effect of SWL on bilateral renal function (26,54,55). The application of 2000 shocks at 24 kV with an unmodified Dornier HM3 lithotriptor to one kidney consistently reduces renal blood flow (RBF) and GFR in the treated kidney as well as the untreated kidney (Fig. 4). At one-hour post-SWL, the fall in RBF was 27% for the young adult animals and 50% in the juvenile pigs. By four hours post-SWL, RBF returned to baseline in the young adult pigs, but was still significantly reduced in the juvenile pigs. GFR followed a similar course but was reduced to a lesser extent than RBF. In the untreated kidney, a significant reduction in RBF was demonstrated at one-hour post-SWL. Therefore, the major

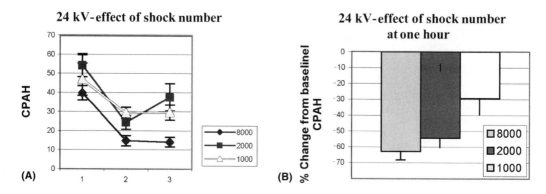

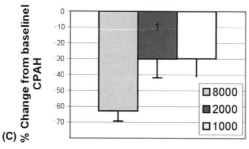

FIGURE 4   Para-aminohippurate (PAH) clearance in treated pig kidney after one and four hours post-shock wave lithotripsy (SWL) treatment with 2000 shocks at 24 kV. (**A**) All three dosage levels induce a significant fall in PAH clearance at one hour post-SWL. (**B**) The 8000 shock treatment induced a greater fall in PAH clearance compared to the 1000 shock dose. (**C**) At four hours post-SWL, the 1000 and 2000 shock doses show similar changes while the 8000 shock dose shows a persistent reduction in PAH clearance. *Abbreviation*: CPAH, clearance of para-aminohippurate. *Source*: From Ref. 188.

change in renal function appears to be a result of vasoconstriction, and smaller kidneys may be at increased risk for side effects.

Acute changes in renal function have also been documented using radionuclide studies to measure effective renal plasma flow (ERPF) and creatinine clearance. Kaude et al. (31) found an immediate decrease in effective plasma flow as measured by renal scans in 30% of kidneys treated with a clinical dose of SWL (1800 shock waves). The decrease in ERPF and/or a delay in contrast excretion in unobstructed SWL-treated kidneys has been confirmed by other investigators (31,51,56–58). Transient reductions in intrarenal blood flow at F2 have also been observed (59–62).

Risk Factors for Acute Renal Injury

Risk factors for shock wave-induced acute renal injury are related to patient factors as well as the characteristics of the lithotripter used and the parameters of treatment. Knapp et al. (28) found that patients with pre-existing hypertension (HTN) were at increased risk of developing a perinephric hematoma following SWL. Kostakopoulos et al. (63) reported a similar finding in a study of 4247 SWL treatments performed using the Dornier HM3 and HM4 lithotriptors in which patients with pre-existing HTN and especially those with poor control had a significantly increased incidence of perinephric hematoma.

Certainly patients with thrombocytopenia or coagulopathy are at increased risk of bleeding complications. While irreversible coagulopathy is an absolute contraindication to SWL, patients with bleeding diatheses have undergone safe treatment with SWL when the coagulopathy was sufficiently corrected (64,65). Other factors thought to contribute to an increased risk of hematoma following SWL include age, diabetes mellitus (DM), coronary artery disease, and obesity (66). Dhar et al. (67) examined results using the Storz Modulith SLX electromagnetic lithotripter (Karl Storz, Culver City, California, U.S.A.), and found that the probability of developing a subscapsular hematoma increased 1.67 times for every 10 year increase in patient age.

Animal studies have suggested that the number of shock waves administered and the rate of administration influence the degree of renal injury (54,68–71). Thomas et al. (72) demonstrated that the administration of over 1500 shocks induced a fall in renal plasma flow. Similar findings by Orestano et al. (73) revealed that fewer than 2500 shocks produced changes in renal function that totally resolved by 30 days post-SWL, but a greater dosage of shock waves was associated with more extensive changes in renal function (reduction in clearance, prolonged I-131Hippuran transit) of the treated kidney as well as the contralateral kidney. Therefore, the majority of data collected in animal and human studies suggest that although the kidney and surrounding tissues are vulnerable to the effect of shock wave administration, the microvasculature appears to be at highest risk. Moreover, the risk of injury appears to correlate with the number of shocks administered.

Infection

Infectious complications are fortunately unusual following SWL. The incidence of sepsis has been reported to be less than 1%; however, the rate increases to 2.7% for staghorn calculi (74). Renal trauma and vascular disruption induced by SWL may permit the entry of bacteria into the bloodstream. The incidence of bacteremia has been reported to be as high as 14% (75,76). Active urinary tract infection (UTI) and/or pyelonephritis are contraindications to SWL. Even in the presence of sterile urine, stones may harbor bacteria (77). The fragmentation of these stones by SWL may result in the release of preformed bacterial endotoxins and viable bacteria that increase the risk for sepsis (78–81). A variety of infectious complications have been described following SWL including perinephric abscess, psoas abscess, military tuberculosis, endophthalmitis, and abdominal wall abscess (82–89).

The routine administration of prophylactic antibiotics for SWL has generally been thought to be unnecessary. However, certain clinical and radiographic features may indicate the need for preoperative antibiotics. These include the presence of staghorn calculi, history of struvite stones or UTI, instrumentation or stone manipulation prior to SWL, the presence of an indwelling ureteral stent, catheter or nephrostomy tube, and patients at high risk for infected stones (i.e., urinary diversion). Although prior studies have demonstrated no advantage to routine prophylactic antibiotics in patients without preoperative UTI or infection stones (90–93), a meta-analysis by Pearle and Roehrborn (94) concluded that routine prophylactic antibiotics for all patients undergoing SWL were cost-effective when weighed against the inpatient treatment of urosepsis. While the routine use of prophylactic antibiotics remains controversial, the risk of infectious complications following SWL can be minimized by treating only in the presence of sterile urine and in the absence of distal obstruction.

Stone-Related Complications

Stone-related problems following SWL are usually the result of poor fragmentation. There are several factors that may influence the degree of stone fragmentation and clearance. Grasso et al. (95) reviewed a series of 121 patients who failed an initial SWL treatment, and identified several factors associated with poor stone clearance rates: large renal calculi (mean, 22.2 mm), stones within dependent or obstructed portions of the collecting system, stone composition (mostly calcium oxalate monohydrate and brushite), obesity or a body habitus that inhibits imaging, and unsatisfactory targeting of the stone. The negative effect of increasing stone burden (size and number) on the results of SWL has been reported by many groups using a variety of lithotripters (3,74,96–100). The effect of stone location on stone-free rates following SWL has been demonstrated in a prospective randomized multicenter trial (101). Stone-free rates for lower pole calculi greater than 10 mm were 91% for percutaneous nephrolithotomy (PNL) versus 21% for SWL.

Poor stone fragmentation can result in ureteral obstruction. Steinstrasse ("street of stone") is the term used to describe a column of stones obstructing the ureter (Fig. 5). The risk

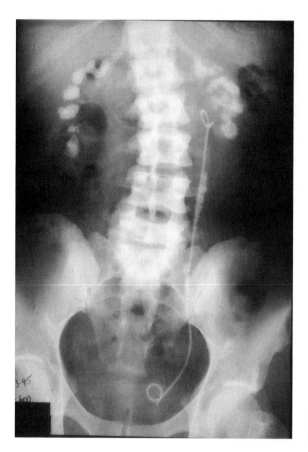

FIGURE 5 Complex steinstrasse following treatment of large left renal calculi by shock wave lithotripsy.

of steinstrasse has been shown to correlate with stone size (102–104). Madbouly et al. (104) reported an overall incidence of steinstrasse of 3.97% in 4634 patients treated with a Dornier MFL 5000 lithotriptor. Stone size and site (>2 cm), renal morphology, and shock wave energy (>22 kV) were significant risk factors for steinstrasse. Steinstrasse may present as renal colic or may even be asymptomatic. This underscores the need for follow-up imaging in all patients treated with SWL to rule out silent obstruction (105,106). Although ureteral stenting has not been shown to improve stone-free rates, the placement of a ureteral stent will prevent obstruction from steinstrasse (107). However, the discomfort associated with a ureteral stent is not trivial (108). PNL may be a better treatment for larger stones at risk for causing steinstrasse following SWL.

Steinstrasse has been treated with a variety of methods (102,109–111). Kim et al. (109) reported successful conservative treatment in 64% of patients presenting with symptomatic steinstrasse (average length of 2.6 cm). In the presence of infection, sepsis, solitary kidney, acute renal failure, or intolerable pain, conservative management is not recommended. The main objective in these cases is to relieve the obstruction. Steinstrasse may be divided into simple and complex categories where simple steinstrasse refers to columns of gravel <5 cm, and complex steinstrasse is defined as a >5 cm column of fragments In patients with simple steinstrasse and no evidence of urosepsis, ureteroscopy (URS) or in situ SWL of the leading fragment may be attempted. To prevent ureteral perforation, ureteroscopic manipulation should be abandoned if a guidewire cannot be passed proximal to the stone fragments. In this case or in the presence of complex steinstrasse and/or urosepsis, placement of a percutaneous nephrostomy tube is the safest method of relieving obstruction. Ureteral peristalsis will permit spontaneous stone passage and resolution of the steinstrasse even in the absence of urine flow.

Extra-Renal Complications

Shock wave-induced injury has been reported in a number of other organs. Injury to the lung parenchyma was recognized by Chaussy (27) and Chaussy and Fuchs (1). Pediatric patients may be particularly at risk for pulmonary contusion as a result of SWL, and shielding of the lungs is necessary in small children (112). The use of SWL in patients with abdominal aortic aneurysms (AAA) is controversial. Some investigators have reported the safety of SWL in these patients (113–116), while others have reported AAA rupture following SWL (117–121). Cardiac arrhythmias have been reported with electrohydraulic spark gap and piezoelectric lithotriptors when the shock waves were not synchronized to the electrocardiogram (122–124). However, recent clinical studies have demonstrated that ungating is safe (125–127). Patients with pacemakers can be safely treated with SWL, but depending on the type of pacemaker, reprogramming may be necessary prior to treatment (128,129).

Gastrointestinal injuries have also been reported including gastric erosion, colonic mucosal injury, duodenal erosion, pancreatitis, ureterocolic fistula, and small bowel perforation (130–136). Acute pancreatitis is associated with a marked rise in serum amylase and lipase levels, and may be more common in patients with underlying liver disease (137). Splenic rupture has also been reported as a complication of SWL (138–140).

A number of animal studies have been performed to investigate the effect of SWL on fertility (141–143). Subsequent human investigation has not shown any long-term gonadal toxicity in males or females. Andreessen et al. (144) noted a decrease in sperm density and motility following SWL that resolved within three months. Vieweg et al. (145) reported that there were no adverse effects on fertility in women treated with SWL for distal ureteral calculi. Of course, pregnancy is an absolute contraindication for SWL.

CHRONIC EFFECTS OF SHOCK WAVE LITHOTRIPSY

The potential long-term effects of SWL are a subject of ongoing research; however, there are data to suggest negative effects on blood pressure and renal function, as well as an increased risk of stone recurrence, brushite stone disease, and DM.

Chronic Renal Injury

The chronic histopathologic changes following SWL have been studied in a few animal models. Newman et al. (146) characterized the morphologic changes found in the canine kidney 30 days following SWL. They reported diffuse interstitial fibrosis, focal areas of calcification, nephron loss, dilated veins, and hyalinized acellular scars running from the cortex to the medulla (Fig. 6). Banner et al. (147) reported mesangial changes in pigs treated with the HM3 or the EDAP lithotriptor. These changes were characteristic of a mesangioproliferative glomerulopathy with deposits of complement (C3) and traces of immunoglobulin G (IgG) in both the treated and untreated kidneys. Again, a correlation between the number of shock waves administered and the size of the resulting scar was observed by Morris et al. (41). In contrast to these studies, Chaussy (27) reported no histologic abnormalities in the dog kidney up to one year post-SWL.

Chronic changes in renal function have also been documented in animal studies. Neal et al. (148) reported a significant decrease in ERPF in infant rhesus monkeys six months following SWL treatment (1500 shocks at 15 kV or 2000 shocks at 18 kV). The long-term effect on renal function in humans following SWL is less clear. Lechevalleir et al. (149) performed single photon emission computed tomography (SPECT) studies pre- and post-SWL (30 days) in 12 patients treated with a piezoelectric lithotriptor. Four of the 12 kidneys treated with SWL demonstrated a greater than 4% loss of local tracer uptake. Williams and Thomas (150) evaluated ERPF in patients 17 to 21 months after SWL, and noted a significant decrease in relative ERPF. Cass et al. (151) reported an average 22% reduction in the estimated GFR in patients with a solitary kidney undergoing SWL. In contrast to this study, Chandhoke et al. (152) did not find any long-term deterioration in renal function, as measured by GFR, following SWL in patients with either a solitary kidney or renal insufficiency.

The long-term effect on renal function after SWL in the pediatric population has also been questioned (114,153–160). Although SWL is generally well tolerated in children, the concern

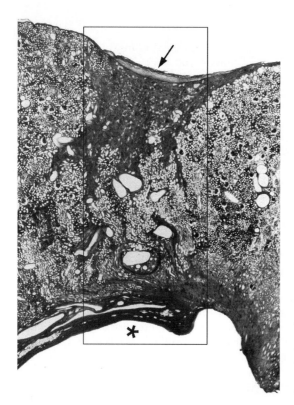

FIGURE 6 Histologic section from a pig kidney treated with 2000 shocks at 24 kV in an unmodified HM3. The acute injury induced at the site of F2 (seen within rectangle) resulted in a scar that extends from the renal capsule (*arrow*) to the renal medulla. The renal papilla is no longer present, being reduced to scar tissue (*asterisk*). *Source*: From Ref. 188.

is that a greater proportion of the kidney is exposed to the effects of shock waves due to its smaller size and the fixed size of the lithotriptor focal area. Corbally et al. (155) noted an immediate 15% decrease in diethyl triamine penta-acetic acid (DTPA)-measured GFR following SWL in pediatric patients. Adams et al. (153) reported the results of SWL in a group of 44 pediatric patients and noted normal renal growth in 14 treated renal units after a mean follow-up time of 23 months. Lottmann et al. (161) assessed the effects of SWL in 15 pediatric kidneys using pre and post-treatment (at least six months) dimercapto-succinic acid (DMSA) renal scans. A DMSA renal scan at six months or longer after SWL revealed no evidence of parenchymal scar. A long-term study (mean nine years) by Lifshitz et al. (162) evaluated actual and predicted renal growth rates in 29 pediatric patients treated with the unmodified HM3 lithotriptor. The treated kidneys were stratified into normal and abnormal groups based on a history of renal surgery, evidence of recurrent infections, and obvious anatomic abnormalities. At treatment, the abnormal group of kidneys seemed to be smaller than expected, whereas the group of normal kidneys was very close to the predicted mean. At follow-up, both groups showed the same trend toward an age-adjusted reduction in renal growth at follow-up. The authors concluded that the alterations in renal growth patterns observed could be secondary to the shock wave injury or to some underlying pathology intrinsic to pediatric kidneys with urolithiasis.

Although SWL has been shown to be efficacious in the pediatric population, conflicting reports exist regarding the long-term renal effects on the growing kidney. Therefore, it is imperative to use the lowest treatment settings (power and number of shocks) that will still achieve stone fragmentation.

Hypertension

Early retrospective studies suggested that SWL may be associated with significant changes in blood pressure (Table 1) (163,164). Lingeman et al. (165) reported that 8.2% of 243 patients who were normotensive at the time of SWL developed an increase in blood pressure requiring antihypertensive medication. The association between SWL and the development of HTN

TABLE 1 Blood Pressure Changes Following Shock Wave Lithotripsy

Reference	Length of study (mo)	Number of shocks		Change in incidence of hypertension	Change in diastolic blood pressure
		Range	Mean		
Liedl et al. 1988 (189)	40	NR	1043	NC	NR
Williams et al. (150)	21	800–2000	1400	↑	↑
Puppo et al. (143)	12	1100–1900	1380	NC	NC
Montgomery et al. 1989 (190)	29	110–3300	1429	↑	NC
Lingeman et al. 1990 (167)		NR	1289	NC	↑
Yokoyama et al. (166)	19	1500–3000	NR	NR	↑
Janetschek et al. (168)	26	2600–3000	2735	↑ (60- to 80-year-old age group)	↑ (60- to 80-year-old age group)
Jewett et al. 1998 (191)	24	NR	4411	NC	NC
Strohmaier et al. 2000	24	NR	NR	↑	↑
Elves et al. 2000 (192)	26.4	NR	5281	NC[a]	NC[a]
Krambeck et al. (169)	228	500–4500	1125	↑	NR

[a]Shockwave lithotripsy-treated patients compared with control group not undergoing treatment.
Abbreviations: NC, no change; NR, not reported; ↑, increased.
Source: From Ref. 187.

is complicated by the fact that the annual incidence of new-onset HTN in untreated men aged 30 to 60 years is 6%. In contrast to this study, a retrospective study by Yokoyama et al. (166) reported an annualized incidence of new-onset HTN of only 0.65% in patients treated with the HM3 for either renal or ureteral calculi. However, there was a statistically significant increase in diastolic blood pressure (DBP) that appeared to correlate with the amount of shock-wave energy administered.

In order to more clearly delineate the relationship between SWL and HTN, Lingeman et al. (167) retrospectively surveyed 961 patients treated at Methodist Hospital of Indiana for nephrolithiasis. The patients were divided into groups based on exposure to SWL (SWL, URS, PNL). The annualized incidence of HTN (2.4%) in the SWL patients did not differ significantly from that in the control patients (4.0%). There was no correlation between the incidence of HTN and the laterality of treatments, the number of shock waves administered, the voltage applied, or the power index. However, there was a statistically significant rise in DBP after treatment with SWL (0.78 mmHg) that was not present in the control group (−0.88 mmHg). A second set of blood pressure measurements was conducted approximately four years after treatment in 749 patients (77.9%). Again, there was no difference in the annualized incidence of new-onset HTN between the groups (2.1% vs. 1.6%). There remained a statistically significant increase in the annualized mean DBP in the SWL-treated patients even after controlling for pretreatment blood pressure, gender, age, time since treatment, direct shock wave exposure to the kidney, and multiple shock wave sessions.

The association between SWL and HTN has also been studied prospectively. Knapp et al. (61) calculated the intrarenal resistive index (RI) in 76 patients treated with a Dornier MFL 5000 lithotriptor. In 15 of 20 patients over 60 years of age, the RI was higher than the upper limit of normal immediately following SWL in the treated kidney but not in the untreated kidney. At 26 months of follow-up in these patients, the RI increased in all nine patients who developed HTN and a strong positive correlation (0.903) between the pathologic RI levels and blood pressure was found. A subsequent study by the same group (168) emphasized the age-dependent risk of developing HTN after SWL. They concluded that patients older than 60 years are at greatest risk for disturbances of renal perfusion, as assessed by RI, and new-onset HTN.

A recent retrospective study by Krambeck et al. (169) with 19 years of follow-up reported a significant increase in the development of HTN in patients who had undergone SWL versus age- and sex-matched controls even after excluding patients with pre-existing HTN. The development of HTN was related to bilateral SWL treatment, but no correlation was found with the total number of shocks or intensity of the SWL treatment. The authors speculate that renal parenchymal or vascular changes may be responsible for the HTN seen in the SWL group, and this effect may be exacerbated by bilateral SWL treatments. The mechanism by which SWL may lead to HTN remains unclear. The renin-angiotensin system has been proposed as a factor in the development of HTN after SWL, but conflicting reports exist as to the importance of its contribution (51,148,170).

Stone-Related Effects

Obvious limitations of interpreting the SWL literature are the different definitions of "stone free" status or "success" rates, and the significance of residual fragments. Carr et al. (171) documented all new stone formation in 298 consecutive patients who initially were determined to be stone free after SWL and compared those findings to 62 patients treated with PNL. Their data showed a significant increase in the rate of new stone formation within one year of SWL treatment compared to PNL. The authors suggested that even the finest residual stone debris remaining after SWL could act as a nidus for subsequent stone growth.

Another observation has been the significant rise in the number of calcium phosphate (CaP) stone formers over the last three decades (172,173). These CaP stone formers underwent a significantly higher number of procedures than the idiopathic calcium oxalate stone formers when adjusted for number of stones and duration of stone disease, and perhaps more intriguing, the brushite stone formers were treated with significantly more SWL procedures. SWL is known to cause damage to the microvessels and collecting duct of the renal papilla, and may induce an abnormality in urinary acidification. Brushite stone formers have considerable pathologic alterations in the renal cortex and papilla including interstitial fibrosis, tubular atrophy, glomerular obsolescence, and deposition of large amounts of hydroxyapatite in the lumens of inner medullary collecting ducts (174).

Diabetes Mellitus

A recent long-term retrospective study by Krambeck et al. (169) has found higher incidence of developing DM in patients who had been treated with SWL for renal and proximal ureteral stones. A structured questionnaire was sent to 578 patients identified by retrospective chart review as being treated with the HM3 lithotriptor from January to December 1985. The questionnaire data from the 288 (58.9%) responders was then compared to age- and sex-matched controls in which urolithiasis was managed nonsurgically. Patients treated with SWL were more likely to have new-onset, medically treated DM at 19 years follow-up ($P < 0.001$) even after controlling for obesity and change in body mass index. The new-onset DM was related to the total number of shocks delivered and the intensity of the SWL treatment. The authors hypothesize that the DM in the SWL group may be the result of damage to pancreatic islet cells, as the pancreas is known to be in the blast path of the Dornier HM3 regardless of the side being treated. As mentioned previously, acute pancreatitis and elevations in pancreatic enzymes have been reported following SWL treatment (137,175). The risk may be greatest with the HM3 lithotriptor as it has the largest focal area; however, study of the long-term adverse effects of newer lithotriptors warrants investigation as these machines are capable of causing tissue damage by generating high pressures at F2 despite smaller focal zones.

STRATEGIES TO REDUCE SHOCK WAVE-INDUCED INJURY

Willis et al. reported a practical way to protect the treated kidney during SWL (176). Prior to giving a clinical dose of 2000 shocks at 24 kV with an unmodified HM3 to the lower pole of a kidney, a pretreatment dose of 100 to 500 shock waves at 12 kV is administered, followed by the full clinical dose to the same site. Under those conditions the normal lesion of about 6% is reduced to about 0.3%, a highly significant change (Fig. 7). This pretreatment protocol substantially limits the renal injury normally caused by SWL, and the threshold for protection may be less than 100 shocks. Although the mechanism of protection is not completely clear, the pretreatment dose of shock waves may induce a significant vasoconstrictive event that works to prevent an incoming stress from shearing the vessel wall, or it may reduce cavitation-induced injury. Other investigators (177–181) have attempted to protect the kidney from SWL injury by the administration of certain drugs including nifedipine, allopurinol, verapamil, and aminophylline. These medications may have a direct action on tubular cells or affect the renal vasculature.

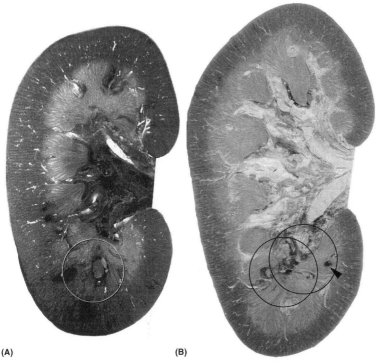

FIGURE 7 (**A**) Digitized image of a pig kidney treated with 2000 shocks at 24 kV. (**B**) Digitized image of a pig kidney treated with 500 shocks at 12 kV followed immediately with 2000 shocks at 24 kV to the same pole. This pretreatment protocol protects the kidney from the predicted lesion induced by 2000 shocks at 24 kV. Arrowhead shows the only site of hemorrhage in the kidney that received the pretreatment protocol. The sites of F2 are signified by an open circle. *Source*: From Ref. 188.

In addition to the protection efforts mentioned before, there are general strategies of shock wave delivery that will improve the outcomes of SWL irrespective of the lithotriptor used. First, treat at low power (12–15 kV), and only increase the power if the stone is not breaking. Second, improved outcomes following SWL have been demonstrated with the use of adequate anesthesia (182,183). This approach allows for proper localization and targeting of the stone for treatment. Slowing the rate of shock wave administration has also been shown to improve the effectiveness of SWL (184–186) Pace et al. (184) reported that treating at a rate of 60 shocks per minute yields better outcomes than at 120 shocks per minute while maintaining an acceptable treatment time. Finally, the lowest treatment settings (power and number of shocks) that will achieve stone fragmentation should be used in an effort to minimize shock wave-induced tissue injury.

CONCLUSION

The awareness that SWL is associated with adverse effects has never been more realized. Investigation into these effects is an important area of ongoing research. A fundamental knowledge of shock wave physics and the potential mechanisms for tissue injury is important in predicting and preventing the acute and chronic complications of SWL. However, the most important factor in avoiding complications is proper patient selection. Long-term prospective clinical trials are still needed to improve our understanding of the chronic effects of SWL.

REFERENCES

1. Chaussy C, Fuchs G. Extracorporeal lithotripsy in the treatment of renal lithiasis. 5 years' experience. J Urol (Paris) 1986; 92:339–343.

2. Chaussy C, Schuller J, Schmiedt E, et al. Extracorporeal shock-wave lithotripsy (ESWL) for treatment of urolithiasis. Urology 1984; 23(5 Spec No):59–66.
3. Drach GW, Dretler S, Fair W, et al. Report of the United States cooperative study of extracorporeal shock wave lithotripsy. J Urol 1986; 135:1127–1133.
4. Sturtevant B. Shock wave physics of lithotriptors. In: Smith AD, Badlani GH, Bagley DH, et al., eds. Smith's Textbook of Endourology. St. Louis, Mosby: Quality Medical Publishing, Inc, 1996:529–552.
5. Zhong P, Preminger GM. Differing modes of shock-wave generation. Semin Urol 1994; 12:2–14.
6. McAteer JA, Bailey MR, Williams JC Jr, et al. Strategies for improved shock wave lithotripsy. Minerva Urol Nefrol 2005; 57:271–287.
7. Cleveland RO, McAteer JA, Muller R. Time-lapse nondestructive assessment of shock wave damage to kidney stones in vitro using micro-computed tomography. J Acoust Soc Am 2001; 110:1733–1736.
8. Eisenmenger W. The mechanisms of stone fragmentation in ESWL. Ultrasound Med Biol 2001; 27:683–693.
9. Sapozhnikov OA, Cleveland RO, Bailey MR, et al. Modeling of stresses generated by lithotripter shock wave in cylindrical kidney stones. In: Chapelon JY, Lafon C, eds. Proceedings of the 3rd International Symposium of Therapeutic Ultrasound. Lyon, France: 2003:323–328.
10. Gracewski SM, Dahake G, Ding Z, et al. Internal stress wave measurements in solids subjected to lithotripter pulses. J Acoust Soc Am 1993; 94(2 Pt 1):652–661.
11. Xi X, Zhong P. Dynamic photoelastic study of the transient stress field in solids during shock wave lithotripsy. J Acoust Soc Am 2001; 109:1226–1239.
12. Coleman AJ, Saunders JE, Crum LA, et al. Acoustic cavitation generated by an extracorporeal shock-wave lithotripter. Ultrasound Med Biol 1987; 13:69–76.
13. Crum LA. Cavitation microjets as a contributory mechanism for renal calculi disintegration in ESWL. J Urol 1988; 140:1587–1590.
14. Vakil N, Everbach EC. Transient acoustic cavitation in gallstone fragmentation: a study of gallstones fragmented in vivo. Ultrasound Med Biol 1993; 19:331–342.
15. Zhong P, Chuong CJ. Propagation of shock waves in elastic solids caused by cavitation microjet impact. I: theoretical formulation. J Acoust Soc Am 1993; 94:19–28.
16. Zhong P, Chuong CJ, Preminger GM. Propagation of shock waves in elastic solids caused by cavitation microjet impact. II. Application in extracorporeal shock wave lithotripsy. J Acoust Soc Am 1993; 94:29–36.
17. Bailey MR, Blackstock DT, Cleveland RO, et al. Comparison of electrohydraulic lithotripters with rigid and pressure-release ellipsoidal reflectors. I. Acoustic fields. J Acoust Soc Am 1998; 104:2517–2524.
18. Bailey MR, Blackstock DT, Cleveland RO, et al. Comparison of electrohydraulic lithotripters with rigid and pressure-release ellipsoidal reflectors. II. Cavitation fields. J Acoust Soc Am 1999; 106: 1149–1160.
19. Lokhandwalla M, Sturtevant B. Fracture mechanics model of stone comminution in ESWL and implications for tissue damage. Phys Med Biol 2000; 45:1923–1940.
20. Lifshitz DA, Williams JC Jr, Sturtevant B, et al. Quantitation of shock wave cavitation damage in vitro. Ultrasound Med Biol 1997; 23:461–471.
21. Zhong P, Zhou Y, Zhu S. Dynamics of bubble oscillation in constrained media and mechanisms of vessel rupture in SWL. Ultrasound Med Biol 2001; 27:119–134.
22. Evan AP, Willis LR, McAteer JA, et al. Kidney damage and renal functional changes are minimized by waveform control that suppresses cavitation in shock wave lithotripsy. J Urol 2002; 168 (4 Pt 1):1556–1562.
23. Lokhandwalla M, McAteer JA, Williams JC Jr, et al. Mechanical haemolysis in shock wave lithotripsy (SWL): II. In vitro cell lysis due to shear. Phys Med Biol 2001; 46:1245–1264.
24. Rigatti P, Colombo R, Centemero A, et al. Histological and ultrastructural evaluation of extracorporeal shock wave lithotripsy-induced acute renal lesions: preliminary report. Eur Urol 1989; 16:207–211.
25. Evan AP, Willis LR, Connors B, et al. Shock wave lithotripsy-induced renal injury. Am J Kidney Dis 1991; 17:445–450.
26. Willis LR, Evan AP, Connors BA, et al. Relationship between kidney size, renal injury, and renal impairment induced by shock wave lithotripsy. J Am Soc Nephrol 1999; 10:1753–1762.
27. Chaussy C. Extracorporeal Shockwave Lithotripsy: New Aspects in the Treatment of Kidney Stone Disease. Basel, Switzerland: S Karger, 1982.
28. Knapp PM, Kulb TB, Lingeman JE, et al. Extracorporeal shock wave lithotripsy-induced perirenal hematomas. J Urol 1988; 139:700–703.
29. Rubin JI, Arger PH, Pollack HM, et al. Kidney changes after extracorporeal shock wave lithotripsy: CT evaluation. Radiology 1987; 162(1 Pt 1):21–24.
30. Baumgartner BR, Dickey KW, Ambrose SS, et al. Kidney changes after extracorporeal shock wave lithotripsy: appearance on MR imaging. Radiology 1987; 163:531–534.
31. Kaude JV, Williams CM, Millner MR, et al. Renal morphology and function immediately after extracorporeal shock-wave lithotripsy. Am J Roentgenol 1985; 145:305–313.

32. Dyer RB, Karstaedt N, McCullough DL, et al. Magnetic resonance imaging evaluation of immediate and intermediate changes in kidneys treated with extracorporeal shock wave lithotripsy. In: Lingeman JE, Newman DM, eds. Shock Wave Lithotripsy 2: Urinary and Biliary Lithotripsy. New York: Plenum Press, 1989:203–205.

33. Lingeman JE, McAteer JA, Kempson SA, et al. Bioeffects of extracorporeal shock-wave lithotripsy. Strategy for research and treatment. Urol Clin North Am 1988; 15:507–514.

34. Lingeman JE, Woods J, Toth PD, et al. The role of lithotripsy and its side effects. J Urol 1989; 141 (3 Pt 2):793–797.

35. Lingeman JE, McAteer JA, Kempson SA, et al. Bioeffects of extracorporeal shock wave lithotripsy. J Endourol 1987; 1:89–98.

36. Jaeger P, Redha F, Marquardt K, et al. Morphological and functional changes in canine kidneys following extracorporeal shock-wave treatment. Urol Int 1995; 54:48–58.

37. Jaeger P, Redha F, Uhlschmid G, et al. Morphological changes in canine kidneys following extracorporeal shock wave treatment. Urol Res 1988; 16:161–166.

38. Seitz G, Pletzer K, Neisius D, et al. Pathologic-anatomic alterations in human kidneys after extracorporeal piezoelectric shock wave lithotripsy. J Endourol 1991; 5:17–20.

39. Karlin GS, Urivetsky M, Smith AD. Side effects of extracorporeal shock wave lithotripsy: assessment of urinary excretion of renal enzymes as evidence of tubular injury. In: Lingeman JE, Newman DM, eds. Shock Wave Lithotripsy II: Urinary and Biliary Lithotripsy. New York: Plenum Press, 1989:3–6.

40. Assimos DG, Boyce WH, Furr EG, et al. Selective elevation of urinary enzyme levels after extracorporeal shock wave lithotripsy. J Urol 1989; 142:687–690.

41. Morris JS, Husmann DA, Wilson WT, et al. Temporal effects of shock wave lithotripsy. J Urol 1991; 145:881–883.

42. Sarica K, Suzer O, Yaman O, et al. Leucine aminopeptidase enzymuria: quantification of renal tubular damage following extracorporeal shock wave lithotripsy. Int Urol Nephrol 1996; 28:621–626.

43. Weichert-Jacobsen K, Stockle M, Loch T, et al. Urinary leakage of tubular enzymes after shock wave lithotripsy. Eur Urol 1998; 33:104–110.

44. Kirkali Z, Kirkali G, Tahiri Y. The effect of extracorporeal electromagnetic shock waves on renal proximal tubular function. Int Urol Nephrol 1994; 26:255–257.

45. Hasegawa S, Kato K, Takashi M, et al. Increased levels of calbindin-D in serum and urine from patients treated by extracorporeal shock wave lithotripsy. J Urol 1993; 149:1414–1418.

46. Jung K, Kirschner P, Wille A, et al. Excretion of urinary enzymes after extracorporeal shock wave lithotripsy: a critical reevaluation. J Urol 1993; 149:1409–1413.

47. Recker F, Hofmann W, Bex A, et al. Quantitative determination of urinary marker proteins: a model to detect intrarenal bioeffects after extracorporeal lithotripsy. J Urol 1992; 148(3 Pt 2):1000–1006.

48. Krongrad A, Saltzman B, Tannenbaum M. Enzymuria after extracorporeal shock wave lithotripsy. J Endourol 1991; 5:209–211.

49. Karlin GS, Schulsinger D, Urivetsky M, et al. Absence of persisting parenchymal damage after extracorporeal shock wave lithotripsy as judged by excretion of renal tubular enzymes. J Urol 1990; 144:13–14.

50. Kishimoto T, Senju M, Sugimoto T, et al. Effects of high energy shock wave exposure on renal function during extracorporeal shock wave lithotripsy for kidney stones. Eur Urol 1990; 18:290–298.

51. Karlsen SJ, Berg KJ. Acute changes in renal function following extracorporeal shock wave lithotripsy in patients with a solitary functioning kidney. J Urol 1991; 145:253–256.

52. Gilbert BR, Riehle RA, Vaughan ED Jr. Extracorporeal shock wave lithotripsy and its effect on renal function. J Urol 1988; 139:482–485.

53. Jaeger P, Constantinides C. Canine kidneys: changes in blood and urine chemistry after exposure to extracorporeal shock waves. In: Lingeman JE, Newman DM, eds. Shock Wave Lithotripsy II: Urinary and Biliary Lithotripsy. New York: Plenum Press, 1989:7–10.

54. Willis LR, Evan AP, Lingeman JE. The impact of high-dose lithotripsy on renal function. Contemp Urol 1999; 11:45–50.

55. Willis LR, Evan AP, Connors BA, et al. Effects of extracorporeal shock wave lithotripsy to one kidney on bilateral glomerular filtration rate and PAH clearance in minipigs. J Urol 1996; 156:1502–1506.

56. Bomanji J, Boddy SA, Britton KE, et al. Radionuclide evaluation pre- and postextracorporeal shock wave lithotripsy for renal calculi. J Nucl Med 1987; 28:1284–1289.

57. Saxby MF. Effects of percutaneous nephrolithotomy and extracorporeal shock wave lithotripsy on renal function and prostaglandin excretion. Scand J Urol Nephrol 1997; 31:141–144.

58. Grantham JR, Millner MR, Kaude JV, et al. Renal stone disease treated with extracorporeal shock wave lithotripsy: short-term observations in 100 patients. Radiology 1986; 158:203–206.

59. Mostafavi MR, Chavez DR, Cannillo J, et al. Redistribution of renal blood flow after SWL evaluated by Gd-DTPA-enhanced magnetic resonance imaging. J Endourol 1998; 12:9–12.

60. Kataoka T, Kasahara T, Kobashikawa K, et al. Changes in renal blood flow after treatment with ESWL in patients with renal stones. Studies using ultrasound color Doppler method. Nippon Hinyokika Gakkai Zasshi 1993; 84:851–856.

61. Knapp R, Frauscher F, Helweg G, et al. Age-related changes in resistive index following extracorporeal shock wave lithotripsy. J Urol 1995; 154:955–958.

62. Nazaroglu H, Akay AF, Bukte Y, et al. Effects of extracorporeal shock-wave lithotripsy on intrarenal resistive index. Scand J Urol Nephrol 2003; 37:408–412.

63. Kostakopoulos A, Stavropoulos NJ, Macrychoritis C, et al. Subcapsular hematoma due to ESWL: risk factors: a study of 4,247 patients. Urol Int 1995; 55:21–24.

64. Streem SB, Yost A. Extracorporeal shock wave lithotripsy in patients with bleeding diatheses. J Urol 1990; 144:1347–1348.

65. Christensen JG, McCullough DL, Cline WA Sr. Extracorporeal shock-wave lithotripsy in hemophiliac patient. Urology 1989; 33:424–426.

66. Newman LH, Saltzman B. Identifying risk factors in development of clinically significant post-shock-wave lithotripsy subcapsular hematomas. Urology 1991; 38:35–38.

67. Dhar NB, Thornton J, Karafa MT, et al. A multivariate analysis of risk factors associated with subcapsular hematoma formation following electromagnetic shock wave lithotripsy. J Urol 2004; 172 (6 Pt 1):2271–2274.

68. Delius M, Enders G, Xuan ZR, et al. Biological effects of shock waves: kidney damage by shock waves in dogs--dose dependence. Ultrasound Med Biol 1988; 14:117–122.

69. Delius M, Jordan M, Eizenhoefer H, et al. Biological effects of shock waves: kidney haemorrhage by shock waves in dogs—administration rate dependence. Ultrasound Med Biol 1988; 14:689–694.

70. Delius M, Jordan M, Liebich HG, et al. Biological effects of shock waves: effect of shock waves on the liver and gallbladder wall of dogs—administration rate dependence. Ultrasound Med Biol 1990; 16:459–466.

71. Willis LR, Evan AP, Connors BA, et al. Shockwave lithotripsy: dose-related effects on renal structure, hemodynamics, and tubular function. J Endourol 2005; 19:90–101.

72. Thomas R, Roberts J, Sloane B, et al. Effects of extracorporeal shock wave lithotripsy on renal function. J Endourol 1988; 2:141–144.

73. Orestona F, Caronia N, Gallo G, et al. Functional aspects of the kidney after shock wave lithotripsy. In: Lingeman JE, Newman DM, eds. Shock Wave Lithotripsy II: Urinary and Biliary Lithotripsy. New York: Plenum Press, 1989:15–17.

74. Lam HS, Lingeman JE, Barron M, et al. Staghorn calculi: analysis of treatment results between initial percutaneous nephrostolithotomy and extracorporeal shock wave lithotripsy monotherapy with reference to surface area. J Urol 1992; 147:1219–1225.

75. Muller-Mattheis VG, Schmale D, Seewald M, et al. Bacteremia during extracorporeal shock wave lithotripsy of renal calculi. J Urol 1991; 146:733–736.

76. Gasser TC, Frei R. Risk of bacteraemia during extracorporeal shock wave lithotripsy. Br J Urol 1993; 71:17–20.

77. Mariappan P, Smith G, Bariol SV, et al. Stone and pelvic urine culture and sensitivity are better than bladder urine as predictors of urosepsis following percutaneous nephrolithotomy: a prospective clinical study. J Urol 2005; 173:1610–1614.

78. McAleer IM, Kaplan GW, Bradley JS, et al. Staghorn calculus endotoxin expression in sepsis. Urology 2002; 59:601.

79. McAleer IM, Kaplan GW, Bradley JS, et al. Endotoxin content in renal calculi. J Urol 2003; 169:1813–1814.

80. Paterson RF, Kuo RL, Lingeman JE. Staghorn calculus endotoxin expression in sepsis. Urology 2003; 62:197–198.

81. Scherz HC, Parsons CL. Prophylactic antibiotics in urology. Urol Clin North Am 1987; 14:265–271.

82. Peiser J, Kaneti J, Lissmer L, et al. Perinephric inflammatory process following extracorporeal shock wave lithotripsy. Int Urol Nephrol 1991; 23:107–111.

83. Davidson T, Tung K, Constant O, et al. Kidney rupture and psoas abscess after ESWL. Br J Urol 1991; 68:657–658.

84. Federmann M, Kley HK. Miliary tuberculosis after extracorporeal shock-wave lithotripsy. N Engl J Med 1990; 323:1212.

85. Greenwald BD, Tunkel AR, Morgan KM, et al. Candidal endophthalmitis after lithotripsy of renal calculi. South Med J 1992; 85:773–774.

86. Westh H, Mogensen P. Extracorporeal shock wave lithotripsy of a kidney stone complicated with Candida albicans septicaemia and endophthalmitis. Case report. Scand J Urol Nephrol 1990; 24:81.

87. Kremer I, Gaton DD, Baniel J, et al. Klebsiella metastatic endophthalmitis: a complication of shock wave lithotripsy. Ophthalmic Surg 1990; 21:206–208.

88. Karamalegos AZ, Diokno AC, Moylan DF. Formation of perinephric abscess following extracorporeal shock-wave lithotripsy. Urology 1989; 34:277–280.

89. Unal B, Kara S, Bilgili Y, et al. Giant abdominal wall abscess dissecting into thorax as a complication of ESWL. Urology 2005; 65:389.

90. Pettersson B, Tiselius HG. Are prophylactic antibiotics necessary during extracorporeal shockwave lithotripsy? Br J Urol 1989; 63:449–452.

25 | Complications of Percutaneous Lithotripsy

C. Charles Wen and Stephen Y. Nakada
Division of Urology, School of Medicine and Public Health, University of Wisconsin, Madison, Wisconsin, U.S.A.

INTRODUCTION

The first documented percutaneous nephrostomy was performed by Thomas Hillier, MD, in 1865; however, it was not until 1955 when Willard Goodwin published his work on percutaneous nephrostomy for hydronephrosis, that percutaneous nephrostomy gained widespread acceptance (1,2). Goodwin's report provided the foundation for minimally invasive renal surgery. More than 20 years later, Ferstrom described the first planned percutaneous pyelolithotomy (3). Stone extraction required fluoroscopic imaging and endoscopic skill to break and remove renal stones. Since then advances in endoscopic equipment including the fiberoptic light source have helped to make percutaneous access to the kidney, a useful route for almost all renal and ureteral surgery involving the upper collecting system.

ANATOMY REVIEW

In order to prevent complications in percutaneous renal surgery the urologist must understand renal anatomy. Below the skin the latissimus dorsi muscle and the erector spinae muscles overlie the intercostals muscles and ribs. Intercostal vessels and nerves run along the costal groove located on the inferior aspect of each rib. Any intercostal access should be obtained immediately above the rib to avoid damage to the neurovascular elements. The upper pole of the left kidney typically extends to the upper border of the 11th rib at the level of the 12th thoracic vertebrae while the top of the right kidney being pushed down by the liver is usually at the first lumbar vertebrae. Deep to the ribs is the diaphragm, which attaches to the inferior border of the 12th rib. Between the diaphragm and the ribs is the parietal pleura which is reflected to the level of the 10th rib in the mid axillary line and usually crosses the 12th rib at its mid-point, making the lateral half of this rib inferior to the pleural margin. The diaphragm comes down to cover the posterior upper pole portions of both kidneys while the middle and lower poles rest on the psoas and quadratus lumborum. The slope of the psoas muscles causes the lower pole of the kidney to tilt anteriorly, this allows for a straight tract along the long axis of the kidney if the posterior upper pole calyx is used for renal access (4). Between the kidneys and muscles is a layer of pararenal retroperitoneal fat which surrounds the perirenal fascia commonly called Gerota's fascia. Gerota's fascia is made of anterior and posterior leaves, which fuse medially, laterally, and superiorly to enclose perirenal fat, adrenal gland, kidney, and ureter. Inferiorly Gerota's fascia remains open and is contiguous with the retroperitoneal fascia (Fig. 1).

The anterior relation of the left kidney include the left adrenal, spleen, stomach, tail of pancreas, jejunum, and splenic flexure of the colon, whereas the right kidney is in association with the right adrenal, liver, duodenum, and hepatic flexure of the colon.

The typical kidney has seven to nine renal papillae each cupped by a corresponding minor calyx. These calyces are usually arranged in two rows with the posterior calyces opening posteriorly and the anterior calyces opening laterally. These minor calyces narrow to an infundibulum before joining other minor calyces to form a major calyx. Typically three major calyces join to form a single renal pelvis, but there can be great variability in calyceal formation. The renal pelvis may also be bifid which results in a narrower pelvis. Care should be taken when treating a bifid system, as the narrow pelvis does not have the same parenchymal backing of a narrow calyceal infundibulum.

The renal artery and vein are typically anterior to the renal pelvis. The artery normally has four to five branches. The earliest branch is the posterior segmental artery. It is the only branch located posterior to the renal pelvis, making it the most susceptible to injury during percutaneous

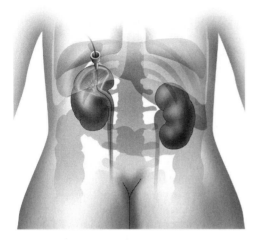

FIGURE 1   Renal anatomy.

procedures, especially when access is too medial. Brödels line is an avascular plane between the anterior and the posterior blood supplies approximately 1 cm from the lateral margin of the kidney on the posterior aspect. When obtaining access to the collecting system a needle path that is posterolateral aimed end-on to a posterior calyx will traverse Brödel's line transparenchymally minimizing risk of injury to major blood vessels (5). The arterial supply of the renal pelvis and ureter also comes from the main renal artery entering from the medial aspect. Any reconstructive surgery should consider the vascular supply, and incisions in the proximal ureter should be made laterally.

Renal anatomical variants are not uncommon, and horseshoe kidney is the most common renal fusion anomaly with an incidence of about 1 in 400 persons worldwide. During development the kidneys fuse at the lower poles and the inferior mesenteric artery halts their ascent. The fusion prevents normal rotation of the kidneys, leaving the renal pelvis anterior and the calyces posterior. The whole vascular supply usually enters medially making injury during percutaneous renal surgery (PRS) and access less likely (6). In horseshoe kidneys upper pole access is favorable, as the upper pole tends to be lower making pleural injury less likely, and their anterior displacement make the shorter upper pole nephrostomy tracts more desirable (Table 1)

PREOPERATIVE IMAGING

Although knowledge of renal anatomy is essential, it is the variations in anatomy that often lead to complications. Therefore, proper imaging is required for preoperative evaluation and surgical planning. Intravenous pyelogram (IVP) is usually sufficient for uncomplicated cases; however, advances in technology and decrease in cost have allowed computed tomography (CT) to be the predominant imaging modality for the upper urinary tract. Although CT offers the

TABLE 1   Indications for Percutaneous Renal Surgery

Percutaneous renal drainage
Whitaker test
Renal cyst aspiration and sclerotherapy
Renal biopsy
Percutaneous nephrostolithotomy
Antegrade endopyelotomy
Percutaneous resection of urothelial cancer
Percutaneous endopyeloplasty
Calyceal diverticulum with or without lithopaxy
Percutaneous infundibuloplasty
Incision or dilation of ureteral stricture
Perfusion chemolysis for nephrolithiasis
Percutaneous cryoablation or radiofrequency ablation

highest sensitivity for identifying renal calculi and masses, due to the axial imaging of CT, some anatomical variants such as a bifid renal pelvis may be more apparent on IVP which images the kidney in the anterior to posterior (AP) view. This can be overcome with the use of three-dimensional reconstructions or coronal slices for CT and magnetic resonance imaging (MRI) as well as coronal slices on MRI. Additionally, CT-urogram as well as MRI urography can be used to enhance evaluation of the collecting system (7).

Preoperative ultrasound can also be used to assess the level of hydronephrosis, and for determining the feasibility of percutaneous access in complicated cases.

Knowledge of the vascular anatomy may be necessary for planning the correction of ureteropelvic junction (UPJ) obstructions, and identifying crossing vessels. CT or MRI angiography can be performed to better, elucidate the renal vasculature. When combined with three-dimensional reconstructions the anatomy becomes easier to interpret (8).

Nuclear imaging studies may be used to determine differential function and assess obstruction. A dimercaptosuccinic acid (DMSA) scan provides percent renal function to assess the prudence of performing renal surgery versus nephrectomy for an impaired kidney (cutoff is generally <20% for adults). Diuretic renography with mercapto acetyl triglycine (MAG3) or diethylene triamine penta-acetic acid (DTPA) can be performed to help determine if a UPJ or ureteral obstruction would benefit from surgical correction.

PREOPERATIVE EVALUATION

Proper preoperative evaluation is the cornerstone to preventing complications. Having accurate knowledge of patient risk factors can allow correction preoperatively and increased caution intra-operatively. The only absolute contraindications to PRS are uncorrected bleeding diathesis, or suspicion of a hydatid fluid collection (9,10). Strong contraindications include active urinary tract infection, and medical comorbidities making patients unfit for surgery (11). Obesity in, and of, itself is not a contraindication for percutaneous surgery; however, modification to the standard technique and equipment may be required, as well as acceptance of higher complication rates in some series (Table 2) (12).

A detailed medical and surgical history along with a physical examination should be performed prior to any procedure. Special attention should be paid to contrast or shellfish allergies, valvular heart disease, surgical implants, respiratory problems, religious beliefs limiting the use of blood transfusions, and prior renal and abdominal surgery. Minimum requirements for preoperative testing include complete blood cell count, coagulation profile including prothrombin time, activated partial thromboplastin time and platelet count, blood urea nitrogen, creatinine, urinalysis, urine culture and blood typing and screening. Chest X ray (CXR) and electrocardiogram should be performed in patients with histories warranting these tests (Table 3).

For elective procedures patient should suspend medications that alter platelet function (e.g., aspirin). Patients with thrombocytopenia should consider correction with platelet transfusion. Patients taking coumadin should have coagulation factors normalized prior to surgery. Although the risk of significant bleeding problems is only 1% to 3%, the possibility of transfusion should be discussed with patients. Routine autologous or designated donor blood is not recommended at our institution.

Active urinary infections should be eradicated with appropriate antibiotic treatment. In patients with indolent or recurrent infections we recommend antibiotic treatment up to 2 weeks prior to PRS to limit the risk of perioperative infections. In patients with infections

TABLE 2   Contraindications to PRS

Absolute
Uncorrected bleeding diathesis
Suspicion of hydatid fluid
Relative
Urinary tract infection
Medical comorbidities precluding appropriate anesthesia
Body habitus

Abbreviation: PRS, percutaneous renal surgery.

TABLE 3 Preoperative Evaluation

History and physical examination
   Allergies (contrast, shellfish)
Discussion with patient regarding procedure, risks and alternatives
Review of available imaging
   Determine if additional preoperative imaging is necessary
Preoperative clearance: ECG, chest radiograph, specialty consultation if indicated
Laboratory testing: CBC, creatinine, BUN, electrolytes, INR, PTT, urine culture, type and screen

Abbreviations: BUN, blood urea nitrogen; CBC, complete blood count; INR, International Normalized Ratio; PTT, partial thromboplastin time.

associated with urinary obstruction, drainage should be considered prior to complex interventions.

PERCUTANEOUS RENAL ACCESS
Positioning and Anesthesia

General endotracheal intubation is the preferred method of anesthesia for most PRS due to the length of procedure and prone positioning. Shorter procedures may be performed with only epidural anesthesia. If regional anesthesia is utilized, a T-6 vertebral level is required for upper tract instrumentation. Local anesthesia and intravenous sedation has been reported (13).

Ureteral Catheter Placement

Prior to percutaneous access a 5 Fr open-ended catheter can be placed in a retrograde fashion to the level of the UPJ, and left in. This catheter can be used to inject contrast and air into the renal collecting system to define the posterior calyces.

Percutaneous Renal Access

At our institution a team approach is used for PRS. The urologist and uroradiologist discuss and plan the appropriate access route for each case. This is particularly beneficial as the radiologists are familiar with the patient in the rare instance that angiography and embolization is needed.

To briefly review our technique, a radiopaque object and fluoroscopic imaging is used to locate the desired calyx at the level of the skin after a ureteral access catheter has been inserted cystoscopically. An 18 g × 7–15 cm percutaneous entry needle with baseplate is directed into the renal parenchyma on end expiration using biplanar fluoroscopy. To avoid colonic injury percutaneous access should be medial to the posterior axillary line. A 21 g × 15 cm needle is advanced through the percutaneous entry needle to access the calyx. Position can be confirmed with urine aspiration and contrast injection. A 0.018 in wire is then advanced through the 21 g needle guided into the ureter or coiled in the collecting system. The percutaneous entry needle and the 21 g needle are then removed in a "pinch-pull" fashion. An 11 blade is then used to make a small incision in the skin and a 6 Fr access catheter with 4 Fr inner sheath is advanced over the wire using Seldinger technique. When the radiopaque marker for the 4 Fr inner sheath reaches the renal collecting system, the 6 Fr access catheter is advanced forward off of the stiff 4 Fr inner sheath, and the inner sheath is then removed. The 0.018 in wire can then be exchanged for a 0.35 in × 150–180 cm, Teflon-coated stiff guidewire, which is advanced down to the bladder. If there is difficulty directing the wire into the ureter, straight or angled nitinol-coated wires, and angled angiographic catheters can be used to direct the wire into the ureter. After confirmation of the guidewire in the bladder with fluoroscopy the 6 Fr access catheter can be exchanged for a 6.5 Fr × 37 cm introducer catheter, and a second 0.35 in × 150–180 cm, Teflon coated stiff guidewire can be placed and secured to the patient (safety wire).

Tract Dilation

With the patient properly anesthetized the skin incision is lengthened adjacent to the guidewire, and a 30 Fr 12 cm balloon dilator is passed over the guidewire under fluoroscopic guidance until the radiopaque marker is in the calyx. Proper balloon positioning is critical. Overaggressive balloon placement may tear a narrow calyceal infundibulum or displace a renal stone into the parenchyma or renal pelvis causing collecting system perforation. Alternatively, insufficient depth of balloon placement can lead to partial parenchymal dilation and bleeding. With the balloon in position it is inflated with saline-diluted contrast until the waist has disappeared and the balloon is rigid to touch. Care should be taken not to exceed the burst pressure of the ballon (17 atm for the Nephromax balloon) The 30 Fr nephrostomy sheath is then advanced over the balloon in a corkscrew fashion and the balloon is completely deflated and removed over the guidewire. At our institution balloon dilators are preferred over Teflon fascial dilators. Reported transfusion rates after Teflon fascial dilation range from 16% to 25% compared to balloon dilation 10% to 13% (14,15).

Some urologists have advocated a "Miniperc" procedure using 11 to 15 Fr access sheaths which have shown favorable results in regard to bleeding (16,17). Average estimated blood loss using mini percutaneous nephrostolithotomy has ranged from 25 to 83 cc compared to standard nephrostomy access 800 cc (17–20). The benefit in pediatric cases is clearer with smaller anatomy and instruments; however, indication for use of smaller access sheaths may be limited in adult cases in which PRS is usually reserved for larger stone burden or procedures which require larger instruments. In addition, animal studies have not shown an advantage to using smaller access sheaths based on renal scarring alone (21).

Most surgeons today leave a percutaneous nephrostomy drain following PRS; however, tubeless percutaneous procedures where renal drainage is provided only by an internalized ureteral stent has been described. Complication rates compared with standard PRS were comparable. Tubeless PRS does not appear to increase urinoma or transfusion rates (22).

At our institution a small caliber re-entry malecot percutaneous nephrostomy tube is placed at the end of PRS allowing for a second look nephroscopy postoperatively if necessary for 24 hours. If further surgical intervention is unnecessary the nephrostomy tube is either removed or replaced with a small pigtail nephrostomy tube or a ureteral stent depending on the antegrade drainage from the kidney.

COMPLICATIONS
Pleura

The primary risk of supracostal access for PRS is puncture of pleura and lung. An infracostal approach should be used when possible; however, a supracostal approach is often ideal for upper pole access which may be necessary for treating complex renal calculi and other intrarenal and ureteral pathology. The advantages of accessing the upper pole are direct access to upper pole calyx, UPJ and proximal ureter, good exposure of calyceal contents, and renal pelvis and the ability to operate along the long axis of the kidney allowing for less torque from a rigid nephroscope.

The upper pole of both kidneys lies anterior to the 11th and 12th ribs. Supra-12th rib access is usually transthoracic but extrapleural whereas supra 11th rib access is transthoracic and transpleural. Violation of the parietal pleura is usually clinically insignificant and identification of the inferior border of the lung on fluoroscopy during supracostal access is essential in avoiding injury to the lungs.

Complication rate of a supracostal approach is threefold greater than that of a subcostal approach with reported complication rates of 23% to 100% and 1% to 13% for supra 11th and supra 12th rib respectively (4,23). The risk of pulmonary injury is twofold greater on the right side than on the left-hand side (24).

Subclinical pneumothorax or pleural effusion may be observed with serial chest radiographs; however, signs of respiratory deterioration or increased size of pneumothorax or effusion may require placement of a thoracostomy tube (Fig. 2) (25).

Liver and Spleen

Preoperative imaging may suggest hepatomegaly and splenomagaly which may influence percutaneous access for PRS. A preoperative prone CT can help determine the safety of upper pole access. Rarely US or CT fluoroscopy may be necessary to perform percutaneous access

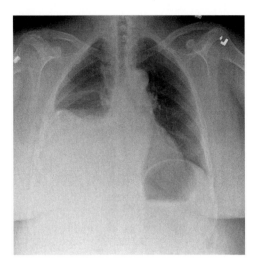

FIGURE 2 Hydrothorax.

safely. In these cases it may be advisable to perform lower pole access with a combined retrograde approach (26).

Injury to the liver during PRS is unlikely (24). Transhepatic percutaneous access is usually
without sequelae, and injury to major intrahepatic vessels after track dilation is the greatest risk.
If transhepatic access is diagnosed removal of the percutaneous nephrostomy tube with collecting
system decompression using an indwelling ureteral stent and foley catheter drainage minimizes
the risk of renobiliary fistula formation. If significant bleeding is encountered, balloon tamponade
of the track can temporize bleeding and angiographic embolization can be performed.

Splenic injury is also a rare event during PRS (27). It can lead to significant internal
bleeding requiring emergent splenectomy for uncontrollable hemorrhage (28). Suspicion for
splenic injury may arise intraoperatively in patients who are hemodynamically unstable with a
relatively clear visual field during PRS. Intraoperative abdominal ultrasound or postoperative
CT can confirm the diagnosis (29).

Colon

Injury to the colon during PRS is a rare event and is usually due to transcolonic percutaneous
renal access. Early detection is the key to successful treatment. Patients at risk for colonic injury
include those with prior abdominal surgery where colonic adhesions are more likely and those
with a history of constipation or other causes of colonic distension. Colonic injury is more likely
on the left hand side (colon more likely to be retrorenal on left), or with lower pole and excessively lateral renal access. Subtle symptoms of colonic injury include fever, leukocytosis,
abdominal tenderness, and ileus (30,31). More obvious symptoms include blood per rectum,
pneumoperitoneum, and gas or feces from the percutaneous nephrostomy (PCN) tube (31,32).

Intraoperative diagnosis is usually made after injection of contrast reveals colonic
enhancement. Delayed diagnosis is usually made on postoperative imaging, either antegrade
nephrostogram or CT scan confirming transcolonic passage of the PCN tube.

Once identified, treatment includes triple antibiotic therapy (ampicillin, gentamycin, metronidazole), bowel rest, and separation of the gastrointestinal and urinary tracts. This can be
accomplished by draining the colon and then decompressing the renal collecting system with a
PCN tube or internal ureteral stent and foley catheter. If the injury is identified intraoperatively
the PCN tube can be withdrawn into the lumen of the colon to allow the medial colonic injury
to heal (33,34). After imaging studies confirm no renal extravasation the Foley catheter can be
removed and the PCN tube is further withdrawn to lie in the pericolonic space to allow for the
lateral colonic injury to heal.

Alternatively, if identification of a colonic injury is delayed, the PCN tube should be removed
and a penrose drain be placed into the pericolonic space under fluoroscopic guidance (31). The
pericolonic drain can then be removed three to seven days later followed by discontinuation of

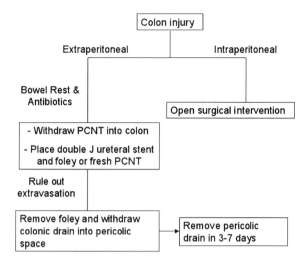

FIGURE 3 Management of colonic injury.

antibiotics 1 week later. Intraperitoneal colonic perforation or peritonitis warrants open surgical intervention (32). Generally, if a delayed diagnosis of colonic injury is made, a general surgical consult is wise (Fig. 3).

Duodenum and Jejunum

Duodenal and jejunal injury is extremely rare in PRS. Intraoperative diagnosis is by visualization of enteric fluid or enteric mucous membrane folds. Postoperative diagnosis is by CT scan revealing retroperitoneal collection associated with renoduodenal fistula (35). Open surgical repair is the classic approach for duodenal trauma; however, nonoperative management with bowel rest, nasogastric suction, with or without percutaneous duodenal drainage, and renal collecting system drainage has been described (36).

Energy Sources and Equipment Problems—Renal Trauma

Care should be taken when using energy sources. Inadvertent misdirection can result in equipment damaging leading to retained fragments, or renal trauma. In addition, the advent of new energy sources has made aggressive manipulation completely unnecessary in PRS.

A case of a ruptured plastic nephrostomy sheath was reported resulting in significant bleeding requiring transfusion. Stones that do not easily fit into the nephrostomy sheath should be further fragmented (37).

Electrohydraulic (EHL) energy can be used to fragment stones; however, the emitted spark is also capable of damaging the telescope or the collecting system. The EHL probe should always be placed in direct contact with the stone to prevent complications (38).

Ultrasound energy can be used to disintegrate most stones. Continuous flow irrigation helps to cool the tip of the probe; however, when irrigation is held, the tip can become very hot risking injury to endothelium.

Pneumatic lithotripsy can be used in conjunction with ultrasonic energy or on its own. It requires direct contact with the stone and may cause a backward movement of the stone during fragmentation. Use of pneumatic energy should be avoided in delicate tissue.

Laser energy can be used to fragment stones as well as treat renal transitional cell carcinoma (TCC). Although laser penetration depth is shallow, inadvertent laser discharge on endothelium can lead to bleeding making visualization difficult.

Contrast Allergy

Contrast reactions occur in less than 0.2% of PRS. Patients with known contrast allergies can be treated with preoperative steroids. If a reaction develops during a procedure treatment includes antihistamines, H1 and H2 blockers, steroids and epinephrine if needed (39).

Hemorrhage

Bleeding during PRS can occur during needle passage, tract dilation, nephroscopy, or postoperatively. Intraoperative bleeding can usually be limited with the nephrostomy sheath to allow for completion of the procedure. It is important to remember that bleeding from PRS can be brisk and the large instrument diameters and irrigation make underestimation of blood loss more likely.

Renal venous bleeding including renal vein injury is usually treatable with placement and clamping of a large diameter (24–28 Fr) PCN tube to allow for pelvicalyceal tamponade (40). There have been reports of renal vein perforation. A technique described to control this involves inflating a council-tip catheter in the renal pelvis at the site of renal vein perforation and confirming adequate tamponade by the lack of further extravasation of contrast medium into the vein (34,41). The PCN tube should be left in place for two to four days, and removal should be over a guidewire under fluoroscopy to allow for rapid re-insertion should bleeding recur.

Significant arterial bleeding is usually from segmental arteries as the smaller interlobular arteries are surrounded by parenchyma allowing for tamponade. Arterial bleeding can be differentiated from venous bleeding with its brighter color. Unlike venous bleeding, arterial bleeding is more likely to be resistant to conservative treatments. Initial management should control active bleeding with a clamped nephrostomy tube or a tamponade balloon (Kaye—36 Fr, 15 cm). If bleeding persists, angiography and embolization should be performed. Angioembolization is also indicated if bleeding persists postoperatively after replacement of initial blood loss, or if sudden hemorrhage occurs especially if the nephrostomy tube has been removed (Fig. 4) (42).

Late postoperative hemorrhage (after seven days) is most often caused by arteriovenous fistulas or ruptured pseudoaneurysm. Initial management is with angiography and embolization; however, if embolization fails, the next step is partial or total nephrectomy (41,42).

Loss of Material Outside the Urinary Tract

Extrarenal loss of stone fragments may occur with renal pelvis or ureteral perforation, or through the percutaneous access track. In general, loss of stone fragments is not problematic and aggressive attempts to retrieve lost fragments should be avoided (43).

Occasionally fragments can be embedded submucosally within the ureter creating symptomatic obstruction. These fragments tend to be less than 4 mm from the ureteral lumen and often require surgical treatment. Fragments greater than 4 mm from the ureteral lumen tend not to obstruct and do not require further treatment (44).

Retained Material

Retained foreign bodies are usually iatrogenic in nature resulting from broken equipment. Foreign bodies should be removed to prevent infection, granulomatous reaction, or stone formation. If discovered after PCN tube removal, initial attempts at retrieval should be made

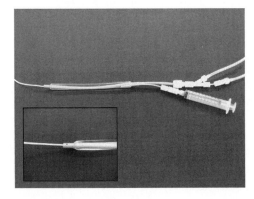

FIGURE 4   Kaye tamponade balloon.

with ureteroscopy. If discovered prior to PCN tube removal a second look nephrostomy can be performed. This procedure is well tolerated without anesthesia and involves flexible nephroscopy through the established nephrostomy track after a guidewire has been placed down to the bladder. Nitinol baskets or flexible graspers can be used to remove foreign body or residual stone fragments. Replacement of the PCN tube is often unnecessary, and if concern for drainage persists, an indwelling ureteral stent can be placed antegrade.

Stricture

UPJ obstruction is a rare complication of PRS (28,45,46). Trauma with or without retained stone fragments is the reported etiology (47). If there is question of a UPJ obstruction an antegrade nephrostogram can be obtained at the time of PCN tube removal. If drainage is delayed a small diameter loop PCN tube is left in place for two to three weeks to allow for possible postoperative edema to resolve. This can be followed by a Whitaker test to confirm obstruction.

Complete distal ureteral obstruction unrelated to ureteral calculi has been reported, following PRS with resolution after prolonged percutaneous drainage (48).

Infundibular stricture is another rare complication of PRS (49). Diagnosis is usually made by imaging revealing calyceal dilation behind the infundibulum with possible urinoma. Treatment involves percutaneous drainage of the infected calyx and retrograde or antegrade infundibulotomy.

Fistulas

Renocutaneous fistula is a rare complication following PRS. Risk factors include prolonged percutaneous drainage, untreated urinary tract infection, ureteral obstruction, radiation history, and poor nutrition status. Diagnosis is suspected with persistent drainage from the nephrostomy track and confirmed by imaging or checking drainage creatinine level. The initial treatment consists of antibiotics and decompressing the renal collecting system with an indwelling stent and foley catheter drainage. If a urinoma is present this should be drained percutaneously. Surgical intervention may be warranted if nonoperative measures fail to heal the fistula. In cases associated with TCC a biopsy should be considered.

The incidence of nephropleural fistula after supracostal access has been as high as 2.3% above the 12th rib and 6.3% above the 11th rib (25). Postoperative chest pain or shortness of breath after PRS through a supracostal approach should raise suspicion for nephropleural fistulas. Retrograde pyelography with confirmation of a fistulus tract is diagnostic, and treatment is usually conservative with renal collecting system decompression and a thoracostomy tube placed on suction initially. Thoracostomy tube can be removed after resolution of effusion or pneumothorax off suction. Persistent fistulas or loculated effusions may require thoracoscopy with decortication and possible sclerosis. Early consultation with a thoracic surgeon is recommended.

Nephrocolonic fistula and colocutaneous fistula are also rare complications of PRS (50). Initial treatment mirrors that of colonic injury during PRS including bowel rest, antibiotics, renal decompression, and colonic drainage. Indolent cases may require surgical intervention.

MEDICAL COMPLICATIONS
Infection and Urosepsis

Preoperative urinalysis and culture are necessary to rule out urinary tract infection prior to elective PRS. If infection is suspected the patient should be treated with a course of antibiotics prior to surgery, and the procedure is deferred until sterile urine is achieved.

Prevention of infection involves administering perioperive antibiotics, low-pressure irrigation, and postoperative renal drainage when appropriate. In patients whose preoperative urine cultures are sterile, single dose aminoglycoside or fluoroquinolones are recommended for routine antibiotic prophylaxis (51). For patients at high risk of endocarditis antibiotic combinations active against streptococci and enterococci are recommended (ampicillin 2.0 g plus gentamicin 1.5 mg/kg within 30 minutes preoperatively, ampicillin 1.0 g 6 hours later. Substitute vancomycin 1.0 g for ampicillin in patients with penicillin allergies) (52). Special considerations should also be made for patients who have compromised immune systems or patients with prosthetic devices (53,54).

Patients with negative urine cultures preoperatively who are maintained on perioperative antibiotics do not necessarily require immediate bacteriologic evaluation if hemodynamically stable (55). Patients who experience fever, tachycardia, tachypnea, or leukocytocis should be monitored closely and may benefit from perioperative antibiotics. Complicated patients including those with compromised immune systems, history of recurrent infections, ureteral obstruction, retained infection stone fragments, urinary extravasation, or positive cultures from the upper tract should receive postoperative antibiotics. The incidence of urosepsis after PRS is 1% to 2%. Patients with infected urine from the renal pelvis or infected renal stones are at a fourfold greater risk for developing urosepsis (56). Treatment of urosepsis includes renal decompression, aggressive fluid resuscitation, invasive monitoring in an intensive care setting, and broad-spectrum antibiotics. Cultures obtained from the upper tract are superior to voided urine for guiding antibiotic therapy (56).

Intravascular Fluid Overload

Intravascular fluid overload is uncommon during PRS. Risk factors include vascular perforation, prolonged operative times, use of hypotonic solutions, high-pressure irrigation, medical comorbidities including patients with congestive heart failure and chronic renal insufficiency. The key to avoiding this complication is understanding the risks and practicing good surgical techniques. Treatment should start with diuretics.

Extravasation of Fluid

Fluid extravasation following PRS may occur when a shallow access sheath becomes dislodged from the renal collecting system. Extravasation can also occur following injury to the renal collecting system. The management of extravasation usually involves percutaneous renal drainage postoperatively. If a significant amount of fluid is noted intra-operatively it is possible to drain the fluid using the nephroscope perirenally, however caution must be exercised to protect renal access in the form of the safety wire. Postoperative identification of a urinoma can be followed by ultrasound and may warrant percutaneous drainage.

Air Embolism

Incremental injections of 5 to 7 cc of air into the renal collecting system via a ureteral catheter can help delineate the posterior calyces for precise nephrostomy access. Although the normal collecting system has a capacity of approximately 10 cc, air embolism secondary to positive pressure air pyelograms have been reported both before and after initial attempts at calyceal access (57,58). Signs suggesting air embolism include oxygen desaturation, decreased end-tidal carbon dioxide, hypotension, and bradycardia. When air embolism is suspected the procedure should be halted and any routes for further air entry should be sealed. The patient should be placed supine in trendelenburg position and if possible with the right side up. Cardiopulmonary resuscitation should be initiated. A right internal jugular central line may confirm diagnosis with aspiration of foamy blood and be used to evacuate air from the right atrium.

Deep Venous Thrombosis and Pulmonary Embolism

The incidence of venous thromboembolism in percutaneous renal surgery is <1% to 3% (Table 4) (51,59,60). Prevention starts with identification of patients at risk. For uncomplicated patients early postoperative mobilization is probably all that is necessary. For patients at higher risk including those with advanced age and malignancy, graduated elastic stockings and intermittent pneumatic compression stockings may be warranted (61). Routine prophylaxis with low-dose unfractionated heparin or low molecular weight heparin is not indicated and may increase the risk of hemorrhage.

If deep vein thrombosis is diagnosed postoperatively, management is directed at preventing a thromboembolic event. Standard therapy with anticoagulation immediately after surgery may result in bleeding which can lead to further complications. Placement of a vena

TABLE 4 Complications from Percutaneous Renal Surgery

Complication	%
Overall complication rate	4–8
Fever	23–25
Bleeding requiring transfusion	2.3–23
Extravasation	1–7
Transient ureteral obstruction	6
Hydro/hemothorax	<1–2.1
Infundibular stenosis	2
Sepsis	<1–1.25
Pneumothorax	<1
Urinoma	<1
Contrast allergy	<1
Bowel perforation	<1
Renal pelvic laceration	<1
Ureteral avulsion	<1
Ureteropelvic junction or ureteral stricture	<1
Nephropleural or nephrocutaneous fistula	<1
Deep venous thrombosis with or without pulmonary embolus	<1

caval filter can prevent major thromboembolic complications until the nephrostomy track has had time to heal. When anticoagulation is started, monitoring for bleeding should be continued until the patient is stable at therapeutic doses.

Management of acute pulmonary embolism (PE) in the early postoperative period is a challenge as early anticoagulation and thrombolytic therapy for massive PE may be lifesaving. Careful monitoring for bleeding in an intensive care setting is warranted.

Radiation Exposure

Urologists are routinely exposed to radiation during endoscopic cases. Percutaneous nephrolithotomy has the highest radiation exposure to urologists, up to ten times the fluoroscopy time (62). Most of the radiation received by the surgeon comes from scatter from the patient. The radiation dose to the surgeon's legs is usually the highest and increases with closer proximity to the beam. Studies have shown that the estimated annual radiation exposure for urologists is well below the threshold dose for deterministic effects of ionizing radiation (62). Regardless, the as low as reasonably achievable (ALARA) principle should be used when operating fluoroscopy. Minimizing radiation exposure involves wearing lead aprons, thyroid shields and lead impregnated glasses, minimizing fluoroscopy time, collimating the beam (to narrow the field), keeping the image intensifier close to the patient, and keeping the surgeon's hands outside of the beam.

CONCLUSION

Percutaneous renal surgery remains an integral part of the endourologists' armamentarium. It remains the gold standard approach for staghorn stones and calyceal diverticular disease, while its use in the treatment of UPJ obstruction and transitional cell carcinoma continue to expand with the advent of new technology. PRS has also expanded to include the treatment of renal cell carcinoma with ablative therapies. Although percutaneous access is a relatively safe route for renal surgery, awareness for potential complications will lead to early detection and treatment, which is the cornerstone of successful postoperative management.

REFERENCES

1. Bloom DA, Morgan RJ, Scardino PL. Thomas Hillier and percutaneous nephrostomy. Urology 1989; 33:346–350.
2. Goodwin WE, Casey WC, Woolfe W. Percutaneous trocar (needle) nephrostomy in hydronephrosis. JAMA 1955; 157:891.

3. Ferstrom I, Johansson B. Percutaneous pyelolithotomy: a new extraction technique. Scand J Urol Nephrol 1976; 10:257–259.

4. Gupta R, Kumar A, Kapoor R, et al. Prospective evaluation of safety and efficacy of the supracostal approach for percutaneous nephrolithotomy. BJU Int 2003; 90:809–813.

5. Sampaio FJB. Surgical anatomy of the kidney. In: Smith AD, Badlani GH, Bagley DH, et al., eds. Smith's Textbook of Endourology. St Louis, MO: Quality Medical, 1996:153–184.

6. Yahoannes P, Smith AD. The endourological management of complications associated with horseshoe kidney. J Urol 2002; 168:5–8.

7. Kawashima A, Glockner JF, King BF. CT urography and MR urography. Radil Clin North Am 2003; 41:945–961.

8. Herts BR. Role of three-dimensional imaging in surgical planning for kidney surgery. BJU Int 2005; 95:16–20.

9. Rizvi SAH, Naqvi SAA, Hussain Z, et al. The management of stone disease. BJU Int 2002; 89:62–68.

10. Gerzof SG, Johnson WC, Robbins AH, et al. Expanded criteria for percutaneous abscess drainage. Arch Surg 1985; 120:227–232.

11. Holman E, Khan AM, Pásztor I, et al. Simultaneous bilateral compared with unilateral percutaneous nephrolithotomy. BJU Int 2002; 89:334–338.

12. Pearle MS, Nakada SY, Womack JS, et al. Outcomes of contemporary percutaneous nephrostolithotomy in morbidly obese patients. J Urol 1998; 160:669–673.

13. Dalela D, Goel A, Singh P, et al. Renal capsular block: a novel method for performing percutaneous nephrolithotomy under local anesthesia. J Endourol 2004; 18:544–546.

14. Davidoff R, Bellman G. Influence of technique of percutaneous tract creation on incidence of renal hemorrhage. J Urol 1997; 157:1229–1231.

15. Safak M, Gogus C, Soygur T. Nephrostomy tract dilation using a balloon dilator in percutaneous renal surgery: experience with 95 cases and comparison with the fascial dilator system. Urol Int 2003; 71:382–384.

16. Helal M, Black T, Lockhart J., et al. The Hickman peel-away sheath: alternative for pediatric nephrostolithotomy. J Endourol 1997; 11:171–172.

17. Jackman SV, Hedican SP, Docimo SG, et al. Miniaturized access for pediatric percutaneous nephrolithotomy. J Endourol 1997; 11:133.

18. Jackman, SV, Docimo SG, Cadeddu JA, et al. The "mini-perc" technique: a less invasive alternative to percutaneous nephrolithotomy. World J Urol 1998; 16:371–374.

19. Chan DY, Jarrett TW. Mini-percutaneous nephrolithotomy. J Endourol 2000; 14:269.

20. Stoller ML, Wolf JS, St Lezin MA. Estimated blood loss and transfusion rates associated with percutaneous nephrolithotomy. J Urol 1994; 152:1977–1981.

21. Traxer O, Smith TG, Pearle MS, et al. Renal parenchymal injury after standard and mini percutaneous nephrostolithotomy. J Urol 2001; 165:1693–1695.

22. Bellman GF, Davidoff R, Candela J, et al. Tubeless percutaneous renal surgery. J Urol 1997; 157:1578–1582.

23. Munver R, Delvecchio FC, Newman GE, et al. Critical analysis of supracostal access for percutaneous renal surgery. J Urol 2001; 166:1242–1246.

24. Hopper KD, Yakes WF. The posterior intercostal approach for percutaneous renal procedures: risk of puncturing the lung, spleen, and liver as determined by CT. Am J Roentgenol 1990; 154:115–117.

25. Lallas CD, Delvecchio FC, Evans BR, et al. Management of nephropleural fistula after supracostal percutaneous nephrolithotomy. Urology 2004; 64:241–245.

26. Landman J, Venkatesh R, Lee DI, et al. Combined percutaneous and retrograde approach to staghorn calculi with application of the ureteral access sheath to facilitate percutaneous nephrolithotomy. J Urol 2003; 169:64–67.

27. Kondas J, Szentgyorgyi E, Vaczi L, et al. Splenic injury: a rare complication of percutaneous nephrolithotomy. Int Urol Nephrol 1994; 26:399–404.

28. Roth RA. Beckmann CF. Complications of extracorporeal shock-wave lithotripsy and percutaneous nephrolithotomy. Urol Clin North Am 1988; 15:155–166.

29. Routh WD, Tatum CM, Lawdahl RB, et al. Tube tamponade: potential pitfall in angiography of arterial hemorrhage associated with percutaneous drainage catheters. Radiology 1990; 174:945–949.

30. Buchholz N. Colon perforation after percutaneous nephrolithotomy revisited. Urol Int 2004; 72:88–90.

31. Gerspach JM, Bellman GC, Stoller ML, et al. Conservative management of colon injury following percutaneous renal surgery. Urology 1997; 49:831–836.

32. Vallancien G, Capdeville R, Veillon B, et al. Colonic perforation during percutaneous nephrolithotomy. J Urol 1985; 134:1185–1187.

33. LeRoy AJ, Williams HJ, Bender CE. Colon perforation following percutaneous nephrostomy and renal calculus removal. Radiology 1985; 155:83–85.

34. Paul EM, Marcovich R, Lee BR, et al. Choosing the ideal nephrostomy tube. BJU Int 2003; 92:672–677.

35. Neto ACL, Tobias-Machado M, Vaz Juliano R, et al. Duodenal damage complicating percutaneous access to kidney. Sao Paulo Med J 2000; 118:116–117.

36. Culkin DJ, Wheeler JS, Canning JR. Nephro-duodenal fistula: a complication of percutaneous nephrolithotomy. J Urol 1985; 134:528–530.
37. Ugras M, Gunes A, Baydinc C. Severe renal bleeding caused by a ruptured renal sheath: case report of a rare complication of percutaneous nephrolithotomy. BMC Urol 2002; 2:1–4.
38. Fitzpatrick. Operative Urology. Chapter 10. Surgery for Calyceal and Pelvic Stones. Philadelphia, PA: Krane, Siroky, Fitzpatick, 2000.
39. Coleman CC, Kimura Y, Reddy P. Complications of nephrostolithotomy. Sem Intervent Radiol 1984; 1:70–74.
40. Goel MC, Robert JG. Percutaneous resection of renal transitional carcinoma: venous injury and its conservative management. Urol Int 2001; 67:170–172.
41. Gupta M, Bellman G, Smith D. Massive hemorrhage from renal vein injury during percutaneous renal surgery: endourological management. J Urol 1997; 157:795–797.
42. Kessaris DN, Bellman GC, Pardalidis NP, et al. Management of hemorrhage after percutaneous renal surgery. J Urol 1995; 153:604–608.
43. Evans CP, Stoller ML. The fate of the iatrogenic retroperitoneal stone. J Urol 1993; 150:827–829.
44. Grasso M, Liu JB, Goldberg B, et al. Submucosal calculi: endoscopic and intraluminal sonographic diagnosis and treatment options. J Urol 1995; 153:1384–1389.
45. Segura JW, Patterson DE, LeRoy AJ, et al. Percutaneous removal of kidney stones: review of 1,000 cases. J Urol 1985; 134:1077–1081.
46. Lang EK. Percutaneous nephrostolithotomy and lithotripsy: a multi-institutional survey of complications. Radiology 1987; 162:25–30.
47. Dretler SP, Young RH. Stone granuloma: a cause of ureteral stricture. J Urol 1993; 150:1800–2.
48. Culkin DJ, Wheeler JS Jr, Canning JR. Distal ureteral obstruction complicating percutaneous nephrolithotomy. Urology 1987; 30:364–368.
49. Buchholz NP. Double infundibular obliteration with abscess formation after percutaneous nephrolithotomy. Urol Int 2001; 66:46–48.
50. Neustein P, Barbaric ZL, Kaufman JJ. Nephrocolic fistula: a complication of percutaneous nephrostolithotomy. J Urol 1986; 135:571–573.
51. Dogan HS, Sahin A, Cetinkaya Y, et al. Antibiotic prophylaxis in percutaneous nephrolithotomy: prospective study in 81 patients. J Endourol 2002; 16:649–653.
52. Dajani AS, Taubert KA, Wilson W, et al. Prevention of Bacterial Endocarditis: recommendations by the American Heart Association. Circulation 1997; 96:358–366.
53. Kingston R, Kiely P, McElwain JP. Antibiotic prophylaxis for dental or urological procedures following hip or knee replacement. J. Infect 2002; 45:243–245.
54. Olson ES, Cookson BD. Do antimicrobials have a role in preventing septicaemia following instrumentation of the urinary tract? J Hosp Infect 2000; 45:85–97.
55. Cadeddu JA, Chen R, Bishoff J, et al. Clinical significance of fever after percutaneous nephrolithotomy. Urology 1988; 52:48–50.
56. Mariappan P, Smith G, Bariol SV, et al. Stone and pelvic urine culture and sensitivity are better than bladder urine as predictors of urosepsis following percutaneous nephrolithotomy: a prospective clinical study. J Urol 2005; 173:1610–1614.
57. Cadeddu JA, Arrindell D, Moore RG. Near fatal air embolism during percutaneous nephrostomy placement. J Urol 1997; 158:1519.
58. Varkarakis J, Su LM, Hsu THS. Air embolism from pneumopyelography. J Urol 2003; 169:267.
59. Patel A, Fuchs GJ. Air travel and thromboembolic complications after percutaneous nephrolithotomy for staghorn stone. J Endourol 1988; 12:51–53.
60. Lee WJ, Smith AD, Cubelli V, et al. Complications of percutaneous nephrolithotomy. Am J Roentenol 1987; 148:177–180.
61. Agnelli G. Prevention of venous thromboembolism in surgical patients. Circulation 2004; 110: IV4–IV12.
62. Hellawell GO, Mutch SJ, Thevendran G, et al. Radiation exposure and the urologist: what are the risks? J Urol 2005; 174:948–952.

26 | Complications of Laparoscopic Adrenal Surgery

Aaron Sulman
Medical College of Wisconsin, Milwaukee, Wisconsin, U.S.A.

Louis Kavoussi
Smith Institute for Urology, North Shore-Long Island Jewish Health System, New Hyde Park, New York, U.S.A.

INTRODUCTION

Gagner et al. first described laparoscopic adrenalectomy in 1992 (1). Subsequently, this technique has been applied to treat a variety of adrenal pathology including Cushing's syndrome, Cushing's disease, ectopic adrenocorticotropic hormone (ACTH) syndrome, Conn's adenoma, adrenal incidentalomas, myelolipomas, pheochromocytomas, carcinomas, and metastasis from nonadrenal primaries (2–6). These experiences have demonstrated a clear advantage of laparoscopy with respect to convalescence and postoperative analgesic requirements when compared with open surgery. Indeed in select patients, laparoscopic adrenalectomy can be performed as an ambulatory procedure (7).

Contraindications to laparoscopic adrenalectomy are dictated in part by the experience of the individual surgeon with regard to lesion size, patient body habitus, and prior surgical history (5). Laparoscopic adrenalectomies can be performed by either a transperitoneal or retroperitoneal approach and the choice of technique depends upon surgeon preference as well as specific clinical situations. Patients with a history of extensive intra-abdominal surgery may benefit from a retroperitoneal approach (4,8,9). Obese patients with Cushing's syndrome may be more easily approached from a transperitoneal route as most adipose tissue is located posterior to the gland (4,8). With retroperitoneal access there are fewer anatomical landmarks and a smaller working space (8). As such, a retroperitoneal approach for adrenal masses larger than 7 to 8 cm can be challenging (9).

As with any surgical procedure, laparoscopic adrenal surgery carries a risk of minor and major morbidity. This chapter will focus on potential complications of laparoscopic adrenalectomy. Specific aspects of preoperative and postoperative management will also be addressed.

COMPLICATIONS

Laparoscopic adrenal surgery is more complex than procedures such as pelvic lymphadenectomy, renal biopsy or varicocelectomy, and carries a different portfolio of complications (10). Fahlenkamp et al. reviewed 2407 laparoscopic procedures, classifying them based upon the difficulty of the procedure and noted a direct correlation between complication rate and difficulty level. They also noted a decreasing complication rate with increasing surgeon experience, with a drop from 13.3% during the first 100 procedures to 3.6% (11). Overall complication rates of up to 33% have been noted with adrenalectomy, with a mortality rate of up to 0.9% (2,3,12,13). Terachi et al. noted an 8% complication rate in transperitoneal versus a 12% complication rate in retroperitoneal laparoscopic adrenalectomies (8). Gill et al. noted a 4.7% complication rate with retroperitoneal laparoscopic adrenalectomies (14). Table 1 lists morbidity and mortality rates in several large series of laparoscopic adrenalectomies.

There are size limitations related to laparoscopic adrenalectomy. Most agree that laparoscopy is indicated with adrenal masses smaller than 10 cm (2,15,16). Some support the laparoscopic approach even for lesions ranging from 10 to 12 cm in diameter (9,15). There is a direct correlation between adrenal mass size (≥5 cm) and complication rate, length of hospital stay, and operative time (3).

TABLE 1   Morbidity and Mortality Rates for Laparoscopic Adrenalectomies

Author	Number of cases	Complications (%)	Mortality (%)
Bonjer et al. (2)	111	11	0.9
Henry et al. (29)	169	7.5	0
Lezoche et al. (19)	108	3.7	0.9
David et al. (23)	90	9	1.1
WolzWalz et al. (16)	325	3.4	0
Brunt et al. (13)	527	12	0.9
Terachi et al. (8)	370	9	0
Gonzalez et al. (15)	78	7	0
Fahlenkamp et al. (11)	44	13.6	0
Soulie et al. (67)	52	17.2	0

VISCERAL INJURIES

Organs injured include small and large bowel, liver, spleen, pancreas, gallbladder, and the adrenal gland itself (8,11,13,17–20). Many of these injuries are less common with laparoscopic versus open approaches. In fact, the incidence of splenectomies required for splenic injuries during a laparoscopic adrenalectomy is one-tenth of that noted with open adrenalectomies (13). Magnified laparoscopic vision and the use of gravity for retraction instead of manual retraction contribute to this decreased complication rate (13). While many of these injuries occur with both the transperitoneal and retroperitoneal approach, hepatic injuries are seen primarily with the transperitoneal approach and pancreatic injuries are seen with the retroperitoneal approach. The latter may require open conversion for adequate repair (8). One difficulty specific to retroperitoneal adrenalectomies is the potential for a peritoneal tear. This can result in a diminished working space; however, it does not necessarily require conversion to an open procedure (2). Visceral injuries have been noted in 0.3% to 2.5% of cases (14,11).

Previous surgery in the adrenal area is not an absolute contraindication of laparoscopy but does add difficulty to the procedure, potentially increasing the risk of visceral injury and a retroperitoneal approach may be preferred (4). Colon injuries such as a tear during dissection can be of significant consequence, particularly in immunosuppressed patients with Cushing's disease (19).

Renal injuries can occur during laparoscopic adrenalectomies. In particular, renal perfusion can be compromised by the dissection of the renal vasculature, resulting in upper pole renal ischemia (21,22). Devascularization of the upper pole of the kidney can occur when renal polar arteries are occluded for mobilization of an adrenal tumor (23).

OPEN CONVERSION

Although not necessarily a complication, there is an open conversion rate of 1.9–11.7% (2,4,8,14). The conversion rate for adrenal masses larger than 5 cm is higher (14.2%) than for smaller lesions (2.1%) (3). Conversion rates decrease with increasing surgeon experience (8). A common reason for open conversion is the presence of a vascular injury (2). Bleeding, both major (cause by adrenal vein, renal vein/artery, and inferior vena caval injuries) and minor (persistent venous oozing) are the most frequent reasons for open conversion (13). Another indication is the failure to progress with the surgery or the presence of poorly defined tissue planes (3). Additional reasons for open conversion include visceral injuries, obesity, retroperitoneal fibrosis, unclear anatomy, failure to progress, unsuspected invasion of adjacent structures by adrenocortical carcinoma, peritoneal tears, suboptimal working space, and laparoscopic equipment failure (14,23,24). Because bleeding and other complications are always a possibility, it is important to have the availability of an open laparotomy set as well as two units of cross-matched blood in the event of a need to convert to an open procedure and/or to acutely address severe bleeding during a laparoscopic adrenalectomy (25). Preoperative three-dimensional computed tomography (CT) or magnetic resonance imaging (MRI) can be performed to assess for resectability and for adequate surgical planning and laparoscopic ultrasonography can also be helpful in assessing the adrenal gland's resectability and its spatial relationship to surrounding structures (5). A high suspicion of a primary adrenal malignancy is an indication with some urologists for open conversion as a wider margin of resection is necessary than can be safely obtained laparoscopically (3). In addition, adrenal metastases from other primaries (renal cell carcinoma, lung cancer, colon cancer) are frequently difficult to resect laparoscopically due to the presence of an inflammatory reaction and adherence to surrounding structures such as the liver and vena cava, requiring open conversion (26). Depending upon the experience of the surgeon, these lesions are still, however, resectable, provided that preoperative, intra-operative imaging, and/or intra-operative visualization excludes invasion of adjacent structures (27,28). It is important to maintain open conversion as an option to successfully complete a difficult adrenalectomy when the situation arises (29).

BLEEDING COMPLICATIONS

Laparoscopic adrenalectomies have been shown to result in less than half of the blood loss compared with open adrenalectomies although significant bleeding complications are still encountered (30). Troublesome bleeding can occur when establishing access for a pneumoperitoneum. When bleeding in the abdominal wall vessels is noted, hemostasis can be obtained by electrocautery or by suture ligature, as unaddressed abdominal wall bleeding can result in a subcutaneous hematoma which can later become infected (31). Abdominal wall vessels can bleed with the insertion of the Veress needle or the trocar. This bleeding can be treated with endoscopic coagulation or subsequent circular suture placement (11). A bleeding epigastric vessel can be ligated under laparoscopic guidance by placing a figure 80-prolene suture both proximal and distal to the vessel by passing a Stamey needle in these locations, grasping the suture laparocopically and tying the suture over the skin and over a bolster. Alternatively, a foley catheter can be placed through the sheath and pulled back under traction as a temporizing measure until definitive ligation is done (31). Another option for abdominal wall hemostasis is the fulguration of bleeding by using a roller ball electrode. This is done by inserting a resectoscope through an adjacent working port (31). Endoscopic coagulation requires caution as this is a known etiology of delayed visceral injuries (11). Ultimately, if needed, the skin incision can be extended, cutting down to the bleeding vessels, which can then be suture ligated under direct vision (31).

Significant bleeding can occur during dissection of the adrenal vein and vena cava (11,32,33). These injuries can be caused by Veress needle placement, trocar placement, excessive traction, or other difficulties during dissection of branches of the renal artery and vein, and the vena cava (2,11,32). Fortunately, vessel injuries caused by Veress needle placement are often self-sealing and can, on occasion, be managed with observation (25). Significant bleeding also occurs in cases where surgical clips become dislodged after placement in the course of adrenal gland removal (34). Thermal injury, often from monopolar electrocautery, can contribute to bleeding and while conversion to an open laparotomy may be required to successfully address it from most of the stated causes, these injuries have been fixed by individuals with laparoscopic suturing, endoscopic clipping, and the use of fenestrated forceps (11,32,33). Careful dissection and avoidance of monopolar electrocautery near large vessels can minimize the occurrence of these injuries (33). If an open laparotomy is required, the sheath needs to be left in place as a means of tamponade and as a guide to the injury site. The laparoscope is then torqued toward the anterior abdominal wall. This tents up the wall, allowing an incision directly over the sheath, allowing rapid peritoneal access while minimizing the risks for bowel injury (25). In the case of large adrenal masses, a retroperitoneal approach is advocated as safer as it allows improved visibility at the posterior aspect of the great vessels (3). During the course of dissection, additional bleeding can occur. In addition to major vessel injuries, bleeding can also occur because of injuries of the mesentery or liver. In contrast to major vascular injuries, this can usually be addressed laparoscopically, using direct pressure, loops, or ties (35). At the end of a laparoscopic procedure, it is important to decrease the pneumoperitoneal pressure to 5 mmHg and reinspect for intra-peritoneal bleeding or for an expanding hematoma and to address bleeding as noted using clips, electrocautery, or other means. It is important to inspect the operative area at lower intaperitoneal pressures as higher pressures can tamponade bleeding which can resume at the end of the procedure (31).

A right-sided adrenalectomy carries with it a higher probability of bleeding due to injuring the adrenal vein or inferior vena cava so in the event of a bilateral adrenalectomy, it is advisable to first perform the left adrenalectomy. Therefore, if open conversion is necessary, the patient is more likely to benefit from at least a unilateral laparoscopic approach (15).

Coagulopathy is stated by many to be a contraindication to a laparoscopic adrenalectomy because of the increased risk of bleeding (28). However, when appropriate steps are taken such as pre- and intra-operative desmopressin replacement in patients with disorders such as von Willebrand's syndrome, successful surgery can still be undertaken (19).

METABOLIC COMPLICATIONS

The dynamics of the pneumoperitoneum have the potential for multiple metabolic consequences. Pneumoperitoneum can cause decreased cardiac output, metabolic acidosis, secretion of vasopressin and catecholamines, and decreased urine volume (30). Carbon dioxide absorbed during the procedure causes a decreased blood pH (acidosis) and an increased arterial and carbon dioxide end expiratory pressure which may be poorly tolerated in patients with baseline significant cardiopulmonary pathology (11,36). A tension pneumoperitoneum, occurring with insufflation pressures of greater than 20 mmHg can result in cardiorespiratory compromise (37). In addition, peritoneal CO_2 blebs can form with high intra-peritoneal pressures which cause diffusion of CO_2 into the peritoneum and distort the anatomy (25). Pneumoperitoneum has several effects on the cardiovascular system. It causes an increased central venous pressure and venous resistance as sell as a decreased cardiac stroke volume, an increased arterial resistance, arterial pressure, and systemic venous pressure, resulting in a hyperdynamic state which is a relative contraindication in patients with moderate to severe ischemic heart disease or untreated congestive heart failure (38). In addition, carbon dioxide absorption is increased with pneumoperitoneum and subsequent hypercapnea, combined with peritoneal irritation and subsequent vagal stimulation can lead to cardiac arrhythmias (38). While arrhythmias can be treated with intravenous lidocaine, initial treatment should consist of hyperventilation with 100% oxygen, desufflation of the abdomen, and releasing traction on any organs (39). It is also possible for hypercarbia to cause sympathetic nervous stimulation leading to tachycardia and hypertension (39). Hypertension, if present, can be controlled with vasodilatory agents such as sodium nitroprusside. Subsequent alpha or beta adrenergic blockade can also be used (39). Excess carbon dioxide can usually be eliminated with increased ventilation although this is more problematic in patients with significant pulmonary disease (38). End-tidal carbon dioxide should be monitored and maintained between 35 and 45 mmHg (39).

Longer operative times, particularly those seen with bilateral adrenalectomies result in hypercapnea which is poorly tolerated in patients with hypercortisolism seen in Cushing's syndrome (37). On occasion, this may necessitate conversion to an open procedure for the removal of at least one of the adrenal glands (37). Depending upon the pathology involved, adrenalectomy can also result in the metabolic consequences seen with adrenal insufficiency, the treatment of which is discussed in detail subsequently (15).

Diaphragmatic injury leading to pneumothorax can also be caused during dissection of the superior aspect of the adrenal gland (40). Other causes include barotrauma caused by positive pressure ventilation as well as trocar placement above the 12th rib for a retroperitoneal approach (39). Signs of this include progressive tracheal deviation, decreased breath sounds unilaterally, hypotension, and increased ventilation pressures. When possible, it is confirmed with an upright chest X-ray (39). A pneumothorax of less than or equal to 20% can be managed expectantly. Positive pressure ventilation can cause a pneumothorax to expand, however, risking a tension pneumothorax and subsequent cardiovascular collapse. This is treated initially by placing a large bore needle at the midclavicular line in the second or third intercostal space followed by a chest tube placement in the fourth intercostal space. Furthermore, in the presence of a pneumothorax, nitrous oxide administration can expand it so this gas administration must be terminated (39). Pulmonary emboli have also been reported, requiring subsequent anticoagulation (41).

ADRENAL MALIGNANCIES

There is controversy regarding the safety of a laparoscopic approach for the treatment of adrenal cancer and the argument against this is supported by reports of diffuse peritoneal dissemination noted postoperatively as well as trocar port-site seeding (2,42). Removal of adrenal cortical carcinoma laparoscopically, however, has been shown to be feasible in the presence of organ-confined disease (9,28). Rupture of tumor capsules has been noted during dissection for laparoscopic adrenalectomies (22). One step which can be taken to decrease the risk of intraoperative tumor spillage is to remove the gland intact in an entrapment bag without morcellation (25). In addition, because of the potential for rapid growth rates of adrenocortical carcinoma, obtaining a repeat CT or MRI study immediately preoperatively can prevent commencement of a laparoscopic adrenalectomy where an open, wider excision may be indicated because of interval growth and extension of an adrenal mass (42). A possible contraindication to laparoscopic adrenalectomy is the presence of an adrenal vein tumor thrombus (9).

CUSHING'S-SPECIFIC RISKS

Patients with Cushing's syndrome present unique risk factors because of the hypercortisolism brought about by their disease state. They are more prone to infectious and thromboembolic complications as well as respiratory distress and consequent anesthetic complications related to hypercapnea (37). They are subject to high infection rates, deep vein thrombosis, bleeding tendencies, pulmonary emboli, hypertension, and potentially multi-organ failure (5). Postoperative hypocortisolism can also result in fatal hypoglycemia (43).

NEUROLOGIC INJURIES

Peripheral nerve injuries necessitate preventive measures. The most common injury is a brachial plexus injury which can result from malpositioning. The arms should not be abducted beyond 90° and the use of shoulder braces with patients in Tredelenburg position should be avoided as this exerts pressure on the brachial plexus. Padding of bony prominences can help decrease peripheral nerve injury risks (39).

VISUALIZATION

Most of the complications described above can be avoided with good visualization and in addition to equipment choices, the laparoscope lens can become fogged intra-operatively, causing blurred vision. This can be remedied by using warm, antifogging solution and/or by wiping the lens on the peritoneum or a bowel loop (25).

ADDITIONAL COMPLICATIONS

Additional complications include pleural tear, Addisonian crisis, myocardial infarction, stroke, pneumonia, temporary relaxation of the abdominal wall, and temporary hypesthesia of the abdominal wall, chronic port site pain, multisystem organ failure, and gastrointestinal bleeds (13,16,23,44). Also seen is deep venous thrombosis and pulmonary embolus which should be prophylaxed against with intermittent compression devices and/or heparin therapy (29). Parsons et al. noted an increased incidence of complications to correlate with a higher American Society of Anesthesiologists (ASA) score (17).

PREOPERATIVE, INTRA-OPERATIVE, AND POSTOPERATIVE MANAGEMENT OF PHEOCHROMOCYTOMAS

The only definitive means of curing a pheochromocytoma is through surgical extirpation and in comparison with open approaches, laparoscopic adrenalectomies have been shown to yield more stable hemodynamics intra-operatively (36,45). Prior to performing the adrenalectomy, however, medical therapy is necessary to control blood pressure, restore blood volume, and to control heart rate and arrhythmias (46). Laparoscopic adrenalectomies for pheochromocytomas have the potential to be more complicated than laparoscopic adrenalectomies performed for other reasons with regard to the length of hospital stay and blood loss when compared with other laparoscopic adrenalectomies (12). A complication unique to the management of pheochromocytomas is the presence of intra-operative hypertensive crises (30). Severe hypotension is also a significant issue as a drop in blood pressure following the ligation of the tumor's venous drainage has the potential to be so severe as to precipitate a cardiac arrest (47,48).

Critical in the successful surgical extirpative treatment of this disease is adequate pre, intra, and postoperative medical management. Preoperative assessment for end-organ damage such as catecholamine-induced cardiomyopathy is important (49). Blood pressure is best controlled by preoperative alpha-adrenergic blockade administered for 10 days to 2 weeks preoperatively (16,45,46). Phenoxybenzamine is titrated starting at 10 mg two or three times per day and is increased until either all signs of pressor activity have been suppressed, or until the patient complains of side effects of postural hypotension or a stuffy nose (46). Doses usually vary from 20 to 100 mg per day but have been titrated as high as 300 mg daily (2,30,46,49). Phenoxybenzamine works via a noncompetitive, covalent bond with the alpha-adrenergic receptor, preventing preoperative surges of catecholamine release and should be discontinued 48 hours before surgery (46). Intravenous phentolamine can replace oral phenoxybenzamine 48 hours preoperatively (22). Phenoxybenzamine, however, is a nonselective alpha adrenoceptor antagonist, also blocking alpha-2-adrenoceptors which are important in the negative feedback loop which regulates norepinephrine release. Therefore, normal sympathetic nerve activity can, in this situation, cause accentuated chronotropic and ionotropic effects. The addition of beta-adrenoceptor antagonists can be used to counteract this (46). However, beta-adrenergic blockade also risks exacerbating negative ionotropic effects of catecholamine-induced cardiomyopathy (48). Another potential drawback to phenoxybenzamine is its long duration of action. Postoperatively, patients have somnolence, stuffy nose, headaches, and postural hypotension due to the central and peripheral alpha-2-adrenoceptor blockade (46).

Prazosin and doxazosin are selective alpha-1 antagonists which can avoid the effects that phenoxybenzamine has on the presynaptic blockade of alpha-2-adrenoceptors. The starting dose for prazosin is 1 mg every 8 hours and can be increased to a maximal dose of up to 12 mg daily. Doxazosin is given in once-a-day or twice-a-day dosing and is started at 1 mg and can be titrated up to 16 mg daily (45,46). It's advantage over phenoxybenzamine is that blood pressure returns to normal quickly postoperatively compared with patients given phenoxybenazamine who tend to have more prolonged postoperative hypotension, often refractory to large doses of adrenoceptor agonists and requiring more fluid loading (46). Preoperative alpha blockade results in varying degrees of expansion of the circulating blood volume and the more that the blood volume is increased, the more significant the hypotension is following the removal of the pheochromocytoma (50).

Alpha-blocking agents can be augmented with alpha-methyl-p-tyrosine, a tyrosine hydroxylase inhibitor, which blocks the rate-limiting conversion of tyrosine to dopa in the catecholamine synthetic pathway as this may result in better blood pressure control, less bleeding, and less of a need for intra-operative fluid replacement (50,51). Catecholamine synthesis can be reduced by 40% to 80% (48). This is particularly useful in patients who haved cardiomyopathy, are resistant to phenoxybenzamine, or who have multiple catecholamine-secreting tumors (36).

In the case of arrhythmias, beta-adrenergic blockade (propranolol) is a valuable adjunct (30) although it is crucial that alpha blockade is present first to alleviate an increase in hypertension due to possible adrenergic receptor agonism. Preoperatively, patients can be maintained on their individual antihypertensive treatment up until the day of surgery. Angiotensin-converting enzyme inhibitors, however, need to be discontinued 1 day prior to surgery (52).

Calcium channel blockers are an alternative to this treatment (22). Preoperatively patients can be started on verapramil-SR or nifedipine XL (5). Calcium channel blockers may decrease the catecholamine release from pheochromocytomas (52). If preoperative treatment with alpha 1-adrenergic blocking agents is not carried out, an intravenous infusion of nicardipine, a calcium channel blocker can be started 15 minutes before anesthesia and continued intra-operatively to prevent blood pressure elevations. It is a peripheral and coronary vasodilator with a rapid onset and a short duration of action (52).

Several intra-operative management details are important with these patients. An intra-arterial catheter is used for blood pressure monitoring (12). Monitoring with a pulmonary artery catheter is useful for following cardiac output and systemic vascular resistance (2). Pulmonary artery occlusion pressures are monitored and crystaloid or colloid solutions are given to maintain a pulmonary artery occlusion pressure of between 10 and 12 mmHg in order to prevent any hypovolemia and its resultant hemodynamic effects after treatment with vasodilators. Also of note, pulmonary artery occlusion pressures can be artificially elevated during pneumoperitoneum because of increased intrapleural pressure. Ventilation is adjusted to keep the pulmonary end-tidal carbon dioxide between 32 and 38 mmHg (52).

Anesthetic agents need to be specifically tailored for pheophromocytoma patients. Preoperatively, patients are premedicated with hydroxyzine and alprazolam (46,52). Benzodiazepines are ideal anxiolytics as they decrease catecholamine release whereas opioids can cause histamine release which can stimulate catecholamine release (48). Propofol is a helpful induction agent as the vasodilation it causes can counteract the hypertensive response to endotracheal intubation (48). An anesthetic preference is a sufentanil, fentanyl, and/or propofol infusion combined with inhaled isoflurane (46,52). Fentanyl has the advantage of not causing histamine release (48,49). Vecuronium is the nondepolarizing muscle relaxing agent of choice as it does not release histamine and it does not induce sympathetic stimulation or muscular fasciculations (48,49). Isoflurane is an ideal inhalation agent as it does not sensitize the myocardium to catecholamines (48). Neuromuscular blockade reversal is accomplished with a combination of neostigmine (antimuscarinic effects) and glycopyrolate (cholinergic effects) (48).

Depending upon the anesthesiologists'/urologists' choice, an alpha blockade and if needed, beta blockade is titrated to maintain a systolic blood pressure between 120 and 160 mmHg and to prevent tachycardia (46,52). If beta blockers are used, it is important that the patient first receives sufficient alpha or calcium channel blockade as otherwise, pulmonary edema can result by suppression of beta-adrenoceptor-mediated cardiac sympathetic activity in the absence of adequate arteriolar dilation (46). Elevated circulating epinephrine levels and their resultant tachycardia and possibly arrhythmias are treated with beta blockers (46). Preoperative selective beta-1-adrenoceptor antagonists can be administered orally (atenolol 100 mg daily and bisoprolol 10–20 mg daily). These minimize side effects with the bronchi and peripheral vasculature (46). Intra-operatively, with gland manipulation and when subsequent elevations in blood pressure are anticipated, intravenous phentolamine can be given and isoflurane doses can be adjusted as well. Intravenous labetolol, atenolol, and esmolol can be used to suppress intra-operative tachycardia (12,46,52). Labetalol offers beta blockade and also supplements pre-existing alpha blockade and is dosed at 100 to 400 mg daily (46). Another useful drug for intra-operative adrenergic blockade is magnesium sulfate (46). Metoprolol (50–200 mg daily) and propranolol (40–240 mg daily) are useful nonselective beta bockers but should be used only in patients without a history of peripheral vascular disease or obstructive airway disease (46).

Several intra-operative precautions minimize the risk for hypertensive crises. Minimal manipulation of the adrenal mass and early ligation and transection of the adrenal vein is important (30). It is crucial for the surgeon to be in close communication with the anesthesiologist during the procedure with respect to timing of tumor manipulation and adrenal vein ligation in order to establish proper timing for short-acting antihypertensives, fluid replacement, and changing the depth of anesthesia (36). In addition, pneumoperitoneum during laparoscopic adrenalectomies causes increased cataecholamine release because of hypercapnea and increased intra-abdominal pressure. There is also direct compression of the tumor producing excess catecholamine release and this can be minimized by keeping the abdominal pressure below 10 to 12 mmHg. Kazaryan et al. recommended a pneumoperitoneum of 8 to 9 mmHg (45). A retroperitoneal approach may allow for lower intra-abdominal pressures (36). Epinephrine and norepinephrine levels as well as cardiac output have been documented to increase with creation of pneumoperitoneum and with adrenal gland manipulation. Following adrenalectomy, these factors decrease. Preoperative preparation with alpha and beta blockers as well as intra-operative calcium channel blockers (nicardipine) decrease the magnitude of associated hemodynamic changes (52). Joris et al. found that when patients received adequate fluids postoperatively combined with the above described preoperative and intra-operative medication, the majority were normotensive, without additional treatment on the first postoperative day (52). Adequate fluid therapy with colloids, crystaloids, blood, and vasopressors (epinephrine, phenylephrine, norepinephrine) helps prevent and treat hypotension (5,48,53). In patients with adequate volume expansion and sufficient pharmacotherapy, it is important to have a high index of suspicion for bleeding in the presence of persistent hypotension (48). Compared to open adrenalectomies, however, laparoscopic procedures and hypotensive episodes are less severe (54). Hemodynamic instability in the form of significant hypertension can be managed with nitroprusside infusion although nitroprusside infusion requires frequent dose adjustments (52). Isoflurane is also a potent arteriolar dilator and its titration can negate the need for prolonged nitroprusside infusions (46). Postoperatively, patients require close monitoring in the ICU initially and can subsequently be transferred to a regular inpatient floor (46).

The primary postoperative concern following the excision of a pheochromocytoma is hypotension and this can be difficult to treat even with adrenoceptor agonists and intravenous fluid replacement. This can be the result of pre- and intra-operative adrenoceptor agonists, primarily with the use of long-acting medications such as phenoxybenzamine. In addition, the prolonged catecholamine output from the pheochromocytoma can cause a downregulation of adrenoceptors in the contralateral gland (46). Hypertension can also persist after the pheochromocytoma is removed due to residual high concentrations of vasoactive substances and fluid overload (55). Sapienza and Cavallaro noted that the age-dependent long-term persistence of hypertension in patients greater than 56 years of age and those with long-standing preoperative hypertension are more likely to still be hyperstensive at long-term follow-up after adrenalectomy (56). The presence of a pheochromocytoma can stimulate a reactive insulin increase and following removal of the tumor, hypoglycemia can result and can be exacerbated by pre-operative and intra-operative alpha blockade. Therefore, close monitoring for and treatment of hypoglycemia is crucial during and after surgery (57).

MANAGEMENT OF ADRENAL INSUFFICIENCY

Bilateral and, depending upon the indication, unilateral adrenalectomy can lead to adrenal insufficiency which must be addressed. Patients undergoing adrenalectomy for adenomas were found by Daitch et al. to require a mean length of steroid replacement therapy of 16.8 months prior to patients recovering their hypothalamic-pituitary-adrenal axis, permitting cessation of replacement. Of the patients 53.9% required replacement for over 24 months (43). There is a potential for requiring lifelong replacement therapy in up to 25% of patients (43). Addisonian crises requiring hospital admission occur in up to 32% of patients undergoing bilateral adrenalectomies (58). Symptoms can include anorexia, fatigue, and weight loss as well as a diminished health-related quality of life. There is a potential for an adrenal crisis, presenting with acute abdominal pain, vomiting, severe hypotension, or hypovolemic shock. Glycemic control can also worsen. Glucocorticoid, mineralocorticoid, and possibly dehydroepianrosterone replacement therapy are all important postoperative adjuncts (59). In some situations, Addisonian crises and other sequelae of adrenal insufficiency can potentially be avoided by doing a partial adrenalectomy when acceptable as a surgical option (16).

Mineralocorticoid deficiency, presenting with primary adrenal insufficiency can result in hypotension, prerenal failure, and hypotension because of dehydration and hypovolemia. It can also result in hyperkalemia and hyponatremia (59). Preoperatively, patients undergoing adrenalectomy for Conn's syndrome should be treated with potassium-sparing diuretics and oral potassium replacement (16). Replacement therapy is accomplished with fluorocortosine daily doses of 0.05 to 0.2 mg and its adequacy is measured by monitoring blood pressure, serum sodium, plasma renin, and potassium levels (59,60). Fluorocortisone levels, however, are not titrated to a completely normal plasma renin level as this may lead to a higher incidence of hypertension (60).

Dehydroepiandrosterone is lost in adrenal insufficiency and in women can lead to diminished androgen levels and resultant reduced libido, dry skin, and loss of axillary and pubic hair. Replacing dehydroepiandosterone helps negate these issues and acts as an antidepressant (60). The recommended daily dose is 25 to 50 mg and can be monitored by measuring serum dehydroepiandrosterone sulfate levels (59).

Secondary adrenal insufficiency can cause hypoglycemia (59). If a patient is suspected of adrenal insuffficiency and is critically ill, empiric hydrocortisone replacement is recommended immediately following a random serum cortisol and plasma adrenocorticotropic hormone (ACTH) level being drawn (59). Proper adrenal replacement therapy is critical as reports of mortality from Addisonian crises following bilateral adrenalectomy are still evident (58).

Glucocorticoid replacement is necessary with adrenal insufficiency. In cases of an adrenalectomy for a cortisol-secreting tumor, replacement is given intravenously until oral intake is tolerated (4). Because of their postoperative propensity for glucocorticoid deficiency, patients require intravenous postoperative hydrocortisone 300 to 400 mg as a continuous infusion which is eventually tapered and changed to oral administration (37).

Once oral replacement is tolerated, it is administered in two or three daily doses, with half of the daily dose given in the morning (59,61). Total daily doses include hydrocortisone (10–30 mg) or cortisone acetate (25–37.5 mg) (59,62,63). Higher daily hydrocortisone levels (30 mg) can induce bone loss with long-term therapy. Lower doses (15–20 mg) have been shown to similarly affect quality of life parameters and may be preferable by lessening the risk of bone loss (64). Mitotane, administered for treating adrenal carcinoma, decreases the bioavailability of glucocorticoids and therefore requires that dosing be doubled or tripled. Replacement therapy does need to be monitored although specific plasma ACTH levels and urine cortisol levels are not currently accepted as absolute indicators of adequate dosing. ACTH levels, however, can be measured if patients develop skin hyperpigmentation despite replacement therapy, and urinary cortisol levels are used to assess patient compliance. The best means of monitoring replacement is through clinical judgment, assessing for signs or symptoms of under or over-replacement. Signs of under-replacement include weight gain, truncal obesity, hyperpigmentation, hypotension, hypokalemia, hyperkalemia, and symptoms include fatigue, weakness, insomnia, recurrent infections, and nausea. Evidence of over-replacement includes impaired glucose tolerance, osteoporosis, and obesity (59).

A critical aspect of adrenal replacement therapy is the ability to manage stress dose adjustments in order to avoid the onset of adrenal crises. Patients need to be taught to increase their hydrocortisone dose by 5 to 10 mg prior to strenuous activities and if they experience nausea, the medication can be administered parenterally or rectally. An acute adrenal crisis can be managed by 100 mg of intravenous hydrocortisone with subsequent daily doses of 100 to 200 mg (59). Alternatively, dexamethasone can be administered empirically in the presence of a suspected adrenal crisis as it does not affect subsequent plasma cortisol levels drawn as part of a diagnostic evaluation (65). Patients on adrenal replacement require tripling of their daily dose of hydrocortisone in the face of a febrile illness and they require hydrocortisone dosing of 100 to 200 mg daily when undergoing major surgery (62). They also need to keep an emergency bracelet or card indicating their glucocorticoid requirements (59,66).

CONCLUSION

Advances in the applications of laparoscopy in urologic surgery have been beneficial to patients with many different types of pathology. Adrenalectomy is one procedure that truly allows patients to have an excellent result without being subjected to the same rigors of a major open procedure. The advantages of this represent significant progress in urologic surgery but they are not without the potential for significant complications and have a significant learning curve, estimated at 25 to 50 cases (10,12,23,32). Complication rates decrease with experience but particularly in teaching programs, the complication rate ultimately plateaus due to the constant influx of new, less experienced residents (17). Many complications and operative times are lessened with increasing surgical expertise and with the assistance of a nursing staff and surgical assistant who is familiar with the laparoscopic procedures and the necessary equipment (10,23,24,35,39). A respect for the potential pitfalls of laparoscopic adrenalectomies and the knowledge of how to forsee, prevent, and remedy the unique complications will help support the acceptance of this surgical technique as a durable option representing the standard of care. While complication rates are low, complications do occur and it is important to inform patients not only of the benefits but also of the real possibility for complications so that they are able to make an educated decision as to whether or not to undergo a laparoscopic adrenalectomy (9).

REFERENCES

1. Gagner M, Lacriox A, Bolte E. Laparoscopic adrenalectomy in Cushing's syndrome and pheochromocytoma. N Engl J Med 1992; 327:1033.
2. Bonjer HJ, Sorm V, Berends FJ, et al. Endoscopic retroperitoneal adrenalectomy: lessons learned from 111 consecutive cases. Ann Surg 2000; 232(6):796–803.
3. Hobart MG, Gill IS, Schweizer D, Sung GT, Bravo EL. Laparoscopic adrenalectomy for large-volume (> or =5 cm) adrenal masses. J Endourol 2000; 14(2):149–154.
4. Pisanu A, Cois A, Montisci A, Uccheddu A. Current indications for laparoscopic adrenalectomy in the era of minimally invasive surgery. Chir Ital 2004; 56(3):313–320.
5. Gill IS. The case for laparoscopic adrenalectomy. J Urol 2001; 166(2):429–436.
6. Kadamba P, Habib Z, Rossi L. Experience with laparoscopic adrenalectomy in children. J Pediatr Surg 2004; 39(5):764–767.
7. Gill IS, Hobart MG, Schweizer D, Bravo EL. Outpatient adrenalectomy. J Urol 2000; 163:717–720.
8. Terachi T, Yoshida O, Matsuda T, Orikasa S, et al. Complications of laparoscopic and retroperitoneoscopic adrenalectomies in 370 cases in Japan: a multi-institutional study. Biomed Pharmacother 2000; 54(Suppl. 1):211s–214s.
9. Guazzoni G, Cestari A, Montorsi F, et al. Current role of laparoscopic adrenalectomy. Eur Urol 2001; 40:8–16.
10. Rassweiler JJ, Seemann O, Frede T, Henkel TO, Alken P. Retroperitoneoscopy: experience with 200 cases. J Urol 1998; 160:1265–1269.
11. Fahlenkamp D, Rassweiler J, Fornara P, Frede T, Loening SA. Complications of laparoscopic procedures in urology: experience with 2,407 procedures at 4 German centers. J Urol 1999; 162(3 Pt 1):765–770;discussion 770–771.
12. Kim AW, Quiros RM, Maxhimer JB, El-Ganzouri AR, Prinz RA. Outcome of laparoscopic adrenalectomy for pheochromocytomas vs aldostoronomas. Arch Surg 2004; 139:526–529.
13. Brunt LM. The positive impact of laparoscopic adrenalectomy on complicatons of adrenal surgery. Surg Endosc 2002; 16:252–257.
14. Gill IS, Clayman RV, Albala D, et al. Retroperitoneal and pelvic extraperitoneal laparoscopy: an international perdpective. Urology 1998; 52(4):566–571.
15. Gonzalez R, Smith CD, Mcclusky DA III, et al. Laparoscopic approach reduces likelihood of preioperative complications in patients undergoing adrenalectomy. Am Surg 2004; 70:668–674.
16. Walz MK, Peitgen K, Diesing D, et al. Partial versus total adrenalectomy by the posterior retroperitoneoscopic approach: early and long-term results of 325 consecutive procedures in primary adrenal neoplasia. World J Surg 2004; 28:1323–1329.
17. Parsons JK, Varkarakis I, Rha KH, Jarrett TW, Pinto PA, Kavoussi LR. Complications of abdominal urologic laparoscopy: longitudinal five-year analysis. Urology 2004; 63:27–32.
18. Hawn MT, Cook D, Deveney C, Sheppard BC. Quality of life after laparoscopic bilateral adrenalectomy for Cushing's disease. Surgery 2002; 132(6):1064–1068.
19. Lezoche E, Guerrieri M, Paganini AM, et al. Laparoscopic adrenalectomy by the anterior transperitoneal approach. Surg Endosc 2000; 14:920–925.
20. Varkarakis IM, Allaf ME, Bhayani SB, et al. Pancreatic injuries during laparoscopic urologic surgery. Urology 2004; 64(6):1089–1093.
21. Col V, de Canniere L, Collard E, Michel L, Donckier J. Laparoscopic adrenalectomy for phaeochromocytoma: endocrinological and surgical aspects of a new therapeutic approach. Clin Endocrincol (Oxf) 1999; 50(1):121–125.
22. Col V, de Canniere L, Collard E, Michel L, Donckler J. Laparoscopic adrenalectomy for phaeochromocytoma: endocrinological and surgical aspects of a new therapeutic approach. Clin Endocrinol 1999; 50:121–125.
23. David G, Yoav M, Gross D, Reissman P. Laparoscopic adrenalectomy: ascending the learning curve. Surg Endosc 2004; 18:771–773.
24. Esposito C, Lima M, Mattiolo G, et al. Complications of pediatric urological laparoscopy: mistakes and risks. J Urol 2003; 169:1490–1492.
25. Gill IS, Munch LC, McRoberts. Complications of urologic laparoscopy. Urol Ann 1995; 9:153–165.
26. Gerber E, Dinlenc C, Wagner JR. Laparoscopic adrenalectomy for isolated adrenal metastases. J Soc Laparoendosc Surg 2005; 8:314–319M.
27. Heniford BT, Arca MJ, Walsh M, Gill IS. Laparoscopic adrenalectomy for cancer. Semin Surg Oncol 1999; 16:293–306.
28. Henry JF, Defechereux T, Gramatica L, Raffaelli M. Should laparoscopic approach be proposed for large and/or potentially malignancy adrenal tumors? Langenbeck's Arch Surg 1999; 384: 366–369.
29. Henry JF, Defechereux T, Raffeilli M, Lubrano D, Gramatica L. Complication of laparoscopic adrenalectomy: results of 169 consecutive procedures. World J Surg 2000; 24:1342–1346.
30. Kim HH, Kim GH, Sung GT. Laparocopic adrenalectomy for pheochromocytoma: comparison with conventional open adrenalectomy. J Endourol 2004; 18:251–255.

31. Stanley KE. Management of laparoscopic vascular injuries in urology. Atlas Urol Clin North Am 1993; 1:103–116.
32. Soulie M, Seguin P, Richeux L, et al. Urological complications of laparoscopic surgery: experience with 350 procedures at a single center. J Urol 2001; 165(6 Pt 1):1967.
33. Corcione F, Esposito C, Cuccurullo D, et al. Vena cava injury. A serious complication during laparoscopic right adrenalectomy. Surg Endosc 2001; 15(2):218.
34. Takeda M, Go H, Imai T, Nishiyama T, Morishita H. Laparoscopic adrenalectomy for primary aldosteronism: report of initial ten cases. Surger 1994; 115(5):621–625.
35. Bongard F, Dubecz S, Klein S. Complications of therapeutic laparoscopy. Curr Probl Surg 1994; 31(11):859–925.
36. Del Pizzo JJ, Schiff JD, Vaughan ED. Laparoscopic adrenalectomy for pheochromocytoma. Curr Urol Rep 2005; 6:78–85.
37. Porpiglia F, Flori C, Bovio S, et al. Bilateral adrenalectomy for Cushing's syndrome: a comparison between laparoscopy and open surgery. J Endocrinol Invest 2004; 27:654–658.
38. Wolf JS Jr, Stoller ML. The physiology of laparoscopy: basic principles, complications and other considerations. J Urol 1994; 152:294–302.
39. See WA, Monk TG, Weldon BC. Complications of laparoscopy: strategies for prevention and treatment. In: Clayman RV, McDougall EM, eds. Laparoscopic Urology. St. Louis, MO: Quality Medical, 1993:183–206.
40. Naito S, Uozumi J, Shimura H, Ichimiya H, Tanaka M, Kuazawa J. Laparoscopic adrenalectomy: review of 14 cases and comparison with open adrenalectomy. J Endourol 1995; 9(6):491–495.
41. Undre S, Munz Y, Moorthy K, et al. Robot-assisted laparoscopic adrenalectomy: preliminary UK results. BJU Int 2004; 93:357–359.
42. Porpiglia F, Fiori C, Tarabuzzi R, et al. Is laparoscopic adrenalectomy feasible for adrenocortical carcinoma or metastasis? BJU Int 2004; 94:1026–1029.
43. Daitch JA, Goldfarb DA, Novick AC. Cleveland Clinic experience with adrenal Cushing's syndrome. J Urol 1997; 158:2051–2055.
44. Vargas HI, Kavoussi LR, Bartlett DL, et al. Laparoscopic adrenalectomy: a new standard of care. Urology 1997; 49(5):673–678.
45. Kazaryan AM, Kuznetsov NS, Shulutko AM, Beltsevich DG, Edwin B. Evaluation of endoscopic and traditional open approaches to pheochromocytoma. Surg Endosc 2004; 18:937–941.
46. Prys-Roberts C. Phaeochromocytoma–recent progress in its management. Br J Anaesth 2000; 85(1):44–57.
47. Shupak RC. Difficult anesthetic management during pheochromocytoma surgery. J Clin Anesth 1999; 11(3):247–250.
48. Singh G, Kam P. An overview of anaesthetic issues in phaeochromocytoma. Ann Acad Med 1998; 27(6):843–848.
49. Hull CJ. Phaeochromocytoma: diagnosis, preoperative preparation and anaesthetic management. Br J Anaesth 1986; 58:1453–1468.
50. Iijima T, Takagi T, Iwao Y. An increased circulating blood volume does ot prevent hypotension after pheochromocytoma resection. Can J Aneaesth 2004; 51(3):212–215.
51. Perry RR, Keiser HR, Norton JA, et al. Surgical management of pheochromocytoma with the urse of metyrosine. Ann Surg 1990; 212(5):621–628.
52. Joris JL, Hamoir EE, Hartstein GM, et al. Hemodynamic changes and catecholamine release during laparoscopic adrenalectomy for pheochromocytoma. Anesth Analg 1999; 88(1):16–21.
53. James MFM. Correspondence: Phaeochromocytoma–recent progress in its management. Br J Anesth 2001; 86(4):594–606.
54. Sprung J, O'Hara JF Jr, Gill IS, Abdelmalak B, Sarnaik A, Bravo EL. Anesthetic aspects of laparoscopic and open adrenalectomy for pheochromocytoma. Urology 2000; 55(3):339–343.
55. Johansson H, Brismar B, Hedenstierna G. Hypertensive crisis immediately after complete removal of a phaeochromocytoma. Intensive Care Med 1986; 12(1):56–57.
56. Sapienza P, Cavallaro A. Persistent hypertension after removal of adrenal tumours. Eur J Surg 1999; 165:187–192.
57. Meeke RI, O'Keefe JD, Gaffney JD. Phaeochromocytoma removal and postoperative hypoglycaemia. Anesthesia 1985; 40(11):1093–1096.
58. de Graaf JS, Dullaart RP, Zwierstra RP. Complications after bilateral adrenalectomy for phaeochromocytoma in multiple endocrine neoplasia type 2–A plea to conserve adrenal function. Eur J Surg 1999; 165(9):843–846.
59. Arlt W, Allolio B. Adrenal insufficiency. Lancet 2003; 361:1881–1893.
60. Jadoul M, Ferrant A, De Plaen JF, Crabbe J. Mineralocorticoids in the management of primary adrenocortical insufficiency. J Endocrinol Invest 1991; 14:87–91.
61. Groves RW, Toms GC, Houghton BJ, Monson JP. Corticosteroid replacement therapy: twice or thrice daily? J R Soc Med 1988; 81(9):514–516.
62. Stewart PM. Adrenal replacement therapy: time for an inward look to the medulla? J Clin Endocrinol Metab 2004; 89(8):3677–3678.

63. Kehlet H, Binder C, Blichert-Toft M. Glucocorticoid maintenence therapy following adrenalectomy: assessment of dosage and preparation. Clin Endocrinol 1976; 5(1):37–41.
64. Wichers M, Springer W, Bidlingmaier F, Klingmuller D. The influence of hydrocortisone substitution on the quality of life and paameters of bone metabolism in patients with secondary hypercortisolism. Clin Endocrinol 1999; 50(6):759–765.
65. Henriques HF III, Lebovic D. Defining and focusing perioperative steroid supplementation. Am Surg 1995; 61:809–813.
66. Flemming TG, Kristensen LO. Quality of self-care in patients on replacement therapy with hydrocortisone. J Int Med 1999; 246(5):497–501.
67. Soulie M, Mouly P, Caron P, et al. Retroperitoneal laparoscopic adrenalectomy: clinical experience in 52 procedures. Urology 2000; 56(6):921–925.

27 | Complications of Laparoscopic Radical Prostatectomy

Patricio C. Gargollo and Douglas M. Dahl
Harvard Medical School and Department of Urology, Massachusetts General Hospital, Boston, Massachusetts, U.S.A.

INTRODUCTION

The first reports of laparoscopy were published in the early twentieth century (1). Since then, laparoscopy has been widely implemented and established as an invaluable surgical technique in multiple specialties. The first reported series of transperitoneal laparoscopic radical prostatectomy (LRP) was by Schuessler et al. in 1997 who reported their experience in nine patients. The mean operative time was 9.4 hours and they had three complications (cholecystitis, pulmonary embolism, and a small bowel hernia into a trocar site) (2). They concluded that LRP was feasible but offered no advantage over radical retropubic prostatectomy (RRP) with regard to oncologic outcomes, length of stay (LOS), convalescence, or cosmetic result. The high rate of complications reported in this initial series relegated LRP to relative obscurity in the United States for several years. The Montsouris Institute in Paris, France performed their first LRP in 1998 and reported the first large series of LRP in 65 patients (3). This report re-established LRP as a feasible alternative for the surgical treatment of prostate cancer. Improved surgical training, the establishment of centers specializing in minimally invasive surgery, and the recent addition of robotic-assisted LRP has increased the popularity of this procedure for the treatment of localized prostate cancer. In fact, as of January 1, 2006 there have been over 8000 cases of LRP reported in the literature.

When a radical prostatectomy is planned the first question that arises is which surgical technique should be used? Current technology and surgical training have expanded the urologist's armamentarium in this arena and both the physician and the patient must choose if this procedure should be done open or laparoscopically (with or without robotic assistance). Although LRP is a challenging operation, there are various methods for surgeon education which have made skill attainment for this type of operation feasible. These include laparoscopic skills training laboratories, models of the urethrovesical anastomosis, and dedicated mentorship programs run by experienced laparoscopists (4,5).

The current body of scientific evidence has shown that LRP provides equal oncologic and functional outcomes as RRP (6–9). Recent large series of LRP cohorts further suggest that the complication rate may be lower than RRP when the operation is performed by a urologist with extensive laparoscopic experience (10,11). The advantages of minimally invasive surgery benefit both the surgeon and patient. With improved technology and 10–15× magnification LRP provides superior visualization and resolution of anatomical structures and surgical planes when compared with RRP. The maintenance of pneumoperitoneum during the operation has also been theorized to decreased blood loss through venous compression. Minimally invasive techniques in surgery have also led to a decreased LOS, shorter convalescence, and improved cosmesis (Fig. 1). The theoretical disadvantages of LRP over RRP are the lack of tactile feedback, a steep learning curve, and potentially increased initial cost especially for centers not having an established minimally invasive center. In short, although LRP is a technically challenging operation which requires mastery of advanced laparoscopic skills, it can be carried out safely and effectively with excellent oncologic and functional outcomes.

There are complications that are inherent to laparoscopy and there are those that are inherent to the procedure, in this case RRP. The complications discussed here are not exclusive to laparoscopy but rather to radical surgery of the prostate. The etiology, recognition, and management of these complications differ from those of RRP given that the fundamentals of each surgical technique are different. This chapter will cover the most frequently encountered and

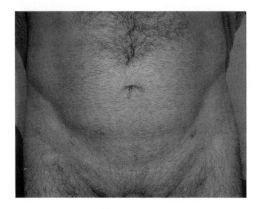

FIGURE 1 Cosmetic result after laparoscopic radical prostatectomy.

described complications of LRP as well as their management. With few exceptions these are the same complications encountered with robotic-assisted LRP.

INTRAOPERATIVE COMPLICATIONS OF LAPAROSCOPY

There are complications related to the technique of laparoscopy regardless of the type of surgery being performed. A thorough review of the physiologic changes that occur during laparoscopy is beyond the scope of this chapter but should be information that is very familiar to the laparoscopic urologist (12). The establishment and maintenance of an adequate working area for LRP involves insufflation of carbon dioxide gas either in the intra- or extra-peritoneal space (depending on the approach used). The increased intra-abdominal pressure is transmitted to the diaphragm, restricting lung volumes and decreasing pulmonary compliance. The same pressure leads to a reduction in cardiac preload and an increase in cardiac afterload and thus an overall decrease in cardiac output. Although these changes do not seem to be clinically significant in healthy patients under standard insufflation pressures (15–20 mmHg), the potential for cardiovascular compromise should always be considered (13,14). Table 1 lists the potential causes for cardiovascular collapse during laparoscopic surgery. The management of these particular complications is covered elsewhere in this text.

SURGICAL TECHNIQUE AT MASSACHUSETTS GENERAL HOSPITAL

At the Massachusetts General Hospital we primarily use an extraperitoneal approach for LRP the details of which have been previously described (15,16). All patients self-administer an oral FLEET® phosphosoda bowel preparation one day before surgery. Upon arrival to the operating room they receive a dose of antibiotics, usually cefazolin (unless they have a documented allergy). We do not use preoperative heparin or anticoagulants but all patients have compression stockings and pneumatic compression boots placed and activated prior to induction of anesthesia. Once anesthesia is induced, the patient is positioned supine with arms tucked at the sides and the legs slightly spread. A pillow is placed behind the knees and the ankles are padded. We

TABLE 1 Causes of Cardiovascular Failure During Laparoscopic Surgery

Vasovagal reflex
Myocardial infarction
Carbon dioxide embolus
Hemorrhage
Diaphragm rupture
Pneumothorax
Pneumomediastinum
Pulmonary embolus
Arrhythmias
Decreased venous return

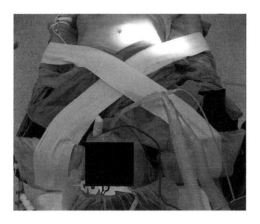

FIGURE 2 Patient positioning. Patients are placed on a vacuum bean bag with the shoulder extensions draped over the shoulders and padded prior to deflation. Care should be taken not to hyperextend the shoulders at this step in positioning as this may cause a brachial plexus injury. Note that the arms are padded and tucked at the patient's side.

use a vacuum bean bag under the patient and drape the shoulder extensions over the patient's shoulders prior to deflating it. The shoulder extensions are then taped in a crossed fashion across the patient's chest and the tape is secured to the operating table (Fig. 2). This allows for the table to be placed in steep Trendelenburg without fear that the patient will not remain securely in position. We make an infraumbilical incision, open the anterior rectus sheath, and develop the preperitoneal working space with the aid of an oval preperitoneal distention balloon (United States Surgical, Tyco Healthcare Group, Norwalk, Connecticut, U.S.A.). We then position our working trocars as shown in Figure 3. The laparoscopic camera and a 0° lens are controlled with the voice-activated AESOP robot (Computer Motion Inc., Bethesda, California, U.S.A.). We do not use a laparoscopic cautery device at any time during the LRP. All dissection is carried out with the 5 mm curved Harmonic Scalpel® (Ethicon Inc., Somerville, New Jersey, U.S.A.) or with laparoscopic scissors. If a pelvic lymphadenectomy is indicated we perform this first. The dissection of the prostate begins with incision of the endopelvic fascia. The dorsal venous complex is then ligated but not transected at this time. The bladder neck is divided and the posterior prostatic space is developed to identify the seminal vesicles which are very carefully dissected free of their attachments. The vasa are identified and divided. The prostatic pedicles are then divided with

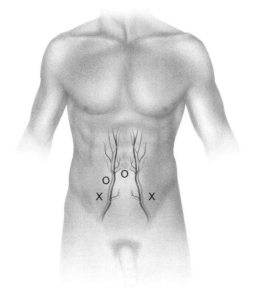

FIGURE 3 Trocar positioning. Three working and one camera port are arranged as shown. O (infraumbilical): Camera Port 12 mm balloon tipped trocar (12 mm Blunt tip trocar; United States Surgical, O (right paramedian): 11 mm working port. X: 5 mm working ports. The inferior epigastric vessels are in close vicinity to these ports and can be injured during trocar insertion or while changing instruments.

the Harmonic Scalpel®. If the neurovascular bundles are to be preserved they are dissected free from the prostatic capsule with laparoscopic scissors. We have previously described the technique of hydrodissection of the neurovascular bundles which we feel is very helpful during this step (17). Denonvilliers fascia is incised and the dissection continues caudad until the apex is clearly visualized. The dorsal vein is divided and the urethra is then divided taking care to preserve as much urethral length as possible. The vesicourethral anastomosis is then performed with six, interrupted 2-0 polyglactin sutures. A 20 Fr Foley catheter is placed and the anastomosis is tested for leaks with saline. A closed suction drain is positioned and the prostate is removed within a laparoscopic bag via the umbilical incision. All patients receive two further doses of intravenous antibiotics. Most patients are discharged home on postoperative day one. The bladder catheter is routinely removed on postoperative day seven.

CHARACTERIZING THE SEVERITY OF COMPLICATIONS

Comparing morbidity among different centers for LRP remains difficult as institutions and surgeons do not define, classify, or record their complications in a standardized fashion. The reporting of complications is further limited in part because of the ambulatory nature of this procedure. That is, small deviations in recovery of function may go unreported or not be recorded by the physician. Lastly, follow-up data may not be available for patients who travel to centers seeking treatment by LRP and subsequently return to their home institutions. Several published studies have aimed to classify the severity of complications of LRP using the Clavien grading classification system (11,18–20). This system offers a convenient and reproducible metric with which to evaluate complications of different techniques of radical prostatectomy. It suffers, however, in that differences in data collection and reporting, and variability in interpretation make comparisons between techniques almost impossible (21). Therefore, in order to truly evaluate and compare the complications experienced during LRP, a standardized, prospective method of data acquisition is necessary and must be established.

PERIOPERATIVE COMPLICATIONS
Injury During Patient Positioning

Patient positioning during LRP requires meticulous attention to detail in order to prevent serious injury. This procedure can be lengthy, especially at the beginning of the learning curve, and potential complications solely related to prolonged extrinsic compression on tissues are not uncommon. As can be seen, the patient is placed supine in steep Trendelenburg with the arms tucked at the sides (Fig. 2). We prefer to use a vacuum bean bag for shoulder and torso support and secure the patient to the bed with wide cloth tape. Care is taken not to hyperextend the shoulders at this time as this can be a cause of brachial plexus injuries. Vallancien et al. reported two patients with such injuries who had transient paresis of the upper limb. These resolved spontaneously in less than one week (22). Some centers place the legs in lithotomy stirrups which can be helpful for accessing the rectum or applying perineal pressure during urethrovesical anastomosis. Care must be taken to adequately pad potential pressure sites to the ulnar and common peroneal nerves. The eyes should also be protected by the anesthesia team as corneal abrasions and conjunctivitis from corneal irritation by saliva have been reported in LRP series (22).

OPERATIVE COMPLICATIONS
Injury During Port Placement

All laparoscopic surgery has in common the need to establish access to the anatomical location of interest through an initial primary port. There are different methods of accomplishing this which have been described and range from the "open" Hasson technique (23) to Veress needle insertion. In a large study of laparoscopic entry access injuries Chandler et al. noted that 75% of initial access injuries involved puncture to the bowel or retroperitoneal vessels (24). Injury during secondary port placement was to abdominal wall vessels in 35% of cases, to the aorta or iliac artery in 30% of cases, and to the small bowel in 10% of cases. In the same study, the authors found that the majority of injuries occurred when using shielded pyramidal and shielded blade trocars. Although the Hasson technique is thought to be the safest approach, it still carries a significant risk of intra-abdominal injury, especially to the small bowel (24,25).

Peripheral Neurologic Injuries

The most frequent cause of neurologic injuries during LRP is by direct damage to nerves or traction injuries from inadequate patient positioning (see above section). Injury to the obturator nerve during pelvic lymphadenectomy is a known complication of both RRP and LRP. During LRP care must be taken to visually identify the obturator nerve prior to ligation and cutting of the inferior aspect of the node bundle. If the nerve is ligated but not cut, removal of the clip is all that is necessary although most of these patients will be symptomatic from the crush injury. Transection of the obturator nerve during LRP can be repaired by reapproximating the nerve sheath with 7-0 polypropylene sutures in interrupted fashion. This situation was reported by Hu et al. with resolution of adductor weakness seen at one month postoperatively (19).

Bowel Complications

Bowel injuries during LRP can occur during trocar placement, during instrument exchange, during tissue dissection, or as a result of thermal injury from electrocautery devices. In LRP the lateral large bowel (sigmoid and cecum) is vulnerable to injury during placement of the lateral ports and when instruments are being changed. Thermal tissue damage from a harmonic scalpel or electrocautery device as well as arcing of the monopolar current to adjacent organs is a common etiology of bowel injury and accounts for more than half of all laparoscopic bowel injuries (26). Inadequate placement and subsequent inadvertent activation of coagulation pedals is also associated with organ injury. Thermal injury can be prevented by maintaining the instruments away from adjacent bowel, keeping in mind that heat diffuses along tissue plains, and assuring that all instruments are insulated properly. The location of the tip of the instrument should be known by both the surgeon and the scrub nurse at all times. The scrub nurse should ensure that all instruments have an intact insulation coating and that all connections are adequate and secure. It has been shown that tissue necrosis occurs when a temperature differential of 30°C is reached for as little as two seconds (27).

The most important aspect regarding bowel injuries is that they need to be identified intraoperatively. Failure to recognize these injuries when they occur can have significant morbidity and mortality. In fact in a large study of laparoscopic entry access injuries Chandler et al. showed that delayed recognition and diagnosis of these injuries along with age greater than 59 years were significant predictors of fatal outcomes (24). They also noted that unrecognized bowel injuries were significantly more likely to cause death than injuries to major retroperitoneal vessels. Early recognition is particularly important as patients with laparoscopic bowel injuries will present with atypical signs and symptoms. Bishoff et al. reviewed their experience as well as the published experience with laparoscopic bowel injuries (26). They noted that this is a rare complication in laparoscopy occurring in approximately 1.3/1000 cases. The majority of injuries (69%) were not recognized intra-operatively and the most common segment of bowel injured was the small bowel (58%) followed by the colon (32%). Of the injuries 50% were caused by thermal injury from electrocautery instruments and 32% from Veress needle or trocar insertion. One of the most interesting and clinically relevant observations raised by this report is that the initial presenting symptom of all patients in their series with unrecognized bowel injury was persistent pain at a single trocar site without significant erythema or purulent discharge. Ileus, nausea, vomiting, fever, leukocytosis, and peritoneal signs were uncommon findings. In fact, all but one patient had leukopenia. Two of three patients with unrecognized colonic injuries died of sepsis.

The exact etiology for the atypical presentation in patients with laparoscopic bowel injury is not known. It has been postulated that the minimally invasive nature of laparoscopy leads to less tissue damage and a less pronounced stimulation of acute phase reactants and inflammatory mediators (28–30).

When a bowel perforation is recognized it should be repaired immediately. A double layer closure should be used for colonic and rectal injuries while a single layer closure is usually sufficient for small bowel injuries (31). Some authors have advocated the repair of serosal abrasions as abscess formation and fistula have been noted at these sites (26).

If a bowel injury is suspected in a postoperative patient abdominal pelvic computed tomography (CT) with oral contrast has been shown to be a reliable method for diagnosis (32). Alternatively, a diagnostic laparoscopy can be performed with high diagnostic accuracy in 92% to 97% of cases (33,34). Any injury noted at laparoscopy can then be immediately repaired either laparoscopically or with open surgery depending on the skill and comfort of the surgeon.

Rectal Injury

Injury to the rectum is a specific type of bowel injury that needs to be considered separately. Rectal injury during LRP has been reported in 0.3% to 3.8% of cases (Table 2) (35). During RRP most rectal injuries occur while transecting the rectourethralis muscle and inadvertently cutting too far into the anterior rectal wall. (9) Most rectal injuries during LRP occur during the dissection of the posterior prostate and Denonvilliers' fascia particularly at the prostatic apex. In fact, in a series of 1000 LRPs, Guillonneau et al. reported 13 rectal injuries, 10 of which occurred during dissection of the posterior surface of the prostate at the apex (36). Anterior traction on the prostate during apical dissection has also been implicated in rectal tear injuries during LRP (18). Lastly, these types of injuries can occur from thermal or electrical injury to the rectum at any point during an LRP. Some have advocated that the most important measure to avoid rectal injury during LRP is to adhere to the posterior prostate surface during dissection and stress the importance of utilizing a rectal probe during LRP (18,37). However, the use of a rectal probe in these two series did not seem to prevent rectal injury as these series had a rectal injury rate of 1.6% and 1.4%. Furthermore, the use of a rectal probe does not seem to increase the rate of intraoperative diagnosis of rectal injury.

There are several methods for identifying rectal injuries during RRP which may be used during LRP. When such an injury is suspected digital rectal examination can be helpful in diagnosis (38). The technique described by Pisters can also be used whereby the pelvis is filled with irrigant and air is insufflated into the rectum. Bubbles in the irrigation fluid confirm a rectal injury (39).

Laparoscopic repairs of rectal injuries incurred during LRP have been described (36,40,41). The main point, as in other bowel injuries, is that these need to be recognized at the time they occur in the operating room in order to minimize morbidity. Once these injuries are diagnosed, either by direct visualization or by some of the techniques listed above, the pelvis needs to be copiously irrigated with saline. The edges of the defect should be clearly identified and closed in two layers (mucosal and serosal) with a 3-0 absorbable suture. The integrity of the repair should be checked with air insufflation as described above. Prior to urethrovesical anastomosis some authors have advocated interposition of the omentum, perirectal, or perivesical fat between the bladder and rectal repair (40). Urethrovesical anastomosis can then be completed with particular emphasis on a watertight closure. One or two suction drains should be placed. Postoperatively the patient is placed on a liquid diet initially and then on a low residue diet. Broad-spectrum antibiotics should be instituted at the time of injury and continued for at least seven days. There is no consensus on when the bladder catheter should be removed in these cases or whether a cystogram should be performed prior to removal and these decisions are really at the discretion of the surgeon. In addition, no clear agreement exists as to whether or not a bowel preparation is needed prior to LRP or whether a bowel preparation has any effect on the outcome of rectal injuries during LRP. In contemporary series there does not seem to be any differences in patient outcomes if a bowel preparation is used or not as long as the rectal injury is recognized and repaired in two layers intraoperatively immediately after it occurs (36,40). Although there is no clear evidence for this, a diverting colostomy should be considered in cases of gross fecal spillage, previous radiation, an urethrovesical anastomosis under tension, or in a patient who is chronically treated with steroids (38,42). The consequences of a missed rectal injury or of inappropriate repair can have significant morbidity and are covered elsewhere (40,43).

It is still unclear if an extraperitoneal approach is safer in terms of rectal injury. Bollens et al. reported one series of 50 patients and encountered no rectal injuries while Rozet et al. had

TABLE 2 Reported Perioperative and Operative Complication Rates for Various Laparoscopic Radial Prostatectomy Series

Author	Approach	Number of patients	Mean operative time (min)	Mean EBL (mL)	Transfusion (%)	Rectal injury (%)	Other bowel injury (%)	Bladder injury (%)	Ureteral injury (%)	Percent conversions
Schuessler 1997 (2)	TP	9	564	583	n/a	0	0	0	0	0
Dahl 2002 (16)	TP	70	274	449	5.7	1.4	1.4	0	0	1.4
Guillonneau 2002 (18)	TP	567	203	380	4.9	1.4	0.5	1.6	0.5	1.2
Eden 2002 (72)	TP	100	245	313	3	1	0	0	0	1
Gregori 2003 (75)	TP	80	218	376	53.75[a]	0	0	0	0	0
Stolzenburg 2005 (47)	EP	700	151	220	0.9	0.6	0	0	0	0
Rozet 2005 (45)	EP	600	173	380	1.2	0.67	0	0	0	0
Gonzalgo 2005 (11)	TP	250	n/a	n/a	2.8	0.8	0	0	0	1.6
Hu 2006 (19)	TP	358	246	200	2.2	1.9	0.3	0	13.4	0.8
Rassweiler 2006[b] (10)	TP and EP	5424	211	n/a	4.1	1.7	0.7	n/a	0.1	2.4

This table shows the reported rates of perioperative and operative complications.
[a]46.25% of patients in this series received their autolgous units only and 6.25% received both autologous and homologous units.
[b]This was a meta-analysis of 18 centers and in this published report items marked n/a were not specifically mentioned.
Abbreviations: EBL, estimated blood loss; EP, extraperitoneal; TP, transperitoneal.

two missed injuries in a series of 600 patients who then presented postoperatively with peritonitis and a rectourethral fistula (44,45). The posterior dissection of the prostate is the same for both approaches and as it is at this time that most of these injuries occur, it does not seem that either approach would have an advantage over the other in this respect.

Bleeding

Some amount of bleeding can be expected for any surgical procedure and at which point operative bleeding becomes a "complication" is subject to debate. Obviously, an unplanned or unrecognized injury to a blood vessel or an injury that requires any additional intervention beyond that planned during a procedure constitutes a complication. During LRP inadvertent injury to vessels usually occurs during trocar placement, during pelvic lymphadenectomy, or during instrument exchange and inadvertent injury to the iliac vessels or the epigastric vessels. Injury to accessory pudendal arteries has also been described (46). The rates of these types of injuries are rare in contemporary series and range from 0% to 1% (Table 2) (11,45,47,48). However, although rare, intraoperative recognition is very important. In a series by Guillonneau et al. epigastric artery laceration/avulsion was reported in only three cases but they were all diagnosed postoperatively and required subsequent operative intervention in one patient and transfusion in all three. They therefore advocate decreasing the insufflation pressure at the end of the operation and removing the trocars under direct vision (18). Bleeding from a trocar site may be stopped with direct electrocautery or clip placement. In the case of injury to a larger anterior abdominal wall vessel or persistent bleeding, repair of the defect using a Reverdin needle, a Carter-Thomason needle, or the EndoClose® device (U.S. Surgical Corp., Norwalk, Connecticut, U.S.A.) is usually sufficient.

A theoretical advantage of minimally invasive surgery is decreased bleeding. This seems to be the case when comparing LRP to RRP, although blood loss during both procedures is difficult to quantify as blood mixes with urine during the case. A more reliable predictor of bleeding as a complication may be blood transfusion rates. Both of these parameters vary widely in reported series with the estimated blood loss (EBL) ranging from 150 to 1100 mL and transfusion rates ranging from 0% to 31% (2,16,37,41,44,48–50). Despite these differences, the average EBL and average transfusion rates for LRP seems, to be less than that of RRP (51). Furthermore, the EBL seems to decrease with the surgeon's experience. In one large series of 550 patients, the average EBL was 380 mL for the whole series and 290 mL for the last 350 patients (48).

The two major sites of bleeding during LRP are the dorsal venous plexus and the prostatic pedicles. Adequate ligation of the former and meticulous hemostasis during pedicle dissection will obviate most serious hemorrhage. The actual degree of bleeding can be underestimated visually by the surgeon secondary to insufflation pressure on venous structures. For this reason it is imperative to decrease the insufflation pressure and examine the field for bleeding prior to the conclusion of the operation. Unrecognized venous bleeding during LRP may lead to pelvic hematoma formation. Although some amount of hematoma may be expected, larger hematomas may lead to recurrent fevers, infection, voiding symptoms, urinary retention, pelvic pain, and anastomotic disruption (52). In these cases we have found it best to drain these hematomas either through a percutaneous approach or through a small infraumbilical incision. Although not technically a bleeding complication, lymphocele is a recognized complication of laparoscopic lymphadenectomy and has been noted to occur in 0.1% to 1% of patients (Table 2) (53). If these become symptomatic or infected, percutaneous drainage is also a good treatment modality.

Ureteral Injury

Ureteral complications have been reported in 0% to 1% of patients undergoing LRP (Table 2) (6,35). The majority of ureteral injuries occur at one of three specific steps in the dissection of the bladder or during vesicourethral anastomosis (18). During LRP, the ureter is usually injured during:

1. Posterior dissection of the vesiculo-deferential junction if the transperitoneal Montsouris technique is used (54) (Fig. 4).

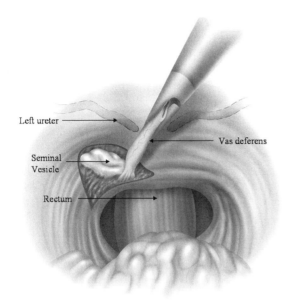

Left ureter

Vas deferens

Seminal
Vesicle

Rectum

FIGURE 4 Sites of ureteral injury during the transperitoneal (TP) approach. This picture represents the TP mobilization of the vas and seminal vesicles. The ureters can be seen represented here by the dashed lines. They course below the peritoneum and thus can be injured during the transperitoneal approach. The two most common injuries occur during posterior dissection of the vesiculo–deferential junction (if the TP Montsouris technique is used) or during dissection of the lateral vesical peritoneum. Injury during the second scenario is especially the case if the dissection is carried too far caudad and it is for this reason the bladder should be mobilized only to the level where the vas deferens crosses the iliac vessels.

2. Dissection of the lateral vesical peritoneum. This is especially the case if the dissection is carried too far caudad and it is for this reason the bladder should be mobilized only to the level where the vas deferens crosses the iliac vessels (Fig. 4).
3. Dissection of the dorsal bladder neck and injury to the ureteral orifices. Patients particularly at risk for these types of injuries are those in which a previous trans-urethral resection of the prostate has been performed or who have a prominent median lobe (Figs. 5 and 6). In these cases the ureteral orifices are close to the transection plane between the bladder and prostate.

In all three of these cases the ureter may be injured directly or indirectly by thermal or electrical injury (22). Another common step during LRP resulting in ureteral injury is suture placement near or through the ureteral orifice at the time of urethrovesical anastomosis resulting in ureteral obstruction (Fig. 7). If the ureteral orifices appear close to the edge of the dorsal bladder neck (Fig. 6) we advocate cannulating the ureteral orifices with 5 Fr. pediatric feeding tubes prior to suture placement. These are left in place during the anastomosis and are removed prior to placement of the ventral sutures (Fig. 8).

Ideally, any ureteral injury should be recognized at the time it occurs. In these cases the ureter can be repaired primarily over a ureteral stent or an ureteroneocystostomy can be performed. Both these techniques have been performed laparoscopically (55,56). If the diagnosis is

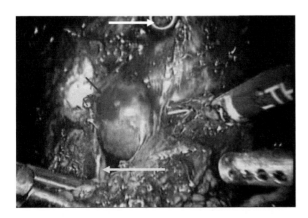

FIGURE 5 Dissection of a large median lobe. This picture shows a patient with a large median lobe undergoing laparoscopic radical prostatectomy. The *top arrow* shows the urethral sound in place. The *middle arrow* shows the large median lobe. The *bottom arrow* shows the ventral lip of the bladder neck. In these cases, the ureteral orifices can be easily damaged and must be identified and preserved when dividing the dorsal bladder neck.

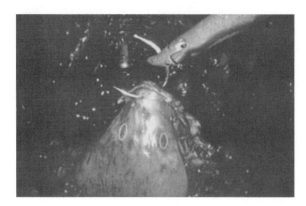

FIGURE 6   Bladder neck after large median lobe dissection. As can be seen, the ureteral orifices (highlighted by two circles) are close to the edge of the bladder neck and are at risk for injury during vesicourethral anastomosis.

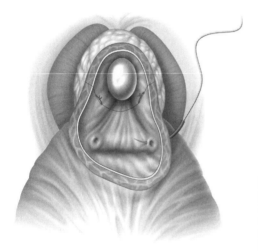

FIGURE 7   Injury to the ureter during vesicourethral anastomosis. Injury to the ureteral orifice can occur during division of the dorsal bladder neck or during suture placement for vesicourethral anastomosis. Depicted here is an anastomotic suture placed in the vicinity of the ureteral orifice. This type of injury can lead to ureteral obstruction.

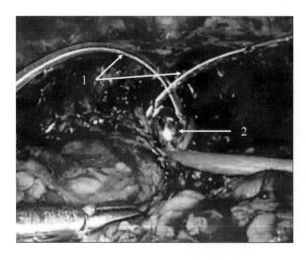

FIGURE 8   Feeding tubes in the ureteral orifices. In cases where the ureteral orifices are close to the bladder neck, we advocate cannulating the ureters with 5 Fr. pediatric feeding tubes during placement of the posterior and lateral sutures. Once these are placed and tied, effortless motion of these tubes within the ureters confirms that there has not been an inadvertent injury with one of the sutures. At this time the tubes are removed and the anterior sutures are placed and tied. *1*, feeding tubes in ureters; *2*, urethral sound.

not made intra-operatively, persistent urinary ascites in the absence of an urethrovesical anastomotic leak should raise suspicion for an occult proximal ureteral injury. Flank pain, hydronephrosis, or creatinine elevation in the absence of urinary ascites is usually indicative of a ureteral orifice or distal ureteral injury. Partial transactions can be handled by endourologic placement of a ureteral stent while complete transactions necessitate ureteroureterostomy or ureteroneocystostomy (57,58). Unrecognized ureteral orifice obstruction or damage will usually require anastomotic revision or temporary percutaneous nephrostomy tube placement.

Bladder Injury

Bladder injuries are rare and occur almost exclusively during dissection of the retrovesical space to gain access to the seminal vesicles or during dissection of the retropubic space during a transperitoneal approach. In their series of 567 patients Guillonneau et al. reported nine bladder injuries all of which occurred during dissection of the retropubic space (18). These were identified intraoperatively and repaired without sequelae. Bladder injury during retropubic dissection is a particular risk if the patient has undergone a previous laparoscopic prosthetic mesh inguinal herniorrhaphy (59).

Conversion Rates

LRP is a technically demanding operation which requires competence in advanced laparoscopic techniques. There is a definite learning curve for this operation and the rate of complications seems to decrease with surgeon experience (10,48). This is very evident if conversion rates are examined. Conversion rates in the literature for LRP range from 0% to 6% depending on the series (6). A multi-institutional study of conversions from LRP to open surgery found a rate of 1.9% (60). The most common steps of the operation requiring conversion in that series were apical and posterior dissection followed by dissection of the bladder neck. Thirty-one percent of the conversions occurred after injury to adjacent organs requiring open repair. As could be expected, the majority (46%) of conversions occurred during the surgeons' first five cases further stressing the steep learning curve of this procedure.

Open conversion is sometimes required if there is a lack of well-defined tissue planes which may occur secondary to previous surgery, previous injury, inflammation or infection. Although previous abdominal surgery is not a contraindication for LRP, certain surgeries, such as hernia repairs with mesh (especially if the mesh is in the properitoneal space), may preclude an extraperitoneal approach and should be approached intraperitoneally as we have previously described (59).

Extraperitoneal vs. Transperitoneal Laparoscopic Radical Prostatectomy and Complication Rates

The introduction of extraperitoneal LRP (EP-LRP) by Raboy in 1997 and later Bollens in 2001 and 2002 established a new technique for LRP. From a complications standpoint the theoretical advantage of an extraperitoneal approach is that there may be less potential for intraperitoneal organ injury. However, in a series of 600 EP-LRPs, Rozet et al. reported no real difference in the incidence of rectal injury or anastomotic leaks between the two approaches (45). The one exception to this was that they encountered no ureteral injuries. Thus, there may be an advantage regarding extravesical ureteral injuries with EP-LRP given that most of these types of injuries seem to occur during the transperitoneal (TP) dissection of the rectovesical space (18). Cathelineau et al. also compared both techniques and found no difference regarding operative, postoperative, or pathological data (61). The authors make a point that EP-LRP may have the advantage of creating a limited potential space for fluid collection and extravasation. Therefore, postoperative anastomotic leaks (or hematomas) can be managed more effectively than in TP-LRP patients as the urinoma is usually contained to the space of Retzius and patients do not develop urinary ascites with resultant ileus. The choice for which approach to use is surgeon dependent and must be based on operator experience and comfort with a particular technique. We have reported previously however that the EP approach is particularly useful in obese patients (62) or in patients who have had precious abdominal surgery (15).

TABLE 3 Reported Postoperative Complication Rates for Various Laparoscopic Radical Prostatectomy Series

Author	Approach	Number of patients	Anastomotic leak (%)	Bladder neck contracture (%)	Ileus (%)	Neuropathy (%)	Hernia at trocar site (%)	Pelvic hematoma (%)	Lymphocele (%)
Schuessler 1997 (2)	TP	9	0	0	n/a	n/a	11	0	0
Dahl 2002 (16)	TP	70	8.6	0	8.6	1.4	0	0	0
Guillonneau 2002 (18)	TP	567	10	n/a	1.1	0.5	0	0.9	0.17
Eden 2002 (72)	TP	100	1	2	1	1	1	1	0
Gregori 2003 (75)	TP	80	7.5	1.25	1.25	0	0	6.25	0
Stolzenburg 2005 (47)	EP	700	n/a	0.25	n/a	0.3	0.14	0.9	1
Rozet 2005 (45)	EP	600	5.16	0.17	n/a	0	0	0.33	0.17
Gonzalgo 2005 (11)	TP	250	n/a	1.2	3.3	0	0	0	0
Hu 2006 (19)	TP	358	13.4	2.2	5.3	0.67	0	0	0.8
Rassweiler 2006[a] (10)	TP and EP	5424	2.4	0.4	n/a	n/a	n/a	0.5	0.4

[a]This was a meta-analysis of 18 centers and in this published report items marked n/a were not specifically mentioned.
Abbreviations: EP, extraperitoneal; TP, transperitoneal.

POSTOPERATIVE COMPLICATIONS
Anastomotic Complications

Urine leak from the urethrovesical anastomosis can be observed as an early or late complication and is the most common complication of LRP seen in up to 13% of patients (Table 3). Persistent, high volume drainage from the closed suction drain early in the postoperative course can lead to reflex ileus from urinary ascites with concomitant elevation of the serum creatinine. This can especially be observed if the TP approach is used. The best method to prevent a leak from the anastomosis is to ensure intravesical positioning of the bladder catheter and to test the anastomosis for water-tightness with saline irrigation intra-operatively. If a leak is detected postoperatively this should be managed by continuing the closed suction drain and bladder drainage until the leak closes. Guillonneau et al. reported an anastomotic leak in 57 out of 567 patients (10%). Forty-six of these healed spontaneously by continuing suction drainage prolonging bladder drainage for an average of 12 days. One patient required operative intervention (18). In 11 patients they noted a delayed leak after their bladder catheters were removed. These patients presented with urinary retention and abdominal pain and were treated with replacement of the bladder catheter for 1 week without subsequent sequelae.

Bladder neck contracture is usually a late complication of LRP and has been reported in approximately 0.5% to 2% of patients. Some authors have stated that there may be an association between bladder neck contractures and a running suture technique for the urethrovesical anastomosis (63). As there have been no prospective randomized trials comparing a running suture anastomosis to an interrupted anastomosis as related to bladder neck contracture, this cannot be proved at this time. The management and treatment of bladder neck contractures is covered elsewhere in this text.

Ileus

Ileus can occur after RRP or LRP and has been noted to occur in 1% to 8.6% of patients undergoing these procedures (Table 3). It is difficult to evaluate the extent of this complication as centers define ileus differently. Most ileus is associated with urinary ascites and resolution of anastomotic leaks as well as medical management with or without nasogastric tube placement usually suffices as therapy in these cases. Two entities must be excluded when a patient has postoperative ileus. The first is a small bowel hernia at a trocar site causing a small bowel obstruction. (11) The second is an unrecognized bowel injury leading to ileus. This second complication can be fatal and must be recognized and treated immediately.

Thromboembolic Complications

Deep venous thrombosis and pulmonary embolus are infrequent but serious complications of RRP and LRP. Perioperative prophylaxis with low molecular weight heparin and/or pneumatic compression stockings as well as early postoperative ambulation have decreased the frequency of these complications even further. Early series of RRP reported the rate of these complications to be as high as 5% (64). Current LRP series report the frequency of these complications at 0% to 1% (Table 4). In cases where thromboembolic events were reported, patients were usually bedridden for prolonged periods of time usually because of an initial, primary complication (bleeding, peritonitis, anastomotic leak) (48).

Positive Surgical Margins

The main objective of radical prostatectomy is the complete removal of the cancerous gland with subsequent reconstruction of the genitourinary system. Therefore, a positive margin should be considered as a complication. There are various definitions in the literature of what should be considered a positive surgical margin and this makes comparison between different series and different techniques difficult. However, when examining the oncologic results from published LRP series there seems to be no difference from those reported in RRP series (Table 5) (65–72). Brown et al. examined a series of 60 sequential LRPs versus 60 sequential RRPs. There was no significant difference in pathologic stage or grade and they found similar positive margin rates (17% for LRP and 20% for RRP) (8). An interesting observation was made

TABLE 4 Thromboembolic Complications and Mortality Rates

Author	Approach	Number of Patients	DVT (%)	Pulmonary Embolus (%)	Myocardial Infarction (%)	CVA (%)	Death (%)	Percent Overall Complications
Schuessler 1997 (2)	TP	9	0	11	0	0	0	33
Dahl 2002 (16)	TP	70	0	0	1.4	0	0	20
Guillonneau 2002 (18)	TP	567	0.35	0	0	0	0	17.1
Eden 2002 (72)	TP	100	0	0	0	0	0	8
Gregori 2003 (75)	TP	80	0	0	1.25	1.25	1.25	30
Stolzenburg 2005 (47)	EP	700	0.9	0	0.14	0.14	0	14.9
Rozet 2005 (45)	EP	600	0	0.17	0	0	0	11.2
Gonzalgo 2005 (11)	TP	250	0.4	0.4	0.4	0	0	15.4
Hu 2006 (19)	TP	358	0	0	0	0	0	19.7
Rassweiler 2006[a] (10)	TP and EP	5424	0.6	0	n/a	n/a	n/a	8.9

This table shows the reported rates of thromboembolic events and mortality as well as the overall complication rates for various published series.
[a]This was a meta-analysis of 18 centers and in this published report items marked n/a were not specifically mentioned.
Abbreviations: CVA, cerebrovascular accident; DVT, deep venous thrombosis; EP, extraperitoneal; TP, transperitoneal.

by Salomon et al. who examined positive margin location for LRP, RRP, and perineal prostatectomy patients (PRP) (73). Although the overall positive margin rate was not significantly different between the three techniques, each approach had a specific high-risk location of positive margins. For RRP most positive margins were at the apex while PRP had a higher incidence at the bladder neck; LRP margins were mostly positive posterolaterally. Hoznek et al. make the point that the rate of positive margins mostly depends on patient selection and the surgeon's experience rather than on the surgical approach used (74).

Urinary Incontinence and Impotence

Perhaps the two most feared complications of radical prostatectomy from a patient's perspective are urinary incontinence and impotence. The magnification and improved visibility inherent to LRP has led to the assumption that this technique may provide better visualization during apical and neurovascular bundle dissection. Whether this translates to better patient outcomes related to these two functional parameters is still debatable. The main problem is that there are

TABLE 5 Oncologic Outcomes for Contemporary Laparoscopic Radical Prostatectomy and Retropubic Prostatectomy Series

References	Patients (n)	Positive surgical margins (%)		Greater than 0.2 ng/ml PSA recurrence (pT2/pT3) (%)		Clinical progression (%)	
		pT2	pT3	3 yrs	5 yrs	3 yrs	5 yrs
LRP							
Salomon et al. 2002 (71)	137	21.9	40.8	9.6/43.2	n/a	n/a	n/a
Roumeguere et al. 2003 (75)	85	7.8	45.7	8.6/11.4	n/a	n/a	n/a
Guillonneau et al. 2003 (9)	1000	15.5	31.1	11.0/33.0	n/a	n/a	n/a
Rassweiler et al. 2005 (6)	500	7.4	31.8	4.8/28.4	10.5/31.8	4.1	9.8
Poulakis et al. 2006 (66)	255	7	27	n/a	n/a	n/a	n/a
Open RRP							
Catalona et al. 1998 (67)	1778		20.9	7.5/21.3	10.0/31.3	n/a	4.5
Huland et al. 2001 (68)	789	14.9	36.5	6.8/27.7	7.7/44.1	n/a	n/a
Han et al. 2001 (69)	2494	n/a	26.4	15.0/25.0	25.0/40.0	n/a	4
Hull et al. 2002 (70)	1000	n/a	12.8	4.4/14.7	5.1/24.7	n/a	10.1
Salomon et al. 2002 (71)	264	16.4	44.3	6.8/42.0	n/a	n/a	n/a

Abbreviations: LRP, laparoscopic radical prostatectomy; n/a, not stated in the publication; PSA, prostate specific antigen; RRP, retropubic prostatectomy.

TABLE 6 Continence Rates in Contemporary Laparoscopic Radical Prostatectomy and Retropubic Prostatectomy Series

References	Approach	Patients (n)	Continence rate at 12 months (%)
Lepor et al. 2004 (75)	RRP	500	92.1
Artibani et al. 2003 (76)	RRP	50	64
	EP	71	40
Guillonneau et al. 2002 (18)	TP	550	82.3
Salomon et al. 2002 (71)	TP	235	90
Rassweiler et al. 2004 (7)	TP	500	83.6
Stolzenburg et al. 2004 (84)	EP	300	89.6
Erdogru et al. 2004 (78)	TP	53	84.9
	EP	53	86.4
Eden et al. 2004 (79)	TP	100	90
	EP	100	96

Continence was defined in these series as no need for protection or pads at any time.
Abbreviations: EP, extraperitoneal; RRP, radical retropubic prostatectomy; TP, transperitoneal.

no precise definitions of impotence or incontinence in the literature. Furthermore, centers have obtained their outcomes data by widely different methods including questionnaires, telephone interviews, or surgeon assessment. Lastly, continence and potency rates will be higher if the patient population is highly selected (younger and with less co-morbidities). Here we present the published data for both these parameters in contemporary series (10,65,75–84). Table 6 shows urinary continence rates for RRP and LRP defined as no need for any pads or "protection." Table 7 shows the sexual potency rates. As can be seen, the rates of potency and continence are comparable for both techniques, especially when the mean patient age is considered. Essentially, postoperative results regarding continence and sexual potency are multifactorial and depend on preoperative function, co-existing disease, and social habits (tobacco and drug use). The fundamental principles of meticulous tissue handling and avoiding electrocautery during the neurovascular dissection hold true for both RRP and LRP and should minimize injury to these structures hopefully resulting in optimal potency and continence rates.

Mortality

Mortality after LRP is negligible (Table 4). Evaluation of multiple contemporary series, totaling over 8000 patients, revealed only one postoperative death from a cerebrovascular accident 35 days after the procedure (85). It has been suggested by some authors that the low mortality may be due to the decreased blood loss seen with LRP (18). This, in turn, may lead to a decrease

TABLE 7 Sexual Potency Rates in Contemporary Laparoscopic Radical Prostatectomy and Retropubic Prostatectomy Series

References	Approach	Patients (n)	Follow-up (mos)	Mean patient age (yrs)	Potency (%)	Definition	Nerve sparing
Walsh et al. 2000 (80)	RRP	64	18	57	86	Intercourse	Bilateral
Stanford et al. 2000 (81)	RRP	1291	18	62.9	44	Intercourse	Bilateral
Katz et al. 2002 (82)	TP	143	12	64	87.5	Erections	Bilateral
Su et al. 2004 (83)	TP	177	12	n/a	76	Intercourse	Bilateral
Eden et al. 2004 (79)	TP	100	12	62	61	Erections	n/a
	EP	100	12		82	Erections	n/a
Romeguere et al. 2003 (65)	RRP	33	12	63.9	54.5	n/a	Bilateral
	TP	26	12	62.5	65.2	n/a	Bilateral
Rassweiler et al. 2006 (10)	TP and EP	5824	12	64	52.5	n/a	Bilateral

All of the data in these series was collected by questionnaires. It should be noted that this data is confounded by the different collection techniques, the definition of potency and the technique of nerve sparing (bilateral or unilateral). Data not stated in the publications is labeled n/a.
Abbreviations: EP, extraperitoneal laparoscopic radical prostatectomy; RRP, radical retropubic prostatectomy; TP, transperitoneal laparoscopic radical prostatectomy.

TABLE 8 American Society of Anesthesiologists' Physical Status Classification

Class 1	A normal healthy patient
Class 2	A patient with mild systemic disease
Class 3	A patient with severe systemic disease
Class 4	A patient with severe systemic disease that is a constant threat to life
Class 5	A moribund patient who is not expected to survive without the operation
Class 6	A declared brain-dead patient whose organs are being removed for donor purposes

in cardiovascular events (notably myocardial infarction and cerebrovascular accidents). Furthermore, it seems likely that the implementation of routine prostate specific antigen testing has led to prostate cancer diagnosis in younger and healthier men who would be less prone to having serious cardiovascular complications. Mortality rates as related to American Society of Anesthesiologists (ASA) classification were evaluated by Dillioglugil et al. in a consecutive series of 472 patients undergoing RRP (86). Sixteen percent of these patients were ASA class 3 (Table 8) (87). This group included the only reported deaths in the series (2), a threefold increase in major complications, prolonged hospital stay, greater need for ICU admissions, and a higher frequency of blood transfusions. Although patient ASA class and complications after LRP have not been specifically evaluated, the observations by Dillioglugil et al. need to be considered.

SUMMARY

Although the complications encountered during LRP are similar to those of RRP, the etiology, recognition, and treatment of these complications is different. The laparoscopic surgeon needs to be familiar with the physiologic changes which occur during insufflation of the working space with carbon dioxide. Establishing and maintaining accesses during laparoscopy as well as the specialized instrumentation required for the procedure carry with them specific risks of organ injury. Early recognition of intra-operative injuries and expedient intervention is crucial to minimize postoperative morbidity. Lastly, although the rate of complications can be expected to be higher early during a surgeon's experience, the rates decrease with familiarity with the procedure and improved proficiency. Fundamentally, there seems to be no difference between RRP and LRP in regard to complication rates, oncologic outcomes, or postoperative functional status.

REFERENCES

1. Lau W, Leow CK, Li AK. History of endoscopic and laparoscopic surgery. World J Surg 1997; 21:444–453.
2. Schuessler WW, Schulam PG, Clayman RV, Kavoussi LR. Laparoscopic radical prostatectomy: initial short-term experience. Urology 1997; 50(6):854–857.
3. Guillonneau B, Cathelineau X, Barret E, Rozet F, Vallancien G. Laparoscopic radical prostatectomy. Preliminary evaluation after 28 interventions. Presse Med 1998; 27(31):1570–1574.
4. Menon M, Shrivastava A, Tewari A, et al. Laparoscopic and robot assisted radical prostatectomy: establishment of a structured program and preliminary analysis of outcomes. J Urol 2002; 168(3):945–949.
5. Fabrizio MD, Tuerk I, Schellhammer PF. Laparoscopic radical prostatectomy: decreasing the learning curve using a mentor initiated approach. J Urol 2003; 169(6):2063–2065.
6. Rassweiler J, Schulze M, Teber D, et al. Laparoscopic radical prostatectomy with the Heilbronn technique: oncological results in the first 500 patients. J Urol 2005; 173(3):761–764.
7. Rassweiler J, Schulze M, Teber D, Seemann O, Frede T. Laparoscopic radical prostatectomy: functional and oncological outcomes. Curr Opin Urol 2004; 14(2):75–82.
8. Brown JA, Garlitz C, Gomella LG, et al. Pathologic comparison of laparoscopic versus open radical retropubic prostatectomy specimens. Urology 2003; 62(3):481–486.
9. Guillonneau B, el-Fettouh H, Baumert H, et al. Laparoscopic radical prostatectomy: oncological evaluation after 1,000 cases a Montsouris Institute. J Urol 2003; 169(4):1261–1266.
10. Rassweiler J, Stolzenburg J, Sulser T, et al. Laparoscopic radical prostatectomy – the experience of the german laparoscopic working group. Eur Urol 2006; 49(1):113–119.
11. Gonzalgo ML, Pavlovich CP, Trock BJ, Link RE, Sullivan W, Su LM. Classification and trends of perioperative morbidities following laparoscopic radical prostatectomy. J Urol 2005; 174(1):135–139; discussion 9.

12. Bird VG, Winfield H.N Laparoscopy in urology: physiologic considerations. In: Fallon B, ed. Hospital Physician, Urology Board Review. Wayne, PA: Turner White Communications, Inc., 2002.
13. Curlik M, Lofti, MA, Gomella LG. Anesthetic considerations of laparoscopy. In: Gomella L, Kozminski M, Winfield HN. Laparoscopic Urologic Surgery. New York: Raven Press, 1994.
14. Richter B, Kloppik E. Anesthesiological problems in laparoscopy. In: Fahelkamp D, Loening SA, Winfield HN, eds. Advances in Laparoscopic Surgery. Oxford: Blackwell Science, 1995:33–37.
15. Brown JA, Rodin D, Lee B, Dahl DM. Transperitoneal versus extraperitoneal approach to laparoscopic radical prostatectomy: an assessment of 156 cases. Urology 2005; 65(2):320–324.
16. Dahl DM, L'Esperance JO, Trainer AF, et al. Laparoscopic radical prostatectomy: initial 70 cases at a U.S. university medical center. Urology 2002; 60(5):859–863.
17. Gargollo P, McGovern FJ, Lee BC, Dahl DM. Hydrodissection of the Neurovascular Bundles During Laparoscopic Radical Retropubic Prostatectomy: A New Technique. In: American Urological Association. San Francisco, CA, 2004.
18. Guillonneau B, Rozet F, Cathelineau X, et al. Perioperative complications of laparoscopic radical prostatectomy: the Montsouris 3-year experience. J Urol 2002; 167(1):51–56.
19. Hu JC, Nelson RA, Wilson TG, et al. Perioperative complications of laparoscopic and robotic assisted laparoscopic radical prostatectomy. J Urol 2006; 175(2):541–546; discussion 6.
20. Clavien PA, Sanabria JR, Strasberg SM. Proposed classification of complications of surgery with examples of utility in cholecystectomy. Surgery 1992; 111(5):518–526.
21. Dahl DM. Comment on: Classification and trends of perioperative morbidities following laparoscopic radical prostatectomy by Gonzalgo et al. J Urol 2005; 174:139.
22. Vallancien G, Cathelineau X, Baumert H, Doublet JD, Guillonneau B. Complications of transperitoneal laparoscopic surgery in urology: review of 1,311 procedures at a single center. J Urol 2002; 168(1):23–26.
23. Hasson HM. A modified instrument and method for laparoscopy. Am J Obstet Gynecol 1971; 110(6):886–887.
24. Chandler JG, Corson SL, Way LW. Three spectra of laparoscopic entry access injuries. J Am Coll Surg 2001; 192(4):478–490; discussion 90–91.
25. Penfield AJ. How to prevent complications of open laparoscopy. J Reprod Med 1985; 30(9): 660–663.
26. Bishoff JT, Allaf ME, Kirkels W, Moore RG, Kavoussi LR, Schroder F. Laparoscopic bowel injury: incidence and clinical presentation. J Urol 1999; 161(3):887–890.
27. Saye WB, Miller W, Hertzmann P. Electrosurgery thermal injury. Myth or misconception? Surg Laparosc Endosc 1991; 1(4):223–228.
28. McMahon AJ, Baxter JN, O'Dwyer PJ. Physiological and metabolic responses to open and laparoscopic cholecystectomy. Br J Surg 1993; 80(3):402.
29. McMahon AJ, O'Dwyer PJ, Cruikshank AM, et al. Comparison of metabolic responses to laparoscopic and minilaparotomy cholecystectomy. Br J Surg 1993; 80(10):1255–1258.
30. Jakeways MS, Mitchell V, Hashim IA, et al. Metabolic and inflammatory responses after open or laparoscopic cholecystectomy. Br J Surg 1994; 81(1):127–131.
31. Nezhat C, Nezhat F, Ambroze W, Pennington E. Laparoscopic repair of small bowel and colon. A report of 26 cases. Surg Endosc 1993; 7(2):88–89.
32. Cadeddu JA, Regan F, Kavoussi LR, Moore RG. The role of computerized tomography in the evaluation of complications after laparoscopic urological surgery. J Urol 1997; 158(4):1349–1352.
33. Burova RA, Tronin R, Nesterenko Iu A, Grinberg AA. Laparoscopy in the differential diagnosis of acute abdomen. Khirurgiia (Mosk) 1994 (3); 16–20.
34. Bauer JJ, Schulam PG, Kaufman HS, Moore RG, Irby PB, Kavoussi LR. Laparoscopy for the acute abdomen in the postoperative urologic patient. Urology 1998; 51(6):917–919.
35. Trabulsi EJ, Guillonneau B. Laparoscopic radical prostatectomy. J Urol 2005; 173(4):1072–1079.
36. Guillonneau B, Gupta R, El Fettouh H, Cathelineau X, Baumert H, Vallancien G. Laparoscopic [correction of laproscopic] management of rectal injury during laparoscopic [correction of laproscopic] radical prostatectomy. J Urol 2003; 169(5):1694–1696.
37. Rassweiler J, Sentker L, Seemann O, Hatzinger M, Rumpelt HJ. Laparoscopic radical prostatectomy with the Heilbronn technique: an analysis of the first 180 cases. J Urol 2001; 166(6):2101–2108.
38. Borland RN, Walsh PC. The management of rectal injury during radical retropubic prostatectomy. J Urol 1992; 147(3 Pt 2):905–907.
39. Pisters LL, Wajsman Z. A simple test for the detection of intraoperative rectal injury in major urological pelvic surgery. J Urol 1992; 148(2 Pt 1):354.
40. Katz R, Borkowski T, Hoznek A, Salomon L, de la Taille A, Abbou CC. Operative management of rectal injuries during laparoscopic radical prostatectomy. Urology 2003; 62(2):310–313.
41. Turk I, Deger S, Winkelmann B, Schonberger B, Loening SA. Laparoscopic radical prostatectomy. Technical aspects and experience with 125 cases. Eur Urol 2001; 40(1):46–52; discussion 53.
42. Haggman M, Brandstedt S, Norlen BJ. Rectal perforation after retropubic radical prostatectomy: occurrence and management. Eur Urol 1996; 29(3):337–340.

43. Dafnis G, Wang YH, Borck L. Transsphincteric repair of rectourethral fistulas following laparoscopic radical prostatectomy. Int J Urol 2004; 11(11):1047–1049.
44. Bollens R, Vanden Bossche M, Roumeguere T, et al. Extraperitoneal laparoscopic radical prostatectomy. Results after 50 cases. Eur Urol 2001; 40(1):65–69.
45. Rozet F, Galiano M, Cathelineau X, Barret E, Cathala N, Vallancien G. Extraperitoneal laparoscopic radical prostatectomy: a prospective evaluation of 600 cases. J Urol 2005; 174(3):908–911.
46. Secin FP, Karanikolas N, Touijer AK, Salamanca JI, Vickers AJ, Guillonneau B. Anatomy of accessory pudendal arteries in laparoscopic radical prostatectomy. J Urol 2005; 174(2):523–526; discussion 6.
47. Stolzenburg JU, Rabenalt R, Do M, et al. Categorisation of complications of endoscopic extraperitoneal and laparoscopic transperitoneal radical prostatectomy. World J Urol 2006; 24:1–6.
48. Guillonneau B, Cathelineau X, Doublet JD, Baumert H, Vallancien G. Laparoscopic radical prostatectomy: assessment after 550 procedures. Crit Rev Oncol Hematol 2002; 43(2):123–133.
49. Raboy A, Ferzli G, Albert P. Initial experience with extraperitoneal endoscopic radical retropubic prostatectomy. Urology 1997; 50(6):849–853.
50. Hoznek A, Salomon L, Olsson LE, et al. Laparoscopic radical prostatectomy. The Creteil experience. Eur Urol 2001; 40(1):38–45.
51. Salomon L, Sebe P, De la Taille A, et al. Open versus laparoscopic radical prostatectomy: part I. BJU Int 2004; 94(2):238–243.
52. Davidson PJ, van den Ouden D, Schroeder FH. Radical prostatectomy: prospective assessment of mortality and morbidity. Eur Urol 1996; 29(2):168–173.
53. Lang GS, Ruckle HC, Hadley HR, Lui PD, Stewart SC. One hundred consecutive laparoscopic pelvic lymph node dissections: comparing complications of the first 50 cases to the second 50 cases. Urology 1994; 44(2):221–225.
54. Guillonneau B, Vallancien G. Laparoscopic radical prostatectomy: the Montsouris technique. J Urol 2000; 163(6):1643–1649.
55. Modi P, Goel R, Dodiya S. Laparoscopic ureteroneocystostomy for distal ureteral injuries. Urology 2005; 66(4):751–753.
56. Reddy PK, Evans RM. Laparoscopic ureteroneocystostomy. J Urol 1994; 152(6 Pt 1):2057–2059.
57. Armenakas NA. Current methods of diagnosis and management of ureteral injuries. World J Urol 1999; 17(2):78–83.
58. Nezhat C, Nezhat FR. Ureteral injuries at laparoscopy: insights into diagnosis, management, and prevention. Obstet Gynecol 1990; 76(5 Pt 1):889–890.
59. Brown JA, Dahl DM. Transperitoneal laparoscopic radical prostatectomy in patients after laparoscopic prosthetic mesh inguinal herniorrhaphy. Urology 2004; 63(2):380–382.
60. Bhayani SB, Pavlovich CP, Strup SE, et al. Laparoscopic radical prostatectomy: a multi-institutional study of conversion to open surgery. Urology 2004; 63(1):99–102.
61. Cathelineau X, Cahill D, Widmer H, Rozet F, Baumert H, Vallancien G. Transperitoneal or extraperitoneal approach for laparoscopic radical prostatectomy: a false debate over a real challenge. J Urol 2004; 171(2 Pt 1):714–716.
62. Brown JA, Rodin DM, Lee B, Dahl DM. Laparoscopic radical prostatectomy and body mass index: an assessment of 151 sequential cases. J Urol 2005; 173(2):442–445.
63. Remzi M, Klingler HC, Tinzl MV, et al. Morbidity of laparoscopic extraperitoneal versus transperitoneal radical prostatectomy versus open retropubic radical prostatectomy. Eur Urol 2005; 48(1):83–89; discussion 9.
64. Lieskovsky G, Skinner DG, Weisenburger T. Pelvic lymphadenectomy in the management of carcinoma of the prostate. J Urol 1980; 124(5):635–638.
65. Roumeguere T, Bollens R, Vanden Bossche M, et al. Radical prostatectomy: a prospective comparison of oncological and functional results between open and laparoscopic approaches. World J Urol 2003; 20(6):360–366.
66. Poulakis V, Ferakis N, Dillenburg W, Vries R, Witzsch U, Becht E. Laparoscopic radical prostatectomy using an extraperitoneal approach: Nordwest hospital technique and initial experience in 255 cases. J Endourol 2006; 20(1):45–53.
67. Catalona WJ, Ramos CG, Carvalhal GF. Contemporary results of anatomic radical prostatectomy. CA Cancer J Clin 1999; 49(5):282–296.
68. Huland H. Radical prostatectomy: options and issues. Eur Urol 2001; 39(suppl 1):3–9.
69. Han M, Partin AW, Pound CR, Epstein JI, Walsh PC. Long-term biochemical disease-free and cancer-specific survival following anatomic radical retropubic prostatectomy. The 15-year Johns Hopkins experience. Urol Clin North Am 2001; 28(3):555–565.
70. Hull GW, Rabbani F, Abbas F, Wheeler TM, Kattan MW, Scardino PT. Cancer control with radical prostatectomy alone in 1,000 consecutive patients. J Urol 2002; 167(2 Pt 1):528–534.
71. Salomon L, Levrel O, Anastasiadis AG, et al. Outcome and complications of radical prostatectomy in patients with PSA <10 mg/ml: comparison between the retropubic, perineal and laparoscopic approach. Prostate Cancer Prostatic Dis 2002; 5(4):285–290.
72. Eden CG, Cahill D, Vass JA, Adams TH, Dauleh MI. Laparoscopic radical prostatectomy: the initial UK series. BJU Int 2002; 90(9):876–882.

73. Salomon L, Anastasiadis AG, Levrel O, et al. Location of positive surgical margins after retropubic, perineal, and laparoscopic radical prostatectomy for organ-confined prostate cancer. Urology 2003; 61(2):386–390.
74. Hoznek A, Menard Y, Salomon L, Abbou CC. Update on laparoscopic and robotic radical prostatectomy. Curr Opin Urol 2005; 15(3):173–180.
75. Lepor H, Kaci L, Xue X. Continence following radical retropubic prostatectomy using self-reporting instruments. J Urol 2004; 171(3):1212–1215.
76. Artibani W, Grosso G, Novara G, et al. Is laparoscopic radical prostatectomy better than traditional retropubic radical prostatectomy? An analysis of peri-operative morbidity in two contemporary series in Italy. Eur Urol 2003; 44(4):401–406.
77. Salomon L, Anastasiadis AG, Katz R, et al. Urinary continence and erectile function: a prospective evaluation of functional results after radical laparoscopic prostatectomy. Eur Urol 2002; 42(4): 338–343.
78. Erdogru T, Teber D, Frede T, et al. Comparison of transperitoneal and extraperitoneal laparoscopic radical prostatectomy using match-pair analysis. Eur Urol 2004; 46(3):312–319; discussion 320.
79. Eden CG, King D, Kooiman GG, Adams TH, Sullivan ME, Vass JA. Transperitoneal or extraperitoneal laparoscopic radical prostatectomy: does the approach matter? J Urol 2004; 172(6 Pt 1):2218–2223.
80. Walsh PC, Marschke P, Ricker D, Burnett AL. Patient-reported urinary continence and sexual function after anatomic radical prostatectomy. Urology 2000; 55(1):58–61.
81. Stanford JL, Feng Z, Hamilton AS, et al. Urinary and sexual function after radical prostatectomy for clinically localized prostate cancer: the Prostate Cancer Outcomes Study. JAMA 2000; 283(3): 354–360.
82. Katz R, Salomon L, Hoznek A, et al. Patient reported sexual function following laparoscopic radical prostatectomy. J Urol 2002; 168(5):2078–2082.
83. Su LM, Link RE, Bhayani SB, Sullivan W, Pavlovich CP. Nerve-sparing laparoscopic radical prostatectomy: replicating the open surgical technique. Urology 2004; 64(1):123–127.
84. Stolzenburg JU, Truss MC, Bekos A, et al. Does the extraperitoneal laparoscopic approach improve the outcome of radical prostatectomy? Curr Urol Rep 2004; 5(2):115–122.
85. Gregori A, Simonato A, Lissiani A, Bozzola A, Galli S, Gaboardi F. Laparoscopic radical prostatectomy: perioperative complications in an initial and consecutive series of 80 cases. Eur Urol 2003; 44(2):190–194; discussion 4.
86. Dillioglugil O, Leibman BD, Leibman NS. Risk factors for complications and morbidity after radical retropubic prostatectomy. J Urol 1997; 157:1760.
87. Sidi A, Lobato EB, Cohen JA. The American Society of Anesthesiologists' Physical Status: category V revisited. J Clin Anesth 2000; 12(4):328–334.

28 | Complications of Robotic Prostatectomy

Mani Menon and Akshay Bhandari
Vattikuti Urology Institute, Henry Ford Health System, Detroit, Michigan, U.S.A.

INTRODUCTION

Since its introduction to the United States in 2001, robotic prostatectomy has gained wide acceptance among patients as a preferred treatment for localized prostate cancer. Over five years, the number of centers offering robotic prostatectomy has expanded from 1 to over 300, and the numbers of cases performed annually from 100 to 35,000. It is commonly assumed that minimally invasive surgery in general is associated with less morbidity and complications than open surgery. However, there are no randomized trials that compare outcomes of open and laparoscopic radical prostatectomy, much less of robotic radical prostatectomy. For a complex oncologic/reconstructive procedure such as radical prostatectomy, individual surgeon skills and experience have been shown to affect outcomes. Thus, the concept of randomization may be intrinsically problematic for procedures that are highly correlated with individual skills.

The complication rates from retropubic radical prostatectomy performed in centers of excellence are low and range from 6% to 10% (1,2). However data from the analysis of population-based registries yield a complication rate of around 30%:20% medical and 10% surgical (3,4). This may be expected with a surgical procedure in which there is significant bleeding, and indirect effects on homeostasis. The published literature relating to the complications of laparoscopic prostatectomy have been based on the analysis of single and multi-center database (5–7). The situation is even more tenuous for robotic prostatectomy, where the literature is based on single—institution studies of small numbers of patients, or where the literature is based on the analysis of the initial experience from three institutions (5,8–13).

We started our robotic prostatectomy program in 2001 and have performed over 2700 robotic prostatectomies as of this writing. We have published our surgical technique vattikuti institute prostatectomy (VIP) in its various iterations (14,15). Complications rates for the first 200 and subsequent 300 cases have also been published (9,10). As the literature addressing the complications of robotic prostatectomy is sparse, we have drawn heavily upon our own experience in preparing this chapter (Table 1). The numbers in parentheses after each complication are the complications that we have had in our own series and may not reflect the experience of other centers.

The complications of robotic surgery are conceptually no different from those of conventional laparoscopy. While the excellent visualization that is integral to robotics allows for a more precise dissection and enhanced visualization of tissue planes, the technology also has intrinsic drawbacks. For example, the primary surgeon is not scrubbed, and does not even touch the patient. All maneuvers that are directly in contact with the patient are performed by the patient-side surgeon, usually surgical house staff or mid-level providers. The console surgeon thus does not have the ability to directly control these moves, nor to obtain exposure. Thus, the surgical assistants are more critical to the success of the operation than for open or even conventional laparoscopic radical prostatectomy. Team building and a structured operative plan are more critical to robotic than to laparoscopic or open prostatectomy.

INTRAOPERATIVE COMPLICATIONS
Anesthesia-Related Complications (0.1%)

While robotic surgery and laparoscopy share most of the general anesthetic complications of open surgery, certain anesthesia-related complications are unique to laparoscopy and robotics. Insufflation of carbon dioxide raises the intra-abdominal pressure which causes an increase in intra-thoracic pressure and vascular resistance, both systemic and pulmonary and therefore

TABLE 1 Perioperative Complications of Robotic Prostatectomy in 1233 Patients

Mean hospital stay (d)	1.1
% Discharged home in 48 h	97.6%
% Unscheduled post-operative visits	5.8%
Complications	No. patients (%)
Urinary retention	27 (2.2)
Postoperative anemia, blood transfusion	19 (1.5)
Urinoma—CT-guided drainage	12 (0.9)
Postoperative ileus	12 (0.9)
Hematuria	6 (0.5)
Rectal injury	6 (0.5)
Thromboembolism	4 (0.3)
Stitch abscess	4 (0.3)
Bowel injury	3 (0.2)
Anastomotic disruption—re-exploration	3 (0.2)
Port site hernia	2 (0.2)
Pelvic abscess	1 (0.1)
Lymphocele	1 (0.1)
Renal hematoma	1 (0.1)
Negative exploration	1 (0.1)
Bronchial edema—reintubation	1 (0.1)
Total medical	13 (1.0)
Major medical	5 (0.4)
Minor medical	8 (0.6)
Total surgical	91 (7.3)
Major surgical	14 (1.1)
Minor surgical	77 (6.2)
Total complications	104 (8.4)

Abbreviation: CT, computed tomography.

increased blood pressure and decreased cardiac output. Sinus bradycardia is frequently encountered and could be multifactorial because of carbon dioxide insufflation, increased vagal response due to stretching of the peritoneal structures, steep trendelenburg position, and hypercapnia. Bradycardia is usually managed successfully by administering atropine, desufflating the abdomen, and reversing the Trendelenburg position. In extremely rare cases asystolic cardiac arrest may develop. In general, one should avoid excessive intra-abdominal pressures (>20 mmHg).

Appropriate volume resuscitation can be challenging and fluid administration should be carefully monitored specifically during the learning curve when the operative times are in excess of three hours. Inability to accurately measure urine output during radical prostatectomy adds to the challenge. Severe facial edema can develop secondary to fluid overload in the steep Trendelenburg position. We report one case of bronchial edema requiring emergent re-intubation during our initial experience.

We have also observed a small incidence of corneal abrasions in some of our patients. Although not associated with any long-term sequelae in our experience, corneal abrasions can be a cause of great pain and distress in the postoperative period. They could be related to several factors. These include lagophthalmos (failure of eyelids to close properly) leading to corneal drying and direct trauma related from the disposable pulse oximeter probe that is usually placed on the patients' index finger. The injury is supposed to occur when the patient emerges from anesthesia and rubs their eye with their index finger with the probe attached. This complication can be minimized by properly covering the eyes with an eye patch and placing the probe of the pulse oximeter on another finger.

Access-Related Complications (0.3%)

Little information exists about the prevalence of access-related complications unique to laparoscopic, much less robotic prostatectomy. Much more is written about access-related complications of non-urologic laparoscopic surgery. They could range from minor bleeding to major vascular catastrophe. Basic laparoscopic skills are an essential requirement prior to initiating a robotic prostatectomy program. Robotic prostatectomy is a team effort in which patient-side assistants and console surgeon work as an individual unit. The patient-side assistants need to be adequately educated with regard to prevention, recognition as well as management of possible complications. Establishing pneumoperitoneum and inserting the working trocars remain the most crucial steps of laparoscopy. Various techniques are currently used to obtain laparoscopic access to the abdominal cavity. However, none of them entirely obviate the possibility of intraoperative complications caused by trocars and needles. Most surgeons use five to six ports for robotic prostatectomy that includes the 3-4 robotic ports and 1-3 assistant ports (12–15). We use the closed technique of establishing access where the peritoneal cavity is punctured blindly with the Veress needle, followed by insufflation of carbon dioxide. Thereafter, the first trocar, which is often placed near the umbilicus, is introduced blindly into the peritoneal cavity. Subsequent ports are placed under vision. The open technique described by Hasson (16) is another technique to obtain laparoscopic access. While it is suggested that the open technique might be safer and may minimize the incidence of access-related injuries, there have been no studies to support this claim (17). The open technique is considered to be more time consuming and may be compromised by leakage of carbon dioxide as well. Another alternative is to use an optical trocar to enter the abdomen under direct view (18).

Subcutaneous Emphysema and Carbon Dioxide Embolism (0%)

The incidence of subcutaneous emphysema is poorly reported. Subcutaneous emphysema could be caused by either improper placement of the Veress needle or due to leakage of carbon dioxide around ports. Leakage around port occurs when incisions are too large and this allows the intraabdominal carbon dioxide to leak around the ports and track along the subcutaneous tissue planes. Longer operative times and greater number of ports also predispose to subcutaneous emphysema (19). Subcutaneous emphysema may involve a limited area or can extensively track all the way up to the neck and compromise oxygenation. Once discovered, it can be managed by placing a purse-string suture around the port site and also decreasing the intra-abdominal pressure. To minimize the incidence of subcutaneous emphysema, the surgeon should limit the incision size to the size of the port being placed and also avoid multiple passes through the peritoneum while placing ports. In our experience the incidence of subcutaneous emphysema has been very low and we have had no associated complications.

Although very rare, carbon dioxide embolism is an extremely lethal complication of laparoscopy. It is almost invariably caused by insufflation of carbon dioxide following puncture of a blood vessel or organ with the Veress needle (20,21). Carbon dioxide embolism is associated with acute onset of bradycardia and hypotension. It should be suspected if there is an abrupt decline in oxygen saturation and a sudden increase in end-tidal carbon dioxide followed by a rapid decrease. Management is immediate desufflation of peritoneum, turning the patient to left lateral decubitus while still in Trendelenburg position, and hyperventilation with 100% oxygen. This complication can be avoided by simply confirming correct placement of the Veress needle prior to initiating insufflation.

Vascular Injuries (0%)

According to reports in the literature, the incidence of trocar and Veress needle-related vascular injury is low, ranging from 0.03% to 0.2% (22–24). The majority of vascular injuries that have been reported during laparoscopy occur during abdominal entry and are caused either by the first trocar or Veress needle (25,26). In a large collective series of trocar injuries it was found that 83% of the serious vascular injuries occur during the placement of the first trocar (27). The aorta and common iliac vessels are most frequently involved. Injury to the inferior epigastric vessels can also occur during assistant port placement. We recommend port placement under proper transillumination in a dark room to prevent injury to the inferior epigastric artery or other muscular branches to the abdominal wall. Adhering to these guidelines, we have been able to avoid major vascular injuries to date. In our experience lifting the anterior abdominal wall with the help of towel clips may help with Veress needle placement in obese individuals. While this claim has not been supported by the literature, we continue to use this maneuver in select cases (28).

Visceral Injuries (0.3%)

Intra-abdominal organs may be injured during Veress needle or port placement. Both solid and hollow visceral organs can be potentially injured. We have experienced one case of renal hematoma from placing a Veress needle in a patient with left-sided pelvic kidney. A small hematoma was noted upon introducing the endoscope. It was observed for sometime intra-operatively and was not seen to be expanding. We therefore proceeded with the prostatectomy. The patient developed gross hematuria that resolved on post-operative day two. However, the hemoglobin levels remained stable and the patient did not require blood transfusion. Careful review of imaging studies like computed tomography (CT) scans when available preoperatively can alert against such anatomical anomalies. Where patients have a pelvic kidney, a renal transplant or tortuous or dilated abdominal vessels, consideration should be given to the Hasson approach.

Bowel injuries are associated with a high morbidity and mortality rate. A recent review of laparoscopy-related bowel injuries reported a low cumulative incidence of 0.4% (29). The small bowel was most frequently affected and approximately 40% of the bowel injuries were access related and caused by either a trocar or a Veress needle. Approximately 70% of laparoscopy-induced bowel injuries are seen in patients with adhesions or previous laparotomy (29).

Two of the three bowel injuries in our series occurred during extensive lysis of adhesions in patients with prior abdominal surgery. Two were unrecognized at the time of surgery. In the third patient, access was obtained through a minilaparotomy, because of a history of multiple previous laparotomies. A small serosal injury was repaired primarily in two layers. This patient had multiquadrant abdominal adhesions, and these were taken down only as far as needed to place the ports. After open port placement, the robot was docked and the prostatectomy completed. All three patients presented with persistent abdominal pain and ileus. They underwent exploratory laparotomy: all had bowel injury. In two the injury was probably the result of instrument passage. In the third, the patient had developed ileus, secondary to partial lysis of adhesions, and the serosal stitches had pulled out. However, over 30% of our patients had previous abdominal surgery, and the overall incidence of iatrogenic injury to the bowel, even in this subgroup was <1%. Nevertheless, it may be advisable to restrict robotic prostatectomy to patients who have not had abdominal surgery, during the learning phase of the surgical team. Currently, we recommend a radical perineal prostatectomy in patients with multiple previous laparotomies or a history of a ruptured viscous. We will, however, perform robotic surgery if the patient insists and accepts the risk of complications.

Injury to the urinary bladder is also a potential complication that can arise from placing a Veress needle in a distended bladder. Placing a Foley catheter and ensuring complete bladder drainage will prevent this complication. Similarly, we place an oro-gastric tube in all patients prior to proceeding to decompress the stomach and therefore reduce the risk of gastric injuries.

Vascular Complications (Access Unrelated) (0.1%)

The majority of vascular injuries in radical prostatectomy occur during pelvic lymphadenectomy (30,31). Injury to the external iliac artery and its complete laparoscopic repair has been recently described (30). Proper knowledge of anatomy and possible anatomical anomalies can minimize the majority of these complications. We perform pelvic lymphadenectomy in almost all our patients and have never experienced any form of vascular injury as a direct cause of surgical dissection. We have had to re-explore one patient for bleeding from an accessory obturator artery probably from an injury caused by a suture needle. Barring this we have not encountered any major vascular catastrophe. The stereotactic vision along with the precision of the robotic instruments due to tremor filtering and motion scaling prevents inadvertent movements and therefore results in a low incidence of vascular injuries, if the surgical team appreciates the anatomy.

Rectal Injury (0.5%)

The reported rate of rectal injury in laparoscopic radical prostatectomy is from 1% to 3.3% (32–37). We had six patients (0.5%) with rectal injury. Patel et al. (12) have also reported a similar incidence of rectal injury in 200 patients undergoing robotic prostatectomy.

In our patients, rectal injury occurred during posterior apical dissection. Five of six patients had aggressive apical cancer, and underwent planned wide excision of periprostatic tissues, in an attempt to obtain maximum cancer clearance. All rectal injuries in our series were identified intraoperatively and primarily repaired in two layers in a meticulous fashion. We close the inner mucosal and outer seromuscular layers with a running #3-0 Vicryl suture. It is of utmost importance to ensure a water-tight vesicourethral anastomosis in these individuals. There is no evidence that a longer duration of Foley catheterization is indicated if the quality of anastomosis is good. Anal dilation was performed in all patients. Patients were kept on a clear liquid diet for 72 hours and received broad-spectrum antibiotic coverage postoperatively.

Five of six patients were discharged within 72 hours, without complications. One patient developed a recto-vesical fistula that needed a temporary diverting colostomy and delayed repair of the fistula. This patient had locally extensive carcinoma and histologic evidence of serosal involvement of the rectum. The patient was non-compliant with his bowel preparation and gross fecal spillage was noted at the time of injury. In patients with aggressive local disease we now routinely order complete bowel preparation preoperatively. While we have not used a rectal bougie routinely during the posterior dissection, Guillonneau and Vallancien (38) have found this helpful during laparosopic prostatectomy. It has been speculated that the loss of haptic feedback with the robot may contribute to rectal injury; the incidence of this complication is too low to confirm this.

Ureteral Injury (0%)

Guillonneau and Vallancien (38) reported a 0.5% incidence of ureteral injury with the Montsouris technique (37,38). In this technique, the rectovesical cul-de-sac is opened initially and the seminal vesicles and vasa are dissected out before the anterior peritoneum is opened. While this has worked well in many surgeons' hands, the posterior dissection is performed in a confined space with limited visibility. While we initially used this approach, we have found it slightly more difficult to appreciate variations in adnexal anatomy. In patients with lateral lobe hypertrophy of the prostate, the vasa are displaced laterally, and initially may be confused with the ureters. With the VIP technique, the bladder is "dropped" first, the bladder neck is transected, and the seminal vesicals are approached after this. This approach is similar to open surgery, and offers a broader field for seminal vesicle dissection. With the VIP technique, we have not experienced any ureteral injuries hitherto. Several large open radical prostatectomy series (1,2,39) have also reported a very low incidence of ureteral injuries.

POSTOPERATIVE COMPLICATIONS
Postoperative Anemia and Blood Transfusion (1.5%)

Blood loss in robotic prostatectomy is significantly lower than with open radical retropubic prostatectomy. Our average, blood loss is 142 cc. This compares favorably with published laparoscopic series. Other robotic prostatectomy series report a similar blood loss (12,40). This can be attributed to pneumoperitoneum and the superior vision at a high magnification afforded by the da Vinci endoscope. In general, blood loss can be minimized with careful attention to anatomical detail and operating in the correct anatomical planes which is more readily offered by the eyes of the robot. In our entire series there have been no intraoperative blood transfusions and the postoperative transfusion rate is 1.5%.

Bleeding from the dorsal vein complex is one important cause of postoperative hematomas. We therefore emphasize good intra-operative control of dorsal vein complex. As our technique has evolved, we now place the dorsal vein stitch after completing apical dissection and transection of urethra. Lowering the pnuemoperitoneum and application of perineal pressure helps us identify the bleeding sinuses. We have yet to explore any patient for bleeding from the dorsal vein complex.

Our operative technique has evolved to incorporate more complex nerve-sparing techniques. We now routinely release the prostatic fascia anteriorly (veil of Aphrodite nerve-sparing) and use thermal coagulation sparingly. The plane of dissection is between the prostatic capsule and the prostatic venous plexus. If these vessels are not meticulously coagulated, they can retract and go into spasm. Analysis of our operative videotapes has demonstrated this convincingly. When the vessels go out of spasm, they can re-bleed and result in a pelvic hematoma. Patients on anticoagulation or anti-platelet agents, those with bleeding diatheses, with prostates >100 cc in volume, those who undergo "athermal" robotic prostatectomy, and those who undergo wide excision of periprostatic tissues are also at a higher risk for developing postoperative bleeding.

Patients on aspirin, chronic anticoagulation with warfarin, and anti-thrombotic agents should be asked to discontinue these medications at least five days prior the procedure and for a similar time following the surgery after proper clearance from their primary care physician or cardiologist. Particularly troublesome is the "cryptic alcoholic" with impaired liver function. It is best to avoid surgery in such individuals. A cystogram should be obtained routinely in such patients. A sausage shaped bladder is a tell-tale sign of a postoperative hematoma. The catheter should be left in for a minimum of two weeks in such patients, even in the absence of contrast extravasation. Patients with pelvic hematomas can sometimes develop a delayed leak (even with a cystogram that shows no extravasation early on). One major complication in patients with postoperative anemia requiring blood transfusion has been the formation of an organized pelvic hematoma causing partial or complete disruption of the urethrovesical anastomosis. We have seen this on three occasions. These patients were re-explored robotically. The urethro-vesical sutures were taken down, clot was evacuated, bleeding points were coagulated, and the anastomosis was re-done.

Urinary Retention (2.2%)

Urinary retention immediately after catheter removal was the most common cause of deviation from "ideal" course in our series. In our initial experience, we were removing Foley catheters at one to four days postoperatively. The urinary retention rate in these patients was 4.7%. We attributed this to the presence of edema at the urethrovesical anastomosis. We have become more sanguine, leave catheters in for an average of seven days and have noticed a significant decrease in urinary retention (0.9%).

Patients should be observed in the office after the catheter is removed and not discharged until they have urinated. In case of delayed urinary retention, an assistant should place a gloved finger in the rectum to support the urethrovesical anastomosis. The surgeon should then pass a well lubricated Foley catheter into the bladder. This is successful in the vast majority of cases. A flexible cystoscopy should be performed and a guide wire passed into the bladder, only as a second resort.

Urinary Leak and Postoperative Ileus (2%)

We use a modification of the von Velthoven running stitch for urethrovesical anastomosis (41). At the conclusion of the procedure we test our anastomosis for leaks with instillation of normal saline. Any leak is repaired with additional interrupted sutures. Even with such precautions, about 2% of patients developed symptomatic postoperative leaks, which have been our most disturbing complication. While the leak itself can easily be handled with a CT-guided drain, the effect on the patient is quite dramatic. Because we use an intra-peritoneal approach, patients with urinary leaks develop urinary peritonitis. Such patients present with severe pain, abdominal distension, and hypoactive bowel sounds, mimicking a bowel injury. The differentiation between a urinary leak and bowel injury is critical in these patients, as the treatment is vastly different. While half of these patients were managed conservatively with a nasogastric tube and bowel rest, patients with urinomas needed percutaneous drain placement and prolonged Foley catheterization. In our series 1% of patients required this intervention.

Following surgery, a closed suction drain is left in the region of the urethrovesical anasto-mosis, and is removed only when the drainage is less than 100 cc per 8 hours. As the operation is performed in the Trendelenburg position and the surgical site is irrigated repeatedly with saline, much of the fluid collects under the diaphragm. As the patients ambulate, this fluid will egress through the suction drain. If the drainage remains high, creatinine levels should be obtained in the fluid. If it approximates serum levels, the drain can be removed. If the patient presents with abdominal pain for more than 24 hours, a serum creatinine should be obtained.

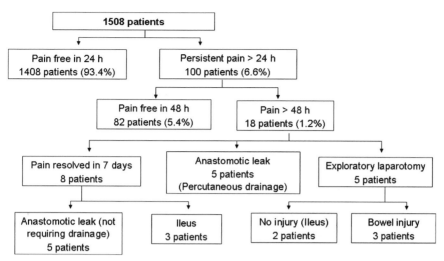

FIGURE 1   Analysis of complications based on postoperative pain following robotic radical prostatectomy.

Any elevation above baseline levels is an indication of urinary absorption. A CT cystogram should be obtained as an emergency and any fluid collection should be drained percutaneously (Fig. 1). Usually, this results in dramatic improvement in the patients' symptoms. If the patient does not improve immediately, he should be re-imaged and re-drained, even if the collection appears to be smaller. In one of 2752 cases, we have had to place three separate drains. Patients with urinary peritonitis appear desperately ill, but recover dramatically with drainage. Patients with an unrecognized bowel perforation are desperately ill and will not recover unless the injury is repaired. Figure 2 shows our algorithm for treating patients with unexplained postoperative pain that lasts >48 hours.

Port Site Hernias (0.2%)

It is felt that port site hernia is usually confined to port sites >10 mm in adults. We use non-cutting 12 mm trocars. These radially expanding trocars dilate and separate tissue, thus causing less tissue trauma while entering the abdominal wall. The non-cutting trocars are associated with a lower incidence of port site bleeding as well as port site hernias (42). On the other hand, the robotic 8 mm trocars are cutting trocars.

Two of the six ports that we use are 12 mm ports. One port is placed periumbilically for the endoscope and the other one is placed in the right anterior to mid-axillary line approximately 3 to 4 cm above the iliac crest. The periumbilical port site is extended to deliver the prostate and the fascia is closed with interrupted non-absorbable sutures. Using meticulous

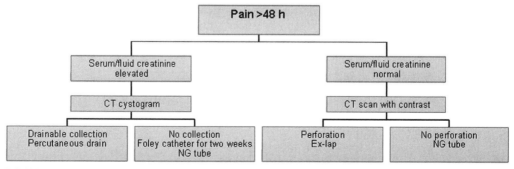

FIGURE 2   Treatment algorithm for patients with unexplained postoperative pain >48 hours following robotic radical prostatectomy. *Abbreviations*: CT, computed tomography; NG, nasogastric tube.

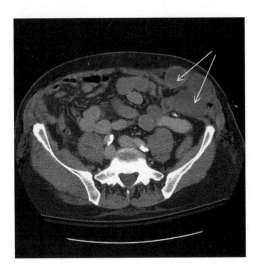

FIGURE 3 Computed tomography scan of the abdomen in a patient with port site herniation of multiple bowel loops (*arrow*).

technique and taking adequate fascial bites, herniation or wound dehiscence can be minimized. We do not routinely close fascia on the other 12 mm trocar site given its location. Patients with port site hernias usually present with severe pain localized to the trocar site associated with nausea and signs of ileus. An acute abdominal series may be indicative of an ileus; however, an abdominal CT scan with contrast is the most definitive study, which will show the bowel protruding above the fascia (Fig. 3). Interestingly these patients initially present with leukopenia rather than leukocystosis (43). A high index of suspicion is necessary to diagnose this entity as patients may rapidly deteriorate due to acute cardiopulmonary collapse secondary to sepsis.

We have experienced two port site hernias and both of these were at the 8 mm robotic trocar sites. One patient needed small bowel resection with primary anastomosis whereas the other patient underwent reduction of hernia with closure of defect with no bowel resection. We have recently started using 5 mm robotic instruments, and hope that we will never see another port site hernia.

Thromboembolic Complications (0.3%)

Although there is a decreased venous return secondary to increased intra-abdominal pressures in patients undergoing laparoscopy, there is no evidence to suggest a higher risk of deep vein thrombosis (DVT) in these patients when compared with open surgery. On the contrary, we have noticed a 0.3% incidence of DVT and/or pulmonary embolism (PE) in our series. This is significantly lower than that reported for radical retropubic prostatectomy (2). We attribute this low incidence to several factors. The average time to ambulation is significantly less with minimally invasive surgery. We encourage all patients to ambulate the evening of surgery. All our patients receive prophylactic doses of subcutaneous heparin in the perioperative period along with the use of pneumatic sequential compression devices for DVT prophylaxis. In addition, given the intraperitoneal nature of our technique, the incidence of significant lymphoceles and thus DVT is significantly less when compared with radical retropubic prostatectomy. Despite using identical DVT prophylactic measures, the incidence of reported thromboembolic complications is 2% to 3% for radical retropubic prostatectomy (2). Most patients present with persistent tachycardia, shortness of breath, and low-grade temperatures in the immediate postoperative period. A PE protocol CT scan is usually diagnostic of PE. Once diagnosed the treatment is immediate anticoagulation initially with heparin and then long term with warfarin.

DELAYED COMPLICATIONS

Among patients with a minimum follow-up of three months, 10 developed (0.5%) anastomotic or meatal strictures requiring dilation (two) or internal urethrotomies (eight). One patient whose Foley catheter was accidentally pulled into the prostatic fossa, has unresolved urethral strictures after multiple internal urethrotomies and requires intermittent self dilation. Six (0.3%) patients have developed incisional hernias at the umbilicus and three have developed inguinal hernias. Three patients have developed Peyronies disease, and have lost erectile function that they had regained after surgery. One additional patient has complained of a decrease in penile length.

The two most commonly reported delayed complications of open radical prostatectomy are incontinence and impotence, however. Indeed many surgeons do not report them as complications. There are no published data (other than ours) on delayed complications from robotic prostatectomy (44). At 12 months of follow-up, 95.2% of the patients were socially continent (0-1 pad), 84% had total urinary control (0 pad), 8% used a security liner, and 0.8% were totally incontinent. Of patients who had total control, 25% achieved this within 24 hours of catheter removal, 50% within four weeks, and 90% within three months. Our data suggest that while the overall continence rates at 12 months are comparable to those reported in open radical prostatectomy series from centers of excellence, the median time to achieve urinary control appears to be lower in patients undergoing robotic prostatectomy. These results may be related to superior visualization that allows for a precise apical dissection and limited trauma to the periurethral striated sphincter.

Similarly, robotic prostatectomy allows for a precise dissection of neurovascular bundles. We have published our technique of preserving the prostatic fascia, the Veil of Aphrodite nerve-sparing surgery (45,46). When performed in patients with no preoperative erectile dysfunction [sexual health inventory for men (SHIM)>21], intercourse was reported in over 90% at 12 months, although only 50% were back to baseline function without medication (46). Analysis of our data confirms that at all levels of preoperative erectile function, patients undergoing a veil nerve-sparing surgery had better potency outcomes than patients undergoing conventional nerve-sparing prostatectomy.

COMPLICATIONS OF ROBOTIC PROSTATECTOMY: A PERSONAL PERSPECTIVE

These are observations from looking after over 2500 patients over five years, and starting one of the first robotic programs in the world. Thus, this section is opinion-based medicine (mostly) rather than evidence-based medicine. Therefore, it can be ignored totally. When we started our program, the primary goal was to perform a gentler, safer operation than the sophisticated, finely developed open radical prostatectomy. Did we accomplish this? When we compare our complication rates with those of a large population based-study of patients undergoing open radical prostatectomy, the serious complication rate was lower by about 90% (1.5% vs. 11.68%) (47). The major difference was in the medical complication rate suggesting that minimally invasive surgery is indeed just that. However, the differences are not so dramatic when our results are compared with those of other centers of excellence. We doubt that we can perform a randomized trial comparing the two treatment options. Randomized trials are wonderful for comparing drug treatments. Are they equally good for comparing surgical techniques where individual surgeon skills are so important? To wit, is it not possible that a surgeon who is good at open radical prostatectomy may not be good at robotics, and vice versa. As a fall back, we analyzed hospital discharge records of all patients who underwent open prostatectomy or robotic prostatectomy at our hospital. Our clinical care pathway for prostatectomy calls for patients to be discharged within 48 hours after surgery. In this study, 40% of patients undergoing open and 97% of patients undergoing robotic prostatectomy met the clinical pathway target of discharge within 48 hours. Eleven percent and 1% of patients undergoing open prostatectomy and robotic prostatectomy, respectively, required a hospitalization of >7 days, demonstrating the presence of significant complications. These numbers strongly suggest that, at least at our institution, robotic prostatectomy was associated with a 90% decrease in complication rates, as reflected by length of stay greater than seven days.

The other side of the story is that when a robotic prostatectomy patient develops a complication, he looks much sicker than an open prostatectomy patient with a complication. In our own experience, persistent pain is the first indication that something is not right. VIP patients without complications have very little pain, and it is the rare patient who cannot be discharged within 24 hours. (Most of them start complaining about hospital food within 24 hours, and would rather be home!) A patient who has pain greater than 24 hours after surgery has a harrowing experience. His expectations for pain control are so high that he is terrified about what may be happening to him. To the surgeon, there are no physical signs that point to where the problem is. We analyzed the postoperative outcomes of patients with unexplained pain after robotic prostatectomy (Fig. 1). Of 1508 patients, 100 had pain persisting after 24 hours. Of these, the pain subsided spontaneously in 82 patients within 48 hours and they had an uncomplicated postoperative course. We assumed that these patients simply had lower pain thresholds and/or higher expectations from surgery. Of the 18 patients with pain lasting >48 hours, 10 developed complications that required intervention (percutaneous drainage or exploratory laparotomy). We now consider persistent pain at 48 hours as an ominous symptom and investigate this aggressively. We will obtain a CT scan with contrast and a CT cystogram as an emergency and drain any fluid collection that is detected. If patients appear to have the faintest suggestion of a bowel problem, they undergo exploratory laparotomy (Fig. 2).

CONCLUSION

Robotic radical prostatectomy is not perfect: there is a low immediate complication rate, a few patients are incontinent, and many more, impotent. However, the blood loss is lower and adverse events appear to occur in far fewer patients than with open prostatectomy. When complications do occur, the robotic prostatectomy patients appear very ill. Persistent pain after 48 hours is the harbinger of a potential problem, and should spur aggressive investigation. Patients with urinary peritonitis should be treated with percutaneous drainage: others should be explored to rule out a bowel injury. The relative safety of the procedure should not result in expanding indications for radical prostatectomy, nor should it condone a relaxation of vigilance in the operating room. Robotic radical prostatectomy is still a radical prostatectomy… a major procedure with potentially major complications!

REFERENCES

1.   Lepor H, Nieder AM, Ferrandino MN. Intraoperative and postoperative complications of radical retropubic prostatectomy in a consecutive series of 1,000 cases. J Urol 2001; 166(5):1729–1733.
2.   Catalona WJ, Carvalhal GF, Mager DE, Smith DS. Potency, continence and complication rates in 1,870 consecutive radical retropubic prostatectomies. J Urol 1999;162(2):433–438.
3.   Alibhai SM, Leach M, Tomlinson G, et al. 30-day mortality and major complications after radical prostatectomy: influence of age and comorbidity. J Natl Cancer Inst 2005; 97(20):1525–1532.
4.   Bianco FJ Jr, Riedel ER, Begg CB, Kattan MW, Scardino PT. Variations among high volume surgeons in the rate of complications after radical prostatectomy: further evidence that technique matters. J Urol 2005; 173(6):2099–2103.
5.   Hu JC, Nelson RA, Wilson TG, et al. Perioperative complications of laparoscopic and robotic assisted laparoscopic radical prostatectomy. J Urol 2006; 175(2):541–546.
6.   Arai Y, Egawa S, Terachi T, et al. Morbidity of laparoscopic radical prostatectomy: summary of early multi-institutional experience in Japan. Int J Urol 2003; 10(8):430–434.
7.   Soulie M, Salomon L, Seguin P, et al. Multi-institutional study of complications in 1085 laparoscopic urologic procedures. Urology 2001; 58(6):899–903.
8.   Menon M, Tewari A, Peabody JO, et al. Vattikuti Institute prostatectomy, a technique of robotic radical prostatectomy for management of localized carcinoma of the prostate: experience of over 1100 cases. Urol Clin North Am 2004; 31(4):701–717.
9.   Bhandari A, McIntire L, Kaul SA, Hemal AK, Peabody JO, Menon M. Perioperative complications of robotic radical prostatectomy after the learning curve. J Urol 2005; 174(3):915–918.
10. Tewari A, Srivasatava A, Menon M, Members of the VIP Team. A prospective comparison of radical retropubic and robot-assisted prostatectomy: experience in one institution. BJU Int 2003; 92(3):205–210.
11. Rassweiler J, Hruza M, Teber D, Su LM. Laparoscopic and robotic assisted radical prostatectomy—critical analysis of the results. Eur Urol 2006; 49(4):612–624.
12. Patel VR, Tully AS, Holmes R, Lindsay J. Robotic radical prostatectomy in the community setting—the learning curve and beyond: initial 200 cases. J Urol 2005; 174(1):269–272.
13. Ahlering TE, Skarecky D, Lee D, Clayman RV. Successful transfer of open surgical skills to a laparoscopic environment using a robotic interface: initial experience with laparoscopic radical prostatectomy. J Urol 2003; 170(5):1738–1741.
14. Tewari A, Peabody J, Sarle R, et al. Technique of da Vinci robot-assisted anatomic radical prostatectomy. Urology 2002; 60(4):569–572.
15. Menon M, Hemal AK, VIP Team. Vattikuti Institute prostatectomy: a technique of robotic radical prostatectomy: experience in more than 1000 cases. J Endourol 2004; 18(7):611–619.

16. Hasson HM. Open laparoscopy: a report of 150 cases. J Reprod Med 1974; 12(6):234–238.
17. Briel JW, Plaisier PW, MeijerWS, Lange JF. Is it necessary to lift the abdominal wall when preparing a pneumoperitoneum? A randomized study. Surg Endosc 2000; 14:862–864.
18. String A, Berber E, Foroutani A, Macho JR, Pearl JM, Siperstein AE. Use of the optical access trocar for safe and rapid entry in various laparoscopic procedures. Surg Endosc 2001; 15(6):570–573.
19. Murdock CM, Wolff AJ, Van Geem T. Risk factors for hypercarbia, subcutaneous emphysema, pneumothorax, and pneumomediastinum during laparoscopy. Obstet Gynecol 2000; 95(5):704–709.
20. Scoletta P, Morsiani E, Ferrocci G, et al. Carbon dioxide embolization: is it a complication of laparoscopic cholecystectomy? Minerva Chir 2003; 58(3):313–320.
21. Cobb WS, Fleishman HA, Kercher KW, Matthews BD, Heniford BT. Gas embolism during laparoscopic cholecystectomy. J Laparoendosc Adv Surg Tech A 2005; 15(4):387–390.
22. Bonjer HJ, Hazebroek EJ, Kazemier G, Giuffrida MC, Meijer WS, Lange JF. Open versus closed establishment of pneumoperitoneum in laparoscopic surgery. Br J Surg 1997; 84:599–602.
23. Hashizume M, Sugimachi K. Needle and trocar injury during laparoscopic surgery in Japan. Surg Endosc 1997; 11:1198–1201.
24. Mac CC, Lecuru F, Rizk E, Robin F, Boucaya V, Taurelle R. Morbidity in laparoscopic gynecological surgery: results of a prospective single-center study. Surg Endosc 1999; 13:57–61.
25. Catarci M, Carlini M, Gentileschi P, Santoro E. Major and minor injuries during the creation of pneumoperitoneum. A multicenter study on 12,919 cases. Surg Endosc 2001; 15(6):566–569.
26. Schafer M, Lauper M, Krahenbuhl L. Trocar and Veress needle injuries during laparoscopy. Surg Endosc 2001; 15(3):275–280.
27. Champault G, Cazacu F, Taffinder N. Serious trocar accidents in laparoscopic surgery: a French survey of 103,852 operations. Surg Laparosc Endosc 1996; 6(5):367–370.
28. Briel JW, Plaisier PW, Meijer WS, Lange JF. Is it necessary to lift the abdominal wall when preparing a pneumoperitoneum? A randomized study. Surg Endosc 2000; 14(9):862–864.
29. van der Voort M, Heijnsdijk EA, Gouma DJ. Bowel injury as a complication of laparoscopy. Br J Surg 2004; 91(10):1253–1258.
30. Safi KC, Teber D, Moazen M, Anghel G, Maldonado RV, Rassweiler JJ. Laparoscopic repair of external iliac-artery transection during laparoscopic radical prostatectomy. J Endourol 2006; 20(4):237–239.
31. Lazzeri M, Benaim G, Turini D, Beneforti P, Turini F. Iatrogenic external iliac artery disruption during open pelvic lymph node dissection: successful repair with hypogastric artery transposition. Scand J Urol Nephrol 1997; 31(2):205–207.
32. Hoznek A, Salomon L, Olsson LE, et al. Laparoscopic radical prostatectomy—the Crete´il experience. Eur Urol 2001; 40:38–45.
33. Turk I, Deger S, Winkelmann B, Schonberger B, Loening SA. Laparoscopic radical prostatectomy–technical aspects and experience with 125 cases. Eur Urol 2001; 40:46–53.
34. Rassweiler J, Sentker L, Seeman O, Hatzinger M, Rumpelt HJ. Laparoscopic radical prostatectomy with the Heilbron technique: an analysis of the first 180 cases. J Urol 2001; 166:2101–2108.
35. Bollens R, Vanden Bossche M, Roumeguere T, et al. Extraperitoneal laparoscopic radical prostatectomy: results after 50 cases. Eur Urol 2001; 40:65–69.
36. Gill IS, Zippe CD. Laparoscopic radical prostatectomy technique. Urol Clin North Am 2001; 28: 423–436.
37. Guillonneau B, Vallancien G. Laparoscopic radical prostatectomy: the Montsouris technique. J Urol 2000; 163(6):1643–1649.
38. Guillonneau B, Vallancien G. Laparoscopic radical prostatectomy–the Montsouris experience. J Urol 2000; 163:418–422.
39. Lepor H, Kaci L. Contemporary evaluation of operative parameters and complications related to open radical retropubic prostatectomy. Urology 2003; 62(4):702–706.
40. Farnham SB, Webster TM, Herrell SD, Smith JA Jr. Intraoperative blood loss and transfusion requirements for robotic-assisted radical prostatectomy versus radical retropubic prostatectomy. Urology 2006; 67(2):360–363.
41. Van Velthoven RF, Ahlering TE, Peltier A, Skarecky DW, Clayman RV. Technique for laparoscopic running urethrovesical anastomosis: the single knot method. Urology 2003; 61(4):699–702.
42. Bhoyrul S, Payne J, Steffes B, Swanstrom L, Way LW. A randomized prospective study of radially expanding trocars in laparoscopic surgery. J Gastrointest Surg 2000; 4(4):392–397.
43. Bishoff JT, Allaf ME, Kirkels W, Moore RG, Kavoussi LR, Schroder F. Laparoscopic bowel injury: incidence and clinical presentation. J Urol 1999; 61(3):887–890.
44. Menon M, Shrivastava A, Kaul S, et al. Vattikuti Institute prostatectomy: contemporary technique and analysis of results. Eur Urol 2007; 51(3):648–658.
45. Kaul S, Bhandari A, Hemal A, Savera A, Shrivastava A, Menon M. Robotic radical prostatectomy with preservation of the prostatic fascia: a feasibility study. Urology 2005; 66(6):1261–1265.
46. Kaul S, Savera A, Badani K, Fumo M, Bhandari A, Menon M. Functional outcomes and oncological efficacy of Vattikuti Institute prostatectomy with Veil of Aphrodite nerve-sparing: an analysis of 154 consecutive patients. BJU Int 2006; 97(3):467–472.
47. Lu-Yao GL, Albertsen P, Warren J, Yao SL. Effect of age and surgical approach on complications and short-term mortality after radical prostatectomy—a population-based study. Urology 1999; 54(2): 301–307.

29 | Complications of Transurethral Surgery

Miguel Srougi and Alberto A. Antunes
Division of Urology, University of Sao Paulo Medical School, Sao Paulo, Brazil

INTRODUCTION

Despite the introduction of new alternatives for the management of benign prostatic hyperplasia (BPH), including new pharmacologic agents and minimally invasive techniques, transurethral resection of the prostate (TURP) remains in 2007, the gold standard for definitive treatment of the disease (1). Following TURP more than 90% of the patients report normal or improved voiding and recent studies with patients followed for more than 10 years have shown sustained clinical and urodynamic improvement in almost all symptomatic patients (2). There are no or only few similar data on durability for any other instrumental treatment for BPH, including open prostatectomy.

During the last decade, transurethral prostatic surgery underwent significant technical improvements (Table 1) with marked decrease in the incidence of post-treatment complications (1). The aim of this chapter is to review the intra- and postoperative complications of two main techniques—transurethral incision of the prostate (TUIP) and TURP.

TRANSURETHRAL INCISION OF THE PROSTATE

Transurethral incision of the prostate is a simple procedure described for the first time by Guthrie in 1834 (3) and later popularized by Orandi (4,5). Although it was less employed in the past, TUIP has been revived by virtue of the increased interest in minimally invasive techniques for the treatment of BPH.

The advantages of this technique are the absence of significant bleeding and irrigation fluid absorption, the short surgical time and a lower incidence of postoperative bladder neck sclerosis when compared with TURP for small glands. Furthermore, about 90% of the patients who undergo TUIP have their ejaculatory function preserved (6). On the other hand, among its disadvantages, TUIP is not effective for patients with prominent median lobe or for those with a markedly enlarged prostate gland. Additionally, no tissue is obtained for pathological analysis (7).

TUIP must be considered as an alternative and effective option to TURP in patients with small prostates. A recent randomized trial compared the results of TUIP versus TURP in 100 patients with prostate weighing less than 30 g. There were similar reductions in daytime and nighttime voiding frequency, increase in the maximal urinary flow rates and equivalent reduction in the linearized passive urethral resistance index. The authors concluded that TUIP is effective and safe for patients with small prostates (8). However, it is important to emphasize the lack of data on its long-term effectiveness (9).

Surgical Tips to Decrease Complications

In order to avoid surgical complications following TUIP, two technical maneuvers seem to be relevant. Less bleeding is seen when one incision at the 6 o'clock position or three incisions in a "Y" configuration are made. Incisions at the 12, 5 and 7 o'clock positions carry higher risks of periprostatic venous plexus injury and profuse bleeding (Fig. 1). Furthermore, incisions with Collin's knife or cold urethrotome are preferred to a loop incision if preservation of ejaculatory function is aimed.

Postoperative Complications

The incidence of complications after TUIP is low, with bleeding and the need for blood transfusions occurring in 0.4% to 2.4% of patients (10–12), retrograde ejaculation in about 10% of them and reoperations for recurrent obstructive symptoms in 5% to 27% of the cases (Table 2).

TABLE 1 Outcomes Following Surgical Treatment of Benign Prostatic Hyperplasia

Variable	Bladder neck incision	Transurethral resection	Open surgery
Patient improvement (%)	78–83	75–96	94–99
Symptoms improvement (%)	73	85	79
Surgical complication (%)	2–33	5–31	7–43
Severe incontinence (%)	0–1	0.7–1.4	0.3–0.7
Reoperations (%)	5–27	9–11	1–4
Impotence (%)	4–24	3–35	5–39
Retrograde ejaculation (%)	6–55	25–99	36–95
Hospitalization (days)	1–3	2–5	5–10
Complete recovery (days)	7–21	7–21	21–28
Costs (USD)	7500	9700	11,800

Source: From Ref. 6.

A recent meta-analysis that compared TUIP with TURP after a minimum follow-up of six months showed that while the re-intervention rates clearly favored TURP to TUIP (2.6% vs. 15.9%), TUIP provided superior results regarding retrograde ejaculation (65.4% vs. 18.2%) and blood transfusion rates (8.6% vs. 0.4%) (12).

TRANSURETHRAL RESECTION OF THE PROSTATE

Transurethral resection of the prostate is one of the most frequent surgical procedures performed in medical practice, preceded only by operations for cataract (13). It is considered the best method for BPH treatment and compared to open surgery has advantages which outweigh its drawbacks. TURP can be successfully used in the majority of cases, the postoperative recovery is more comfortable for patients, its costs are lower, and it is associated with a low mortality and morbidity rate. This explains why the profile of the surgical treatment of BPH has undergone a worldwide change. Prior to the 1970s, about 60% of prostate interventions were performed by the open approach, whereas at the present time only 5% are carried out in that way (14).

The main limitations of this technique relate to its decreased efficacy in the treatment of large prostates and the higher frequency of later reoperations. However, these shortcomings do not reduce the merits of TURP, as only a minority of symptomatic BPH patients seen in the clinical setting present glands weighing more than 100 g (17).

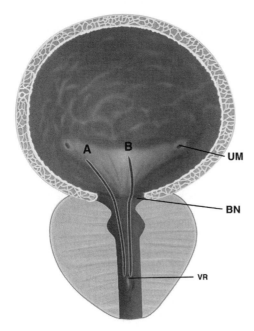

FIGURE 1 Proposed techniques for bladder neck incision. *A*, incision at 6 o'clock (preferable); *B*, incision at 7 o'clock (more bleeding). *Abbreviations*: BN, bladder neck; UM, ureteral meatus; VR, veru montanum.

TABLE 2 Clinical Outcome After Transurethral Incision of the Prostate

| Reference | Patients | Symptom score | | Urinary flow | | Normal ejaculation (%) | Reoperation (%) |
		Preoperative	Postoperative	Preoperative	Postoperative		
Orandi (5)	66	—	—	8.2	13.7	69	11
Christensen et al. (15)	49	16.0	4.0	7.8	12.7	87	10
Sirls et al. (10)	41	12.5	6.9	10.3	15.3	89	10
Riehmann et al. (16)	61	15.0	6.0	9.0	16.0	65	21

Surgical Tips to Decrease Complications
Selection of Patients

Large prostates do not preclude a TURP, but the procedure takes longer, which increases the incidence of surgical complications. However, instead of adopting limits of weight to determine the choice between open and transurethral techniques, it seems more appropriate to establish time limits for the surgical procedure. A specialist who excises 0.5 g/min of prostate should not undertake TURP on glands with more than 40 g, but another surgeon who removes 1.0 to 1.5 g/min may deal efficiently with prostates up to 100 to 120 g. Generally speaking, TURP should be limited to 90 minutes at the most or, if possible, to 60 minutes.

Irrigation System

To avoid an excessive irrigation fluid absorption, the irrigant bags or reservoir systems must be kept 40 to 50 cm above the level of the bladder. The use of non-ionic isotonic solutions such as 4% glucose, 1.5% glycine, 2.7% sorbitol, or 0.5% mannitol reduce the incidence of the so-called TUR syndrome (see below), but do not completely prevent its occurrence. This explains why distilled water is still used in some centers. However, when water is employed, the procedure should be discontinued if large venous sinuses are entered or if there is large perforation of the prostatic capsule. Regardless of the type of irrigant fluid used, it is prudent to administer 20 to 40 mg of furosemide IV to the patient when the surgery lasts longer than 60 minutes.

Electrosurgical System

Electrosurgery is based on the therapeutic use of heat generated within a tissue when it is transversed by an electric current. Depending on the amount of energy applied, on the wave form of the electric current, and on the extent of the area involved, local effect such as tissue coagulation or cutting may be obtained. The coagulation effect is obtained when the electrical current raises tissue temperature to 100°C to 150°C. On the other hand, cutting is achieved when the energy applied rapidly raises the local temperature to 200°C.

During electrosurgery, electric current courses between the active electrode and the neutral electrode or earth-plate (Fig. 2). The smaller the area of the electrode, the greater will be the energy density and local heating. Thus, to perform electrosurgery, active electrodes must have minute dimensions (scalpel blade or resection loop) and a wide earth-plate must be employed, such that the increase in the temperature will only occur to a significant degree at the active extremity.

It is essential that the surgeon should be familiar with these fundamentals in order to decrease complications during TURP. The earth-plate must be not only wide to allow heat dissipation, but it must also be applied to the patient's thigh or leg so that the current will be propagated from the active electrode distally to the lower members. Plates placed on the thorax or upper arms make electric current travel close to the heart, with the risk of disturbing cardiac electrophysiology.

Surgical Technique

Although the use of 27 Fr resectoscope makes TURP faster, this wider sheath increases the incidence of urethral strictures. Thus 27 Fr resectoscope should only be used in prostates weighing more than 60 to 70 g.

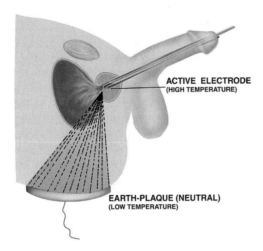

ACTIVE ELECTRODE
(HIGH TEMPERATURE)

EARTH-PLAQUE (NEUTRAL)
(LOW TEMPERATURE)

FIGURE 2   During electrosurgery high temperatures are generated at the active electrode and no heating occurs in the wide earth-plaque.

Prior to TURP care should be taken to reduce the incidence of urethral stricture. The resectoscope insertion should be preceded by a full meatotomy, involving the entire navicular fossa using a fine scalpel and two incisions at 6 and 12 o'clock positions (Fig. 3). Local bleeding, that can initially be significant, is self limited and subsides before the end of surgery. Furthermore, when 27 Fr resectoscope is used, a visual urethrotomy using a Sackse knife and involving the entire bulbar and penile urethra should be performed at the 12 o'clock position.

The urethra must be lubricated with glycerin instead of an anesthetic gel such as lydocaine or liquid vaseline. Lydocaine gel has no insulating properties, which increases the risk of thermal lesion of the urethra. Moreover, it dries rapidly, thus leaving the urethra without lubrication. Liquid vaseline adheres to the cystoscopic lens and disturbs endoscopic vision during the procedure.

Several tactics are applied for endoscopic resection of the prostate and in almost all of them surgery starts at the level of the median lobe, which is removed together with the prostate floor. This stage calls for special attention, as excessive removal of bladder neck between the 5 and 7 o'clock positions may disconnect the bladder from the prostatic capsule in its posterior half (Fig. 4). Should this happen, there is an increased risk of large fluid leakage and greater systemic absorption of the irrigating fluid. Furthermore, this posterior defect sometimes hinders the correct insertion of the foley catheter at the end of the surgery. The catheter can slip into the opened defect and end up behind the bladder, with obvious undesirable consequences. Whenever large posterior bladder neck perforation is seen during TURP (Fig. 4), the Foley's catheter should be inserted into the bladder under direct vision with the help of a guide-wire or after transrectal digital upward pressure applied on the prostate. Rising of the prostatic floor will allow the catheter to pass through the bladder neck correctly.

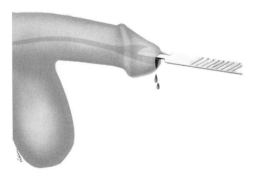

FIGURE 3   Dorsal and ventral meatotomy to avoid meatus stricture.

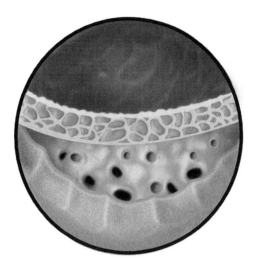

FIGURE 4   Disconnection of posterior half of bladder neck from the prostatic capsule.

Excessive hemostasis of the prostatic fossa may cause necrosis and later sloughing of damaged tissue, with secondary and significant bleeding. This complication can be prevented when coagulating current is kept at the lowest effective level and by using point cauterization of transected vessels.

Extensive cauterization of the bladder neck has also been blamed as the main cause of bladder neck sclerosis. Despite this reasoning, it is most likely that contracture of bladder neck results from large posterior bladder neck perforation as described before, in patients with small prostates (Fig. 4). In such cases, alpha-adrenergic hyperactivity is frequently found and promotes excessive bladder neck closure with subsequent sclerosis. Prevention of this undesirable complication is probably attained with the use of alpha-adrenergic blockers during one or two months following TURP in patients with small glands and large posterior detachment of bladder neck from the prostatic capsule.

In some patients there is profuse bleeding during the TURP procedure, secondary to the transection of arterial vessels or large venous sinuses. In the former case, careful hemostasis is almost always sufficient to control the problem and this task is facilitated by asking the anesthesiologist to increase the patient's blood pressure at the end of the procedure. Arterial bleeding can be more pronounced in patients with preoperative urinary infection or urinary retention and is associated with a congested gland. Some authors have shown that preoperative treatment with finasteride or flutamide may reduce this complication (1).

Entering large venous sinuses may also lead to significant bleeding and this complication must be suspected during the procedure when the irrigation fluid becomes hemorrhagic at the end of bladder emptying. Bleeding from the venous sinuses can be controlled by local electrofulguration but sometimes hemostasis cannot be accomplished. In this situation, the operation must be discontinued and the best move is to insert a Foley catheter in the bladder, inflate the balloon with 60 mL of water and put the catheter under traction for four to six hours. This maneuver, although less effective for arterial bleeding is extremely helpful to control venous bleeding (Fig. 5).

Bladder Drainage and Immediate Postoperative Care

Although some surgeons preclude continuous bladder irrigation after TURP, it is routinely employed by most urologists. Usually the bladder is drained with a 20 Fr Foley catheter and it is important to fix this catheter to the abdomen and not to the thigh of the patient. Beyond preventing scarification and urethral stricture at the penoscrotal angle, fixing the catheter to the abdominal wall keeps it stable during the immediate postoperative period. When the catheter is held in the thigh, it may be pulled under abrupt movements of the awakening patient, with undue pressure over the bladder neck. In addition, the Foley balloon can slip back into prostatic

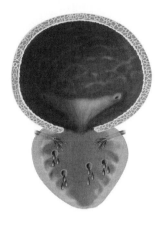
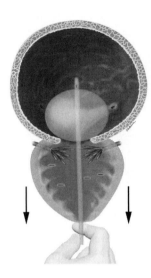

FIGURE 5 Traction applied on the Foley catheter shrinks the prostatic capsule and can stop bleeding from open venous sinus but has less hemostatic effect in opened arterial trunks.

fossa impairing the drainage of the irrigant fluid. Consequently, acute distention of the bladder and prostate capsule can ensue, increasing local bleeding, promoting clot formation and further obstructing the catheter. A vicious cycle is established, which can severely compromise early patient outcome.

Postoperative Complications

Further surgical procedures are necessary in 2% to 15% of the patients who undergo TURP and this rate is much higher than those seen after open surgery, where it happens in 1.8% to 4.5% of cases (18). Reoperation to treat new prostatic growth is rarely needed in patients adequately treated, as urethral obstruction related to prostate regrowth takes 10 to 20 years to occur (19). In the majority of cases, further surgery is performed to remove residual glandular tissue left behind or to repair strictures either of the urethra or bladder neck.

According to the available data morbidity rates associated with TURP have fallen in the recent years, being presently around 20% (15). As infectious control and perioperative patient care have also improved, the severity of the complications following TURP is now lower than it was in the past. For this reason patients presently undergoing TURP are able to leave hospital earlier, usually one or two days following the procedure.

TUR Syndrome

The excessive absorption of the irrigant fluid during TURP may lead to two dreadful complications. The first is represented by intravascular hemolysis especially when water is used for irrigation. The use of nonhemolytic solutions, such as 1.5% glycine, 4% glucose or 0.5% manitol, which have the same serum osmolarity, attenuates this problem. However, if there is no opening of venous sinuses during the operation, absorption of fluid is negligible and consequently distilled water can be used safely.

Another consequence of the excessive absorption of the irrigation fluid is the so-called water intoxication syndrome, seen even when nonhemolytic solutions are employed. This event, which occurs in as many as 10% of patients, arises when more than 1000 mL of the fluid is absorbed within a short period of time (20). The volume of absorbed fluid can be as much as 4 L and results either from direct vascular entry when large venous sinuses are opened or following retroperitoneal reabsorption of extravasated fluid when the prostatic capsule has been extensively perforated.

Patients with the TUR syndrome may develop cardiovascular, neurologic and renal abnormalities. The first manifestations are bradicardia, hypertension, rapid breathing and anxiety. As the syndrome develops, these patients may show restlessness, mental confusion, vomiting, coma, and arterial hypotension, culminating with seizures and cessation of breathing.

When the acute disturbs are overcome, respiratory or renal insufficiency may occur. From the physiopathologic view, these manifestations seem to result from the association of dilutional hyponatremia, low serum osmolarity, and hyperammonemia, the later as a consequence of the metabolism of glycine, when it is used as the irrigant solution.

A recent randomized trial examined the frequency of the TUR syndrome by comparing 1.5% glycine and 5% glucose solutions in 250 patients. Only five patients (2%) developed the TURP syndrome, all in the glycine group, but this incidence was not statistically significant when compared with that of glucose group. A high serum glycine level was associated with the TUR syndrome and there was no difference between the two groups in serum levels of sodium, potassium, urea, creatinine, osmolarity, calcium, hematocrit and albumin (20).

The treatment of the TUR syndrome is based on the administration of intravenous diuretics, hypertonic sodium chloride solution (200 mL of 3% NaCl), and immediate discontinuation of the procedure. On the other hand, this syndrome can be prevented by keeping the irrigant fluid bags or chamber no more than 40 cm above the bladder level and by proper recognition of large venous sinuses opening, or significant perforation of the prostatic capsule. When these later events occur, the procedure must be terminated and the perivesical space must be drained through a small suprapubic incision when substantial irrigant fluid extravasation is suspected.

Postoperative Bleeding

Severe bleeding associated with TURP is reported to range from 6% to 20% and may take place in the immediate postoperative (the first few hours) or the later postoperative (1–4 week) period.

Copious bleeding may occur soon after operation and is frequently triggered off by reopening of large venous sinuses or arteries located mainly at the bladder neck. This event is complicated by clot obstruction of the catheter, which causes acute bladder distension, pain, patient agitation, increase in blood pressure, and more bleeding. Still more significantly, acute distention of the prostatic capsule promotes bursting of all fulgurated vessels, which in turn leads to new sources of bleeding. It is essential to interrupt this sequence of events, and this is done by complete evacuation of clots and promoting free bladder irrigation. When this is unattainable in the patient's bed, the procedure must be performed in the operating room under anesthesia. An endoscopic examination can identify the source of bleeding, but very often clot removal from the bladder is followed by cessation of bleeding and its anatomical origin is rarely identified.

Cold irrigant solutions can be employed when there is moderate arterial bleeding and have some therapeutic value. When the bleeding is related to large opened venous sinuses, this maneuver may be followed by fluid absorption and risk of patient hypothermia.

Severe bleeding can occur one to four weeks after TURP in about 1% to 3% of patients and is caused by excessive cauterization of the prostatic fossa, with late sloughing of prostatic tissue. Reinstallation of bladder irrigation or even surgical evacuation of the clots may be necessary in some cases, although, as already mentioned, endoscopic examination of the prostatic fossa only occasionally reveals the source of bleeding.

Urinary Retention

Between 3% and 9% of patients who undergo TURP are unable to void after Foley removal, and this may be related to the presence of residual obstructing prostatic tissue, to local pain associated with spasm of the external sphincter or to bladder failure (1).

Apical glandular tissue may persist after TURP and block the urethra at the level of verumontanum. The presence of these residual masses, generally located immediately before the external sphincter at the 2 to 10 o'clock positions, should be borne in mind when the patient is unable to void after an additional three to five days of bladder catheterization. Once this diagnosis is suspected endoscopic exploration and resection of the residual tissue should be undertaken. Sphincter spasm and edema at the level of the external sphincter arising from local trauma or pain may also cause immediate urinary retention. Bladder catheterization for a short period and use of nonsteroidal anti-inflammatory drugs almost always overcome this problem.

Detrusor muscle failure is the main cause of persistent urinary retention after adequate TURP (1). This problem is particularly common in patients with aging bladder, long-standing bladder distension, diabetes, and in those undergoing pelvic tumor resections. The majority of patients with hypotonic bladder recover detrusor tonus within a few weeks after TURP, with reestablishment of normal voiding. Despite some controversy, bladder recovery seems to be facilitated by the administration of 25 to 50 mg of betanecol chloride three or four times a day; however, the patient should be maintained on continuous or intermittent bladder catheterization.

Bacteremia and Urinary Tract Infection

Asymptomatic intraoperative bacteremia is observed in 10% to 20% of TURP patients and is associated either with long-lasting bladder catheterization or pre-existing colonization of the prostate tissue (21). In most instances this complication is devoid of major consequences and subsides spontaneously.

The true incidence of urinary tract infection (UTI) following TURP is unknown. According to Grabe (19), in a review of the relevant literature the reported frequency of UTI in these patients ranges from 6% to 70% and this high variation is explained by heterogeneous patient populations evaluated. Although the role of antimicrobial prophylaxis in this setting is controversial, the routine use of these agents during and after TURP probably reduces the incidence of UTIs. Aside from this debate, there are some situations where the use of antimicrobial drugs is mandatory. They include those patients with increased risk for complicated UTIs (uremia, diabetes, neurogenic bladder, and immunosuppression) or with associated diseases that may be aggravated by UTI (cardiac valvopathies, neurologic diseases).

About 30% of the infections that occur after TURP are caused by gram-positive microorganisms, which represents a higher incidence than that seen in uncomplicated UTIs. For this reason prophylactic treatment of noninfected patients who will undergo TURP should be undertaken with antimicrobial drugs active against both gram-negative and gram-positive agents. First- and second-generation cephalosporines and quinolones should be considered for these cases. For infected patients, antibacterial treatment must be considered with third-generation quinolones, aminoglycosides- or third-generation cephalosporins. In such cases, the treatment should be started 1 week before surgery and maintained for 10 to 14 days after catheter removal.

Urinary Incontinence

Urinary incontinence associated with extreme urgency occurs in 30% to 40% of patients following removal of Foley catheter is related to pre-existing bladder instability and improves spontaneously within a few days or weeks (1). Patients who remain with urge incontinence can be treated with anti-cholinergics but the long-term outcome is unpredictable and most of times gloomy.

Stress urinary incontinence can also be seen following TURP, rarely lasts for more than 8 weeks and is related to damage of the external urethral sphincter. In most instances this damage results from mechanic trauma caused by the resectoscope sheath or by excessive cauterization of the prostatic apex with secondary scarring at the level of the membranous urethra. Endoscopic examination of affected patients shows a fibrous ring that impairs urethral closure and gives rise to urinary incontinence. For the same reason, many of these patients cannot also open adequately the urethra during voiding, making them partially obstructed as well as incontinent. More rarely lesion of the external sphincter arises from its accidental resection during operation.

Those patients with slight urinary stress incontinence can be successfully treated with sertraline, 50 mg once daily, imipramine 25 to 75 mg once daily, or ephedrine sulfate, 25 to 50 mg three times a day. The later, by virtue of its vasoconstrictive action, should be avoided in patients with high blood pressure or coronary disease. When the stress urinary incontinence is severe and persistent, medical treatment is ineffective and the patients have to be treated surgically. Periurethral injections of bulky agents can alleviate or cure the less severe symptomatic patients (22,23). To improve the clinical results with this technique, the bulky agent must be injected circumferentially in the area of the external sphincter and a suprapubic urinary diversion (cystostomy) must be maintained for five to six days. On the other hand, the AMS 800 artificial urinary sphincter is highly effective and recommended for patients with severe stress incontinence following TURP (24).

Urethral Strictures

Between 4% and 29% of the patients who have undergone TURP develop urethral strictures related to three main causes: mechanic or thermal trauma caused by the resectoscope, severe urethritis or trauma due to the Foley catheter, and urethral ischemia in patients with chronic arterial insufficiency (25). Urethral strictures are more common when surgery takes longer or when the 27 Fr resectoscope is used. Most of these strictures are located in the fossa navicularis, the urethra at penoscrotal angle and membranous urethra.

Careful handling of the Foley catheter reduces the incidence of urethral strictures. The latex used to manufacture these catheters may cause varying degrees of irritation of the urethra. A number of reports have described acute purulent urethritis or urethral strictures after the use of certain makes of catheters or different lots from the same brand. Therefore, urologists should avoid changing the make of Foley catheters to which they are familiar, and whenever possible, use silicone-coated ones, which causes less urethral irritation. Furthermore, Foley catheters, once installed, should be fixed in the abdominal wall to avoid catheter kinking and scarification of the urethra at the penoscrotal angle, resulting in local fibrosis and stricture.

Some reports suggest that nonsteroidal anti-inflammatory agents given immediately after catheter removal and maintained for two to three weeks following TURP can prevent urethral strictures. In this regard a recent randomized trial showed that at 1 year, urethral strictures were observed respectively in 0% and 17% of patients receiving and not receiving cyclooxygenase-2 (COX-2) inhibitor agent. The treated group also showed greater improvement in the peak urinary flow rate at the first follow-up month (25).

The treatment of urethral strictures related to the TURP is based on the same principles that guide the treatment of strictures from other causes. It is worth to emphasize, however, that strictures of the membranous urethra should be dealt with great care to avoid definitive damage of the external sphincter. This makes endoscopic urethrotomy unadvisable in this subset of patients; the procedure can successfully solve the obstructive problem but is associated with a high risk of urinary incontinence. These patients are better treated with gentle and gradual catheter dilation of the narrowed urethra.

Bladder Neck Sclerosis

Bladder neck sclerosis occurs in approximately 3% of the patients who undergo TURP and is usually diagnosed four to eight weeks after surgery. Although it has been repeatedly stated that this complication results from excessive local cauterization, it is most likely caused by the detachment of posterior bladder neck from the prostate capsule in patients with small glands. Alpha-adrenergic hyperactivity, common in patients with small hyperplastic prostates, produces a sustained postoperative contraction of the bladder neck, which ends up with bladder neck sclerosis.

The treatment of bladder neck sclerosis is undertaken by means of a Y-shaped incision with a Collins or cold knife. However, recurrence of the obstruction is seen in 30% to 50% of patients managed exclusively with bladder neck incisions. Taking in to account the physiopathologic mechanism involved with bladder neck sclerosis, surgical incision should be followed by the use of an alpha-adrenergic blocker for 60 to 90 days in order to keep the bladder neckwide open.

A recent retrospective study tested the efficacy of performing TURP followed by transurethral incision of the bladder neck as opposed to only TURP. Among 1135 patients with a mean follow-up of 37.9 months, the incidence of bladder neck sclerosis was 12.3% in the TURP group and only 6% in patients treated with the combined technique. Moreover, bladder neck contracture was completely prevented when TURP and bladder neck incision was performed in patients with prostate weight greater than 30 g. Multivariate analyses showed that gland weight and surgical technique were the significant risk factors for bladder neck sclerosis (7).

Impotence

Erectile dysfunction has been described in some patients undergoing TURP. In a large study published by Mebust, 3.5% of patients reported new onset of erectile dysfunction after TURP (15). The same finding was reported in other series, but the causative role of the surgical procedure in the etiology of this complication has not been well established. It is worth remembering that around 5% of elderly men who underwent various non-urologic abdominal operations developed postoperative sexual dysfunction (15). Furthermore, in some patients, factors other than TURP itself may give rise to this complication, including postoperative depression, new medications, anxiety related to retrograde ejaculation, as well as the process of aging itself (26).

Despite the controversy that surrounds the etiology of post-TURP sexual dysfunction, it is possible that in some patients there exists a causal relationship between these two events. Thermal damage of the cavernous neurovascular bundles due to their proximity to the prostatic capsule can explain this association. Therefore, all patients who are to undergo TURP should be advised about the uncertainty and the rare occurrence of sexual dysfunction following the procedure.

Mortality

Surgical mortality after TURP is quite low, being around 0.1% (16). This figure seems to be lower than that observed after open prostatectomy, which is associated with a postoperative mortality rate of 1.7% to 2.9%.

Three recent studies have shown that patients who underwent TURP presented higher later mortality than those treated with open surgery. In one of these studies, Roos et al. (27) analyzed the records of more than 58,000 patients who underwent TURP or open prostatectomy in Canada, England, and Denmark. The long-term assessment of these patients showed that the death risk after TURP was about 1.5 times greater than that seen following open surgery. This finding was confirmed by Malenka et al. (28) and by Meyhoff (18), although no obvious explanations for these observations were given.

The main causes of patient deaths in the Roos and Meyhoff studies were myocardium infarct and chronic lung disease. Therefore, it has been suggested that the differences in mortality rates following the two procedures resulted from case selection, being possible that TURP was used in higher risk patients, with more comorbidity factors (16). Another explanation raised was that TURP is usually recommended for patients with smaller glands who perhaps have higher sympathetic activity. This abnormal physiologic state would favor not only bladder outlet obstruction but would also increase the incidence of cardiovascular complications. Favoring the first explanation is a study of Concato et al. (29) where patients underwent TURP or open surgery and were stratified in groups of equivalent comorbidity. Following adjustments identical rates of late mortality were found after following the two procedures.

This report and a more recent study that compared patients treated with TURP or kept under clinical surveillance (30) indicate that TURP is not associated in the long-term run with higher mortality risk.

REFERENCES

1. Rassweiler J, Teber D, Kuntz R, Hofmann R. Complications of transurethral resection of the prostate (TURP). Incidence, management, and prevention. Eur Urol 2006; 50:969–980.
2. Thomas AW, Cannon A, Bartlett E, Ellis-Jones J, Abrams P. The natural history of lower urinary tract dysfunction in men: minimum 10-year urodynamic follow-up of transurethral resection of prostate for bladder outlet obstruction. J Urol 2005; 174:1887–1891.
3. Effert P, Ackermann R. Surgical prostatectomy. In: Chisholm GD, ed. Handbook on Benign Prostatic Hyperplasia. New York: Raven Press, 1994:95–114.
4. Orandi A. Transurethral incision of the prostate. J Urol 1973; 110:229–231.
5. Orandi A. Transurethral incision of the prostate compared with transurethral resection of the prostate in 132 matching cases. J Urol 1987; 138:810–815.
6. Mebust WK. BPH: patient care policies/guidelines. AUA Update Ser 1993; 12:226–231.
7. Lee YH, Chiu AW, Huang JK. Comprehensive study of bladder neck contracture after transurethral resection of prostate. Urology 2005; 65:498–503.
8. Tkocz M, Prajsner A. Comparison of long-term results of transurethral incision of the prostate with transurethral resection of the prostate in patients with benign prostatic hypertrophy. Neurourol Urodyn 2002; 21:112–116.
9. Yang Q, Peters TJ, Donovan JL, Wilt TJ, Abrams P. Transurethral incision compared with transurethral resection of the prostate for bladder outlet obstruction: a systematic review and meta-analysis of randomized controlled trials. J Urol 2001; 165:526–532.
10. Sirls LT, Ganabathi K, Zimmern PE, et al. Transurethral incision of the bladder neck and prostate. J Urol 1993; 150:1615–1621.

11. Edwards LE, Bucknall FE, Pitam MR, et al. Transurethral resection of the prostate and bladder neck incision: a review of 700 cases. Br J Urol 1985; 57:168–171.
12. Madersbacher S, Marberger M. Is transurethral resection of the prostate still justified? BJU Int 1999; 83:227–237.
13. Mebust WK. Transurethral prostatectomy. AUA Update Ser 1994; 13:142–147.
14. Steg A, Ackerman R, Gibbons R et al. Surgery in BPH. In: Cockett ATK, Aso Y, Chatelain C, eds. The International Consultation on Benign Prostatic Hyperplasia (BPH). Paris: World Health Organization, 1991:201–21.
15. Christensen MM, Aagaard J, Madsen PO. Transurethral resection versus transurethral incision of the prostate. Urol Clin North Am 1990; 17:621–630.
16. Riehmann M, Knes JM, Heisey D, et al. Transurethral resection versus incision of the prostate: a randomized prospective study. Urology 1995; 45:768–775.
17. Neal DE. Prostatectomy-an open or closed case. Br J Urol 1990; 66:449–454.
18. Meyhoff AH. Transurethral versus transvesical prostatectomy. Scand J Urol Nephrol 1987; 102(Suppl.):1–26.
19. Grabe M. Perioperative antibiotic prophylaxis in urology. Curr Opin Urol 2001; 11:81–85.
20. Collins JW, Macdermott S, Bradbrook RA, Keeley FX Jr, Timoney AG. A comparison of the effect of 1.5% glycine and 5% glucose irrigants on plasma serum physiology and the incidence of transurethral resection syndrome during prostate resection. BJU Int 2005; 96:368–372.
21. Hofer DR, Schaeffer AJ. Use of antimicrobials for patients undergoing prostatectomy. Urol Clin North Am 1990; 17:595–600.
22. Kabalin JN. Treatment of post-prostatectomy stress urinary incontinence with periurethral polytetrafluoroethylene paste injection. J Urol 1994; 152:1463–1466.
23. Kageyama S, Kawabe K, Suzuki K, et al. Collagen implantation for post-prostatectomy incontinence: early experience with transrectal ultrasonographically guided method. J Urol 1994; 152:1473–1475.
24. Martins FE, Boyd SD. Artificial urinary sphincter in patients following major pelvic surgery and/or radiotherapy: are they less favorable candidates? J Urol 1995; 153:1188–1193.
25. Sciarra A, Salciccia S, Albanesi L, Cardi A, D'Eramo G, Di Silverio F. Use of cyclooxygenase-2 inhibitor for prevention of urethral strictures secondary to transurethral resection of the prostate. Urology 2005; 66:1218–1222.
26. Aitwein JE, Keuler U. Potency and prostatectomy. Prospectives 1991; 1:1–4.
27. Roos NP, Wennberg JE, Malenka DJ, et al. Mortality and reoperation after open and transurethral resection of the prostate for benign prostatic hyperplasia. N Engl J Med 1989; 320:1120–1124.
28. Malenka DJ, Ross N, Fischer ES, et al. Further study of the increased mortality following transurethral prostatectomy: a chart-based analysis. J Urol 1990; 144:224–228.
29. Concato J, Horowitz RI, Feinstein AR, et. al. Problems of comordibity in mortality after prostatectomy. JAMA 1992; 267:1077–1082.
30. Wasson JH, Reda DJ, Bruskewitz RC, et al. A comparison of transurethral surgery with watchful waiting for moderate symptoms of benign prostatic hyperplasia. N Engl J Med 1995; 332:75–79.

30 | Complications of Minimally Invasive Treatments for Lower Urinary Tract Symptoms Secondary to Benign Prostatic Hyperplasia

Brian T. Helfand and Kevin T. McVary
Department of Urology, Feinberg School of Medicine, Northwestern University, Chicago, Illinois, U.S.A.

INTRODUCTION

Benign prostatic hyperplasia (BPH) is the most common benign tumor in the aging male population. In fact, autopsy data estimate that the presence of histologic BPH may be as high as 70% in men by their seventh decade of life (1). Treatment intervention for clinical BPH is most commonly directed toward the alleviation of bothersome lower urinary tract symptoms (LUTSs). In addition, treatment intervention is also indicated for the relief of acute urinary retention (AUR) as well as other morbidities caused by BPH [e.g., recurrent urinary tract infections (UTIs), bladder stones, etc.] (2,3).

Most commonly, men experiencing mild to moderate LUTS from BPH are treated with pharmacotherapeutic agents as a first-line therapy (4). Outcomes of these therapies suggest that they have efficacy in reducing the severity of LUTS (4,5). However, when choosing this treatment, patients must understand the requirement to adhere to a strict medication schedule for their lifetime and the potential side effects of the medications. They must also be aware that the outcomes for these treatments are not as efficacious, or as reliable, as surgical intervention. Despite these inadequacies, patients often choose medications over surgery because of the perceived reduced risk of adverse events and the desire to avoid surgery.

Surgical therapy is an attractive alternative to patients who experience moderate to severe obstructive or irritative voiding symptoms, who have failed medical therapy, or who choose not be managed medically. Surgical therapy for BPH has proven long-term efficacy (6). Patients are oftentimes enthusiastic if they are offered a one-time method to treat LUTS secondary to BPH, provided that the method offers reduced risk and allows an efficacy equal to that of medical therapy. Therefore, surgical intervention has an intrinsic attractiveness.

Transurethral resection of the prostate (TURP) is currently considered to be the "gold standard" surgery treatment for the management of BPH (7–10). However, TURP is still associated with significant morbidities and complications including bleeding, transurethral resection (TUR) syndrome, incontinence, urethral strictures, retrograde ejaculation, and erectile dysfunction (ED) (8–9). In addition, TURP is associated with relatively long hospital stays, which adds to the cost of TURP. These complications and healthcare costs associated with prolonged hospitalization have sparked a movement to develop alternative surgical procedures for the treatment of BPH that are durable, cost-effective, and associated with few morbidities. In the last 20 years, less invasive surgical therapies have been investigated as these treatment alternatives. There are two types among the new modalities for the treatment of BPH—one group includes true "minimally invasive therapies" that use the thermal effects of different sources of energy to reduce obstructing prostatic tissue while the second group encompasses improvements on standard surgical endoscopic techniques. To be preferred over TURP, these new less invasive procedures must achieve a significant subjective and objective success in the majority of cases, have long-lasting results, as well as significantly reduce the morbidity that has historically been associated with open surgery and TURP.

Despite the promise of these new minimally and less invasive techniques, their evolution and application must be viewed with some caution as these procedures have their own set of morbidities and associated problems. This chapter will review many of the current minimally invasive techniques for the treatment of BPH and evaluate their success, morbidities, and mortalities compared to TURP. For convenience, the morbidities and mortalities associated with these procedures are divided into intra-operative, peri-operative (within the first 30 days following the procedure) and postoperative complications (after 30 days).

GENERAL PREOPERATIVE CONSIDERATIONS

As with other surgical procedures, men undergoing surgical management of BPH may have a host other significant medical problems that may complicate anesthesia or promote bleeding. Overall cardiac and respiratory function must be taken into consideration prior to surgery, as dramatic circulatory fluctuations and fluid shifts have been observed with TURP and many of the other minimally invasive procedures.

Azotemia may also contribute to preoperative risk, and as such, preoperative bladder drainage should be performed to relieve urinary retention secondary to outlet obstruction, especially if upper tract damage has occurred. A sufficient period of time must be allotted prior to surgery in order to allow serum creatinine to stabilize (9,10).

At the time of surgery, concurrent bladder pathology, including bladder stones, may be managed intraoperatively (11–17). However this intervention may lead to premature termination of the procedure, and may require a repeat operation.

While the indications for preoperative antibiotics have been extensively reviewed, their usage continues to remain somewhat controversial (18). Although rare, peri-operative sepsis has historically been the leading cause of death from TURP. Other infectious complications, including bacteriuria and epididymitis, have been reported. This has not been extensively studied for many of the newer minimally invasive surgery therapies. However, for TURP, prior studies of infected patients randomized to treatment or no treatment demonstrated a significant decrease in postoperative bacteriuria, sepsis, and length of hospital stay (19–23). Significant differences were noted with a single preoperative dose of aztreonam or gentamicin (24,25). However, another study examining the use of preoperative pipercillin only significantly lowered three-day incidence of bacteriuria, with no effect on three-week incidence (26–36).

In the United States, the majority of TURP procedures are performed using spinal anesthesia (77%). Spinal anesthesia has a decreased tendency to produce respiratory suppression in comparison with general anesthesia, and as such is considered to be a safer option (9). Additionally, as spinal anesthesia permits the patient to remain awake during the procedure, the physician may be alerted to early mental status changes and complaints of abdominal discomfort which may herald the onset of the TUR syndrome. Prior studies have also demonstrated a significant reduction in operative blood loss with the use of spinal anesthesia (37,38). While there are no current multi-center studies involving large numbers of patients for many of the newer minimally invasive techniques, it is generally agreed upon that either spinal anesthesia or local anesthesia is preferred over general anesthesia for these same reasons. It should be noted that most of the newer minimally invasive procedures [e.g., transurethral microwave thermotherapy (TUMT), transurethral needle ablation (TUNA)] can be performed under local anesthesia, IV sedation or transperineal prostate block. These sedations are advantageous in that they are associated with decreased cardiovascular risks.

THE GOLD STANDARD: TRANSURETHRAL RESECTION OF THE PROSTATE

In order to critically evaluate the success of any new technique it is essential to have a reference standard for comparison. Currently, TURP serves as the standard for the treatment of BPH (10). Yet, many studies have indicated that the TURP procedure is associated with many complications and morbidities including intra-operative bleeding, TUR syndrome, urethral stricture, bladder neck contracture, cardiovascular disorders, and perforation (8,10–15). Within the past decade, improvements in operative techniques, video endoscopy, anaesthetic care, and intraoperative monitoring of fluid and electrolytes have significantly decreased the rates of morbidity and mortality associated with TURP (16).

Transurethral resection of the prostate requires urethral catheterization for 24 to 48 hours, and a hospital stay ranging from one to three days (17). In addition, for at least four weeks after

TURP, the patient should restrict physical activity, including avoiding strenuous activity, sudden motions, driving, heavy lifting, and sexual intercourse. Patients should also be aware of potential intra-operative complications which occur at a frequency ranging from 2% to 30 %, with an average closer to 3%, depending on surgeon experience (18–20). These immediate complications include a mortality rate significantly less than 0.2%, usually related to intra-operative myocardial infarction and cardiovascular compromise (12). It has been found that there is an increased risk of many of these complications with increased resection time (>90 min).

The most common intra-operative complication associated with TURP is hemorrhage requiring transfusion in approximately 2% to 25% of patients depending on surgeon experience and institution (20–22). The amount of blood loss is also related to the mass of the gland excised, the duration of the procedure, the mass of prostatic tissue excised, and patients' vital signs. Severe intra-operative hemorrhage leading to significant shock occurs in less than 1% of cases and may be a result of clotting abnormalities or related to tissue plasminogen activator released from the prostate tissue. In these cases, active fibrinolytics can be used to minimize blood loss. It should be noted that the Veterans Affairs Cooperative Study, one of the largest and most comprehensive studies conducted on TURP to date, reported a transfusion rate of 4% to 5%, although the estimated national frequency is closer to 8% (20,21). The average change in hemoglobin associated with TURP is between 1.5 and 2.5 g/dL (17,23). Although transfusion is associated with minimal risks, it represents a significant morbidity as many patients have a general aversion toward receiving blood products. Other intra-operative complications associated with TURP include a 1% to 2% risk of developing a deep venous thrombosis (DVT) (17,30) and less than 1% risk of developing a pulmonary embolism (17,30). Treatment options for these patients include anticoagulation therapy and other possible supportive therapies depending on their stability. If anticoagulation therapy is contraindicated due to the risk of bleeding or other medical problems, then an inferior vena cava filter should be considered.

Transurethral resection of the prostate has been associated with a relatively small risk (0–2%) of sustaining a urethral or bladder injury (17,20,31). For example, bladder perforation complicated approximately 1% of cases. Most perforations are extraperitoneal and result in suprapubic, inguinal or periumbilical pain in the awake patient. Intraperitoneal perforation is far less common, but more serious. In these cases, the patient experiences generalized abdominal pain and may complain of radiation to the shoulder. Pallor, sweating, peritoneal signs, nausea, and vomiting may be present. Management consists of immediate laparotomy and correction of the defect. The treatment of urethral perforation includes termination of the procedure if it is noticed intra-operatively. This should be stopped only after hemostasis is achieved and the resected tissue is removed. A urethral catheter should be inserted. Suprapubic drainage of the retroperitoneum may be indicated to minimize further fluid resorption. Prostatic capsule perforation has also been reported in a small percentage of cases (~1–2%) during TURP. The symptoms are similar to extraperitoneal bladder perforation. Similarly, if extravasation is suspected, the operation should be terminated once hemostasis is achieved and a urethral catheter should be placed. Another rare intra-operative complication associated with TURP is damage to the urethral orifices. This usually occurs in the setting of trigonal hypertrophy, as the orifices are displaced toward the prostate, putting them at risk during prostatic resection. To avoid such trauma, indigo carmine may be used to visualize the orifices.

A unique complication associated with the TURP procedure is the TUR syndrome (24). This syndrome is believed to result from the hyponatremia and hypervolemia and hyperammonemia caused by metabolism of absorbed glycine present in the nonconductive irrigative fluids used during TURP. The TUR syndrome comprises a constellation of symptoms which begin intra-operatively. These include hypotension, bradycardia, confusion, nausea, and vomiting. The condition may occasionally be associated with a loss of vision (25,26). The incidence of the TUR syndrome has not been definitely established, but ranges from 1% to 7% (27,28). It should be noted that within recent years bipolar electrosurgical generators and electrodes that can be used with saline instead of glycine for irrigation have been introduced to minimize the occurrence of the TUR syndrome (29). The treatment of the TUR syndrome may necessitate input from a team of specialists including, apart from the urologist and anesthesiologist, an intensive care therapist, neurologist, cardiologist and opthalmologist. In addition to general supportive therapy, it is mandatory to combat associated hypotension, hyponatremia, hypo-osmolarity, and anuria. The initial management of fluid overload and hyponatremia involves stopping IV fluids and commencing fluid restriction. Furosemide should be given to promote diuresis. Hyponatremia-causing encephalopathy requires more rapid correction than achieved by fluid restriction and diuresis alone. In these cases, hypertonic saline solutions (1.8%, 3%, 5%) should be used to increase the serum sodium level by 1 mmol per hour, not to exceed an increase of more than 20 mmol in the first 48 hours. Sodium levels should be checked every few hours. Therapy with hypertonic saline should be stopped when the sodium level is between 124 and 132 mmol/L. Rapid correction has been implicated in the formation of central pontine myelinolysis. Convulsions associated with the TUR syndrome should be acutely treated with a benzodiazepine. In general, patients with these disorders or other mental status changes will require admission and close monitoring in an intensive care unit.

Improvements in surgical technique and anesthesia have greatly improved the morbidities and mortalities associated with TURP (16). However, despite these improvements, TURP is still associated with some mortality within the peri-operative period. As TURPs are usually performed in an elderly population, this mortality rate may be related to other pre-existing conditions. However, the mortality rate in patients following TURP was higher than for those treated by open prostatectomy (12). The reason for this is unknown and may be related to inaccurate assessment of the severity of illness in previous studies (32). Despite this, it has been reported that there is a mortality rate of approximately 0.2% to 0.5% within 30 days after undergoing TURP (16,17,33,34). Causes of death following the procedure include sepsis, myocardial infarction, stroke, septicemia, massive pulmonary embolism, and problems related to multi-system disease.

Patients typically remain with an indwelling catheter for approximately two to five days after undergoing TURP. After removal of the indwelling catheter, urinary retention has been reported in up to 30% of patients, with an average of ~5% (20). Almost all patients experience transient hematuria and irritative voiding symptoms after the procedure (19,35). Other peri-operative complications include clot retention, transient incontinence, and dysuria (Table 1).

Long-term complications of the TURP procedure have been described in a number of retrospective and prospective studies (39–44). These complications include re-treatment. However, the frequency of re-treatment has been challenging to classify as patients may go to another treating physician or move locations. However, the estimated secondary procedure rate after TURP is as high as 20% (24,45). However, it should be noted that this percentage includes patients who had secondary treatments with either surgical therapy (e.g., repeat TURP, open prostatectomy, etc.) or medical therapy (e.g., alpha-adrenergic antagonists, 5α-reductase inhibitors, etc.). Additional long-term complications include urinary incontinence, bladder neck contractures, and urethral strictures (Table 1).

Transurethral resection of the prostate has been reported to cause some form of sexual dysfunction in many patients (46). For example, nearly 75% of men experience retrograde ejaculation and ~2% to 13% of men experience ED after TURP (47,48) However, the numbers of new-onset ED have to be evaluated with some criticism as ED is positively correlated with BPH progression and advancing age (49,50). Therefore, many of the cases of ED reported after TURP may not have been due to the procedure itself, but rather due to the cumulative incidence of ED that occurs in any population. This possibility is supported by the fact that there is a 5% rate of new-onset ED following hernia and cholecystectomy surgeries.

It should be known that there are contraindications to TURP that could minimize associated complication rates. These contraindications also generally apply to all of the minimally invasive prostatic surgeries mentioned hereinafter. Contraindications include, but are not limited to, active urinary infection and known or suspected prostate or urothelial cancer. Patients with neurogenic bladder voiding dysfunction should have their underlying neurogenic problem evaluated and treated prior to surgery. The presence of renal failure, coronary artery disease, and cerebrovascular disease should be noted prior to the consideration of surgery, as these factors increase the risk of complications associated with surgery.

MINIMALLY INVASIVE SURGICAL THERAPY: TRANSURETHRAL MICROWAVE THERMOTHERAPY

Newer modalities for the treatment of BPH have been aimed to provide a one-time minimally invasive surgical therapy (MIST) that is associated with fewer complications than TURP

TABLE 1 Reported Incidence of Complications following TURP

Complication	Incidence (%)
Intraoperative complications (~3%)	
Transurethral resection syndrome	1–7
Bleeding requiring transfusion	8
Deep venous thrombosis	1–2
PE	<1
Urethral injury	0–2
Bladder injury	0–2
Mortality	<0.2
Perioperative complications	
Irritative voiding symptoms	15–100
Clot retention	3–20
Dysuria	2–16
Urinary retention	2–8
Transient hematuria	4–7
Urinary tract infection	6–20
Transient incontinence	1–4
Septicemia	0–5
Epididymo-orchitis	3–5
Proctitis	<1
Bladder spasm	1–2
Mortality	<0.5
Long-term complications	
Retrograde ejaculation	75–85
Erectile dysfunction	2–13
Retreatment (TURP)	3–8
Urinary incontinence	1–3
Urethral stricture	1–2
Bladder neck contracture	1–3
Meatal stricture	~1
Chronic urinary tract infection	~1
Chronic dysuria	<1
Chronic urinary retention	<1
Chronic prostatitis	<1
Hematospermia	<1
Hematuira	<1

Abbreviations: PE, pulmonary embolism; TURP, transurethral resection of the prostate.

(51–54). One such MIST that has been used in this regard is TUMT. TUMT uses a urethral catheter device to apply heat to the prostatic tissue causing necrosis and relief of bladder outlet obstruction. Temperatures greater than 45°C are necessary to destroy prostatic parenchyma, a process which was termed "thermotherapy" (55). Unfortunately, the urethral temperature for pain threshold is also approximately 45°C. Therefore, low-energy TUMT (LE-TUMT) devices that incorporate urethral cooling instrumentation were developed to allow for these elevated temperatures. To enhance outcomes further, high-energy TUMT (HE-TUMT) machines capable of achieving prostatic temperatures greater than 70°C were developed to cause thermoablation and thermocoagulation of prostatic tissue. Today, several different LE- and HE-TUMT devices are in use around the world, including the Targis (Urologix, Inc., Minneapolis, Minnesota, U.S.A.), Prostatron (Technomed Medical Systemt, Lyons, France), Prolieve (Boston Scientific/Microvasive, Boston, Massachussetts, U.S.A.assachusetts) Prostalund (Lund Instruments AB, Lund, Sweden), Prostcare (Bruker Medical, Wissembourg, France), Urowave (Dornier MedTech America, Kennesaw, Georgia, U.S.A.), PRIMUS U+R (Tecnomatix, Monheim, Germany), and the LEO Microthermer (Laser Electro Optics, London, U.K.).

Both LE-TUMT and HE-TUMT have efficacy in the treatment of BPH. However, the improvement in uroflowmetry induced by HE-TUMT is more pronounced compared with LE-TUMT (51,56). This improvement in maximum urinary flow (Q_{max}) may be a tradeoff for greater irritative symptomatology and longer duration of catheterization [see below, (57)]. While the improvements in irritative urinary symptoms after either LE-TUMT or HE-TUMT have not quite reached those associated with TURP, significant improvements in urinary symptoms have been reported for long time periods. Overall, TUMT has been associated with fewer complications than TURP and thus TUMT should be critically evaluated for its morbidities and durability in treating LUTS secondary to BPH.

One of the major advantages of TUMT is that it can be performed in one hour or less as an outpatient procedure without any general or spinal anesthesia. However, despite the avoidance of inpatient hospitalization, TUMT is still associated with morbidities. Reports of overall complications vary, and range from 0% to 38%, based on the study and the investigators' criteria for complications. As with TURP, the morbidities associated with TUMT can be divided into intra-operative, peri-operative, and postoperative complications. The most common intra-operative complication is pain during the procedure. While TUMT is usually well tolerated by patients, most patients perceive a mild feeling of perineal warmth and a slight sensation of urinary urgency during the procedure. This is due to the urethral pain threshold at temperatures >45°C (58). Approximately 5% to 7% of patients report significant perineal discomfort during the procedure (59). Treatment for these discomforts is usually alleviated by momentary interruption of microwave emission. However, pain medication can be administered before the procedure to minimize these discomforts even further.

An intra-operative advantage of the TUMT procedure is the significant decrease in blood loss and frequency of transfusions compared with TURP. For example, a meta-analysis study demonstrated a mean blood loss of approximately 300 cc after TURP compared with no blood loss after TUMT. In addition, this study demonstrated a trend toward a reduced risk of secondary hemorrhage after TUMT compared to TURP (60,61). Therefore, transfusion and blood loss do not appear to be significant risks for minimally invasive heat-based therapy such as TUMT. In addition, because of the nature of the procedure, TUR syndrome is not considered to be a risk.

The TUMT device was designed to minimize contact with non-prostatic tissues. In addition, cooling fluid circulating through the urethral catheter protects the urethra and surrounding tissues from overheating by automatically controlling microwave energy output based on information supplied by thermo-sensors placed posterior to the prostate within the rectum. However, because of the use of heat application as well as the anatomical location of the prostate, other non-prostatic tissues are still at risk for injury during TUMT. Recently, the risk of serious injuries from microwave thermotherapy has been reported by the U.S. Food and Drug Administration (FDA) (62). This report included a description of 10 instances of fistula formation and six instances of clinically significant tissue damage to the penis/urethra that have required colostomies, partial amputation of the penis, and/or other interventions (63). Fistula formation is generally treated by primary surgical closure with omental interposition. In addition, minor bladder and urethral injuries/perforations have been reported in up to 5% of patients undergoing TUMT (64,65). (Fig. 1). These injuries have been due to either malfunctioning or misplacement of the thermo sensors and/or catheter. As with other urethral and bladder injuries, catheter drainage of the urethra and bladder is the appropriate treatment.

Peri-operative complications associated with TUMT have also been investigated. Compared with TURP, urinary retention occurs in a significantly increased number of patients following TUMT. This is presumed due to the edema and inflammation of the lower urinary tract following the procedure. In fact, between 15% and 30% of patients will require an indwelling urinary catheter secondary to AUR following TUMT (20). The duration of catheterization following TUMT ranges from two days to two weeks depending on the device used and protocol used (51). Indwelling catheterization increases the risk for UTIs following TUMT (~10–15%). The risk of UTIs may also be increased by the fact that the necrotic tissue that remains in the prostatic fossa after TUMT may permit bacterial colonization. Despite these factors, it has been demonstrated that the occurrence of UTIs following TUMT is not significantly greater than following TURP. For example, it has been described that approximately 15% of patients undergoing TURP and 13% of patients undergoing TURP experience UTIs within the first 30 days following treatment (66,67). Post-procedure irritative voiding symptom rates are almost two-fold increased in patients undergoing TUMT compared with patients undergoing TURP (20). Other peri-operative complications include transient urinary incontinence (1–3%) and epididymo-orchitis (<1%) after TUMT (68).

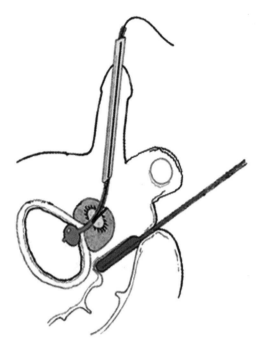

FIGURE 1   Injuries associated with transurethral microwave thermotherapy (TUMT). The image depicts the correct positioning of TUMT. However, injuries can occur secondary to malfunctioning or misplacement of the TUMT device (*dark grey*) or rectal thermosensor. Therefore, these devices should be placed under direct (*black*) visualization. In addition, balloon location should be confirmed at the start of the procedure and repositioned if there is a problem. These steps, along with compliance with the manufacturer's guidelines, should minimize the rates of penile/urethral injuries and fistula formation that have been associated with TUMT.

The long-term complications associated with TUMT have also been investigated (Table 2). Overall, TUMT is associated with significantly lower postoperative frequencies of urinary incontinence, bladder neck contractures, and urethral strictures compared with TURP (20). For example, multiple randomized control trials have demonstrated that the rates of urethral stricture and bladder neck contracture were approximately 0% to 2% in patients who underwent TUMT and between 5% and 16% in patients who underwent TURP (45,67,69). Stress or urge urinary incontinence is a very infrequent complication of TUMT (56,59). The overall rates of secondary treatment for recurrence of LUTS related to BPH are higher for LE-TUMT compared to HE-TUMT. This may be related to the increased improvement in Q_{max} by HE-TUMT (51). TUMT also has a higher re-treatment rate compared with TURP. For example, it has been described that at one year post-TUMT, ~8% of patients initiate medical or surgical therapy for

TABLE 2   Reported Incidence of Complications Following Transurethral Microwave Thermotherapy

Complication	Incidence (%)
Intraoperative complications	
Bleeding requiring transfusion	<1
Urethral injury	5
Bladder injury	5
Perioperative complications	
Irritative voiding symptoms	28–74
Urinary retention	15–30
Urinary tract infection	10–15
Transient urinary incontinence	1–3
Epidiymo-orchitis	<1
Long-term complications	
Retrograde ejaculation	0–28
Erectile dysfunction	1–3
Retreatment (transurethral resection of the prostate)	8–17
Urethral stricture	0–2
Bladder neck contracture	0–2

BPH symptoms (63). Another study reported that by two years after treatment with TUMT, 46.9% of patients were using medical therapy with an alpha-adrenergic antagonist and 17.6% of patients elected for re-treatment with TURP (70).

As mentioned above, it is difficult to demonstrate a causality between MIST and changes in sexual and erectile function. Despite this, it has been reported that changes in sexual function occur in approximately 17% of men following TUMT compared to 36% with TURP (71). One of the most common adverse effects after TUMT is retrograde ejaculation. This is reportedly observed in 48% to 90% of patients after TURP and between 0% and 28% of patients after TUMT (71). ED after TURP or TUMT is rare in a patient good pretreatment erectile function, but it commonly is observed in patients with prior erectile difficulties. Low-energy TUMT protocols have a lower incidence of ED compared to high-energy protocols but at the expense of better urinary results. Francisca et al. reported no change in sexual performance after low-energy TUMT when compared to a sham procedure in 147 patients, while Arai et al. reported a 26.5% rate of ED for TURP and a rate of 18.2% with TUMT using a high-energy protocol (72,73).

Similar to TURP, there is an increased mortality associated with TUMT. For example, the risk of acute myocardial infarction is slightly increased following TUMT. In an approximately four-year follow-up of 888 patients who underwent TURP compared to 478 patients who underwent TUMT, both treatments had a higher incidence of acute myocardial infarction compared with the general population, especially more than two years after therapy (71). More patients died from cardiovascular disease after both therapies than in the general population, which suggests that the presence of BPH disease or the surgical treatment for BPH may accelerate the progression of cardiac risk factors. Alternatively, LUTS secondary to BPH and cardiovascular disease may share previously unrecognized risk factors (i.e., autonomic hyperactivity).

Guidelines have been issued by the U.S. FDA to minimize the risk of complications and appropriately select patients that would be ideal candidates for TUMT (62). These guidelines include a recommendation to pay close attention to the instructions and specifications of the TUMT device being used. For example, it is important to ensure that the prostate is the eligible size indicated for the system being used so that thermotherapy is not applied to non-prostatic tissues (i.e., prostates <25 gm or a prostatic urethral length of less than three cm respond poorly to TUMT, as do patients with glands greater than 100 gm or patients with a prominent median bar). In addition, close attention should be paid to the placement of the urethral catheter and rectal temperature sensor using acceptable methods (e.g., direct visualization, ultrasound imaging) both prior to treatment and other specified times consistent with the manufacturer's recommendations. Catheter balloon location within the bladder should be confirmed at the start of the procedure by ultrasound and re-positioned if there is a problem. The TUMT device should be attended during the entire procedure and attention should be paid for signs of dislodgement. In addition, the patient should not have experienced prior radiation therapy to the pelvic area to minimize the risk of rectal fistula formation. In order to enable the patient to express that he is experiencing discomfort it is also recommended to avoid over-sedation.

Other contraindications specific to TUMT are evolving as the technology changes and outcomes are studied further. Patients with a history of TURP or pelvic trauma should not undergo TUMT because of potential alterations in pelvic anatomy and potential damage to other non-prostatic tissues. Moreover, it is recommended that patients with penile prosthesis, severe urethral stricture disease, Leriche syndrome/severe peripheral vascular disease, or an artificial urinary sphincter should avoid TUMT. Patients with pacemakers and defibrillators need clearance from their cardiologist concerning turning their pacemakers preoperatively.

MINIMALLY INVASIVE SURGICAL THERAPY: TRANSURETHRAL NEEDLE ABLATION

Another technique currently approved for treating patients with symptoms of BPH uses high-frequency radio waves to cause thermal injury to the prostate. TUNA uses interstitial low-level radio frequency energy to produce a temperature above 100°C (74). A special 22-Fr cystoscope incorporates two retractable needles that deliver low-energy radio frequency (490 kHz) power to a well-demarcated region of the prostate. The needles have adjustable shields to protect the urethra from thermal injury. The needle placement during the TUNA procedure is directly visualized. In addition, accuracy in needle placement is also enhanced by the fact that the TUNA catheter can be rotated to place the needles in specific locations within the prostatic parenchyma. Taken together, this visualization and flexibility of the TUNA catheter permit the customization of treatment to desired areas of the prostate and it allows for the preservation and protection of the urethral mucosa and surrounding tissues.

Improvement in LUTS and resolution of bladder outlet obstruction after TUNA is believed to occur because of reabsorption of the necrotic prostatic tissue and subsequent scar formation (75). Some studies have suggested that alpha-adrenergic nerve ablation may also contribute to improvement in LUTS because of necrosis of nerves within the prostate after TUNA (76). Clinically this procedure has been associated with approximately 50% decrease in American Urological Association-International Prostate Symptom Score (AUA-IPSS) score and approximately 70% improvement in maximum urinary flow rate (77). Taken together, TUNA appears to be more effective than medical therapy, but less effective and durable than TURP in the treatment of BPH (20). However, as discussed below, the complication rates after undergoing TUNA are significantly lower compared with TURP which may be a tradeoff between the procedures.

Transurethral needle ablation can be performed under local anesthesia, IV sedation, or transperineal prostate block. Therefore, similar to TUMT and the other MISTs, TUNA does not require spinal or general anesthesia, does not require an additional hospital stay, and is performed as an outpatient procedure. In addition, the lack of general sedation also significantly decreases the length of the procedure time to approximately 30 minutes (78).

Few intra-operative complications have been reported for TUNA. By far, the most common intra-operative complication reported is a burning sensation both during and after the procedure (79). Treatment discontinuation can be expected to occur in a relatively small percentage of patients (~1%) because of this discomfort (79). However, like TUMT, discomfort can be managed with pain medications. Another intra-operative complication of TUNA is bleeding which occurs in less than 1% of patients. However, it should be noted that TUNA, and most of the other MISTs, avoids significant intra-operative bleeding due to the coagulation induced by the heat produced during the procedure. This is demonstrated by the fact that the average drop in hemoglobin is less than 0.9 mg/dL for patients undergoing TUNA compared with a 2-mg/dL drop in hemoglobin in patients undergoing TURP (80). In fact, the current AUA guidelines do not consider transfusion to be a risk after TUNA (21).

The overall incidence of peri- and postoperative complications following TUNA is approximately 25% (Table 3), a rate that is significantly lower than TURP (52). Almost all patients undergoing TUNA are discharged with an indwelling catheter for approximately two to three days postoperatively. Given the sizable protocol-driven nature of post-treatment catheterization, the real rate of AUR following TUNA is not known. In addition, most patients should be informed that they will experience mild dysuria for one to two weeks and mild hematuria for the first two to three days following the procedure (77,81,82). Perineal pain has been reported in almost half of patients after TURP, and a small percentage of these patients will necessitate pain medications for approximately fivedays postoperatively (83). Other complications within the first sixweeks following TUNA include prolonged urinary retention, UTIs, significant hematuria, dysuria, epidiymo-orchitis, clot retention, and prostatitis (77,81–86). Deep vein thrombosis is a rare complication and occurs in less than 2% of patients after TUNA (82). Anticoagulation should be started unless otherwise medically contraindicated. Compared to TURP, the overall incidence of these adverse effects in groups of patients undergoing TUNA is significantly decreased. For example, TUNA was associated with a three times lower risk of hematuria than was TUNA (61). The decreased incidence of peri-operative complications is also supported by the results obtained from a multi-center clinical trial in which more than 120 men with BPH were randomized to either TUNA or TURP. Patients who had TUNA experienced a significantly decreased number of peri-operative complications (Fig. 2).

Long-term complications reported after TUNA include urethral strictures (1–2%), bladder neck contracture (1–5%), chronic prostatitis (<1%), and urinary incontinence (<1%) (77,82–84). Treatment failure, because of recurring LUTS associated with BPH, has been reported in up to 30% of patients within fiveyears after treatment (20,63,81). However, on average, approximately 20% to 25% of patients will necessitate a secondary surgical procedure within three years after undergoing TUNA. Of all patients requiring some form of secondary intervention, less than

TABLE 3 Reported Incidence of Complications Following
Transurethral Needle Ablation

Complication	Incidence (%)
Intraoperative complications	
Urethral burning sensation	50–100
Severe pain requiring abortion of procedure	<1
Urethral injury	0
Bladder injury	0
Perioperative complications	
Irritative voiding symptoms	55–100
Perineal pain	~50
Urinary retention	10–40
Urinary tract infection	8–14
Dysuria	6–7
Epidiymo-orchitis	1–5
Clot retention	1–2
Prostatitis	1–2
Deep venous thrombosis	<2
Long-term complications	
Retrograde ejaculation	<1
Erectile dysfunction	1–3
Retreatment (transurethral resection of the prostate)	5
Urinary incontinence	1–3
Urethral stricture	1–2
Bladder neck contracture	1–5
Chronic prostatitis	<1
Urinary incontinence	<1
Retreatment	20–30

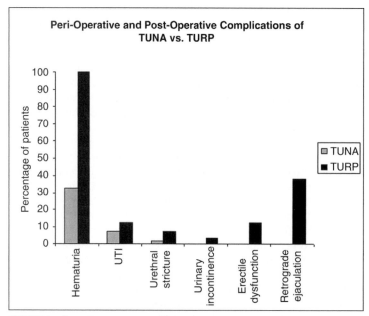

FIGURE 2 Complications reported from a prospective, randomized, multicenter 1-year clinical trial comparing TUNA to TURP are presented above (86). The data support that TUNA is associated with a decreased incidence of both peri-operative and postoperative complications. *Abbreviations*: TUNA, transurethral needle ablation; TURP, transurethral resection of the prostate; UTI, urinary tract infection.

10% require additional medical treatment (i.e., 5α-reductase inhibitor, α-adrenergic antagonist), less than 5% required a second TUNA, and less than 15% required a TURP (63,81).

Sexual and ED have also been evaluated postoperatively in patients after TUNA. In one prospective, randomized study, sexual function was assessed in patients who were sexually active before undergoing TUNA. At one year after TUNA, approximately 8% of patients had no interest in sex. However, 35% of patients who reported no interest in sex before therapy had an interest in sexual activity after TUNA (77). Unlike TURP, retrograde ejaculation is a rare complication of TUNA and occurs in less than 1% of patients (63,77). It should be noted that retrograde ejaculation has been reported in one-third of patients if the bladder neck is heated (63,82,87). ED after TUNA has also been reported infrequently (63).

The ideal candidate for TUNA is a gentleman who demonstrates LUTS secondary to BPH, a prostate of 100 g or less, and predominantly lateral lobe prostate enlargement (20). Therefore, to chose the ideal patient and thereby minimize the risks associated with TUNA, it is recommended that patients undergo a pre-TUNA transrectal ultrasound (TRUS) to evaluate prostate volume. Every patient should also undergo a TRUS measurement of the prostate to determine the maximal transverse width of the prostate. TRUS can also demonstrate prostatic calculi which may make heating difficult and increase the required time for treatment (74). Additionally, cystoscopy will help estimate prostate morphology, assist in determining the duration of therapy, and whether the bladder neck requires treatment. The presence of an enlarged median lobe is not a contraindication to TUNA. However, aggressive therapy to the bladder neck may theoretically increase the risk of retrograde ejaculation (77).

MINIMALLY INVASIVE SURGERIES: TRANSURETHRAL ELECTROVAPORIZATION OF THE PROSTATE

Transurethral electrovaporization of the prostate (TUEVP) is a modification of existing transurethral technology and has been viewed as one of the most promising alternatives to TURP. TUEVP has been shown to decrease the AUA symptom score by ~60% to 85% and more than double the mean Q_{max} (88–91). One prospective randomized control trial suggested that these effects are durable and associated with a relatively low recurrence of LUTS related to BPH (23). Taken with the fact that TUEVP is associated with a relatively low rate of complications, TUEVP is a viable alternative to TURP.

The TUEVP technique is a modification of TURP in which obstructing prostatic tissue is vaporized instead of being removed in chips and pieces. The TUEVP procedure uses a modified electrode, instead of the conventional loop used in TURP. This special electrode permits for the simultaneous vaporization, desiccation, and coagulation of prostatic tissue using radio-frequency electrical current (92–94). Bleeding is reduced because the electrode creates a tissue defect surrounded by a rim of coagulated tissue in which blood vessels and lymphatics are sealed off. This lack of intra-operative bleeding maintains a constant and clear field of view, and thus contributes to decreased complications involving non-prostatic tissues. Damage to surrounding tissues is also prevented during TUEVP because there are no chips of prostatic tissue produced which obstruct the floor of resection. Furthermore, visibility is also maintained by a constant circulation of glycine irrigant. Taken together, TUEVP utilizes a modification of the technology developed for TURP, which provide long-lasting clinical benefits.

Transurethral electrovaporization of the prostate is not completely free from complications. For example, TUEVP is still a transurethral procedure that requires general or spinal anesthesia and lasts for approximately 45 to 60 minutes. These factors increase the likelihood of intra-operative myocardial events and other complications. As with all other procedures involving general or spinal anesthesia, preoperative cardiac clearance and evaluation of medical risk should be obtained. Increased anesthesia requirements also necessitate a hospital stay, with an average postoperative hospital course of approximately one to four days (43,88). Other intra-operative complications that have been reported with TUEVP include a 0% to 5% risk of prostatic capsule perforation or damage to bladder mucosa (95). Management of these complications is as described for the other MISTs. Because TUVP involves electrodesiccation of the prostatic tissue during the procedure, blood transfusions are rarely required and are not considered to be a substantial risk [<1%; (20,88)].

The TUR syndrome can occur anytime; irrigation and glycine solutions are used during a procedure, but has not been reported during TUEVP (96). As mentioned above, a zone of desiccation develops below the vaporized tissue during TUEVP. This zone is believed to prohibit any dangerous irrigant re-absorption and significantly minimizes the occurrence of the TUR syndrome (92). Therefore, TUEVP is advantageous in that the TUR syndrome is not considered to be a substantial risk. Management of the TUR syndrome is described above and should address the hypotension, hyponatremia, hypo-osmolarity, and anuria (see above).

Peri-operative and postoperative complications occur in approximately 33% to 43% of patients undergoing TUEVP (88). By far the most common peri-operative complication is irritative voiding symptoms that occur in 15% to 25% of patients within the first one to two weeks following TUEVP (97). Other complications that occur within the first three months include AUR (6–23%), clot retention (0–5%), and epididymitis (0–1.4%; (21,23,88,97–102). A urinary catheter is required for approximately one to four days following TUEVP (95,98,101). This, along with damage to the prostatic tissue predisposes to UTIs, which occur in 0% to 18% following TUEVP (98,101). A re-hospitalization rate for complications such as urinary or clot retention has been reported in up to 5% to 7% of patients (97).

Treatment failure requiring a re-operation for LUTS or urinary retention secondary to BPH occurs in 4% to 7% of patients within the first year postoperative after TUEVP. A meta-analysis of five different prospective randomized control trials demonstrated that this rate is not statistically different from those reported for TURP [Fig. 3, (97)]. Other postoperative complications reported following TUEVP include a 3% to 18.6% incidence of urinary incontinence, 0% to 4.2% incidence of bladder neck sclerosis/contracture, and a 0% to 4% risk of urethral stricture (23,89,97,98) (2003 #22). Approximately 74% to 92% of patients experience retrograde ejaculation and 0% to 14% of patients report new ED/impotence after TUEVP (93,98,101) (2000). Results from prospective randomized controlled trials have demonstrated that the rates of bladder neck contracture are significantly lower for TUEVP than TURP [3–5% for TURP vs. 0–4.2% TUEVP; Fig. 3, (97)]. In addition, it was found that there is a trend toward a decreased frequency of retrograde ejaculation and ED after TUEVP compared with TURP (97).

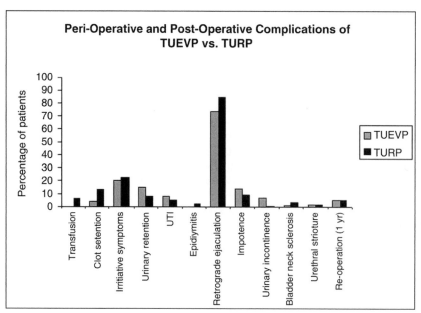

FIGURE 3   Peri-operative and post-operative complications of TUEVP versus TURP. The data presented in the graph are the results of a meta-analysis of five different prospective randomized trials comparing TUEVP to TURP. The data suggest that there is a significantly higher rate of blood transfusion, clot retention, epididymitis, and bladder neck sclerosis following TURP compared to TUEVP. Impotence and urinary incontinence is higher in the TUEVP groups. *Abbreviations*: TUEVP, transurethral electrovaporization of the prostate; TURP, transurethral resection of the prostate; UTI, urinary tract unfection.

As mentioned above, TUEVP uses modifications of existing electrosurgical technology. This is a major advantage as no additional technical skills have to be learned to perform TUEVP successfully. Overall, few additional precautions to minimize complications following TUEVP have been issued. However, one recommendation to minimize the occurrence of bladder neck contractures is to avoid the use of coagulating current at the prostatic apex (97). Taken together, TUEVP is an excellent alternative to TURP in that it has clinical efficacy and low morbidity. However, additional studies involving large numbers of patients and longer follow-up periods are warranted.

MINIMALLY INVASIVE SURGERIES: LASER THERAPIES

One of the less invasive alternative treatments developed to treat BPH involves the use of laser energy to remove obstructing prostatic tissue. Many different systems utilizing laser technologies to treat BPH have evolved over the past decade. To date, four different types of lasers have been used for this purpose—holmium:yttrium-aluminum-garnet (Ho:YAG), neodymium:YAG (Nd:YAG), potassium titanyl phosphate:YAG (KTP:YAG), and the diode laser (99). The laser energy can be delivered through a right-angled fiber (side-firing), bare fiber (end-firing), contact tips or an interstitial fiber (99).

It has been found that laser energy removes obstructing prostatic tissue by causing tissue coagulation (at 60–70°C), vaporization (>100°C), by excision of the tissue, or by a combination of these techniques. The extent of coagulation and vaporization can be varied by adjusting a number of settings including the power setting, wavelength, and exposure time (100). The coagulation technique produces a coagulative necrosis deep within the prostatic tissue. This results in a secondary tissue slough into the urethra for several weeks after treatment (101). In contrast, the higher temperatures created in the vaporization technique produce immediate tissue ablation at the surface of the prostate with a lesser degree of both penetration and secondary tissue slough (99). Both laser methods have been utilized to remove prostatic adenoma and have varying clinical efficacies. Overall, laser technologies are continuously evolving in an attempt to minimize morbidities while increasing symptom improvement durability.

Holmium Laser Resection of the Prostate and Holmium Laser Enucleation of the Prostate

Holmium laser resection of the prostate (HoLRP) technology became popularized in 1994 when the high-powered Ho:YAG laser became commercially available (102,103). HoLRP utilizes the Ho:YAG laser for the incision, ablation, and resection of the prostate with the goal of relieving symptoms related to BPH in a relatively bloodless and minimally invasive manner. Technically, HoLRP involves an end-firing laser fiber to precisely resect large pieces of prostatic tissue (104). Normal saline is used to dissipate thermal energy delivered by the holmium laser. The laser is also used to cut the resected tissue into smaller pieces before their release into the bladder (105,106). These prostatic pieces are then removed with a modified resectoscope loop (104). This is the rate-limiting step in HoLRP. This has led to development of a technique known as holmium laser enucleation of the prostate (HoLEP). HoLEP enables dissection of the intact median and lateral lobes from the prosatic capsule utilizing a method similar to HoLRP. However, once enucleation of the prostatic lobes is achieved, a mechanical morcellator is used to remove the large resected pieces of prostate tissue (107,108).

An advantage of the HoLRP and HoLEP techniques is that they can be used to precisely remove large amounts of prostatic tissue in a fashion similar to TURP. In fact, studies have demonstrated that the short-term clinical outcomes, as measured by symptom relief score and maximum urinary flow rate, are similar between holmium laser resection techniques and TURP (105). As mentioned above, the coagulative ability of the holmium laser effectively seals tissue planes and provides hemostasis, which makes HoLRP and HoLEP relatively bloodless procedures. Therefore, concomitant blood transfusions are relatively rare [<1%, (20)]. In addition, in a fashion similar to TUEVP, the plane created by the holmium laser also decreases fluid absorption during the procedure. Thus, the TUR syndrome is not considered to be an intra-operative risk associated with either HoLRP or HoLEP (20).

In general, HoLRP or HoLEP are associated with significantly longer intra-operative times compared with TURP (~60–130 min vs. ~30–60 min) because of the removal of prostatic chips. However, because the morcellator used in HoLEP was specifically designed to improve the efficiency of tissue removal, HoLEP is a shorter procedure than HoLRP (109). Current data suggest that the overall intra-operative and peri-operative complication rates associated with HoLRP and HoLEP are significantly decreased compared to TURP (40,110). As general or spinal surgery is required for this procedure, most patients require a 1- to 2-day postoperative hospital course, which is similar to TURP (105,111). The average length of indwelling catheterization after HoLRP or HoLEP is zero to three days (40). However, urinary catheterization is not a requirement and is generally not part of protocols, as one study demonstrated that 89% of patients could be discharged after an overnight stay without an indwelling catheter (111).

Intra-operative complications associated with HoLRP or HoLEP are relatively rare. However, the most common intra-operative complication associated with either HoLRP or HoLEP is damage to other non-prostatic tissues. For example, capsular perforation can occur in up to 1% to 2% of patients while the surgeon attempts to separate the surgical capsule and prostatic adenoma (20,105). A 0% to 1% risk of creating a false passage within the bladder neck has also been reported during the enucleation process (112). Management of these cases includes stopping the procedure and placing a urethral catheter. Complications of HoLRP and HoLEP have also been reported during the morcellation process and include a 1% to 2% incidence of bladder mucosal engagement and bladder injury by the morcellator blades, and a 1% to 2% incidence of difficulty extracting retained prostatic pieces (20,105,113). Treatment for these cases also includes bladder drainage through urinary catheter. Peri-operative complications include transient hematuria, dysuria and irritative voiding symptoms in the first 48 to 72 hours postoperatively, UTIs, clot retention, and re-catherization secondary to urinary retention (see Table 4). In addition, paraphymosis, prostatitis, and penile deviation (<1%) have been reported in the peri-operative period (105,111,114,115). One death from septicemic shock in the peri-operative period was reported in a case report series (105) and prophylactic antibiotics should be considered. Cardiopulmonary complications occurring during the peri-operative period include clot retention, pulmonary embolus, pulmonary edema, thrombophlebitis, deep vein thrombosis, and myocardial infarction. It is important to not that these are rare complications (<1%) and generally occur more frequently after TURP (114–116).

Postoperative complications (>3 months postoperatively) have been reported after undergoing HoLRP or HoLEP include a 1% to 3% incidence of urethral strictures. Meatal strictures have been reported in up to 4% of patients [Table 5; (40,114,116,117)]. The most common locations of these strictures occur at the level of the membranous urethra, bulbar urethra at the penoscrotal junction and fossa navicularis. Patients usually present postoperatively with

TABLE 4   Reported Incidence of Complications Following Transurethral Electrovaporization of the Prostate

Complication	Incidence (%)
Intraoperative complications	
Prostatic capsule perforation/damage to bladder mucosa	0–5
Blood transfusion	<1
Perioperative complications	
Irritative voiding symptoms	24.5–48.6
Urinary retention	7.8–18.7
Urinary tract infection	6.1–12.3
Dysuria	6–7
Long-term complications	
Retrograde ejaculation	74–92
Erectile dysfunction	0–14
Retreatment (transurethral resection of the prostate)	4–7
Urinary incontinence	3–18.6
Urethral stricture	0–4
Bladder neck contracture	0–4.2

TABLE 5 Reported Incidence of Complications Following Various Laser Techniques for the Treatment of Benign Prostatic Hyperplasia

	Holmium laser resection of the prostate (%)	Visual laser ablation of the prostate (%)	Interstitial laser coagulation (%)
Intraoperative complications			
Blood transfusion	<1	<1	<1
Transurethral resection syndrome	<1	<1	<1
Capsular performation	1–2	NR	NR
Bladder injury	1–2	NR	NR
Perioperative complications			
Irritative voiding symptoms/dysuria	10–70	10–100	15–70
Transient hematuria	20–30	0–16	80–100
Urinary retention	5–8	20–30	15–35
Urinary tract infection	15–20	4–15	5–35
Clot retention	2–8	0–5	<1
Epidiymo-orchitis	1–5	2–3	1–5
Prostatitis	<1	<1	<1
Long-term complications			
Retrograde ejaculation	60–80	27–33	2–15
Erectile dysfunction	2–13	3–5	1–2
Retreatment	NR	5–16	0–15
Urethral stricture	1–3	0–2	1–5
Meatal stricture	1–4	1–2	NR
Bladder neck contracture	1–5	4–5	<1

obstructive symptoms. Most of these cases of urethral and meatal strictures can be treated with single office sound dilation or urethrotomy under direct visualization. Only rarely will open urethroplasty be necessary. Stricture formation may be prevented by minimizing urethral trauma during the course of operative intervention. Bladder neck contractures occur in approximately 1% to 5% of patients postoperatively and usually require surgical intervention (20). Postoperative mortality rates have only been reported in a few clinical trials (114–116), and no significant difference was detected between HoLRP and TURP at 12, 24, or 48 months postoperatively. To date, there are few studies that directly compare the rates of re-treatment for symptoms related to BPH between HoLRP/HoLEP and TURP. One retrospective study suggested that there was no difference in re-operation rates for urinary retention between the holmium laser procedures and TURP at 12 months postoperatively (105). However, the durability of HoLRP and HoLEP still remains to be determined.

Few studies have investigated the effects of HoLRP or HoLEP on sexual function. In one randomized control trial, no significant difference could be detected in rates of retrograde ejaculation between HoLRP and TURP patients (114–116). This study also reported no significant difference in the rates of new-onset ED after HoLRP and TURP. However, this still has to be studied in greater detail.

Overall, HoLRP and HoLEP appear to be superior to TURP in terms of the incidence of complications such as blood transfusions, postoperative duration of catheterization, and length of hospital stay. However, holmium laser surgeries still have some morbidities including intraoperative trauma to other surrounding tissues, hematuria, urethral strictures, and bladder contractures. Ways to minimize these complications include a thorough evaluation and assessment of prostate size and morphology before surgery. In addition, as with many of the other surgical treatments for BPH, increased experience is also associated with decreased complications. This is particularly relevant as some experts claim that HoLEP and HoLRP procedures have a higher learning curve than laser procedures that use an Nd:YAG laser (118). As described above, morcellator injuries to the bladder because of careless operation during HoLEP have been reported; distending the bladder can prevent the bladder mucosa from being drawn into the blades (119). Taken together, holmium laser technologies are a promising alternative to TURP. However, further multi-center randomized control studies, involving large numbers of patients over a long time period, are still required to fully evaluate the durability, efficacy, and morbidities associated with these technologies.

Visual Laser Ablation of the Prostate

During the early 1990s, the Nd:YAG laser was utilized to develop a technique which has been termed visual laser ablation of the prostate (VLAP). VLAP relies on the application of laser energy to coagulate prostatic tissue. As with other coagulative laser techniques, the tissue eventually becomes necrotic and sloughs off over the following weeks after the procedure, relieving the bladder neck obstruction. The details of the VLAP technique include the use of a simple quartz laser fiber with a distal metallic reflecting mechanism to deflect the Nd:YAG laser beam at a right angle (side-firing) into the prostatic parenchyma. Although VLAP has been extensively studied, the evidence evaluating its efficacy in the treatment of BPH is difficult to summarize statistically because investigators have used various approaches to this procedure (20). For example, the number of treatments per patient, energy used, and method of delivery have been inconsistent between studies (120,121). A few trials have directly compared VLAP to TURP (110,122–125). One multi-center randomized control trial conducted in the United States at six investigational sites found that the AUA symptom score improved by 13.3 points in the TURP group and by 9.0 points in the VLAP group, and the peak urinary flow rate improved by 7.0 mL/s in the TURP group and by 5.3 mL/s in the VLAP group. While the improvement in AUA symptom score was statistically improved in patients who had TURP compared with VLAP, VLAP patients still reported an average of 78.2% improvement in their quality of life score up to one year after undergoing the procedure (122). Further long-term studies suggest that VLAP does not have the durability of TURP (113). However, because of the lower morbidity rate, VLAP technology is still considered a viable therapy for the treatment of BPH.

VLAP is usually performed under either general or spinal anesthesia and therefore usually demands a hospital stay. However, as VLAP employs a coagulative technique which minimizes blood loss, it has been associated with a statistically shorter hospitalization compared with TURP (122). In fact, there have been relatively few reports of blood transfusions after undergoing the procedure (122,126). One meta-analysis concluded that there was a 91% reduction in the risk of blood transfusion after VLAP compared with TURP (61). This is also supported by the fact that there is little change in the peri-operative hematocrit levels following VLAP (61). This minimal blood loss is also advantageous in that it permits VLAP to be performed on patients who are on full anticoagulation therapy or have abnormal coagulation indices because of hematologic disorders (127,128). Another intra-operative advantage is that VLAP does not induce any significant change in serum sodium levels and thus does not predispose toward the TUR syndrome (20).

Peri-operative complications are summarized in Table 5 (60,122). One of the most common sequela after VLAP is irritative voiding symptoms. As prostate coagulation leads to delayed necrosis and sloughing of tissue for weeks after the procedure, it is not surprising that many patients experience these irritative urinary symptoms and urinary retention after the procedure. For example, one study described that post-treatment urinary retention requiring re-catheterization occurred in approximately 30% of patients treated by VLAP (122). Other studies have reported that dysuria occurs almost in 100% of patients immediately postoperatively, and in up to 10% to 15% at one year (89,113,122,129). Perineal pain (1–4%), hesitancy (1–2%), and dribbling (1–2%) (122) have also been reported. Thus, it is recommended that urinary catheterization after VLAP should be for up to seven days postoperatively. UTIs, due to laser damage to the lower urinary tract or to indwelling catheterization occur in 4% to 8% of patients (113,122).

Long-term postoperative complications after VLAP include a urethral stricture rate of 0–1.8%, meatal stenosis rate of 1% to 2%, and a bladder neck contracture rate of 4% to 5% [Table 5; (61,122)]. New-onset ED has been reported in 3% to 5% after VLAP. Once again, this may or may not be a direct consequence of the procedure as the onset of ED is confounded by age factors. The retrograde ejaculation rate varies from 27% to 33% and is thus less frequent compared to TURP. The rate of surgical re-treatment for recurrent LUTS or AUR is significantly higher for VLAP compared with TURP. One study found that 38% of VLAP patients, compared with 16% of TURP patients, required further surgical treatment for BPH at three years (113).

Recommendations have been made in an attempt to minimize morbidities and to lower the re-treatment rate associated with VLAP. For example, it has been found that patients with large prostates (>80 g) are not ideal candidates for VLAP because they require multiple treatments to remove a sufficient amount of the prostate tissue. In addition, patients with chronic UTI or bacterial prostatitis are also not good candidates because coagulated tissue may become infected (130). Overall, the VLAP technique is associated with a low number of serious morbidities (i.e., those requiring intervention) compared with TURP. However, the major disadvantage of VLAP compared to TURP is the relatively slow resolution of symptoms postoperatively and the extended need for urinary catheter drainage. VLAP is still associated with a relatively high rate of dysuria, prolonged catheterization, and UTIs. Therefore, alternatives utilizing vaporizing laser technologies with the Nd:YAG laser are currently being investigated as alternatives.

Interstitial Laser Coagulation

Interstitial laser coagulation (ILC) is another laser therapy for the treatment of BPH that generates coagulation necrosis inside the prostatic tissue rather than at its surface (131,132). To this end, ILC can be performed using a transurethral approach or a percutaneous (perineal) approach (133). The more common transurethral approach is performed with standard cystoscopy, a solid-state diode laser, and a special fiber-optic laser delivery system. Under direct visualization, the laser fiber is introduced directly into the prostate through a small puncture in the prostatic urethra. The fiber can be introduced as deeply and as often as necessary to effectively coagulate any amount of tissue at any desired location. Low-power thermal energy is then delivered through the fiber and is used to ablate prostatic tissue (133). Relief of LUTS is considered to be secondary to the necrosis of the obstructing prostatic adenoma. Many studies have been published to suggest that ILC is associated with minimal morbidity with reasonable efficacy. However, the reported degree of urinary symptom relief as well as the increase in maximum urinary flow rate post-ILC vary considerably between studies. For example, the subjective improvement in AUA symptom score after ILC ranges from 50% to 300% while the increase in maximum urinary flow rate also spans 5 to greater than 10 mL/s (134,135).

Intra-operative complications have been rarely reported with ILC [Table 5; (134,136)]. This is due to the relatively short time period of the operation (30–40 min) as well as to the fact that ILC can be performed under either local (e.g., peri-prostatic block), regional (e.g., spinal), or general anesthesia. Thus, because general or spinal anesthesia is not required, ILC is considered to be a true minimally invasive procedure that can be performed on an outpatient basis (137). Most patients (>90%) tolerate the procedure without any difficulty. However, many patients experience discomfort during the procedure, and pain medications can be used for relief (138,139). As with the laser technologies mentioned above, blood transfusion is not considered to be a risk factor associated with ILC because of the method of laser coagulation. In addition, the TUR syndrome and lowering of serum sodium levels do not occur with ILC (136).

In the peri-operative period after ILC, irritative voiding symptoms are frequently reported and occur in up to 50% of patients (134,136). Sometimes these symptoms have been reported for periods up to 3 months (129). In addition, many of these patients experience urinary retention secondary to the edema and inflammation from ILC. Therefore, postoperative urinary catheterization is often required for time periods up to 1 month (134,140). This catheterization period is significantly longer than for TURP (141), and predisposes to UTIs which are present in as many as 35% of patients after ILC (136). Transient mild hematuria is observed in almost all patients during the first postoperative days (136). Perineal pain and discomfort are also reported for approximately 2 weeks in more than 70% of patients. Approximately, one-quarter of these patients will continue to experience this discomfort for up to one month postoperatively (142). This pain can be managed with oral pain medications.

Long-term complications arising from ILC include bladder neck contractures (<1%) and urethral strictures (1–5%). Management of these includes office sound dilation or internal urethrotomy. Other postoperative complications include new-onset ED (1–2%) and retrograde ejaculation (2–15%) (63,134,136). The frequency of retrograde ejaculation after ILC depends on the intra-operative aggressiveness at the level of the bladder neck (134). Unfortunately, very few studies have addressed the long-term outcome of ILC because most of the reports are based on 12-month follow-up data. However, at 1 year of follow-up, the rate of surgical re-treatment ranges from 0% to 15% (136). One long-term study evaluating the success of ILC at three years found that approximately 40% of patients required re-treatment for symptoms related to BPH (143). Thus, while the durability of ILC does not rival TURP, the incidence of serious morbidities is significantly decreased.

MINIMALLY INVASIVE SURGERIES: EMERGING THERAPIES—TRANSURETHRAL ETHANOL ABLATION

As discussed above, within the past decade urologists have been on a relentless search to develop a durable treatment associated with few morbidities for the treatment of BPH. One of the MISTs that has recently emerged among the treatment alternatives to TURP is transurethral ethanol ablation (TEAP). Under this method, ethanol is injected into the hyperplastic prostate where it acts as a sclerosing agent causing necrosis of the adenoma. While the concept of injection of agents into the prostate is not new (144), it was not until the past decade when ethanol became a plausible treatment for BPH (145). As ethanol exposure to other non-prostatic sites causes tissue damage, the needle used in TEAP is designed to minimize backflow and extravasation of the ethanol solution. The amount of ethanol injected is determined by the volume of the prostate as assessed by TRUS scans (146). The efficacy of TEAP has been reported on in the short term (147,148), and long-term follow-up is currently undergoing final-phase clinical studies. The initial studies suggest that TEAP increases Q_{max} by 45% and decreases AUA symptom scores by over 50% (146,148,149). Thus, while not as efficacious as TURP, TEAP has the potential to relieve urinary symptoms related to BPH.

The TEAP procedure is generally performed as an outpatient procedure because it is carried out under local anesthetic, which involves a transrectal guided peri-prostatic block combined with oral analgesics. The surgeon should be aware that if local anesthetic is used, more than 70% of patients can experience mild to moderate pain during the procedure (150).

Ethanol can destroy structures other than the prostate if delivered incorrectly. Therefore, care should be taken to maintain a distance of greater than 1 cm from the bladder neck and the verumontanum to avoid damage to the internal sphincter or bladder and retrograde ejaculation. Furthermore, continuous irrigation should be used to dilute any ethanol backflow, and the bladder should be emptied after each injection (146). Despite these advisories, ethanol-induced bladder necrosis has been reported in 1% to 2% of patients undergoing TEAP (151). Treatment for this damage is usually managed by insertion of a urethral catheter for time periods up to two to three weeks. Other complications associated with TEAP include irritative voiding symptoms (21–26%) and the need for re-catheterization secondary to AUR in 10% to 18% of patients (146). Based on this, the protocol usually indicates placement of a urinary catheter for at least 48 hours post-TEAP. Uncomplicated hematuria has been reported in 5% to 16% of patients. Other peri-operative morbidities associated with TEAP include UTIs (7–25%), epididymitis (1–4%), and chronic prostatitis (5–6%). Preliminary studies suggest that the rates of urinary incontinence, urethral strictures, retrograde ejaculation, and ED are all less than 5% (146,148–151). Management of these complications is identical to those discussed above.

To date, TEAP appears to be a reasonable and promising alternative to TURP. Data regarding long-term outcomes after TEAP are not yet available and must be reviewed before TEAP can be a viable option to TURP. However, as TEAP can be performed as a single short treatment in an outpatient setting with clinical efficacy and minimal complications, it gives TEAP the potential to be an alternative for the treatment of BPH.

MINIMALLY INVASIVE SURGERIES: EMERGING THERAPIES—WATER-INDUCED THERMOTHERAPY

Another emerging minimally invasive therapy for the treatment of bladder outlet obstruction secondary to BPH is water-induced thermotherapy (WIT). The goal of WIT is to produce heat-induced coagulative necrosis and secondary ablation of the prostatic adenoma (152,153). The thermal energy used in WIT is derived from heated water which is circulated in a closed loop system within a specially designed catheter. As with TEAP, WIT is an emerging technology and therefore has had very few studies evaluating its efficacy and morbidities. However, initial studies suggest that WIT has clinical efficacy in reducing the frequency of LUTS as well as increasing the Q_{max} (154,155).

One of the major advantages promised by the WIT procedure is the alleviation of [systemic analgesia or sedation. Topical lidocaine jelly (2%) is believed to provide sufficient analgesia (154,155) and oral or intravenous pain medication is usually not indicated. Patients often report a sensation of moderate burning accompanied by urgency during the procedure. However, these symptoms are transient and disappear without intervention or stopping the procedure (156).

Adverse outcomes following WIT are similar to many of the other minimally invasive procedures. These complications include epididymitis (3–4%), hematuria (20–25%), transient impotence (1–2%), transient urge incontinence (2–3%), UTI (30–35%), urethral pain (4–5%), and proctitis (<1%). AUR requiring re-catheterization occurs in 10% to 15% of patients after WIT (154). WIT shares the disadvantages of most other thermal-based MISTs in that post-procedural catheterization is required for the high incidence of dysuria and irritative symptoms (11–12%) which occur because of tissue sloughing, edema, and inflammation (154).

As mentioned above, few studies are available that report on the durability of WIT. A few studies suggest that WIT requires re-treatment in 5% to 6% of patients at one year (154). One study reported that this rate went to greater than 11% by three years postoperatively (157). The effect of WIT on sexual function in the short term has been described and data suggest that WIT is not a risk factor for new-onset ED or retrograde ejaculation. Interest in sex, sexual activity, and other measures was not affected by WIT in these studies (154,156,158). Of course, as it is an emerging therapy for the treatment of BPH, WIT requires further evaluation in regard to its durability and morbidities. Long-term studies involving large numbers of patients will reveal the future possibilities of WIT.

CONCLUSIONS

Transurethral resection of the prostate is currently considered to be the gold standard treatment for patients with BPH, the most common benign tumor in elderly men. However, while the efficacy and durability of TURP have been proved time and again, so have the associated morbidities. TURP is associated with a relatively high rate of bleeding requiring transfusion, urethral stenosis, and retrograde ejaculation. In addition, TURP has its own unique complication of the TUR syndrome. Therefore, alternative therapies have been developed in an attempt to outcompete TURP.

These new alternative, less invasive therapies employ a variety of thermal-based therapies (i.e., MISTs) as well as utilize new variations on older surgical techniques. The goals of these alternative treatment options should include outcomes where benefits outweigh the side effects, which are acceptable to the patients, and are cost effective.

It is important to understand that the less invasive treatments for BPH do not necessarily aim to achieve results similar to TURP. This is a tradeoff for their decreased incidence of side effects and adverse outcomes. Thus, there is a fine balance between clinical efficacy and morbidities. Less invasive procedures, such as the ones described above, offer a wide range of clinical improvements as well as have unique complication profiles. Then how does one decide which patient is to receive which treatment? The answer to this question is continually evolving. However, a complete assessment of the patient is necessary to cater the correct treatment option. For example, relatively younger patients may be more suited for a TURP as they may be able to avoid many of the morbidities and require a durable procedure. Alternatively, elderly patients with extensive cardiovascular and medical histories would be better fit for minimally invasive procedures such as TUMT, TUNA, or WIT as no spinal or general analgesia is required. The goals of these MISTs may not include complete resolution of BPH symptoms, but rather relieve their prostatic obstruction, and improve their quality of life.

Less invasive alternatives to TURP are continuously evolving. Many more studies of their long-term outcomes, morbidities, and mortalities have to be determined. To this end, multi-center randomized control trials involving large number of patients studied over many years are required to answer questions such as the durability of the procedure, long-term costs in terms of recurrence, and the need for re-operation. While TURP is still considered to be the gold-standard treatment for BPH, its competition in the form of minimally invasive surgeries is coming closer to overthrowing its reign.

MANAGEMENT OF COMMON SURGICAL COMPLICATIONS (QUICK REFERENCE TO COMMON PROBLEMS)

Transurethral surgery is predisposed to a unique set of possible complications not seen with other forms of surgery. These complications can be secondary to either the technical aspects of the various procedures themselves, or to their respective side effects. As such, vigilance is required to recognize and prevent these problems before they result in significant sequelae.

Introduction of the Resectoscope/Instrumentation

In order to minimize intra-operative and postoperative complications, the resectoscope must be introduced into the bladder with minimal trauma to the urethra and surrounding structures. Certain pre-existing medical conditions may pose an obstacle to the ease of introduction. Phimosis may preclude entry of resectoscope, in addition to inadequate aseptic preparation of the glans itself. This may lead to severe urethritis, stricture formation, and possible postoperative sepsis secondary to trapped secretions and poor urethral catheter drainage. In these cases, circumcision may be warranted prior to further surgical intervention.

Meatal stenosis may pose difficulties to resectoscope/instrument entrance. In addition, it may lead to severe urethral mucosal trauma if the instrument is forced into the bladder, leading to postoperative meatal stricture formation. This may be avoided with preoperative calibration of the urethra to define the degree of stenosis, which can usually be alleviated with ventral meatotomy. Only rarely is internal urethrotomy or perineal urethrostomy required.

Intraoperative Hemorrhage

The presence of intra-operative hemorrhage can compromise visualization, and therefore hinder tissue resection during transurethral surgery. In the presence of a normal coagulation profile, the source of such intra-operative bleeding originates from either open venous sinuses or an unindentified arterial source.

The bladder neck usually constitutes the primary source of arterial bleeds, as it houses the prostatic division of the inferior vesical arteries. When exposed, these pulsatile bleeding vessels must be immediately fulgurated. It would also be prudent to re-examine this site at the termination of the procedure to prevent delayed identification of a postoperative hemorrhage site. Caution should be taken during fulguration as to prevent damage to surrounding structures or perforation of bladder or urethral mucosa. Intra-operative venous bleeding can generally be managed with cauterization. Additionally, contraction of the prostatic capsule itself during the course of resection will aid in tamponading this bleeding. In the setting of venous sinus bleeding, a different course of action must be undertaken. In this setting, further cauterization may only serve to intensify the degree of bleeding, as the vessel defect will be exacerbated.

To avoid such instances, care should be taken to resect prostatic tissue in smooth planes, avoiding deep bites that can result in such complications. If one still opens a venous sinus during the course of the procedure, several considerations must be taken into account. The main risk to the patient stems from increased absorption of irrigating fluid rather than the hemorrhage itself. As such, one must avoid increasing irrigating fluid to improve visualization in the setting of venous sinus hemorrhage. In these situations, a resectoscope can be used to tamponade the bleeding site, and thereby improve visualization. Additionally, the placement of urethral catheter balloon can provide additional hemostasis.

Trauma to Landmarks

The ureteral orifices may be damaged in the setting of trigonal hypertrophy, as the orifices are displaced toward the prostate, putting them at risk during prostatic resection and or during the processes of prostatic energy application. The adenomatous tissue itself may also o orifices, as can advanced trabeculation with diverticula. Under these circumstances, resection or fulguration occurs, stricture formation with subsequent obstruction, and phrosis can occur. To avoid such trauma, indigo carmine may be used to visualize the ......ces.

To avoid inadvertent trauma to the external sphincter, visualization of the vermontanum must be maintained. The apex of the prostate lies adjacent to the veromontanum, and residual tissue here may result in postoperative voiding dysfunction. The anterior most portion of the adenomatous tissue can be found at the level of the verumontanum. Often at this location, resection can be extended too far distally, and care must be taken to avoid this potential pitfall.

Urethral Perforation

Perforation of the urethra or the prostate itself can occur at any time during the course of tissue resection, from unintentional manipulation of the resectoscope or instrument used for minimally invasive surgery. The risk of perforation is further increased in the presence of established urethral strictures or false passages. To avoid this complication, the resectoscope or instrument should be passed under direct vision.

Deep tissue resection at the level of the bladder neck can also result in perforation, as this area is not protected by a large amount of adenomatous tissue. Resection must therefore be performed with a partially filled bladder with particular care to limit resection to adenomatous tissue.

Lateral and anterior perforation of the bladder neck can result in significant extravasation of irrigating fluid. It is often difficult to visualize perforations at these sites, but the absence of fluid return and diminished maneuverability of the resectoscope should raise suspicions of these complications. Other signs of perforation include elevation and compression of the lateral borders of the bladder with poor visualization of the bladder neck. This may cause the posterior wall of the bladder and trigone to appear more distant.

Late signs include decreased bladder capacity with increased intravesical pressure, and decreased visualization. In addition, patients may experience TUR syndrome (see below) with nausea, vomiting, abdominal pain, mental status changes, hypotension, tachycardia, diaphoresis, and dypsnea. Physical signs include abdominal rigidity and tenderness.

With the advent of TUR syndrome, the procedure should be terminated, albeit, once hemostasis is achieved and resected tissue has been removed. A urethral catheter should be inserted. Suprapubic drainage of the retroperitoneum may be warranted to minimize further fluid absorption.

Failure to recognize the circular fibers of the prostatic capsule may result in perforation of this structure, which produces symptoms similar to perforation at the level of the bladder neck. However, additional bleeding from exposure of a venous sinus can occur at this location. In this scenario, resection should be completed, and the patient should be managed as detailed above.

Intraperitoneal extravasation can occur with bladder perforation during TUR. This will result in an abnormal irrigating pattern, with more irrigating fluid entering the bladder than that recovered. Symptoms are similar to the aforementioned extraperitoneal extravasation, but are far more prominent. In such cases, laparatomy and peritoneal drainage should be limited to patients exhibiting respiratory compromise, or in cases of suspected bowel trauma. Less acute scenarios may be managed with catheter drainage and diuretics.

TUR Syndrome

Excessive absorption of irrigating fluid during the course of transurethral surgery may result in the TUR syndrome. Increased operative duration, increased bladder pressure, and perforation of venous sinuses can all lead to fluid overload. The constellation of hypertension, bradycardia, restlessness, muscle twitching, disorientation, visual disturbances, seizures, and vascular collapse marks this clinical syndrome.

Early recognition of these symptoms permits early management, and thus one may avoid the full spectrum of the syndrome. Treatment may be initiated with a small suprapubic incision with insertion of a Penrose drain to permit fluid drainage. To mobilize fluid that has already been absorbed, one may administer hypertonic saline (200–500 mL of 1.8–5% solution) with intravenous furosemide (40–100 mg Lasix). Central venous pressure and urine output must be carefully monitored with the addition of hypertonic saline, as it adds more volume to an already taxed circulatory system. Serum electrolytes and osmolarity should be monitored closely after the onset of the syndrome is recognized. Patients with end-stage renal disease may present with symptomatic hyponatremia even in the absence of serum hypo-osmolality. In these cases, dialysis may be warranted to elevate serum sodium and reduce the osmolar gap produced by absorbed sorbitol.

Replacement with 5% dextrose/0.5 N saline can be used to manage this syndrome. With hourly urine output less than 250 mL/h, the entire amount of fluid loss should be replaced. With outputs ranging from 250 to 500 mL/h, fluid replacement should be two-thirds of this volume. Outputs in excess of 500 mL/h should be replaced with one-half of the hourly volume. Total fluid replacement should not be 1500 to 2000 mL less than the total urine output. Frequent measurement of both serum and urine electrolytes will be necessary.

A variety of irrigating solutions are available for use during transurethral surgery, each with its own risks of predisposing select patients to the TUR syndrome (Table 6). All these solutions are both hypo-osmolar and acidic.

Improved visualization may be noted with the use of distilled water, secondary to lysis of red cells. However, this may lead to excessive hemolysis and hemoglobinemia with renal failure. Patients with impaired liver function are at particular risk when glycine solutions are utilized for irrigation. The fluid is metabolized by the liver to ammonia, resulting in hyperammonemia and subsequent encephalopathy. The use of sorbitol should be avoided in diabetic patients as it is metabolized to glucose resulting in hyperglycemia. Additionally, sorbitol may also be metabolized to lactate, producing a significant lactic acidosis.

The use of mannitol, and iso-osmolar irrigating solution, may result in significant intravascular volume expansion, which may be exacerbated by the osmotic effects of the absorbed mannitol itself. The manifestations of the TUR syndrome may be even more apparent in these cases as mannitol is not evenly distributed throughout the body's fluids, intensifying the hypervolemic changes. Additionally, the use of mannitol may lead to a profound diuresis, which may pose difficulties for fluid replacement.

The use of each irrigating fluid, with its potential advantages and disadvantages, must be limited in certain clinical situations. Adjustment of the mechanics of resection itself is the most effective method of reducing the likelihood of the TUR syndrome.

Peri- and Postoperative Complications
Peri-Operative Fever
Fever following transurethral surgery may suggest the presence of bacteremia. Antibiotics may be given preoperatively in patients with existing UTIs, prior indwelling catheterization, and

TABLE 6 Irrigating Solutions Used During Transurethral Surgery

Solution	Osmolality (mOsm/L)	Advantages	Disadvantages
Distilled water	0	Improved visibility	Hemoglobinemia; hyponatremia; hemolysis; TUR syndrome
Sorbitol (3.3%)	165–180	Less likelihood of TUR syndrome unless massive fluid overload	Hyperglycemia (metabolized to glucose); possible lactic acidosis; risk to diabetics
Glycine (1.5%) (aminoacetic acid)	200	Same as sorbitol	Hyperammonemia (ammonia is metabolic by-product) in patients with hepatic dysfunction
Mannitol (5%)	275	Isomolar solution	May cause massive diuresis; possible acute intravascular volume expansion if absorbed intravenously

Abbreviation: TUR, transurethral resection.

prior instrumentation. If these measures are taken preoperatively, a change in antibiotics following the development of a postoperative fever is not indicated.

If prophylactic antibiotics have not been used, bacteriuria can be prevented by undertaking several measures. For example, a closed drainage system should be used, and frequent catheterization and continuous bladder irrigation should be avoided. If continuous bladder irrigation is necessary postoperatively for clot irrigation, acetic acid (0.125–0.25%) may be added to the irrigating solution to prevent bacterial colonization.

Acute prostatitis and pyelonephritis are rare in the peri-operative period. Acute epididymitis, however, may be observed especially if an indwelling catheter has been in place for an extended period of time.

Peri-operative staphylococcal urethritis may occur between 4 and 5 days postoperatively, most often secondary to use of an indwelling catheter. Treatment may be instituted by removal of the indwelling catheter and the use of antibiotics (penicillin or cephalexin).

Shock

With fever and bacteremia, hypovolemic shock may develop. The most common cause of septic shock in this setting is prior infection with *Escherichia coli*, *Klebsiella*, *Bacteriodes*, or *Pseudomonas*, any of which can gain access to the bloodstream during resection or in the postoperative period.

Patients will present with fever, rigors, and altered mental status. Additional signs include hypotension, oliguria, decreased central venous pressure, decreased cardiac output, tachycardia, metabolic acidosis, respiratory alkalosis, and occasional disseminated intravascular coagulation. Further complications include respiratory distress syndrome, acute renal failure, and heart failure.

Septic shock in the elderly may present more subtly, with fever only presenting after electrolyte and fluid disturbances are severe enough to produce cardiogenic shock. Patients with prior coronary artery disease are at particular risk, and may present with cardiac arrhythmias, and therefore strict cardiac monitoring is warranted in these patients. Treatment includes the rapid administration of intravenous fluids, broad-spectrum antibiotics, and correction of electrolyte abnormalities.

Bacterial Cystitis

Bacterial contamination may lead to peri-operative cystitis, which is amenable to antibiotic treatment. In diabetic patients, cystitis may be secondary to yeast colonization in the presence of indwelling catheterization and antibiotic treatment. These patients require administration of antifungal medications including amphotericin B or 5-fluocytosine to eradicate the infection. To circumvent this complication altogether in at risk patients, early removal of indwelling catheters is necessary.

Irritative Symptoms

Following many of the MISTs mentioned above, patients may experience urinary frequency, urgency, dysuria, occasional urge incontinence, and weak urinary stream. These symptoms are often limited in duration, often abating after 6– 8 weeks postoperatively. Therefore, patients presenting with these postoperative complaints require only reassurance. The following issues however mandate further attention and treatment.

If irritative symptoms persist for greater than six months postoperatively, evaluation for a neoplasm of the bladder or upper urinary tract must be undertaken. Persistent hematuria also requires similar investigation. If further evaluation is unremarkable, revealing only inflammatory changes in the remaining prostatic tissue or trigone, patients may be amenable to conservative therapy (antispasmodics).

Inadequate Resection

Patients with residual obstructive tissue following minimally invasive surgery will present with either symptoms of continuous or intermittent obstruction. This usually requires repeat resection of the residual tissue for symptomatic relief. To avoid this complication at the time of the initial intervention, the surgeon should be thorough in the removal of adenomatous tissue at the apex, the anterior region, and bladder neck.

Abnormal Urinary Sediment

Abnormal urinary sediment may persist for several months following TUR secondary to slough-ing of residual necrotic tissue. This will be indicated by the presence of white blood cells and red blood cells upon examination of urine. However, the presence of white blood cells in the urinary sediment more than three months after surgery may be indicative of an underlying infection.

Incontinence

Incontinence following transurethral surgery may be due to multiple etiologies including inflammation, neoplasm, residual tissue, or intrinsic weakness of the external sphincter or detrusor instability. Evaluation in any of these circumstances includes urinalysis, urine culture, cystourethroscopy, and urodynamic studies.

The most common type of incontinence presenting after prostatic resection is urge incon-tinence. It is seen in the presence of inflammatory or infectious mucosal lesions, neoplasms, or calculi. In the early postoperative period, incontinence may be secondary to the healing prostatic fossa. Thus symptoms that persist beyond two months postoperatively require further evaluation for the aforementioned causes.

Stress incontinence may occur if the external sphincter or tissue adjacent to the verumon-tanum has been damaged. Furthermore, damage to the external sphincter may result in scar-ring with subsequent urethral stricture formation. If such stricture formation prevents complete closure of the sphincter mechanism, incontinence will result. This may be prevented with ure-thral sound dilation; however, care must be taken to avoid undermining the bladder neck and creating false passages. If necessary, direct vision urethrotomy may be utilized. In the setting of minor stress incontinence, patients may be amenable to exercises to enhance the voluntary closure of the external sphincter.

Patients who are not amenable to these measures may require some form of catheteriza-tion. Indwelling catheterization may be preferable in the elderly who may not tolerate external collection devices. In some instances a suprapubic catheter may be the best option. Additionally, several surgical options have been developed to treat urinary incontinence.

Bladder Neck Contracture

Bladder neck contracture following TUR is secondary to the resection of the bladder neck during the course of operative intervention. Contracture may be managed by transurethral inci-sion. Rarely open Y-V plasty may be necessary to alleviate symptoms.

Functional bladder neck obstruction may occur following resection due to neurogenic dysfunction. This may be differentiated from anatomic obstruction with the use of pharmaco-logic agents (alpha-blockers) which will provide relief. Detrusor hypertrophy, secondary to a spastic neurogenic bladder, will often be observed in these cases.

Urethral Stricture

Depending on the surgical intervention used, patients may develop a postoperative urethral stricture. The most common locations are at the level of the membranous urethra, bulbar ure-thra at the penoscrotal junction, and fossa navicularis. Patients will present with progressive obstructive symptoms. They can be managed with urethral dilation or internal urethrotomy under direct visualization. Only rarely will open urethroplasty be necessary.

Stricture formation may be prevented by minimizing urethral trauma during the course of operative intervention. If warranted, strictures of the meatus or fossa navicularis may be avoided by meatomtomy prior to resection.

If a stricture is identified prior to resection, internal urethrotomy is necessary before resec-tion can be undertaken. Catheter selection can also minimize the formation of postoperative strictures. Silastic catheters are less traumatic to the urethral mucosa, and may be beneficial in select cases. Additionally, when placed, the catheter should not place tension on either the blad-der neck or the urethra at the penoscrotal junction, in order to minimize contracture and stric-ture formation.

Perineal Pain

Perineal pain is a rare postoperative complication following prostatic surgery. This pain may mimic that of prostatitis; however, a bacterial origin is not often seen. The symptoms may be secondary to scarring and stenosis of the ejaculatory ducts following tissue resection, which may result in painful orgasm. Therefore, care should be taken to avoid resection in this area.

Symptoms may be amenable to conservative treatment with sitz baths and analgesics. Patients can also be reassured that symptoms will gradually resolve with time. In general, antibiotic therapy is usually not indicated.

REFERENCES

1. Garraway WM, Collins GN, Lee RJ. High prevalence of benign prostatic hypertrophy in the community. Lancet 1991; 338(8765):469–471.
2. Bosch JL, Hop WC, Kirkels WJ, Schroder FH. The International Prostate Symptom Score in a community-based sample of men between 55 and 74 years of age: prevalence and correlation of symptoms with age, prostate volume, flow rate and residual urine volume. Br J Urol 1995; 75(5):622–630.
3. Bosch JL, Hop WC, Kirkels WJ, Schroder FH. Natural history of benign prostatic hyperplasia: appropriate case definition and estimation of its prevalence in the community. Urology 1995; 46(3 Suppl. A):34–40.
4. Chapple CR. Pharmacological therapy of benign prostatic hyperplasia/lower urinary tract symptoms: an overview for the practising clinician. BJU Int 2004; 94(5):738–744.
5. Clifford GM, Farmer RD. Medical therapy for benign prostatic hyperplasia: a review of the literature. Eur Urol 2000; 38(1):2–19.
6. Detailed diagnoses and procedures, national hospital discharge survey, 1987. Vital Health Stat 1989; 100:295.
7. Warres HL. Urethral stricture following transurethral resection of the prostate. J Urol 1958; 79: 989–993.
8. Doll HA, Black NA, McPherson K, Flood AB, Williams GB, Smith JC. Mortality, morbidity and complications following transurethral resection of the prostate for benign prostatic hypertrophy. J Urol 1992; 147(6):1566–1573.
9. Mebust WK, Holtgrewe HL, Cockett AT, Peters PC. Transurethral prostatectomy: immediate and postoperative complications. A cooperative study of 13 participating institutions evaluating 3,885 patients. J Urol 1989; 141(2):243–247.
10. Bruskewitz RC, Christensen MM. Critical evaluation of transurethral resection and incision of the prostate. Prostate Suppl 1990; 3:27–38.
11. Varkarakis J, Bartsch G, Horninger W. Long-term morbidity and mortality of transurethral prostatectomy: a 10-year follow-up. Prostate 2004; 58(3):248–251.
12. Roos NP, Wennberg JE, Malenka DJ, et al. Mortality and reoperation after open and transurethral resection of the prostate for benign prostatic hyperplasia. N Engl J Med 1989; 320(17):1120–1124.
13. Meyhoff HH, Nordling J. Long term results of transurethral and transvesical prostatectomy. A randomized study. Scand J Urol Nephrol 1986; 20(1):27–33.
14. Bruskewitz RC, Larsen EH, Madsen PO, Dorflinger T. 3-year followup of urinary symptoms after transurethral resection of the prostate. J Urol 1986; 136(3):613–615.
15. Chilton CP, Morgan RJ, England HR, Paris AM, Blandy JP. A critical evaluation of the results of transurethral resection of the prostate. Br J Urol 1978; 50(7):542–546.
16. Lu-Yao GL, Barry MJ, Chang CH, Wasson JH, Wennberg JE. Transurethral resection of the prostate among Medicare beneficiaries in the United States: time trends and outcomes. Prostate Patient Outcomes Research Team (PORT). Urology 1994; 44(5):692–698; discussion 698–699.
17. Schatzl G, Madersbacher S, Lang T, Marberger M. The early postoperative morbidity of transurethral resection of the prostate and of 4 minimally invasive treatment alternatives. J Urol 1997; 158(1):105–110; discussion 110–111.
18. Kuntz RM, Ahyai S, Lehrich K, Fayad A. Transurethral holmium laser enucleation of the prostate versus transurethral electrocautery resection of the prostate: a randomized prospective trial in 200 patients. J Urol 2004; 172(3):1012–1016.
19. Tuhkanen K, Heino A, Aaltomaa S, Ala-Opas M. Long-term results of contact laser versus transurethral resection of the prostate in the treatment of benign prostatic hyperplasia with small or moderately enlarged prostates. Scand J Urol Nephrol 2003; 37(6):487–493.
20. AUA guideline on management of benign prostatic hyperplasia (2003). Chapter 1: diagnosis and treatment recommendations. J Urol 2003; 170(2 Pt 1):530–547.
21. Wasson JH, Reda DJ, Bruskewitz RC, Elinson J, Keller AM, Henderson WG. A comparison of transurethral surgery with watchful waiting for moderate symptoms of benign prostatic hyperplasia. The Veterans Affairs Cooperative Study Group on Transurethral Resection of the Prostate. N Engl J Med 1995; 332(2):75–79.
22. Yang Q, Peters TJ, Donovan JL, Wilt TJ, Abrams P. Transurethral incision compared with transurethral resection of the prostate for bladder outlet obstruction: a systematic review and meta-analysis of randomized controlled trials. J Urol 2001; 165(5):1526–1532.

23. Hammadeh MY, Madaan S, Hines J, Philp T. 5-year outcome of a prospective randomized trial to compare transurethral electrovaporization of the prostate and standard transurethral resection. Urology 2003; 61(6):1166–1171.

24. Hahn RG. The transurethral resection syndrome. Acta Anaesthesiol Scand 1991; 35(7):557–567.

25. Barletta JP, Fanous MM, Hamed LM. Temporary blindness in the TUR syndrome. J Neuroophthalmol 1994; 14(1):6–8.

26. Khan-Ghori SN, Khalaf MM, Khan RK, Bakhameez HS. Loss of vision: a manifestation of TURP syndrome. A case report. Middle East J Anesthesiol 1998; 14(6):441–449.

27. Rhymer JC, Bell TJ, Perry KC, Ward JP. Hyponatraemia following transurethral resection of the prostate. Br J Urol 1985; 57(4):450–452.

28. Hahn RG. Transurethral resection syndrome from extravascular absorption of irrigating fluid. Scand J Urol Nephrol 1993; 27(3):387–394.

29. Bishop P. Bipolar transurethral resection of the prostate–a new approach. AORN J 2003; 77(5): 979–983.

30. Donat R, Mancey-Jones B. Incidence of thromboembolism after transurethral resection of the prostate (TURP)–a study on TED stocking prophylaxis and literature review. Scand J Urol Nephrol 2002; 36(2):119–123.

31. van Melick HH, van Venrooij GE, Eckhardt MD, Boon TA. A randomized controlled trial comparing transurethral resection of the prostate, contact laser prostatectomy and electrovaporization in men with benign prostatic hyperplasia: analysis of subjective changes, morbidity and mortality. J Urol 2003; 169(4):1411–1416.

32. Concato J, Horwitz RI, Feinstein AR, Elmore JG, Schiff SF. Problems of comorbidity in mortality after prostatectomy. JAMA 1992; 267(8):1077–1082.

33. Malenka DJ, Roos N, Fisher ES, et al. Further study of the increased mortality following transurethral prostatectomy: a chart-based analysis. J Urol 1990; 144(2 Pt 1):224–227; discussion 228.

34. Koshiba K, Egawa S, Ohori M, Uchida T, Yokoyama E, Shoji K. Does transurethral resection of the prostate pose a risk to life? 22-year outcome. J Urol 1995; 153(5):1506–1509.

35. Olapade-Olaopa EO, Solomon LZ, Carter CJ, Ahiaku EK, Chiverton SG. Haematuria and clot retention after transurethral resection of the prostate: a pilot study. Br J Urol 1998; 82(5):624–627.

36. Montorsi F, Naspro R, Salonia A, et al. Holmium laser enucleation versus transurethral resection of the prostate: results from a 2-center, prospective, randomized trial in patients with obstructive benign prostatic hyperplasia. J Urol 2004; 172(5 Pt 1):1926–1929.

37. Knopf HJ, Weib P, Schafer W, Funke PJ. Nosocomial infections after transurethral prostatectomy. Eur Urol 1999; 36(3):207–212.

38. Iversen P, Madsen PO. Short-term cephalosporin prophylaxis in transurethral surgery. Clin Ther 1982; 5(Suppl. A):58–66.

39. Morris MJ, Golovsky D, Guinness MD, Maher PO. The value of prophylactic antibiotics in transurethral prostatic resection: a controlled trial, with observations on the origin of postoperative infection. Br J Urol 1976; 48(6):479–484.

40. Gujral S, Abrams P, Donovan JL, et al. A prospective randomized trial comparing transurethral resection of the prostate and laser therapy in men with chronic urinary retention: The CLasP study. J Urol 2000; 164(1):59–64.

41. Chacko KN, Donovan JL, Abrams P, et al. Transurethral prostatic resection or laser therapy for men with acute urinary retention: the ClasP randomized trial. J Urol 2001; 166(1):166–170; discussion 170–171.

42. Norby B, Nielsen HV, Frimodt-Moller PC. Transurethral interstitial laser coagulation of the prostate and transurethral microwave thermotherapy vs transurethral resection or incision of the prostate: results of a randomized, controlled study in patients with symptomatic benign prostatic hyperplasia. BJU Int 2002; 90(9):853–862.

43. Gupta NP, Doddamani D, Aron M, Hemal AK. Vapor resection: a good alternative to standard loop resection in the management of prostates >40 cc. J Endourol 2002; 16(10):767–771.

44. Horninger W, Unterlechner H, Strasser H, Bartsch G. Transurethral prostatectomy: mortality and morbidity. Prostate 1996; 28(3):195–200.

45. Floratos DL, Kiemeney LA, Rossi C, Kortmann BB, Debruyne FM, de La Rosette JJ. Long-term followup of randomized transurethral microwave thermotherapy versus transurethral prostatic resection study. J Urol 2001; 165(5):1533–1538.

46. Roos NP, Ramsey EW. A population-based study of prostatectomy: outcomes associated with differing surgical approaches. J Urol 1987; 137(6):1184–1188.

47. Brookes ST, Donovan JL, Peters TJ, Abrams P, Neal DE. Sexual dysfunction in men after treatment for lower urinary tract symptoms: evidence from randomised controlled trial. BMJ 2002; 324(7345): 1059–1061.

48. McCohnell DD, Barry MS, Bruskehjr, et al. Benign Prostatic Hyperplasia: Diagnosis and Treatment. Clinical Practice Guidelines No. 8, Human Service. Public Health Service Agency for Healh Care Policy and Research Rockville, MD, 1994.

49. Korenman SG. Epidemiology of erectile dysfunction. Endocrine 2004; 23(2–3):87–91.

50. McVary KT, McKenna KE. The relationship between erectile dysfunction and lower urinary tract symptoms: epidemiological, clinical, and basic science evidence. Curr Urol Rep 2004; 5(4):251–257.

51. Rubeinstein JN, McVary KT. Transurethral microwave thermotherapy for benign prostatic hyperplasia. Int Braz J Urol 2003; 29(3):251–263.

52. Yerushalmi A, Servadio C, Leib Z, Fishelovitz Y, Rokowsky E, Stein JA. Local hyperthermia for treatment of carcinoma of the prostate: a preliminary report. Prostate 1982; 3(6):623–630.

53. Yerushalmi A, Fishelovitz Y, Singer D, et al. Localized deep microwave hyperthermia in the treatment of poor operative risk patients with benign prostatic hyperplasia. J Urol 1985; 133(5):873–876.

54. Sapozink MD, Boyd SD, Astrahan MA, Jozsef G, Petrovich Z. Transurethral hyperthermia for benign prostatic hyperplasia: preliminary clinical results. J Urol 1990; 143(5):944–949; discussion 949–950.

55. Brehmer M, Baba S. Transurethral microwave thermotherapy: how does it work? J Endourol 2000; 14(8):611–615.

56. de la Rosette JJ, D'Ancona FC, Debruyne FM. Current status of thermotherapy of the prostate. J Urol 1997; 157(2):430–438.

57. De la Rosette JJ, Francisca EA, Kortmann BB, Floratos DL, Debruyne FM, Kiemeney LA. Clinical efficacy of a new 30-min algorithm for transurethral microwave thermotherapy: initial results. BJU Int 2000; 86(1):47–51.

58. Ohigashi T, Baba S, Ohki T, Nakashima J, Murai M. Long-term effects of transurethral microwave thermotherapy. Int J Urol 2002; 9(3):141–145.

59. de la Rosette JJ, Laguna MP, Gravas S, de Wildt MJ. Transurethral microwave thermotherapy: the gold standard for minimally invasive therapies for patients with benign prostatic hyperplasia? J Endourol 2003; 17(4):245–251.

60. Wheelahan J, Scott NA, Cartmill R, et al. Minimally invasive laser techniques for prostatectomy: a systematic review. The ASERNIP-S review group. Australian Safety and Efficacy Register of New Interventional Procedures—Surgical. BJU Int 2000; 86(7):805–815.

61. Wheelahan J, Scott NA, Cartmill R, et al. Minimally invasive non-laser thermal techniques for prostatectomy: a systematic review. The ASERNIP-S review group. BJU Int 2000; 86(9):977–988.

62. Feigal D. Safety alert- serious injuries from microwave thermotherapy for benign prostatic hyperplasia, 2000. (Accessed March 5, 2007, at http://www.fda.gov/cdrh/safety/bph.html).

63. Tunuguntla HS, Evans CP. Minimally invasive therapies for benign prostatic hyperplasia. World J Urol 2002; 20(4):197–206.

64. Floratos DL, Aarnink RG. Predictors of treatment outcome for high-energy transurethral microwave thermotherapy. J Endourol 2000; 14(8):643–649.

65. Larson TR, Blute ML, Bruskewitz RC, Mayer RD, Ugarte RR, Utz WJ. A high-efficiency microwave thermoablation system for the treatment of benign prostatic hyperplasia: results of a randomized, sham-controlled, prospective, double-blind, multicenter clinical trial. Urology 1998; 51(5): 731–742.

66. Ahmed M, Bell T, Lawrence WT, Ward JP, Watson GM. Transurethral microwave thermotherapy (Prostatron version 2.5) compared with transurethral resection of the prostate for the treatment of benign prostatic hyperplasia: a randomized, controlled, parallel study. Br J Urol 1997; 79(2): 181–185.

67. Dahlstrand C, Walden M, Geirsson G, Pettersson S. Transurethral microwave thermotherapy versus transurethral resection for symptomatic benign prostatic obstruction: a prospective randomized study with a 2-year follow-up. Br J Urol 1995; 76(5):614–618.

68. Terada N, Aoki Y, Ichioka K, et al. Microwave thermotherapy for benign prostatic hyperplasia with the Dornier Urowave: response durability and variables potentially predicting response. Urology 2001; 57(4):701–705; discussion 705–706.

69. D'Ancona FC, Francisca EA, Witjes WP, Welling L, Debruyne FM, de la Rosette JJ. High energy thermotherapy versus transurethral resection in the treatment of benign prostatic hyperplasia: results of a prospective randomized study with 1 year of followup. J Urol 1997; 158(1):120–125.

70. Hallin A, Berlin T. Transurethral microwave thermotherapy for benign prostatic hyperplasia: clinical outcome after 4 years. J Urol 1998; 159(2):459–464.

71. Rubeinstein JNaM, K.T. E-medicine: Transurethral thermotherapy of the prostate, 2004. (Accessed March 5, 2007, at http://www.emedicine.com/med/topic3070.htm).

72. Arai Y, Aoki Y, Okubo K, et al. Impact of interventional therapy for benign prostatic hyperplasia on quality of life and sexual function: a prospective study. J Urol 2000; 164(4):1206–1211.

73. Francisca EA, d'Ancona FC, Hendriks JC, Kiemeney LA, Debruyne FM, de la Rosette JJ. Quality of life assessment in patients treated with lower energy thermotherapy (Prostasoft 2.0): results of a randomized transurethral microwave thermotherapy versus sham study. J Urol 1997; 158(5): 1839–1844.

74. Chapple CR, Issa MM, Woo H. Transurethral needle ablation (TUNA). A critical review of radiofrequency thermal therapy in the management of benign prostatic hyperplasia. Eur Urol 1999; 35(2): 119–128.

75. Schulman C, Zlotta A. Transurethral needle ablation of the prostate (TUNA): pathological, radiological and clinical study of a new office procedure for treatment of benign prostatic hyperplasia using low-level radiofrequency energy. Arch Esp Urol 1994; 47(9):895–901.

76. Rasor JS, Zlotta AR, Edwards SD, Schulman CC. Transurethral needle ablation (TUNA): thermal gradient mapping and comparison of lesion size in a tissue model and in patients with benign prostatic hyperplasia. Eur Urol 1993; 24(3):411–414.

77. Roehrborn CG, Issa MM, Bruskewitz RC, et al. Transurethral needle ablation for benign prostatic hyperplasia: 12-month results of a prospective, multicenter U.S. study. Urology 1998; 51(3): 415–421.

78. Ramon J, Lynch TH, Eardley I, et al. Transurethral needle ablation of the prostate for the treatment of benign prostatic hyperplasia: a collaborative multicentre study. Br J Urol 1997; 80(1):128–134; discussion 134–135.

79. Campo B, Bergamaschi F, Corrada P, Ordesi G. Transurethral needle ablation (TUNA) of the prostate: a clinical and urodynamic evaluation. Urology 1997; 49(6):847–850.

80. Schatzl G, Madersbacher S, Djavan B, Lang T, Marberger M. Two-year results of transurethral resection of the prostate versus four 'less invasive' treatment options. Eur Urol 2000; 37(6):695–701.

81. Zlotta AR, Giannakopoulos X, Maehlum O, Ostrem T, Schulman CC. Long-term evaluation of transurethral needle ablation of the prostate (TUNA) for treatment of symptomatic benign prostatic hyperplasia: clinical outcome up to five years from three centers. Eur Urol 2003; 44(1):89–93.

82. Rosario DJ, Woo H, Potts KL, Cutinha PE, Hastie KJ, Chapple CR. Safety and efficacy of transurethral needle ablation of the prostate for symptomatic outlet obstruction. Br J Urol 1997; 80(4):579–586.

83. Daehlin L, Gustavsen A, Nilsen AH, Mohn J. Transurethral needle ablation for treatment of lower urinary tract symptoms associated with benign prostatic hyperplasia: outcome after 1 year. J Endourol 2002; 16(2):111–115.

84. Braun M, Mathers M, Bondarenko B, Engelmann U. Treatment of benign prostatic hyperplasia through transurethral needle ablation (TUNA). Review of the literature and six years of clinical experience. Urol Int 2004; 72(1):32–39.

85. Jepsen JV, Bruskewitz RC. Recent developments in the surgical management of benign prostatic hyperplasia. Urology 1998; 51(4A Suppl.):23–31.

86. Bruskewitz R, Issa MM, Roehrborn CG, et al. A prospective, randomized 1-year clinical trial comparing transurethral needle ablation to transurethral resection of the prostate for the treatment of symptomatic benign prostatic hyperplasia. J Urol 1998; 159(5):1588–1593; discussion 1593–1594.

87. Cimentepe E, Unsal A, Saglam R. Randomized clinical trial comparing transurethral needle ablation with transurethral resection of the prostate for the treatment of benign prostatic hyperplasia: results at 18 months. J Endourol 2003; 17(2):103–107.

88. Kaplan SA, Te AE. Transurethral electrovaporization of the prostate: a novel method for treating men with benign prostatic hyperplasia. Urology 1995; 45(4):566–572.

89. McAllister WJ, Gilling PJ. Vaporization of the prostate. Curr Opin Urol 2004; 14(1):31–34.

90. Kupeli B, Yalcinkaya F, Topaloglu H, Karabacak O, Gunlusoy B, Unal S. Efficacy of transurethral electrovaporization of the prostate with respect to standard transurethral resection. J Endourol 1998; 12(6):591–594.

91. Kupeli S, Baltaci S, Soygur T, Aytac S, Yilmaz E, Budak M. A prospective randomized study of transurethral resection of the prostate and transurethral vaporization of the prostate as a therapeutic alternative in the management of men with BPH. Eur Urol 1998; 34(1):15–18.

92. Djavan B, Madersbacher S, Klingler HC, et al. Outcome analysis of minimally invasive treatments for benign prostatic hyperplasia. Tech Urol 1999; 5(1):12–20.

93. Patel A, Fuchs GJ, Gutierrez-Aceves J, Ryan TP. Prostate heating patterns comparing electrosurgical transurethral resection and vaporization: a prospective randomized study. J Urol 1997; 157(1): 169–172.

94. Patel A, Fuchs GJ, Gutierrez-Aceves J. A pilot study of energy utilization patterns during different transurethral electrosurgical treatments of the prostate. Urology 1997; 50(1):138–141.

95. Van Melick HH, Van Venrooij GE, Eckhardt MD, Boon TA. A randomized controlled trial comparing transurethral resection of the prostate, contact laser prostatectomy and electrovaporization in men with benign prostatic hyperplasia: urodynamic effects. J Urol 2002; 168(3):1058–1062.

96. Wang ZL, Wang XF, Li B, et al. Comparative study of transurethral electrovaporization of prostate versus transurethral resection of prostate on benign prostatic hyperplasia. Zhonghua Nan Ke Xue 2002; 8(6):428–430.

97. Patel A, Fuchs GJ, Gutierrez-Aceves J, Andrade-Perez F. Transurethral electrovaporization and vapour-resection of the prostate: an appraisal of possible electrosurgical alternatives to regular loop resection. BJU Int 2000; 85(2):202–210.

98. Kaplan SA, Santarosa RP, Te AE. Transurethral electrovaporization of the prostate: one-year experience. Urology 1996; 48(6):876–881.

99. Fitzpatrick JM. A critical evaluation of technological innovations in the treatment of symptomatic benign prostatic hyperplasia. Br J Urol 1998; 81(Suppl 1):56–63.

100. Boon TA, van Swol CF, van Venrooij GE, Beerlage HP, Verdaasdonk RM. Laser prostatectomy for patients with benign prostatic hyperplasia: a prospective randomized study comparing two different techniques using the Prolase-II fiber. World J Urol 1995; 13(2):123–125.

101. Dixon CM. Lasers for the treatment of benign prostatic hyperplasia. Urol Clin North Am 1995; 22(2):413–422.

102. Chun SS, Razvi HA, Denstedt JD. Laser prostatectomy with the holmium:YAG laser. Tech Urol 1995; 1(4):217–221.

103. Gilling PJ, Cass CB, Cresswell MD, Malcolm AR, Fraundorfer MR. The use of the holmium laser in the treatment of benign prostatic hyperplasia. J Endourol 1996; 10(5):459–461.

104. Le Duc A, Gilling PJ. Holmium laser resection of the prostate. Eur Urol 1999; 35(2):155–160.

105. Tooher R, Sutherland P, Costello A, Gilling P, Rees G, Maddern G. A systematic review of holmium laser prostatectomy for benign prostatic hyperplasia. J Urol 2004; 171(5):1773–1781.

106. Wollin TA, Denstedt JD. The holmium laser in urology. J Clin Laser Med Surg 1998; 16(1):13–20.

107. Gilling PJ, Kennett K, Das AK, Thompson D, Fraundorfer MR. Holmium laser enucleation of the prostate (HoLEP) combined with transurethral tissue morcellation: an update on the early clinical experience. J Endourol 1998; 12(5):457–459.

108. Fraundorfer MR, Gilling PJ. Holmium:YAG laser enucleation of the prostate combined with mechanical morcellation: preliminary results. Eur Urol 1998; 33(1):69–72.

109. Tan AH, Gilling PJ, Kennett KM, Frampton C, Westenberg AM, Fraundorfer MR. A randomized trial comparing holmium laser enucleation of the prostate with transurethral resection of the prostate for the treatment of bladder outlet obstruction secondary to benign prostatic hyperplasia in large glands (40 to 200 grams). J Urol 2003; 170(4 Pt 1):1270–1274.

110. Donovan JL, Peters TJ, Neal DE, et al. A randomized trial comparing transurethral resection of the prostate, laser therapy and conservative treatment of men with symptoms associated with benign prostatic enlargement: The CLasP study. J Urol 2000; 164(1):65–70.

111. Kuo RL, Paterson RF, Kim SC, Siqueira TM Jr, Elhilali MM, Lingeman JE. Holmium laser enucleation of the prostate (HoLEP): a technical update. World J Surg Oncol 2003; 1(1):6.

112. Kuo RL, Kim SC, Lingeman JE, et al. Holmium laser enucleation of prostate (HoLEP): the Methodist Hospital experience with greater than 75 gram enucleations. J Urol 2003; 170(1):149–152.

113. McAllister WJ, Absalom MJ, Mir K, et al. Does endoscopic laser ablation of the prostate stand the test of time? Five-year results from a multicentre randomized controlled trial of endoscopic laser ablation against transurethral resection of the prostate. BJU Int 2000; 85(4):437–439.

114. Gilling PJ, Kennett KM, Fraundorfer MR. Holmium laser resection v transurethral resection of the prostate: results of a randomized trial with 2 years of follow-up. J Endourol 2000; 14(9):757–760.

115. Gilling PJ, Mackey M, Cresswell M, Kennett K, Kabalin JN, Fraundorfer MR. Holmium laser versus transurethral resection of the prostate: a randomized prospective trial with 1-year followup. J Urol 1999; 162(5):1640–1644.

116. Fraundorfer MR, Gilling PJ, Kennett KM, Dunton NG. Holmium laser resection of the prostate is more cost effective than transurethral resection of the prostate: results of a randomized prospective study. Urology 2001; 57(3):454–458.

117. Das A, Kennett K, Fraundorfer M, Gilling P. Holmium laser resection of the prostate (HoLRP): 2-year follow-up data. Tech Urol 2001; 7(4):252–255.

118. Volpe MA, Fromer D, Kaplan SA. Holmium and interstitial lasers for the treatment of benign prostatic hyperplasia: a laser revival. Curr Opin Urol 2001; 11(1):43–48.

119. Paterson RF, Lingeman JE. Holmium laser prostatectomy. Curr Urol Rep 2001; 2(4):269–276.

120. Nau WH, Roselli RJ, Milam DF. Measurement of thermal effects on the optical properties of prostate tissue at wavelengths of 1,064 and 633 nm. Lasers Surg Med 1999; 24(1):38–47.

121. Kabalin JN, Gill HS, Bite G. Laser prostatectomy performed with a right-angle firing neodymium: YAG laser fiber at 60 watts power setting. J Urol 1995; 153(5):1502–1505.

122. Cowles RS III, Kabalin JN, Childs S, et al. A prospective randomized comparison of transurethral resection to visual laser ablation of the prostate for the treatment of benign prostatic hyperplasia. Urology 1995; 46(2):155–160.

123. Sengor F, Kose O, Yucebas E, Beysel M, Erdogan K, Narter F. A comparative study of laser ablation and transurethral electroresection for benign prostatic hyperplasia: results of a 6-month follow-up. Br J Urol 1996; 78(3):398–400.

124. Jung P, Mattelaer P, Wolff JM, Mersdorf A, Jakse G. Visual laser ablation of the prostate: efficacy evaluated by urodynamics and compared to TURP. Eur Urol 1996; 30(4):418–423.

125. Noble SM, Coast J, Brookes S, et al. Transurethral prostate resection, noncontact laser therapy or conservative management in men with symptoms of benign prostatic enlargement? An economic evaluation. J Urol 2002; 168(6):2476–2482.

126. Anson K, Buonaccorsi G, Eddowes M, MacRobert A, Mills T, Watson G. A comparative optical analysis of laser side-firing devices: a guide to treatment. Br J Urol 1995; 75(3):328–334.

127. Kingston TE, Nonnenmacher AK, Crowe H, Costello AJ, Street A. Further evaluation of transurethral laser ablation of the prostate in patients treated with anticoagulant therapy. Aust N Z J Surg 1995; 65(1):40–43.

128. Costello AJ, Shaffer BS, Crowe HR. Second-generation delivery systems for laser prostatic ablation. Urology 1994; 43(2):262–266.

129. Te AE. The development of laser prostatectomy. BJU Int 2004; 93:262–265.

130. Debruyne FM, Djavan B, De la Rosette J, et al. Interventional Therapy for Benign Prostatic Hyperplasia. Vol. 1. Proceedings of the Fifth International Consultation on BPH. Plymouth, UK: Health Publication L, 2001.

131. Hofstetter A. Interstitielle Thermokoagulation (ITK) von Prostatatumoren. Lasermedizin 1991; 7:179.

132. Muschter R, Hessel S, Hofstetter A, et al. Interstitial laser coagulation of benign prostatic hyperplasia. Urologe A 1993; 32(4):273–281.

133. Muschter R, Hofstetter A. Technique and results of interstitial laser coagulation. World J Urol 1995; 13(2):109–114.

134. Muschter R, Whitfield H. Interstitial laser therapy of Benign prostatic hyperplasia. Eur Urol 1999; 35(2):147–154.

135. Muschter R, Hofstetter A. Interstitial laser therapy outcomes in benign prostatic hyperplasia. J Endourol 1995; 9(2):129–135.

136. Laguna MP, Alivizatos G, De La Rosette JJ. Interstitial laser coagulation treatment of benign prostatic hyperplasia: is it to be recommended? J Endourol 2003; 17(8):595–600.

137. Muschter R, Whitfield H. Interstitial laser therapy of benign prostatic hyperplasia. Eur Urol 1999; 35(2):147–154.

138. Zlotta AR, Schulman CC. Interstitial laser coagulation for the treatment of benign prostatic hyperplasia using local anaesthesia only. BJU Int 1999; 83(3):341–342.

139. Daehlin L, Hedlund H. Interstitial laser coagulation in patients with lower urinary tract symptoms from benign prostatic obstruction: treatment under sedoanalgesia with pressure-flow evaluation. BJU Int 1999; 84(6):628–636.

140. Martenson AC, De La Rosette JJ. Interstitial laser coagulation in the treatment of benign prostatic hyperplasia using a diode laser system: results of an evolving technology. Prostate Cancer Prostatic Dis 1999; 2(3):148–154.

141. Lynch WJ, Williams JC. Interstitial laser coagulation technique: clinical research updates. World J Urol 2000; 18(Suppl. 1):S14–S15.

142. Horninger W, Janetschek G, Watson G, Reissigl A, Strasser H, Bartsch G. Are contact laser, interstitial laser, and transurethral ultrasound-guided laser-induced prostatectomy superior to transurethral prostatectomy? Prostate 1997; 31(4):255–263.

143. Floratos DL, Sonke GS, Francisca EA, Kiemeney LA, Debruyne FM, de la Rosette JJ. Long-term follow-up of laser treatment for lower urinary tract symptoms suggestive of bladder outlet obstruction. Urology 2000; 56(4):604–609.

144. Talwar GL, Pande SK. Injection treatment of enlarged prostate. Br J Surg 1966; 53(5):421–427.

145. Plante MK, Bunnell ML, Trotter SJ, Jackson TL, Esenler AC, Zvara P. Transurethral prostatic tissue ablation via a single needle delivery system: initial experience with radio-frequency energy and ethanol. Prostate Cancer Prostatic Dis 2002; 5(3):183–188.

146. Buchholz NN, Andrews HO, Plante MK. Transurethral ethanol ablation of prostate. J Endourol 2004; 18(6):519–524.

147. Martov AG, Pavlov DA, Gushchin BL. Initial results of absolute ethanol chemo-ablation in benign prostatic obstruction treatment. J Endourol 2003; 17(Suppl 1):A157 (abstract).

148. Guttierez J, Gilling P, Schenini M, Grise P, Mentinez J, Hernandez C. Transurethral ethanol albation of the prostate (TEAP): initial long-term report of two prospective multi-center studies. J Urol 2003; 169(Suppl):466 (abstract).

149. Buchholz NPN, Andrews HO. Transurethral ethanol ablation of the prostate (TEAP) in high-risk patients unable to undergo TURP-a feasibility study. Eur Urol 2003; 2:174 (abstract).

150. Plante MK, Anderson R, Badlani G, Rukstalis D. Transurethral ethanol ablation of the prostate using local anesthesia. J Endourol 2003; 17(Suppl 1):A158.

151. Plante MK, Palmer J, Martinez-Sagarra J, Gutierrez J, Gilling P. Complications associated with transurethral ethanol ablation of the prostate for the treatment of benign prostate hyperplasia: a worldwide experience. J Urol 2003; 169(Suppl 2):392 (abstract).

152. Corica FA, Cheng L, Ramnani D, et al. Transurethral hot-water balloon thermoablation for benign prostatic hyperplasia: patient tolerance and pathologic findings. Urology 2000; 56(1):76–80; discussion 81.

153 Corica AG, Qian J, Ma J, Sagaz AA, Corica AP, Bostwick DG. Fast liquid ablation system for prostatic hyperplasia: a new minimally invasive thermal treatment. J Urol 2003; 170(3):874–878.

154. Muschter R. Conductive heat: hot water-induced thermotherapy for ablation of prostatic tissue. J Endourol 2003; 17(8):609–616.

155. Cioanta I, Muschter R. Water-induced thermotherapy for benign prostatic hyperplasia. Tech Urol 2000; 6(4):294–299.

156. Muschter R, Schorsch I, Danielli L, et al. Transurethral water-induced thermotherapy for the treatment of benign prostatic hyperplasia: a prospective multicenter clinical trial. J Urol 2000; 164(5): 1565–1569.
157. Muschter R, Schorsch I, Matalon G, et al. Water induced thermotherapy (WIT): A prospective multicenter study with three year follow up results. J Urol 2001; 165 (suppl):296 (abstract).
158. McVary KT, Rademaker A, Lloyd GL, Gann P. Autonomic nervous system overactivity in men with lower urinary tract symptoms secondary to benign prostatic hyperplasia. J Urol 2005; 174(4 Pt 1):1327–433.

31 | Complications of Minimally Invasive Renal Surgery

Sangtae Park
Department of Urology, University of Washington Medical Center, Seattle, Washington, U.S.A.

Jeffrey A. Cadeddu
Department of Urology, University of Texas Southwestern Medical Center, Dallas, Texas, U.S.A.

INTRODUCTION

Traditional open techniques are increasingly being replaced by minimally invasive surgery for both benign and malignant renal diseases. Patients and their surgeons are enthusiastic about laparoscopy, and its widespread adoption is due to the demonstrated shorter hospitalization, decreased pain medication requirement, and a more rapid return to normal activity (1).

Despite the promise of laparoscopy, the surgeon's enthusiasm must be tempered by a thorough appreciation of the potential complications associated with these modalities. Numerous groups have reported on the learning curve associated with various laparoscopic procedures, demonstrating that complication rates are inversely related to the experience of the surgeon (2). The novice laparoscopist is initially at a disadvantage, due to unfamiliar hand–eye coordination requirements, minimal tactile feedback, and anatomic dissection from a new perspective. The novice renal laparoscopic surgeon should seek out surgical mentorship, attending one of the many laparoscopic courses available. He or she should also gain initial experience performing simpler operations such as renal cyst decortication. For all laparoscopic operations, the surgeon must discuss his or her experience and the potential risks, benefits, and alternatives, including the risk of open conversion with the patients.

In this chapter, we present primary preventive measures for the recognition of, and treatment options for complications arising from minimally invasive renal surgery. This encompasses laparoscopic and percutaneous needle techniques for renal extirpation, ablation, and reconstruction, whereas endourologic techniques and general laparoscopic complications will be addressed elsewhere.

PREOPERATIVE EVALUATION AND PREPARATION

When renal surgery is being planned, a thorough medical history and physical examination are mandatory. Absolute and relative contraindications must be sought during this initial interview. Chronic medical conditions such as coronary disease, pulmonary disease, hypertension, or diabetes mellitus should be optimized in order to maximize surgical outcome. In a review of 399 patients undergoing laparoscopic renal surgery, age more than 65, American Society of Anesthesiology (ASA) score and Charlson comorbidity indices were correlated with surgical complication rates (3). In the multivariate analysis, having >3 medical conditions was an independent predictor of perioperative complications ($p = 0.04$). Blood transfusion rates and hospital lengths of stay were also higher in patients with more comorbid medical conditions.

Absolute contraindications to renal laparoscopy include severe uncorrectable coagulopathy, active peritonitis or abdominal wall infection, possible malignant ascites, and acute intestinal obstruction with bowel dilatation. Relative contraindications include physiologic states that may impair intra-operative success and postoperative recuperation. Carbon dioxide (CO_2) pneumoperitoneum in patients with uncorrected severe chronic obstructive pulmonary disease (COPD) may lead to dangerous hypercarbia and acidemia. Morbidly obese individuals require higher insufflation pressures, with the attendant increased risk of deep venous stasis, decreased pulmonary compliance, higher ventilatory pressures, and impaired visceral perfusion (4).

Morbid obesity also increases the technical difficulty of surgery. Previous abdominal surgery, organomegaly, or a history of peritonitis may increase the risk of vascular or visceral injury caused by intraperitoneal adhesive disease (5). Pregnancy may complicate renal surgery, particularly in the later stages of pregnancy, although laparoscopic nephrectomy has been performed during gestation (6).

If the patient is judged to be fit to undergo renal laparoscopy, bowel preparation with a light mechanical prep will suffice the day before surgery.

Positioning

Patient safety should be the surgeon's utmost concern, and this begins with proper positioning. Wolf et al. reported a 2.7% incidence of neuromuscular injuries upon analyzing over 1600 procedures performed in 15 urologic surgical centers in the United States (7). These included cases of rhabdomyolysis, and sensory and motoneuron deficits. Longer operative time, greater patient weight, and upper urinary tract surgery were associated with higher risk of neuromuscular injuries, although the incidence of the injuries due to laparoscopic procedures was no higher than that reported for similar open operations.

Therefore, the surgeon must be mindful of measures that will protect the most susceptible nerves such as the brachial plexus (8), and femoral, sciatic, and peroneal groups. A modified (30°) lateral decubitus position is commonly used in laparoscopic renal surgery, and duration of elevation of the kidney rest and table flexion should be minimized (9). A survey of laparoscopic urologists in practice after concentrated advanced laparoscopy training (fellowship or residency) revealed a 12% incidence of complications during laparoscopic procedures (10). The most common complication was neuropathy, indicating that careful patient positioning should be considered at least as critical as laparoscopic technical ability.

When postoperative neuromuscular dysfunction is recognized, a neurological consultation may be appropriate. Computed tomography (CT) scanning may also be necessary to rule out retroperitoneal hematoma causing compressive neuropathy. After reversible causes have been eliminated, physical therapy is recommended to prevent muscle atrophy. Patients can be informed that while mild palsies resolve in one to two months, more severe injuries may be permanent or may take several years to resolve.

Patients should be secured using pads, safety belts, or a sturdy tape. This is particularly important because laparoscopic surgeons often use gravity and bed rotation to move mobile viscera away from the surgical field. Orogastric suctioning and urethral catheter placement are strongly recommended before transperitoneal insufflation. Use of lower extremity compression stockings and sequential compressive device is prudent to prevent deep venous thrombosis, in light of decreased venous return from insufflation (11).

Before incision, a "time-out" is prudent to insure correct patient identification, laterality, and to confirm nursing and anesthesia teams' agreement. In terms of the specialized equipment used in renal laparoscopy, it is ultimately the surgeon's responsibility to insure their proper functioning. Consequently, the responsible surgeon should be the most knowledgeable person about the equipments, from the video tower to the suction irrigator, and be ready to solve intra-operative trouble-shooting.

GENERAL CONSIDERATIONS FOR RENAL LAPAROSCOPY

There have been several large series reporting the overall complications associated with urological laparoscopy. While the surgeon can quote these data to patients before minimally invasive renal surgery, some would argue that a discussion of the surgeon's personal experience and results would be more valid. Nevertheless, knowledge of the literature on the incidence and types of complications associated with renal laparoscopy is useful (Table 1).

Parsons et al. reported on 894 laparoscopic procedures performed between 1996 and 2000, of which 94% were renal extirpative or reconstructive (12). The overall complication rate was 13.2%, with 4.7% occurring intra-operatively, 6.7% postoperatively, and 1.8% related to medical comorbidities. The most common intra-operative issue was hemorrhage (2.6%), followed by injury to adjacent organs (1.1%), and bowel injuries (0.8%). In the postoperative setting,

TABLE 1 Summary of Complications from Laparoscopic Renal Surgery

Related to pneumoperitoneum	Hypercarbia, acidosis
	Oliguria
	Ventilation-perfusion mismatch
	Hypertension
	Cardiac arrythmias
	Gas embolism
	Pneumothorax
	Pneumomediastinum, pneumopericardium
	Subcutaneous emphysema
	Venous thrombosis and embolism
Related to positioning	Neurapraxia
	Rhabdomyolysis
	Extremity compartment syndrome
Related to instrumentation	Vascular or visceral injury
	Abdominal wall bleeding
	Trocar site hernia
	Wound infections

neuromuscular complications were the most common (1.3%), followed by hematoma (1.2%), and urine leakage (1%). This series reported a 0.2% mortality rate, a 1.5% open conversion rate, and a 1.5% rate of re-operation, with ASA score being directly correlated to the risk of complication ($p = 0.01$). Clearly, any surgical series of complications must be adjusted for level of difficulty, and accordingly, the authors summarized their data using the "European scoring system" (13) for difficulty of laparoscopic surgery, and 73% of the cases in their series were classified as "difficult" or "very difficult" using this scale.

In a review of over 2400 laparoscopic urological operations, Fahlenkamp et al. reported an 8.2% incidence of complications in 351 patients who had undergone renal extirpative surgery (14). The most common issue was hemorrhage in 1.7% of cases, with injury to adjacent vital structures in 1.1%. As expected, the risk of complication increased when they stratified the 2407 cases into easy, difficult, or very difficult cases (1% when easy, 9.2% when very difficult). Reviews by Vallancien et al. (15) and others (16,17) report results similar to the above-mentioned.

Complications Associated with Abdominal Access

Once proper positioning and equipment function have been confirmed, laparoscopy can be performed via a transperitoneal or retroperitoneal approach, depending on surgeon preference and expertise. Initial access is achieved using closed (Veress), open (Hasson), or visualizing trocar techniques. While these various tools were introduced in order to minimize access-related injuries, their incidence is not nil, and ranges between 0.05% and 2.8% (18). In this study reviewing insurance claims and Food and Drug Administratation (FDA) post-marketing medical device safety reports, there was a 13% risk of mortality after access-related injuries. Bowel and retroperitoneal vascular injuries were the most common, with delayed recognition past 24 hours in almost half the cases of bowel injury. Independent predictors for death were age greater than 60, major vascular injury, and delayed recognition. All forms of trocars were reported, and the authors concluded that no entry technique or device was immune from these potentially devastating injuries.

In terms of access in previously operated abdomens, Seifman et al. reported on 190 patients who underwent transperitoneal renal laparoscopy between 1996 and 2001 (19); 76 (40%) patients had a history of previous abdominal surgery, and in a multivariate logistic model, the authors found that previous abdominal surgery was a significant independent predictor for intra-operative and major complications. In particular, upper midline and ipsilateral scars were associated with increased risk of access-related complications ($p = 0.029$).

Nevertheless, primary prevention of injury is possible if the following principles are used. The closed transperitoneal technique (Fig. 1) (20) uses the Veress needle, and its safety relies on

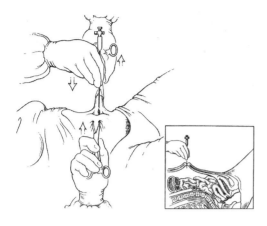

FIGURE 1 The Veress needle is grasped at the shaft and advanced into the peritoneum. The periumbilical skin is elevated with towel clamps to provide counter-traction. *Source*: From Ref. 20.

the blunt, spring-loaded inner obturator which shields the cutting tip. Both reusable and disposable Veress needles are available, and its safety should be verified before use. Confirmation of intraperitoneal placement is made by performing the aspiration and injection test. In this test, a half-filled syringe is aspirated, looking for blood or intestinal succus. If nothing is aspirated, a few drops of fluid are instilled into the Veress, and a characteristic "drop" in the meniscus is observed if the needle is in the correct space. Another test is the advancement test, whereby advancement of the Veress by one or two centimeters should be free of resistance.

Complications may occur when the needle is placed too deep (visceral or vascular injury) or not deep enough (preperitoneal placement). Preperitoneal insufflation can be severe enough to impede the planned renal laparoscopic operation. Other serious complications such as subcutaneous emphysema, pneumomediastinum, and pneumopericardium can occur as a result. Preperitoneal placement is diagnosed by resistance to needle advancement, opening pressures greater than 7 mmHg, and rapidly rising insufflation pressures to greater than 10 mmHg with less than 1 L of instilled gas. If preperitoneal placement is suspected, complete removal of the Veress and a fresh pass are recommended.

The open transperitoneal technique should be employed when significant adhesions from previous operations are suspected. In this technique, a sufficiently large skin incision is made and the fascia and peritoneum are incised under direct vision. The larger skin incision can lead to subcutaneous emphysema and difficulties maintaining pneumoperitoneum. Another alternative reported in the literature is initial retroperitoneoscopic access (21). This allows the surgeon to visualize the posterior peritoneum and safely gain access into the peritoneal space. Further trocars are then placed intraperitoneally under direct vision of the anterior abdominal wall while avoiding adhesions.

Vascular Injury During Access

The great vessels or other smaller vessels may be injured during initial Veress needle or first trocar placement. Once insufflation is successful, initial peritoneoscopy should be aimed at ruling out injuries. A retroperitoneal hematoma may result, which can be expanding or pulsatile in nature. If such a major vascular injury is noted, open conversion should be considered. However, injuries to smaller veins are often self-limiting, with spontaneous clotting commonly occurring. Sudden cardiovascular instability should raise the suspicion of a missed retroperitoneal bleed or gas embolus related to an unrecognized vascular injury.

The inferior epigastric artery and vein can be injured during initial access and trocar insertion. Since these structures travel on the undersurface of the rectus muscle belly, trocar insertion in the midline or lateral to the rectus border is prudent (Fig. 2) (22). Transillumination can sometimes make these vessels visible, allowing the surgeon to avoid injuring them. If laceration is noted, cautery alone is insufficient. A figure-of-eight suture should be placed under videoscopic monitoring and tied over a bolster on the skin or subcutaneously. A fascial closure device is appropriate for this purpose. Another critical point is that these vessels are branches

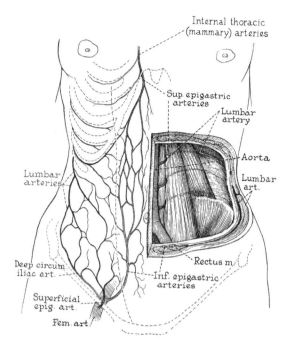

FIGURE 2   Inferior epigatric vessels. They arise from the femoral vessels and travel cephalad along the posterior aspect of the rectus abdominis muscle. *Source*: From Ref. 22.

of the femoral vessel caudally, and the internal mammary artery cranially, therefore, both ends of the cut ends must be ligated for secure hemostasis.

Visceral Injury During Access

During initial access, the likelihood of gastrointestinal and urinary bladder injury is minimized by orogastric and urethral catheter drainage. Management of visceral injuries depends on the organ and type of injury. Bowel injuries caused by Veress insertion can usually be managed conservatively. Management of trocar injury to the bowel depends on its extent and presence of spillage. Suctioning out of intestinal contents followed by primary repair is usually adequate, but more extensive damage may require general surgical consultation.

Hepatic lacerations may respond to cautery or argon beam coagulation, whereas splenic injuries or capsular tears may require additional attention such as cellulose matrix or other commercially available materials. On rare occasions, uncontrolled bleeding may follow injury to these organs, and a general surgical consultation would be wise. Urinary bladder injury with the Veress needle is likely innocuous, but larger insults should be suture-repaired, with urethral catheter drainage for a longer period.

Intra-operatively, some of the most hazardous situations are unrecognized visceral or vascular injuries outside of the laparoscopic field of view. This may occur when stray electric current from the electrocautery unit is conducted to organs outside of the field of view. The chance of this is minimized by insuring good working conditions of the instruments and checking the integrity of insulation in the shaft of the instruments. Reusable metal trocars can also contribute to inadvertent injury if there is contact of the active cautery instrument and the trocar. A further source of injury is during instrument introduction, when rigid metal instruments can perforate the bowel or puncture delicate structures. A key principle in prevention is to introduce the instrument "facing up" towards the anterior abdominal wall, thereby evading important structures outside of the field of view.

In a review by Bishoff et al., a 0.1% to 0.6% incidence of bowel injuries was reported in the urological, gynecological, and general surgical experience (23). In their study, injuries caused by cautery and scissors were each responsible for 50% of bowel injuries, and 69% of cases were unrecognized intra-operatively with delayed laparotomy in 80%. The small bowel was affected most commonly, followed by the colon. The mortality associated with unrecognized bowel injury was 50% in this study (23), underscoring the importance of having a high index of suspicion in the postoperative period, particularly if there are signs such as greater than normal pain at a port-site, distension, diarrhea or leukopenia. While the above-mentioned study reported on transperitoneal operations, in a similar study of 404 retroperitoneal laparoscopic renal operations, bowel injuries occurred in 0.3%, indicating that this approach does not eliminate this complication completely (24). If suspected, early computed tomography has been shown to be a sensitive and specific test in diagnosing these injuries (25).

Physiologic Complications of Insufflation

Corbon dioxide is the most commonly used gas to create pneumoperitoneum. Its solubility in blood minimizes the risk of gas embolism, and its non-flammability allows the use of electrical energy sources intra-abdominally. However, the surgeon must be aware of the potential systemic effects of CO_2 insufflation, and be prepared to lead the surgical and anesthetic teams in the recognition and management of its complications. Cardiac impairment due to decreased venous return may occur but is not often clinically significant and will not be addressed here.

Pulmonary Complications

Carbon dioxide at 15 mmHg pressure in the peritoneum dissolves directly through the visceral peritoneal surfaces, leading to hypercarbia and acidemia. COPD patients are unable to efficiently exchange CO_2, and preoperative room air arterial blood gases are recommended for those with limited pulmonary reserve. Alternatives to CO_2, such as nitrous oxide, helium, and noble gases should be considered (26). Nitrous oxide is flammable, helium is insoluble, and the noble gases are expensive, limiting their widespread use except for select cases. In some with underlying medical conditions such as sickle cell disease, acidemia may precipitate a sickling crisis.

Pneumothorax and pneumomediastinum may develop as a result of iatrogenic diaphragmatic injury or defects in the esophageal, aortic, or caval hiatus. Del Pizzo et al. published a multi-institutional study of 1765 patients who underwent laparoscopic renal surgery (27). The overall incidence of pleural injury was (0.6%) in 10 patients, of which two occurred due to transpleural trocar placement during a retroperitoneoscopic approach. The remainder occurred during kidney dissection, and in each case, the injury was suture-repaired after intra-operative recognition. In two cases, no gross diaphragmatic defect could be seen, but diaphragmatic injury was strongly suspected due to billowing down of the diaphragm. The authors presented a treatment algorithm, requiring close teamwork with the anesthesiologist. If clinically stable, the surgeon should complete the procedure, followed by definitive diaphragmatic repair. This allows unrestricted view of the injury and meticulous repair. If unstable, immediate repair with simultaneous tube thoracostomy to relieve the probable tension pneumothorax is required. Postoperatively, a chest X ray is prudent to rule out a large persistent pneumothorax, which can be present in 10% of cases (27). Mediastinal air on these films is usually self-limited, and rarely causes physiologic compromise. Other methods of diaphragmatic closure include use of the Endostitch device (28) (U.S. Surgical Corp, Stamford, Connecticut, U.S.A.) and gelfoam matrix (29).

INTRA-OPERATIVE BLEEDING

The most common energy source for renal laparoscopy is monopolar electrocautery. Before use, the insulation of electrosurgical instruments is checked by inspecting the surface for defects. The entire uninsulated tip of the cautery device should always be in the laparoscopic visual field during use, to prevent stray electric injury to adjacent viscera or vessels.

Prevention of bleeding during renal laparoscopy is achieved by appropriate traction and counter-traction on the structure of interest and its surrounding connective tissues. Vessels placed on the longitudinal stretch become visible and may be dissected free and cauterized. When greater than 1 to 2 mm in size, other modalities such as clips, ultrasonic shears, or laparoscopic stapling device may be used, depending on the size. As in open surgery, circumferential dissection of the fibroareolar tissues around substantial vessels allows more precise hemostatic maneuvers. A point worth stressing is that metal clips or Hem-o-lok clips (Teleflex Medical,

Limerick, Pennsylvania, U.S.A.) should not be placed too close to the hilum as they may inter-fere with division of the hilar vessels during nephrectomy.

In laparoscopic renal surgery, the most common sites of bleeding are the hilum, adrenal fossa, lateral perirenal attachments, gonadal artery, and gonadal vein. Perhaps more so than in open surgery, laparoscopic renal surgery should not be an endeavor in "discovery," but rather anticipation. Therefore, careful review of the preoperative images will help define the hilar venous and arterial anatomy. The left renal hilum is often more complicated due to the entry of lumbar, adrenal, and gonadal veins. Furthermore, venous variants such as retroaortic or circumaortic veins can be recognized and suitable operations planned. In adrenal-sparing nephrectomy, the renal vein may be transected lateral to the adrenal vein, thereby obviating the need for more extensive dissection of the three branches entering medially. On the right side, the hilar anatomy is usually less complex, although damage to the adrenal vein can certainly lead to significant hemorrhage.

Bleeding from the adrenal fossa can be troublesome but preventable. Upper pole renal vessels can enter via this area, therefore, systematic dissection and coagulation of suprarenal fat are wise. Others prefer to use the harmonic scalpel or even one or two loads of the endo-gastrointestinal anastomosis (endo-GIA) in order to expedite this dissection.

Large renal masses also often have parasitic vessels arising from multiple directions, and can be anticipated by reviewing the cross-sectional images. While clipping individual vessels is reasonable, a quicker strategy may to be use the endo-GIA stapler to control these vessels en bloc. The gonadal vein is usually visible after incising the white line of Toldt and reflecting the colon medially. This vessel should be controlled with clips or staplers. In terms of the gonadal artery, this is often appreciated much better than in open surgery due to lapa-roscopic magnification. This vessel commonly travels parallel, but caudal to the gonadal vein and should be clipped.

If significant bleeding is encountered from any of the above-mentioned sites, specific laparoscopic maneuvers have to be used. Unlike open surgery, blood and clots cannot be cleared away easily and manual compression can be difficult. Furthermore, unrestrained use of suction/irrigation is not possible due to the potential loss of pneumoperitoneum.

The first principle is to have good exposure and visualization of the bleeding source. It is important to remain calm, and the urge to blindly clip and haphazardly cauterize should be suppressed. Temporarily increasing the pneumoperitoneal pressure to 20 to 25 mmHg helps tamponade venous bleeding. Sustained direct pressure using forceps or a rolled up gauze can be very effective. At times, several gauze rolls can be left to tamponade the bleeding site, and if not bleeding excessively, attention can be turned to a different part of the operation. Frequently, after a few minutes of working elsewhere, the venous bleeding points can be examined and they will have thrombosed spontaneously.

If unresponsive to these conservative measures, defining the open vessel by meticulous dissection, followed by judicious clip or cautery use will usually stop bleeding. One should also consider using a commercially-available hemostatic agent, such as Floseal (Baxter, Deerfield, Illinois, U.S.A.), Tisseel (Baxter), thrombin-soaked gelfoam, and argon beam coagulation. If copious bleeding persists despite these maneuvers, consideration should be given to open sur-gical control.

A special instance of severe, life-threatening bleeding can occur due to failure of laparo-scopic stapling devices. Use of endo-thoracic abdominal (endo-TA) staplers spares us from this dreaded complication, because a series of staples are placed without cutting. On the other hand, in the more commonly used endo-GIA staplers, a series of staples are placed on either side of the cut line, and then the tissues are divided. Since these are most commonly used in the renal hilum, their malfunction usually requires rapid conversion to open surgical control. For this reason, it may be prudent for the novice laparoscopic surgeon to have an open surgical set available in the operating room always.

Stapler malfunction can be avoided by including well-informed scrub nurses with a thor-ough knowledge of stapling device loading and reloading in the operation team. Spent car-tridges should be immediately removed from the sterile field. The surgeon must confirm that the staple loads are vascular loads, as larger staples designed for bowel use may not appose the walls of the renal artery or vein, leading to dangerous bleeding.

At the completion of the operation, the operative field should be inspected for bleeding. Desufflation to 5 mmHg will eliminate the tamponading effect of the pneumoperitoneum, revealing any points of venous bleeding. These can be controlled with the above-mentioned maneuvers or by using commercially available hemostatic agents.

SAFE REMOVAL OF SPECIMEN

Renal laparoscopy for malignancy and infection creates a special concern for potential seeding of trocar sites or gross spillage. There are other reasons to advocate routine intact specimen removal. The prognosis and follow up of patients with renal cell carcinoma (RCC) depend on tumor size, stage, grade, microvascular invasion, and completeness of tumor resection (30). The information gathered from accurate histologic analysis is used to prognosticate patients and to formulate stage-dependent surveillance protocols on an individual basis (30). While pathologic analysis does not help identify those who would benefit from currently available adjuvant therapy, individualized adjuvant immunotherapy will be possible in the future.

While morcellation for benign renal conditions seems reasonable, more data are required to confirm the safety of morcellation for suspected RCC. Furthermore, morcellation requires an additional operating room and anesthetic time compared to intact extraction. In the report of Hernandez et al., morcellation was associated with an average of 11 minutes more of operative time (31). If morcellation is chosen, impervious bags are strongly recommended. In a review of port-site metastases after urological laparoscopy, nine cases were reported (32). Four of the cases occurred after morcellation, and two recurrences were potentially preventable, because they occurred in those whose tumors were entrapped in bags not approved for morcellation. Bowel injury has also been reported to occur during morcellation, stressing the need to firmly lift up the bag onto the anterior abdominal wall during morcellation.

PORT-SITE COMPLICATIONS

Both acute and chronic complications can occur with laparoscopic port sites (14–16). In the acute setting, bleeding and bowel herniation can occur. Primary prevention involves removing the trocar under direct vision. Arterial bleeding from a port site is rare but can be detected by removing the trocar under direct vision. If brisk bleeding is present, devices such as a foley catheter under traction through the port or a simple through-and-through figure-of-eight suture will usually suffice. Bowel loops can also acutely herniate into a working trocar site. Again, removal of trocars under direct vision allows the surgeon to insure that no bowel loops "follow" the trocar as it exits the abdominal wall.

Longer term complications include port-site recurrence and hernia formation. Port-site recurrence was studied in an international survey, including over 10,912 laparoscopic cancer operations (33). In their study, seven of 13 (54%) port-site recurrences occurred in patients with urothelial cancer. While the overall occurrence was 0.1%, the risk of recurrence was highest in 559 patients who underwent nephroureterectomy for upper tract transitional cell cancer (0.9%). Another striking finding is that there were four cases of trocar recurrence after simple nephrectomy, and all occurred in patients with unsuspected upper tract urothelial cancer. In a similar analysis, Rassweiler et al. reported on 1098 urologic oncology operations performed laparoscopically (34). This group found a 0.18% rate of port-site recurrence, and risk of recurrence was related to the biological aggressiveness of disease, rather than surgical technical causes.

With regard to port-site hernias, Rumstadt et al. reviewed 2500 laparoscopic cases and found a 0.08% incidence of incisional hernias (35). Current recommendations are that each fascial cutting trocar site requires a fascial stitch, placed either using conventional methods or a fascial closure device. Suture closure of nonbladed trocar sites can be omitted, for ports up to 12 mm in size, but there have been reports of symptomatic hernia formation even when these are used (36). Infection at port sites may be treated with parenteral antibiotics that target skin flora, and occasionally, incision and drainage may be required for subcutaneous collections.

The proponents of hand-assisted laparoscopic surgery have suggested that these operations take less time, while having equivalent overall complication rates, cost, length of stay and convalescence period compared to pure laparoscopy (37). Several groups have reviewed their experience on complications associated specifically with these port sites. Terranova et al. reported on 54 patients who underwent hand-assisted laparoscopic renal surgery (38). Hand-port-specific complications occurred in 9.3%, with three major and two minor events. The major complications included one evisceration, one enterocutaneous fistula, and one incisional hernia, all requiring re-operation. Minor complications included wound infection and skin separation.

COMPLICATIONS ASSOCIATED WITH SPECIFIC PROCEDURES

Minimally invasive renal surgery as practiced currently encompasses extirpative, ablative, and reconstructive methods. In addition to the above-mentioned general complications that may occur, specific complications associated with each operation are reviewed below.

Laparoscopic Nephrectomy

Table 2 summarizes the complications reported by large series of laparoscopic nephrectomy. The most common complications are intra-operative bleeding and injury to adjacent viscera.

Cadeddu et al. reported on 157 patients undergoing laparoscopic nephrectomy for clinical T1 and T2 renal masses (39). In this multi-institutional study, complications occurred in 15 of 157 patients (9.6%). Intra-operatively, there was one death due to presumed pulmonary embolus, six open conversion, and one duodenal injury requiring reoperation. The most common post-operative complication was prolonged ileus in four patients. No port-site or local recurrence was noted at a mean follow up of 19.2 months.

A rare but significant complication is great vessel injury during laparoscopic radical nephrectomy. In a report by McAllister et al., two cases of complete vena caval transection during retroperitoneoscopic nephrectomy were reviewed (40). In both cases, caval reconstruction by vascular surgeons allowed recovery without sequelae. Upon analysis, the authors concluded that a rotated camera on a 30°-angled laparoscope led to disorientation and mistaking the cava for the renal vein.

TABLE 2 Laparoscopic Nephrectomy Complications

Reference	N	Complications	Comments
Ono et al. (61)	103	13% overall 4% open conversion 5% blood transfusion 2% bowel injuries 2% visceral injury	One duodenojejunostomy and one colostomy required
Cadeddu et al. (39)	157	9.6% overall 3% ileus 1% urinary tract infection 1% pulmonary embolus 1% congestive heart failure 1% wound complications 1% duodenal perforation 1% bleeding, with transfusion	
Stifelman et al. (62)	95	12% overall 1% caval injury 1% pneumonia 3% prolonged ileus 3% wound infections 1% incisional hernia 1% bowel obstruction required laparotomy	All cases were hand-assisted
Gill et al. (63)	100	14% overall 2% open conversion 2% postoperative hematoma 2% wound infection 2% vascular injury 2% prolonged ileus 4% cutaneous hyperesthesia	One splenectomy required

Laparoscopic Partial Nephrectomy

Acute or delayed bleeding and postoperative urinary leaks from the resection bed are the most commonly reported urologic complications associated with this technically challenging operation. Complications reported in the larger series are summarized in Table 3. However, in experienced hands, laparoscopic partial nephrectomy (LPN) may not be associated with increased complications when compared to open partial nephrectomy (OPN) or laparoscopic radical nephrectomy (LRN).

Gill et al. compared 100 LPN to 100 OPN performed in a similar time period at the Cleveland Clinic (41). The OPN group had larger masses, more absolute indications for nephron-sparing approach and shorter ischemia time (all $p < 0.05$). However, operative time was shorter, blood loss was less and postoperative analgesic requirements were lower in the LPN group. While the overall complication rates for LPN and OPN were similar, at 16% versus 13%, the LPN group had higher urology-related complications (7% vs. 2%).

In the largest series of laparoscopic partial nephrectomy, Link et al. reviewed the outcomes of 223 patients who underwent laparoscopic partial nephrectomy between 1999 and 2004 (2). The overall complication rate was 10.6%, with bleeding complications in 1.8%, prolonged ileus in 1.8%, urine leakage in 1.4%, and wound infection in 1.4%. In a similar series studying 200 patients, there was a 9.5% of bleeding and a 5% incidence of urinary leakage, all of which resolved with double-J ureteral stenting (42).

Kim et al. compared the results of 35 LRN and 79 LPN operations performed by an experienced senior surgeon (43). In this series of operations performed between 1998 and 2002, the mean tumor size was 2.8 cm for LRN and 2.5 cm for LPN ($p = 0.17$). No difference was found between these groups in terms of overall complications, length of stay, change in creatinine levels, operative time, transfusion rate, or pain medication requirement. However, this study may have not been adequately powered to detect a statistical difference.

Intra-operative bleeding is minimized by renal hilar clamping. However, there is significant variability in the literature regarding routine renal vein clamping, the use of bulldog clamps versus laparoscopic Satinsky clamps, and even in hilar clamping. While the first two issues are still unresolved, hilar clamping is associated with less blood loss and shorter

TABLE 3 Laparoscopic Partial Nephrectomy Complications

Reference	N	Complications	Comments
Ramani et al. (42)	200	33% overall 1% open conversion 10% hemorrhage 5% urine leak 2% transient renal failure 15% pulmonary 5% cardiovascular 2% gastrointestinal 3% musculoskeletal	3% positive surgical margin
Link et al. (2)	217	11% overall 1% open conversion 1% bleeding, with transfusion 1% ureteropelvic junction obstruction 1% wound infection 1% urine leak 1% acute renal failure 2% prolonged ileus	3.5% positive surgical margin
Abukora et al. (64)	78	23% overall 4% open conversion 5% hemorrhage 4% urinary leak 1% ureteral stenosis 1% pulmonary embolus 3% pneumonia 3% splenic injury	

operative time. Guillonneau et al. reported on 12 patients undergoing LPN after clamping and 16 without. Despite the clamping group having larger tumors (2.5 cm vs. 1.8 cm), the operative time was significantly shorter (121 minutes vs. 179 minutes) and blood loss much lesser (270 cc vs. 708 cc) (44).

However, laparoscopic hilar clamping and renorrhaphy have caused vascular complications. Moore et al. reported two cases of renal artery pseudoaneurysm discovered by CT scans performed for decreasing hematocrit and gross hematuria postoperatively (45). Due to the risk of spontaneous perforation, these pseudoaneurysms (2 and 4 cm) required selective angioembolization, with good results.

In order to minimize the risk of urine leakage, some surgeons routinely place a 5 French open-ended ureteral catheter at the outset of the operation (43,46). After tumor excision, dilute indigo carmine is injected into the catheter, allowing targeted suture closure if the collecting system has been violated.

Cryotherapy and Radiofrequency Ablation

With the increasing number of small renal masses being detected, there has been a growing interest in renal ablative surgery as an alternative to partial nephrectomy. While long-term cancer control data have not yet matured, a lot has been learned about safe ablation and potential complications from cryoablation (CA) or radiofrequency ablation (RFA). Percutaneous and laparoscopic approaches are possible with each ablative technique, and each has a unique pattern of complications.

Johnson et al. published a multi-institutional review of complications associated with CA and RFA (47). Four institutions contributed their experience with 133 RFA cases and 139 CA cases. Percutaneous approach was used in 181 and laparoscopy in 90. The overall complication rate was 11%, with 9.2% major and 1.8% minor complications; 87% of complications were directly attributable to ablation, and the most common issue was pain or paresthesia at the probe insertion site. One death occurred due to aspiration pneumonia, of a poor surgical candidate with a history of chronic pulmonary disease, congestive heart failure, and pulmonary histoplasmosis. Most complications were successfully managed conservatively, with only two of 30 patients requiring re-operation. One patient required laparotomy for hemorrhage after percutaneous CA and one delayed nephrectomy for ureteropelvic junction obstruction after laparoscopic RFA.

Radiofrequency Ablation

Minor and major complications can occur with radiofrequency ablation. As this technology relies on conductive heat transfer for killing tumor cells, normal tissues can also be injured. Table 4 summarizes the reports in the literature. The concept of image-guided therapy is

TABLE 4 Radiofrequency Complications

Reference	N	Complications (N)	Comments
Gervais et al. (65) Percutaneous	100	Calyceal obliteration (3) Hemorrhage (4) Ureteral stricture (3) Urine leak (3)	Conservative management Ureteral stent, urethral catheter Nephrostomy tube in one One urinoma drainage and stent
Varkarakis et al. (66) Percutaneous	60	Flank wall laxity (1) Liver hematoma (1) Death due to aspiration pneumonia (1)	14 cases of insignificant perirenal hematoma
Mayo-Smith et al. (67) Percutaneous	36	Hydrocalyx (1)	
Farrell et al. (68) Percutaneous	35	Neuropathy (3)	
Hwang et al. (69) Lap and percutaneous	24	Gross hematuria (2) Ureteropelvic junction obstruction (1)	Open pyeloplasty 9 months postoperatively
Matsumoto et al. (70) Lap and percutaneous	109	Neuropathy (6) Hydrocalyx (1) Lower pole infarct (1) Urine leak (1) Ureteropelvic junction obstruction (1)	

important both in effective targeting of the renal mass and avoiding critical structures such as the pyelocalyceal collecting system and major renal vessels.

Despite careful probe deployment, collecting system and ureteral injury can occur when RFA is performed on masses close to these structures. Calyceal obliteration, infundibular obstruction, urinary leak, and ureteropelvic junction obstruction have all been described. Matsumoto et al. reported on RFA for 109 renal masses. Three major (2.8%) and 10 minor (9%) complications occurred, with prolonged pain at the needle ablation site being the most common minor complication. The major complications were a urine leak, lower pole infarction and a ureteropelvic junction requiring nephrectomy. In a similar review of 100 renal masses on which percutaneous RFA was performed, 23 tumors were adjacent to the collecting system on cross-sectional imaging. After RFA, follow-up imaging demonstrated that the zone of ablation extended to a calyx in 26 of 100 cases, and in three cases (12%), a previously opacified calyx was obliterated. While this radiographic complication was noted, no clinical sequelae were reported in these patients.

Ureteral injury is a potentially serious complication that has a reported incidence of 1% to 3%. In the Gervais et al. series, ureteral stricture occurred when the medial aspect of the tumors were 2 and 4 mm away from the proximal ureter, suggesting that it is prudent to have at least a 5- to 10-mm margin from the proximal ureter for reasons of safety. While retrograde renal cooling has been tested in a porcine RFA model, there have been no reports of its use in clinical practice to prevent this potentially serious complication (48).

Bleeding is another complication that has been reported after RFA. While there were no significant cases of bleeding or transfusion in Matsumoto et al.'s series, Gervais et al. reported gross hematuria in those with masses adjacent to the collecting system. Four of 100 patients had gross hematuria, with resolution after conservative management and no transfusions were required. Central tumors and those adjacent to the collecting system were more likely to lead to this complication.

Bowel injury is possible during RFA because the colon lies anterior to the kidney. In the study by Gervais et al., 21 tumors were ablated even when the bowel was within 1 cm of the tumor. Percutaneous hydrodissection of bowel away from tumor was performed by injecting 50 to 200 cc of saline in the plane between the colon and anterior Gerota's fascia. While this group reported no bowel injuries with this approach, the authors suggest a laparoscopic approach to dissect vital structures away from the expected ablation zone.

Cryoablation

In this technology, freezing of tissues to less than –20°C allows destruction of the neoplasm. Again, the concept of image-guided therapy allows the surgeon to precisely target the neoplasm while avoiding vital intra- and perirenal structures. Nevertheless, potentially serious injuries to vital structures have been reported, and Table 5 summarizes the complications published to date.

TABLE 5   Cryoablation Complications

Reference	N	Complications (N)	Comments
Gill et al. (71) Laparoscopic	56	Splenic hematoma (1) Heart failure (1) Pleural effusion (1) Herpetic esophagitis (1)	
Bachmann et al. (72) Laparoscopic	7	Bleeding (2) Skin frostbite (1)	
Silverman et al. (49) Percutaneous	26	Postoperative bleed (1) Colo-rectal fistula (1)	One unit transfused, percutaneous abscess drainage
Moon et al. (73) Laparoscopic	16	Open conversion (1) Pneumonia (1)	Conversion for failure to progress
Cestari et al. (51) Laparoscopic	37	Renal fracture (3) Postoperative fever (3) Ureteropelvic junction obstruction (1)	One unit transfused, pyeloplasty 8 months postoperatively
Lee et al. (52) Laparoscopic	20	Pancreatic injury (1) Elevated amylase and lipase (5) Atrial fibrillation (1)	Re-exploration, one unit transfused
Shingleton et al. (74) Percutaneous	20	Superficial skin abscess (1)	Incision and drainage

Gill et al. reported their intermediate 3-year results after laparoscopic renal cryoblation in 56 patients. There were two major (splenic hematoma and heart failure) and two minor complications (4% each). Minor complications were postoperative herpetic esophagitis and pleural effusion, with resolution in both cases.

Silverman et al. reported on 26 percutaneous CA cases, with two complications (8%) (49). One was hemorrhage requiring a one unit transfusion, with resolution after conservative management. In another patient, a colo-renal fistula occurred after CA of a 4.6-cm exophytic solid mass. Percutaneous abscess drainage was necessary, and the fistula healed without further intervention. In another report on 20 patients, Lee et al. reported a case of pancreatic injury after laparoscopic cryoablation (50). Persistent abdominal pain and elevated serum amylase and lipase prompted re-exploration, and the patient was discharged on postoperative day 9, when his symptoms resolved, with surgical drains placed around the pancreas.

Renal fracture seems to be a complication unique to cryoablation. Cestari et al. reviewed their experience of 37 patients who underwent laparoscopic cryoablation, and renal fracture occurred in 3 (8%) (51). In two cases, the estimated intra-operative blood loss was 650 and 900 cc, respectively, and other than blood transfusion, no other intervention was reported. The authors did make some hypotheses on the reasons for this complication, such as not inserting the cryoprobe perpendicularly into the tumor, movement of the probe during ablation, and removal of the probe after the second thaw phase, when the tissue has completely thawed. In this same series, one case of ureteropelvic junction obstruction occurred (3%), requiring pyeloplasty eight months after cryoablation.

Laparoscopic Pyeloplasty

This advanced reconstructive operation has been demonstrated to be as durable as open pyeloplasty, with success rates ranging from 88% to 98% (52–55). In addition to the complications associated with laparoscopy in general, some unique complications can occur.

In the largest series to date, Inagaki et al. reported on 147 laparoscopic transperitoneal pyeloplasties between 1993 and 2000 (52). Thirteen patients (9%) had complications, with two bowel injuries (1%) recognized and managed intra-operatively without sequelae. Urinary leakage occurred in three (2%), requiring laparoscopic repositioning of the drainage tube in two, and conservative management in one.

Laparoscopic Donor Nephrectomy

Laparoscopic donor nephrectomy was introduced by Ratner et al. in 1995, and this operation has been increasingly performed, such that kidneys from living donors currently exceed cadaveric sources (56). In terms of approach, hand-assisted, pure laparoscopic, and robot-assisted donor nephrectomy have been reported (Table 6).

Jacobs et al. reported on 738 consecutive laparoscopic living donor nephrectomies at the University of Maryland (57); 96% were left-sided kidneys, with an open conversion rate of 1.6% and blood transfusion rate of 1.2%. Vascular injury was the most common reason for open conversion, and 60% of vascular injuries occurred during the use of the vascular stapler. Major complications occurred in 6.8% of cases and 87% of these were vascular injuries to the great vessels or renal hilar vessels. Thirteen percent of the major complications were bowel injuries, requiring repair and delaying donor nephrectomy. Minor complications occurred in 17.1%, and included injuries to the spleen, liver, juxta-adrenal bleeding, and complications associated with graft extraction. In this series, the incidence of ureteral strictures or necrosis was stratified by year of surgery, and there was a significant decrease over the learning curve, with a rate of 7% initially, down to 2.5% by the sixth year.

In a similar study reviewing 381 cases, Su et al. reported on 381 cases, 95% of which were left-sided (58). Major complications occurred in 7.6%, and minor complications in 8.9%. The open conversion rate was 2.1%, most commonly for renal hilar vessel injury. Re-operation was necessary in seven patients (1.8%), including epigastric vessel injury, incisional hernia, scrotal exploration for ischemic testis, postoperative bleeding and duodenal injury requiring duodeno-jejunostomy. Su et al. examined the temporal trends of these complications by stratifying their series into quartiles of 95 patients. There was a statistically significant decrease ($p \leq 0.05$) in total donor complications, ureteral complications, allograft loss, and vascular thrombosis when the

TABLE 6   Laparoscopic Donor Nephrectomy Complications

Reference	N	Complications	Comments
Leventhal et al. (75)	500	6% overall 1.8% open conversion 1.4% renovascular complications 0.6% splenic capsular tear 0.6% pulmonary 1.2% urinary retention 0.8% wound infection 0.4% chylous ascites	2.8% intraoperative 3.4% postoperative
Posselt et al. (59)	387	5.9% overall 0.3% open conversion 4.7% delayed graft function 4.1% ureteral complications 1.5% transfusion 0.5% bowel injury 2.3% wound infection 0.3% pulmonary embolus	
Jacobs et al. (57)	738	8.8% overall 1.6% open conversion 0.5% delayed graft function 4.5% ureteral complications 1.2% blood transfusions 1.8% major vascular injury 0.3% bowel injuries	

first and last quartiles were compared. Specifically, the total complication rate in the first 95 cases was 21%, whereas a 10.4% rate was observed in the last 96 cases.

Right-sided laparoscopic donor nephrectomies are traditionally not favored because of concerns about inadequate renal vein length, poorer exposure due to the liver and potential caval injury. However, Posselt et al. reported their experience on 387 pure laparoscopic donor nephrectomies, of which 54 (14%) were right-sided (59). They found no difference in blood loss, length of stay and graft complications between left-sided and right-sided donors.

Another complaint patients may have after donor nephrectomy is ipsilateral orchalgia, which has been reported to occur in 9.6% of cases (60). The onset of this symptom is typically around postoperative day five. Nonsteroidal anti-inflammatory drugs are generally prescribed with complete resolution noted in 50% after an average of six months of follow up. In the remainder, persistent pain is reported, with one case of atrophy.

CONCLUSIONS

Minimally invasive renal surgery has truly been an advance in the urological armamentarium. Both benign and malignant renal conditions, ranging from extirpative to reconstructive, can be managed using these techniques.

Urological surgeons can be proud to be able to offer these innovative options, and their patients will continue to benefit from the decreased postoperative pain, shorter convalescence period, and improved cosmesis from these procedures. While the benefits of minimally invasive surgery are clear, the urological surgeon and the patient must be cognizant of the potential life-threatening complications that can occur intra- and postoperatively.

Over the past 15 years, reports of complications associated with these operations have allowed surgeons to improve their techniques in primary prevention and early recognition of these complications. With further research, even more innovative minimally invasive techniques should be possible for surgical renal diseases.

REFERENCES

1. Simforoosh N, Basiri A, Tabibi A, Shakhssalim N, Hosseini Moghaddam SM. Comparison of laparoscopic and open donor nephrectomy: a randomized controlled trial. BJU Int 2005; 95(6):851–855.

2. Link RE, Bhayani SB, Allaf ME, et al. Exploring the learning curve, pathological outcomes and peri-operative morbidity of laparoscopic partial nephrectomy performed for renal mass. J Urol 2005; 173(5):1690–1694.

3. Matin SF, Abreu S, Ramani A, et al. Evaluation of age and comorbidity as risk factors after laparoscopic urological surgery. J Urol 2003; 170(4 Pt 1):1115–1120.

4. Conacher ID, Soomro NA, Rix D. Anaesthesia for laparoscopic urological surgery. Br J Anaesth 2004; 93(6):859–864.

5. Parsons JK, Jarrett TJ, Chow GK, Kavoussi LR. The effect of previous abdominal surgery on urological laparoscopy. J Urol 2002; 168(6):2387–2390.

6. O'Connor JP, Biyani CS, Taylor J, Agarwal V, Curley PJ, Browning AJ. Laparoscopic nephrectomy for renal-cell carcinoma during pregnancy. J Endourol 2004; 18(9):871–874.

7. Wolf JS Jr, Marcovich R, Gill IS, et al. Survey of neuromuscular injuries to the patient and surgeon during urologic laparoscopic surgery. Urology 2000; 55(6):831–836.

8. Shankar S, Vansonnenberg E, Silverman SG, Tuncali K, Flanagan HL Jr. Whang EE. Brachial plexus injury from CT-guided RF ablation under general anesthesia. Cardiovasc Intervent Radiol 2005; 28(5):646–648.

9. Tuncali BE, Tuncali B, Kuvaki B, Cinar O, Dogan A, Elar Z. Radial nerve injury after general anaesthesia in the lateral decubitus position. Anaesthesia 2005; 60(6):602–604.

10. Cadeddu JA, Wolfe JS Jr. Nakada S, et al. Complications of laparoscopic procedures after concentrated training in urological laparoscopy. J Urol 2001; 166(6):2109–2111.

11. Morris RJ, Woodcock JP. Evidence-based compression: prevention of stasis and deep vein thrombosis. Ann Surg 2004; 239(2):162–171.

12. Parsons JK, Varkarakis I, Rha KH, Jarrett TW, Pinto PA, Kavoussi LR. Complications of abdominal urologic laparoscopy: longitudinal five-year analysis. Urology 2004; 63(1):27–32.

13. Guillonneau B, Abbou CC, Doublet JD, et al. Proposal for a "European Scoring System for Laparoscopic Operations in Urology." Eur Urol 2001; 40(1):2–6; discussion 7.

14. Fahlenkamp D, Rassweiler J, Fornara P, Frede T, Loening SA. Complications of laparoscopic procedures in urology: experience with 2407 procedures at 4 German centers. J Urol 1999; 162(3 Pt 1):765–770; discussion 770–771.

15. Vallancien G, Cathelineau X, Baumert H, Doublet JD, Guillonneau B. Complications of transperitoneal laparoscopic surgery in urology: review of 1311 procedures at a single center. J Urol 2002; 168(1):23–26.

16. Soulie M, Salomon L, Seguin P, et al. Multi-institutional study of complications in 1085 laparoscopic urologic procedures. Urology 2001; 58(6):899–903.

17. Madeb R, Koniaris LG, Patel HR, et al. Complications of laparoscopic urologic surgery. J Laparoendosc Adv Surg Tech A 2004; 14(5):287–301.

18. Chandler JG, Corson SL, Way LW. Three spectra of laparoscopic entry access injuries. J Am Coll Surg 2001; 192(4):478–490; discussion 490–491.

19. Seifman BD, Dunn RL, Wolf JS Jr. Transperitoneal laparoscopy into the previously operated abdomen: effect on operative time, length of stay and complications. J Urol 2003; 169(1):36–40.

20. Wetter PA, ed. Prevention and Management of Laparoendoscopic Surgical Complications. 2nd edn. Miami, FL: Society of Laparoendoscopic Surgeons, 2005.

21. Cadeddu JA, Chan DY, Hedican SP, et al. Retroperitoneal access for transperitoneal laparoscopy in patients at high risk for intra-abdominal scarring. J Endourol 1999; 13(8):567–570.

22. Shackelford RT, Zuidema G, ed. Surgery of the Alimentary Tract. 2nd edn. Philadelphia, PA: W.B. Saunders, 1981.

23. Bishoff JT, Allaf ME, Kirkels W, Moore RG, Kavoussi LR, Schroder F. Laparoscopic bowel injury: incidence and clinical presentation. J Urol 1999; 161(3):887–890.

24. Meraney AM, Samee AA, Gill IS. Vascular and bowel complications during retroperitoneal laparoscopic surgery. J Urol 2002; 168(5):1941–1944.

25. Cadeddu JA, Regan F, Kavoussi LR, Moore RG. The role of computerized tomography in the evaluation of complications after laparoscopic urological surgery. J Urol 1997; 158(4):1349–1352.

26. Wolf JS Jr. Clayman RV, McDougall EM, Shepherd DL, Folger WH, Monk TG. Carbon dioxide and helium insufflation during laparoscopic radical nephrectomy in a patient with severe pulmonary disease. J Urol 1996; 155(6):2021.

27. Del Pizzo JJ, Jacobs SC, Bishoff JT, Kavoussi LR, Jarrett TW. Pleural injury during laparoscopic renal surgery: early recognition and management. J Urol 2003; 169(1):41–44.

28. Potter SR, Kavoussi LR, Jackman SV. Management of diaphragmatic injury during laparoscopic nephrectomy. J Urol 2001; 165(4):1203–1204.

29. Bhayani SB, Grubb RL 3rd, Andriole GL. Use of gelatin matrix to rapidly repair diaphragmatic injury during laparoscopy. Urology 2002; 60(3):514.

30. Lam JS, Shvarts O, Leppert JT, Pantuck AJ, Figlin RA, Belldegrun AS. Postoperative surveillance protocol for patients with localized and locally advanced renal cell carcinoma based on a validated prognostic nomogram and risk group stratification system. J Urol 2005; 174(2):466–472; discussion 472; quiz 801.

31. Hernandez F, Rha KH, Pinto PA, et al. Laparoscopic nephrectomy: assessment of morcellation versus intact specimen extraction on postoperative status. J Urol 2003; 170(2 Pt 1):412–415.
32. Tsivian A, Sidi AA. Port site metastases in urological laparoscopic surgery. J Urol 2003; 169(4):1213–1218.
33. Micali S, Celia A, Bove P, et al. Tumor seeding in urological laparoscopy: an international survey. J Urol 2004; 171(6 Pt 1):2151–2154.
34. Rassweiler J, Tsivian A, Kumar AV et al. Oncological safety of laparoscopic surgery for urological malignancy: experience with more than 1000 operations. J Urol 2003; 169(6):2072–2075.
35. Rumstadt B, Sturm J, Jentschura D, Schwab M, Schuster K. Trocar incision and closure: daily problems in laparoscopic procedures—a new technical aspect. Surg Laparosc Endosc 1997; 7(4):345–348.
36. Lowry PS, Moon TD, D'Alessandro A, Nakada SY. Symptomatic port-site hernia associated with a non-bladed trocar after laparoscopic live-donor nephrectomy. J Endourol 2003; 17(7):493–494.
37. Nelson CP, Wolf JS Jr. Comparison of hand assisted versus standard laparoscopic radical nephrectomy for suspected renal cell carcinoma. J Urol 2002; 167(5):1989–1994.
38. Terranova SA, Siddiqui KM, Preminger GM, Albala DM. Hand-assisted laparoscopic renal surgery: hand-port incision complications. J Endourol 2004; 18(8):775–779.
39. Cadeddu JA, Ono Y, Clayman RV, et al. Laparoscopic nephrectomy for renal cell cancer: evaluation of efficacy and safety: a multicenter experience. Urology 1998; 52(5):773–777.
40. McAllister M, Bhayani SB, Ong A, et al. Vena caval transection during retroperitoneoscopic nephrectomy: report of the complication and review of the literature. J Urol 2004; 172(1):183–185.
41. Gill IS, Matin SF, Desai MM, et al. Comparative analysis of laparoscopic versus open partial nephrectomy for renal tumors in 200 patients. J Urol 2003; 170(1):64–68.
42. Ramani AP, Desai MM, Steinberg AP, et al. Complications of laparoscopic partial nephrectomy in 200 cases. J Urol 2005; 173(1):42–47.
43. Kim FJ, Rha KH, Hernandez F, Jarrett TW, Pinto PA, Kavoussi LR. Laparoscopic radical versus partial nephrectomy: assessment of complications. J Urol 2003; 170(2 Pt 1):408–411.
44. Guillonneau B, Bermudez H, Gholami S, et al. Laparoscopic partial nephrectomy for renal tumor: single center experience comparing clamping and no clamping techniques of the renal vasculature. J Urol 2003; 169(2):483–486.
45. Moore CJ, Rozen SM, Fishman EK. Two cases of pseudoaneurysm of the renal artery following laparoscopic partial nephrectomy for renal cell carcinoma: CT angiographic evaluation. Emerg Radiol 2004; 10(4):193–196.
46. Desai MM, Gill IS. Laparoscopic partial nephrectomy for tumour: current status at the Cleveland Clinic. BJU Int 2005; 95(suppl 2):41–45.
47. Johnson DB, Solomon SB, Su LM, et al. Defining the complications of cryoablation and radio frequency ablation of small renal tumors: a multi-institutional review. J Urol 2004; 172(3):874–877.
48. Margulis V, Matsumoto ED, Taylor G, Shaffer S, Kabbani W, Cadeddu JA. Retrograde renal cooling during radio frequency ablation to protect from renal collecting system injury. J Urol 2005; 174(1):350–352.
49. Silverman SG, Tuncali K, vanSonnenberg E, et al. Renal tumors: MR imaging-guided percutaneous cryotherapy—initial experience in 23 patients. Radiology 2005; 236(2):716–724.
50. Lee DI, McGinnis DE, Feld R, Strup SE. Retroperitoneal laparoscopic cryoablation of small renal tumors: intermediate results. Urology 2003; 61(1):83–88.
51. Cestari A, Guazzoni G, dell'Acqua V, et al. Laparoscopic cryoablation of solid renal masses: intermediate term followup. J Urol 2004; 172(4 Pt 1):1267–1270.
52. Inagaki T, Rha KH, Ong AM, Kavoussi LR, Jarrett TW. Laparoscopic pyeloplasty: current status. BJU Int 2005; 95(suppl 2):102–105.
53. Janetschek G, Peschel R, Bartsch G. Laparoscopic Fenger plasty. J Endourol 2000; 14(10):889–893.
54. Soulie M, Salomon L, Patard JJ, et al. Extraperitoneal laparoscopic pyeloplasty: a multicenter study of 55 procedures. J Urol 2001; 166(1):48–50.
55. Turk IA, Davis JW, Winkelmann B, et al. Laparoscopic dismembered pyeloplasty—the method of choice in the presence of an enlarged renal pelvis and crossing vessels. Eur Urol 2002; 42(3):268–275.
56. Schweitzer EJ, Wilson J, Jacobs S, et al. Increased rates of donation with laparoscopic donor nephrectomy. Ann Surg 2000; 232(3):392–400.
57. Jacobs SC, Cho E, Foster C, Liao P, Bartlett ST. Laparoscopic donor nephrectomy: the University of Maryland 6-year experience. J Urol 2004; 171(1):47–51.
58. Su LM, Ratner LE, Montgomery RA, et al. Laparoscopic live donor nephrectomy: trends in donor and recipient morbidity following 381 consecutive cases. Ann Surg 2004; 240(2):358–363.
59. Posselt AM, Mahanty H, Kang SM, et al. Laparoscopic right donor nephrectomy: a large single-center experience. Transplantation 2004; 78(11):1665–1669.
60. Kim FJ, Pinto P, Su LM, et al. Ipsilateral orchialgia after laparoscopic donor nephrectomy. J Endourol 2003; 17(6):405–409.
61. Ono Y, Kinukawa T, Hattori R, Gotoh M, Kamihira O, Ohshima S. The long-term outcome of laparoscopic radical nephrectomy for small renal cell carcinoma. J Urol 2001; 165(6 Pt 1):1867–1870.

62. Stifelman MD, Handler T, Nieder AM, et al. Hand-assisted laparoscopy for large renal specimens: a multi-institutional study. Urology 2003; 61(1):78–82.
63. Gill IS, Meraney AM, Schweizer DK, et al. Laparoscopic radical nephrectomy in 100 patients: a single center experience from the United States. Cancer 2001; 92(7):1843–1855.
64. Abukora F, Nambirajan T, Albqami N, et al. Laparoscopic nephron sparing surgery: evolution in a decade. Eur Urol 2005; 47(4):488–493; discussion 493.
65. Gervais DA, Arellano RS, McGovern FJ, McDougal WS, Mueller PR. Radiofrequency ablation of renal cell carcinoma: part 2, Lessons learned with ablation of 100 tumors. AJR Am J Roentgenol 2005; 185(1):72–80.
66. Varkarakis IM, Allaf ME, Inagaki T, et al. Percutaneous radio frequency ablation of renal masses: results at a 2-year mean followup. J Urol 2005; 174(2):456–460; discussion 460.
67. Mayo-Smith WW, Dupuy DE, Parikh PM, Pezzullo JA, Cronan JJ. Imaging-guided percutaneous radiofrequency ablation of solid renal masses: techniques and outcomes of 38 treatment sessions in 32 consecutive patients. AJR Am J Roentgenol 2003; 180(6):1503–1508.
68. Farrell MA, Charboneau WJ, DiMarco DS, et al. Imaging-guided radiofrequency ablation of solid renal tumors. AJR Am J Roentgenol 2003; 180(6):1509–1513.
69. Hwang JJ, Walther MM, Pautler SE, et al. Radio frequency ablation of small renal tumors:: intermediate results. J Urol 2004; 171(5):1814–1818.
70. Matsumoto ED, Johnson DB, Ogan K, et al. Short-term efficacy of temperature-based radiofrequency ablation of small renal tumors. Urology 2005; 65(5):877–881.
71. Gill IS, Remer EM, Hasan WA, et al. Renal cryoablation: outcome at 3 years. J Urol 2005; 173(6):1903–1907.
72. Bachmann A, Sulser T, Jayet C, et al. Retroperitoneoscopy-assisted cryoablation of renal tumors using multiple 1.5 mm ultrathin cryoprobes: a preliminary report. Eur Urol 2005; 47(4):474–479.
73. Moon TD, Lee FT Jr. Hedican SP, Lowry P, Nakada SY. Laparoscopic cryoablation under sonographic guidance for the treatment of small renal tumors. J Endourol 2004; 18(5):436–440.
74. Shingleton WB, Sewell PE Jr. Percutaneous renal tumor cryoablation with magnetic resonance imaging guidance. J Urol 2001; 165(3):773–776.
75. Leventhal JR, Kocak B, Salvalaggio PR, et al. Laparoscopic donor nephrectomy 1997 to 2003: lessons learned with 500 cases at a single institution. Surgery 2004; 136(4):881–890.

32 | Complications in Ureteroscopy

Brent Yanke and Demetrius Bagley
Department of Urology, Thomas Jefferson University, Philadelphia, Pennsylvania, U.S.A.

INTRODUCTION

In a medical climate increasingly geared toward minimally invasive procedures, ureteroscopy has gained a place as a primary treatment modality for an array of urologic applications including stone disease, ureteropelvic junction (UPJ) obstruction, and upper urinary tract transitional-cell carcinoma (UTTCC). Its modern clinical use was first described in the late 1970s by Lyon et al. as were the first complications (1,2). At that time, the potential hazards of ureteroscopy were foreseen when these authors stated that "disasters, such as perforation of the ureter, are a distinct possibility if care and thought are not practiced." Since that time, several large series have been published on rates and types of complications (3–7). In these more recent reports, overall complication rates have ranged from 8% to 16%.

With increased surgical experience and improvements in endoscopic equipment the number of overall and severe complications has decreased. In their experience of 2735 retrograde ureteroscopy procedures over a 10-year period, Geavlete et al. confirmed that 77% of their complications appeared in the first five years compared to only 23% in the last five years (3). Likewise, Harmon et al. described a reduction in the rate of major complications from 6.6% to 1.5% over time (4). Increased surgeon experience has been associated with a decrease in both the number of intraoperative injuries as well as the number of postoperative complications (5,8). At the same time, smaller semirigid and flexible ureteroscopes have increased the efficacy of treatment while also decreasing risk. Abdel-Razzak and Bagley demonstrated that the 6.9F semirigid ureteroscope precluded the need for dilation of the ureteral orifice, giving a clearer picture for diagnostic purposes (9). In a comparison of conventional rigid ureteroscopes (9.5–11.5F) with small-caliber semirigid ureteroscopes (6–7.5F), Francesca et al. reported a three-fold decrease in complications with the latter instruments (7).

In this chapter, intraoperative complications will be reviewed along with those occurring in the early and late postoperative period. In addition, events will be classified based on their severity. Minor complications make up the majority of incidents encountered during and after ureteroscopy. These can be effectively managed by nonoperative means with minimal sequelae. Major complications constitute injuries that necessitate operative intervention or are life-threatening. In two large series, open surgery was performed in only 0.22% of patients (3,10). Although these complications are clearly rare, they can have enduring effects that contribute to long-term morbidity.

INTRAOPERATIVE COMPLICATIONS
Major Complications
Intussusception

Ureteral intussusception refers to the telescoping of mucosa after circumferential injury weakens the ureteral wall. Reports are infrequent and generally are spontaneous due to a ureteral tumor such as transitional cell carcinoma, polyp, or inverted papilloma (11–13). A small number of iatrogenic causes have been described including retrograde intussusception as a result of repeated ureteroscopy and antegrade intussusception during endopyelotomy (14,15). This complication typically arises during basket extraction of a large stone through a smaller caliber ureter that cannot accommodate the stone and basket together. With the use of larger ureteroscopes earlier, there were also instances of the ureter being dragged proximally as the ureteroscope was advanced.

Intussusception should be suspected when there is difficulty placing a stent after basket deployment or when upper tract obstruction persists after stone retrieval (14). When performed, retrograde ureteropyelography may show the characteristic "bell-shaped" ureter (16). Stent placement over the safety wire can be attempted but generally this is only a temporizing measure as much of the ureter distal to the injury is devitalized. Appropriate treatment entails open or laparoscopic surgical excision of the intussuscepted segment followed by ureteroneocystostomy, ureteroureterostomy or ureteropyelostomy.

Avulsion

Complete avulsion of the ureter is perhaps the most dreaded complication encountered during ureteroscopy. The first report of avulsion using a Dormia basket was reported in 1967 by Hart (17). Luckily, its occurrence is relatively rare with rates of 0% to 0.5% reported in several large series (3,8,10,18). As is the case with intussusception, avulsion generally occurs during forceful removal of a stone through a segment of ureter with a diameter smaller than the stone itself. The proximal third of the ureter is at particular risk as it has less muscle support and contains a thinner layer of mucosal cells than the distal ureter (19). Additional risks for avulsion include the presence of an impacted stone, stone retrieval in a diseased portion of the ureter, and the use of multiple wire baskets (19).

Immediate recognition of the injury usually occurs because either the ureter is seen with the stone as it is extracted from the patient or a portion of the ureter is seen in the bladder during cystoscopy. Infrequently, delayed recognition can be observed in the setting of fevers, flank pain, or a flank mass due to a urinoma or an abscess (20). If this is suspected, retrograde pyelography, computed tomography (CT) urography, or intravenous pyelography (IVP) can be performed. The retrograde pyelogram will reveal extravasation with lack of contrast in the proximal ureter while the CT urogram and IVP will demonstrate a urinoma or extravasation with lack of contrast in the distal ureter.

Prudent use of the basket during stone extraction is the key to ureteral avulsion prevention. Stones should not be extracted with the basket if they are larger than any portion of the ureter distal to the stone. If the stone does not travel easily then basketing should be abandoned and either lithotripsy should be performed or stenting must be considered if significant trauma is present. Vigilance should be employed with proximal stones as well as in cases with the aforementioned risk factors. Improved safety is provided by newer tipless nitinol baskets which can be withdrawn from the ureter more safely than tipped baskets (19). The ability of these baskets to articulate improves stone-releasing capability. Some authors have advocated the use of reversible, wire-pronged graspers that allow release of the stone as a safer alternative to stone basketing (21). In cases of an entrapped basket, excessive force to remove the basket and stone can also result in partial or complete avulsion as well as intussusception. Geavlete et al. reported 19 cases of trapped stone extractors in their series, representing 0.7% of all cases (3). Eighteen were treated by endoscopic means while one required open ureterolithotomy and basket removal. Several approaches have been described to remove entrapped baskets. One method involves fragmentation of the basketed stone using extracorporeal shock wave lithotripsy (ESWL), although this measure may fail if a part of the ureteral wall has been caught within the wires of the basket (19). An entrapped basket can be treated endoscopically by disassembling the basket, removing the ureteroscope, and replacing it alongside the basket (3). Once the stone and basket are in view, lithotripsy can be performed. However, care must be taken to avoid the basket wires if laser is used. In a study testing wire durability to holmium laser application, Honeck et al. found that the average time required to transect a safety wire was 55 to 103 seconds (22). In comparison, they reported that nitinol basket wires were disrupted after only 1 to 4 seconds.

When complete avulsion is encountered, open or laparoscopic repair is the mainstay of treatment. The type of repair is dependent on factors such as location of the avulsion, length of devitalized ureter, patient age and comorbidities, and renal function. With the use of a safety wire, a stent can be placed in order to temporize the situation and provide drainage. However, strictures will subsequently develop requiring further treatment. Distal injuries are best addressed with ureteroneocystostomy. However, longer ureteral defects as well as those in the middle third may require the addition of a psoas hitch, a Boari flap, or a combination of both

(23). Short injuries to the middle third of the ureter can often be repaired by ureteroureterostomy. Proximal avulsions can be treated with ureteroureterostomy or dismembered pyeloplasty if the length of devitalized ureter is short. Often the length of damage is extensive and more complex procedures such as ileal interposition or autotransplantation are required (24). Bluebond-Langner et al. recently described two cases of significant ureteral loss after avulsion in which laparoscopic nephrectomy with renal autotransplantation was successfully performed (25). In rare cases, nephrectomy may be a reasonable option for the patient with good contralateral renal function who is at risk with a more involved repair (26). Finally, delayed recognition of an avulsion injury or an unstable patient may warrant placement of a percutaneous nephrostomy until the time of definitive repair (21).

Minor Complications
Perforation
Although the reported incidence of ureteral perforation has decreased over the last several decades, it remains one of the most common complications. The first perforations were reported by Lyon et al. in the late 1970s (1,2). Early series had perforation rates exceeding 15%. In 1987, Kramolowsky reported perforations in 17% of 142 ureteroscopic procedures (27). In this series, one perforation was caused by patient movement during a cough while under epidural anesthesia. Harmon et al. referred to this incident when stating that general anesthesia with muscle paralysis would aid in preventing ureteral injuries (4). Another early series by Stoller et al. in 1992 reported a similar perforation rate of 15.4% using a larger caliber 12.5F ureteroscope (28).

Development of smaller diameter ureteroscopes had a dramatic impact on reported perforation rates. In 1993, Abdel-Razzak and Bagley published their series of 65 cases where the smaller 6.9F semirigid ureteroscope was used (9). There was only one minor perforation which was due to the use of electrohydraulic lithotripsy (EHL). These authors found a 1.7% perforation rate in 290 procedures using smaller flexible ureteroscopes ranging from 8.5 to 10.5F (29). In a follow-up study, Grasso and Bagley described their experience with small-diameter, actively deflectable, flexible ureteroscopes (18). Using ureteroscopes that were 8F or smaller, there were no perforations in 492 consecutive patients. Recent large series reporting on complications cite perforation rates between 0.5% and 4.7% with the majority at 1% or less (3–6,10).

The evolution of lithotrite modalities available in ureteroscopy has also contributed to its increased safety. Despite early studies reporting no perforations with EHL, the limited safety margin of EHL has clearly been demonstrated (30,31). Direct activation on urothelium causes a punch-like perforation while more extensive tissue damage is produced by the cavitation bubble when the probe is not in direct contact with urothelium (32). Bilen et al. reported perforations in four of 13 patients where EHL was used for disintegration of stones (33). On the other hand, perforation rates for pneumatic lithotripsy have ranged from 0% to 3.4% (34–36). In a comparison of EHL and pneumatic lithotripsy, Hofbauer et al. demonstrated equivalent efficacy but with significantly different perforation rates (17.6% vs. 2.6%, respectively) (37). While the holmium:yttrium aluminum garnet (Ho:YAG) laser does not discriminate between tissue types, it does have a low perforation rate in clinical use. Because holmium laser energy is absorbed within 0.5 mm, ureteral perforation risk is minimal if direct contact with mucosa is avoided (32,38). With the stone positioned between the laser and ureteral mucosa, risk of tissue damage is negligible. Sofer et al. reported one perforation attributable to the laser while treating 598 patients over a seven-year period (32).

All instruments in the ureteroscopic armamentarium have the potential to perforate the ureter. As discussed earlier, ureteroscopes and various lithotrites can cause perforation but other equipments such as guidewires, baskets, balloon dilators, and ureteral catheters can also commonly cause perforations. Regardless of the source, the vast majority of perforations is small and can be managed conservatively with ureteral stent placement for four to six weeks. A safety wire should be placed at the beginning of the procedure to allow stent placement in these situations. If access is lost and a wire or ureteroscope cannot be traversed past the perforation, then the procedure should be terminated and percutaneous nephrostomy with possible antegrade stenting should be considered. In rare cases of large perforations, open or laparoscopic repair may be necessary.

False Passage

False passage describes perforation of the ureteral mucosa and submucosal tunneling of the offending instrument without full penetration through the ureteral wall. Excessive force and improper placement of the ureteroscope, in particular when entering the ureteral orifice, can easily result in a false passage necessitating termination of the procedure. Guidewires, stone retrieval baskets, and lasers are all capable of creating false passages especially in the treatment of urolithiasis. Often, false passages are overlooked and many series fail to comment or report on them (5,6,10). In a series of iatrogenic ureteric injuries, Al-Awadi et al. described 15 false passages (18.3%), making it one of the most common complications in their series (39). If a false passage is not appreciated, a truly disastrous consequence can occur if the ureteroscope is then passed over the misplaced guidewire (40). The ensuing dissection can interfere with ureteral blood supply resulting in necrosis and stricture or, in severe cases, loss of the entire ureter.

A false passage should be suspected when a guidewire does not travel up the ureter smoothly or when there is a lack of coil in the renal pelvis or calyces. If there are concerns of a false passage, an open-ended or dual-lumen ureteral catheter can be passed over the guidewire and a retrograde pyelogram performed. In this case, lack of contrast in the renal pelvis along with tracking of contrast around the collecting system confirms the diagnosis. When this occurs, the guidewire should be removed and replaced. If the false passage is relatively large and obstructing or if several attempts at placement have failed, the ureteroscope may be needed to place the guidewire under direct vision.

These injuries are relatively benign and treatment generally consists of ureteral stenting for two to four weeks. A small false passage can be managed conservatively without a stent if no other indications for stent placement are present (21). Like most complications, adherence to proper technique and safety will make this a rare occurrence. When intubating the ureter with the ureteroscope, the lumen must always be kept in the center of the screen. Passing the ureteroscope over a guidewire can help navigate difficult passageways while balloon dilatation can make narrow ureters easier to traverse. If a guidewire cannot easily pass a point of obstruction, an angled-tip hydromer-coated guidewire should be utilized to bypass the area gently (38). A safety wire is imperative as cases where the ureter is impassable will require a stent.

Extravasation

Ureteral perforations and avulsions can lead to varying amounts of extravasation. Commonly, urine, irrigant, contrast, and blood can travel into the retroperitoneal space but calculi and tumor can also be propelled through the ureter. Information on extravasation is often not reported. In their series of 290 procedures, Abdel-Razzak and Bagley described three cases of extravasation (1.0%) (29). In general, small perforations result in minor amounts of extravasation that are of no clinical significance. However, large disruptions of the ureter can produce considerable collections with detrimental consequences. Lytton et al. described a patient with perforation and urinoma formation that required subsequent drainage (40). These urine collections can become infected necessitating percutaneous or open drainage. During ureteroscopy, extravasation can be demonstrated on retrograde pyelography after perforation or overfilling of the collecting system (Fig. 1).

Stone extravasation is a well-recognized event with a reported incidence of approximately 1% (41,42). This occurs as a result of perforation during lithotripsy followed by extrusion of the stone while engaging the lithotrite or while irrigating. Several authors have confirmed the harmless nature of periureteral stones (41–43). Lopez-Alcina et al. noted 11 occurrences in 1047 consecutive patients treated with pulsed-dye laser lithotripsy (42). With a mean follow-up of 18 months, no evidence of urinary extravasation, infection, or secondary ureteral strictures was found. Evans and Stoller observed five patients with stone extravasation arguing against aggressive ureteroscopic manipulation and stone retrieval (41). They stressed the importance of radiologic documentation and patient understanding of the extra-ureteral stone location in order to avoid future misdiagnosis and mismanagement. Grasso et al. employed a 6F intraluminal ultrasound probe to assess depth and location of extruded stones in 20 patients referred for obstruction from stone fragments (43). They confirmed that stones more than 4 mm from the lumen caused no obstruction and could be left in situ safely. However, they commented that submucosal fragments needed to be removed in order to relieve the obstruction.

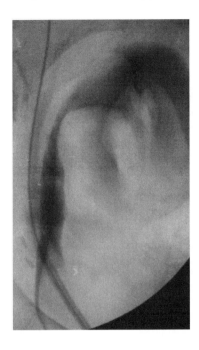

FIGURE 1 Retrograde pyelogram demonstrating extravasation from the collecting system.

The theoretical risk of extraluminal seeding of upper tract neoplasms during biopsy and treatment has been addressed by Lam and Gupta (44). They noted one report of tumor cells found in the submucosal lymphatic and vascular structures in a nephroureterectomy specimen removed immediately after ureteroscopy and biopsy of the neoplasm (45). However, they also refer to several published series reporting no adverse events following perforation during endoscopic management of upper tract tumors. In particular, Hendin et al. confirmed that diagnostic ureteroscopy for UTTCC had no adverse effects on long-term or disease-specific survival (46).

Thermal Injury
Thermal energy is produced by many ureteroscopic devices including lasers, electrocautery, and EHL probes. Heat produced from the EHL probe spark can produce coagulative necrosis leading to perforation when in contact with urothelium (47). The neodymium:YAG (Nd:YAG) laser has a depth of penetration of 5–6 mm. This makes it effective for treatment of upper tract tumors. However, its use in the ureter should be minimized to avoid damage to adjacent organs (38). As mentioned previously, the Ho:YAG laser has a smaller depth of penetration of 0.5 mm. When applied directly to a ureteral tu mor, thermal damage to adjacent tissues is minimized. In an ex vivo model on pig ureters, Santa-Cruz et al. demonstrated that at a depth of 0.5 mm, the Ho:YAG laser was able to perforate in two seconds at a setting of 5 W with only 0.01 kJ delivered (48). However, when placed two mm away from mucosa, the laser was unable to perforate at any energy setting. Several studies have confirmed that judicious use of the Ho: YAG laser during lithotripsy will result in minimal to no risk of thermal damage to adjacent urothelium (49,50). Minimal thermal damage can be managed but more extensive damage will likely need short-term stent placement.

Mucosal Abrasion
Any instrument passed through the ureter can cause mucosal abrasions. The larger the instrument, the more is the friction applied to the ureteral mucosa. Identifiable mucosal abrasions were reported in 0.3% of 2273 patients by Butler et al. (10). They noted that the seven mucosal tears were caused by the ureteroscope itself. Geavlete et al. likewise reported a low incidence in their series with mucosal abrasions being found in 1.5% of patients (3). These lesions generally have no significant consequence. However, mucosal flaps may bleed or obstruct the lumen

thereby decreasing visibility. In most cases, only observation is warranted. If there is considerable bleeding or edema, obstruction may ensue and a ureteral stent should be placed for drainage (21).

Bleeding

Intraoperative causes of bleeding include trauma to the ureteral orifice during ureteroscope insertion, abrasions caused by passage of the guidewire, overdistention of the collecting system, and tissue damage during stone fragmentation and tumor treatment. Most bleeding episodes are minor and have little impact on the case. However, a small blood clot can obscure vision. Occasionally, bleeding is profuse enough to cause termination of the procedure as a result of poor visibility. Geavlete et al. reported three of 2735 total procedures (0.1%) where visibility difficulties secondary to bleeding forced them to halt the procedure and place a ureteral stent (3). In their series of 290 cases, Abdel-Razzak and Bagley reported on three patients that had prolonged bleeding lasting longer than two days (29). None of these patients required blood transfusion.

Acucise endopyelotomy which employs a cutting balloon under fluoroscopic control has been associated with significant bleeding complications (51). Kim et al. described three patients that required blood transfusion after the procedure. Two of these patients underwent angioembolization of lower-pole branching arteries to attain hemostasis. Significantly lower rates of bleeding have been reported during holmium laser endopyelotomy (52). Use of an endoluminal ultrasound can help prevent significant bleeding during direct-vision endopyelotomy (53). Imaging of the periureteral anatomy can lead to the identification of crossing and adjacent vessels. As a result, a safe location for incision can be made.

In most cases, the use of smaller ureteroscopes precludes the need for ureteral orifice dilatation, thereby minimizing bleeding (9). Diagnostic accuracy can also be maintained by avoidance of guidewire trauma to the renal pelvis. Most bleeding is self-limiting but more severe bleeding may lead to clot formation necessitating stent placement. If reasonable hemostasis cannot be achieved, a tamponade balloon catheter may need to be placed. Persistent hemorrhage may necessitate angioembolization or more invasive surgery in extreme cases.

Difficult Access

Inability to traverse the ureter and gain access to the desired location was commonplace in early series. The large and rigid early ureteroscopes often made passage through the ureteral orifice difficult. In a comparison of patients treated between 1982 and 1985 to patients treated in 1992, Harmon et al. showed that success of diagnostic inspections increased from 73% to 98% (4). They attributed most failures in the earlier group to inability to access the upper tract as a result of the size of the endoscope. The development of small-diameter, actively deflectable, flexible ureteroscopes allowed inspection of the entire upper urinary tract with a minimal need for dilatation. Hudson et al. tested varying shaft diameters of flexible ureteroscopes in order to assess the need for ureteric dilatation (54). The rate of failing to pass with no formal dilatation was 37% for the 9.0F, 8.5% for the 8.6F, 5% for the 8.4F and 0.9% for the 7.4F ureteroscope. Using flexible ureteroscopes with an 8.5F tip diameter or less, Grasso and Bagley were able to access the entire intrarenal collecting system in 94% of 492 consecutive cases (18).

Situations preventing access include edema surrounding the stone, narrow or tortuous ureter, stricture, enlarged prostate, or trauma causing obstruction as can be the case with mucosal flaps or false passages. In many cases these circumstances arise as a result of previous surgical intervention or physiologic narrowing of the ureter (3). Soft strictures can be passively dilated with the ureteroscope, coaxial dilators, or dual-lumen catheters. Balloon dilators can also be utilized to open more rigid strictures. If the ureteroscope can still not be passed, a ureteral stent can be placed to allow gradual passive dilatation over several weeks time with definitive treatment thereafter. In some instances, the lumen is completely obliterated by tumor, stricture, or trauma. These patients may be best served by an antegrade approach.

Equipment Breakdown

Due to the complexity of the ureteroscopic equipment, occasional malfunction is inevitable. Carey et al. reported that new flexible ureteroscopes provided 40–48 uses before initial repair was required (55). However, after repair these ureteroscopes averaged only eight uses before needing repair again while older model ureteroscopes averaged between 4.75 and 7.7 uses before repair was needed. Ureteroscope damage can include loss of active deflection, loss of fiberoptic acuity, and shaft destruction. Improper technique such as excessive torque can lead to loss of deflection, bending of the ureteroscope, or fiberoptic destruction. Placement of accessory instruments through a deflected flexible ureteroscope can result in shaft perforation while activating the laser within the ureteroscope can destroy the channel, the optic fiber, or the structure of the shaft. Examples of accessory instrument malfunction include laser fiber fracture, stone basket breakage, and laser unit failure.

Proper inspection and care of instruments are essential in minimizing intraoperative equipment failure. All ureteroscopes should be inspected for damage before the procedure is begun. Standard evaluation includes testing the active defection and confirming optical quality through the eyepiece. The laser unit must be examined and ready for service while the laser fiber is inspected for damage before use. It is essential that additional semi-rigid and flexible ureteroscopes are readily available in case the first ureteroscope is damaged and unusable. Postoperatively, instruments should be properly cleaned, sterilized, and stored.

EARLY POSTOPERATIVE COMPLICATIONS
Major Complications
Infection and Fever

Infectious complications after ureteroscopy can be as mild as a low-grade fever or as serious as septic shock. Instrumentation in the presence of an infected urinary tract can lead to fever and sepsis. However, introduction of a pathogen into a sterile system is also a potential source of infection. In addition, stones and encrusted ureteral stents potentially harbor bacteria that can be spread during treatment.

In their series of 329 consecutive patients, Cheung et al. assessed predictive factors for postoperative events (56). There were no episodes of sepsis but eight (4.2%) patients had postoperative fever treated with intravenous antibiotics. Of note, none of these patients had culture-proven urinary tract infection. Of 2735 ureteroscopic procedures, Geavlete et al. reported 31 patients with postoperative fever or sepsis (1.13%) (3). Unfortunately, fever and sepsis were not distinguished. Schuster et al. identified four of 322 patients (1.2%) with urinary tract infection postoperatively (5). Only one patient was admitted for sepsis.

Several precautions should be taken to minimize the risk of postoperative infection. It is imperative that the preoperative culture is sterile. Any positive urine culture should be treated with appropriate antibiotics and a subsequent negative urine culture should be documented before the procedure. If infection is present in an obstructed collecting system, drainage by retrograde ureteral catheterization or percutaneous nephrostomy has been found to be equally effective (57). Although antibiotic prophylaxis is routinely practiced, its use is controversial. Knopf et al. compared 57 patients receiving a single 250 mg dose of Levofloxacin (Ortho-Mc Neil, Inc., Raritan, New Jersey, U.S.A.) prior to ureteroscopy to 60 patients receiving no prophylaxis (58). Although there were no postoperative symptomatic urinary tract infections in either group, significant bacteriuria was higher in the group without prophylaxis (12.5%) than in the group with prophylaxis (1.8%). They reasoned that single-dose prophylaxis could be beneficial in cases of unexpected intraoperative complications such as ureteral perforation. Finally, low-pressure irrigation should be used in order to prevent elevated intrarenal pressures. In the presence of bacteria, pyelovenous backflow created by elevated intrarenal pressures can lead to bacteremia and sepsis.

Minor Complications
Ureteral Obstruction and Acute Urinary Retention

Causes of postoperative ureteral obstruction include edema, clot, trauma, stone fragments, and stent migration (Fig. 2). Pain is often the manifesting symptom and it is generally recommended that a stent be placed in more complicated cases (56,59,60). Ureteral dilation has been associated with obstruction in clinical and animal models (6,61). Chow et al. recommend stent placement for all procedures involving ureteral dilation or ureteral complications. Stents

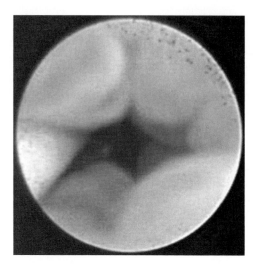

FIGURE 2   Endoscopic view of ureteral edema.

themselves have also been the source of ureteral obstruction. Typically, this is a result of proximal or distal stent migration as well as stent encrustation (Fig. 3). In their series of 329 consecutive patients, Cheung et al. reported five instances of proximal stent migration and 7 instances of distal stent migration (56). They attributed their rather high rate of stent migration to the use of shorter stents in their early procedures. Lam and Gupta recently described 26 patients requiring additional procedures for encrusted stents (62). While 23 patients (88.5%) had successful stent removal in a single session, the need for another procedure underscored the potential difficulties of postoperative ureteral obstruction from a retained stent.

In most cases, postoperative obstruction is self-limiting. Conservative treatment consisting of pain medications or intravenous fluids is generally all that is needed. However, persistent obstruction will often require a shorter duration of stenting. This allows passage of clots and stone fragments, resolution of edema, and healing of trauma. It is important to note that not all ureteral obstruction will be clinically evident. Weizer et al. discovered silent obstruction in seven of 459 patients (2.9%) undergoing ureteroscopy for stone disease (63). All of these patients required secondary ureteroscopy with one patient requiring chronic hemodialysis for renal failure. As a result, these authors recommended imaging within three months for all patients undergoing ureteroscopy for stone disease.

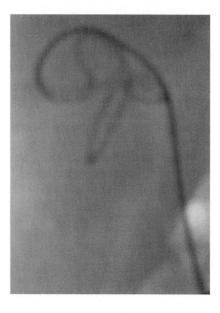

FIGURE 3   Fluoroscopy demonstrating proximal stent migration into the kidney.

Acute urinary retention is likely an underreported consequence of ureteroscopy. It has been cited to occur in <1% of procedures (5,6). Patients at increased risk, especially those with known symptomatic prostatic enlargement, should be considered for short-term postoperative catheterization. Vigilance should also be maintained for postoperative hematuria as clot retention can develop.

Stent Colic

Few topics are more controversial in ureteroscopy than the need for postoperative stenting. Complaints of colic and urinary symptoms frequently accompany stent placement. Many recent prospective trials have argued against the use of stents in uncomplicated cases (59,60,64). In a randomized trial, Byrne et al. (64) compared 38 stented and 22 nonstented procedures. Flank discomfort was significantly less common in the nonstented group on days 0, 1, and 6 (all $p < 0.005$) as was the incident of suprapubic pain on day 6 ($p = 0.002$). Urinary frequency, urgency, and dysuria were similar between the groups on postoperative day 1, but were significantly reduced in the nonstented group on day 6 (all $p < 0.005$). Only one patient in the non-stented group developed obstruction necessitating stenting. Cheung et al. agreed that routine stenting was not necessary after uncomplicated ureteroscopy (60). They stated that ureteral stents increased the incidence of pain and urinary symptoms but did not prevent postoperative urinary sepsis and unplanned medical visits. Severity of preoperative obstruction and intra-operative ureteral trauma were not shown to be determining factors for stenting. Stent placement is recommended for all cases of ureteral trauma. It should also be performed when there is increased risk of obstruction such as from bleeding, edema, previous obstruction, impacted stone, or large treated stone burden.

Vesicoureteral Reflux

Vesicoureteral reflux has been reported to occur in up to 20% of patients after balloon dilation (65). However, even after dilation, reflux has been confirmed to be transitory and low grade (61,65,66). Richter et al. addressed early postoperative reflux in their series of 40 patients (67). Reflux was demonstrated in four patients (10%) by retrograde cystography performed 24 hours after dilation during ureteroscopy. Follow-up cystograms performed 2 weeks later revealed resolution of reflux in all patients. Due to the low incidence and clinical insignificance of vesicoureteral reflux, in particular now that dilation is performed less often, routine postoperative radiographic surveillance is not justified.

LATE POSTOPERATIVE COMPLICATIONS
Major Complication
Ureteral Stricture

Ureteral stricture can present months to years after ureteroscopy. In most large series, incidence ranges from 0% to 3.3% (3,4,6,29,56,68,69). The most recent of these series has reported stricture rates of <1%. One postoperative stricture was discovered by Harmon et al. in their series of 209 procedures (0.5%) (4). They compared this to a stricture rate of 1.4% in an earlier series citing the use of smaller ureteroscopes, ureteral orifice dilation, and postoperative ureteral stenting as responsible for the decline. Trauma from instrumentation with larger ureteroscopes likely contributed to the development of ureteral strictures in early series (21). However, ureteral perforation has persisted as a risk factor for stricture formation. In a study of 42 patients with impacted ureteral stones treated by pneumatic lithotripsy, Brito et al. reported the development of seven ureteral strictures (16.6%) (70). One stricture developed in the 34 patients without ureteral perforation while six strictures developed in the eight patients with ureteral perforation.

The treatment of impacted stones can lead to perforations with subsequent embedding of stone fragments submucosally. Grasso et al. presented 20 patients referred after previous treatment failed to clear fragments or relieve obstruction (43). Using endoluminal ultrasound, they noted that multiple, small fragments embedded in the mucosa were often associated with subsequent stricture. They advocated removal of submucosal fragments within the wall of the ureter in order to relieve obstruction and avoid consequent stricture formation. Dretler and Young were the first to describe the stone granuloma as a cause of persistent symptomatic ureteral strictures (71). They evaluated five patients with ureteral strictures refractory to endourological methods of management and discovered embedded particles of calcium oxalate associated with macrophages and foreign body giant cells in four of them. These patients required more aggressive operative intervention in order to avoid stricture recurrence.

The ureteral access sheath has been a useful adjunct in flexible ureteroscopy. Although its use over a long duration may put the patient at risk of ischemic injury, increased risk of ureteral stricture development has not been seen (72).

Higher stricture rates have been observed with UTTCC treatment. Chen and Bagley summarized several series and reported 12 strictures in 139 patients (8.6%) (38). Due to the significantly smaller depth of penetration with the Ho:YAG laser, its use is associated with a decreased stricture rate compared to the Nd:YAG laser making it the treatment of choice in the ureter. At the same time, the Nd:YAG laser leads to less scarring than electrofulguration making it the more prudent treatment modality in the renal pelvis.

In cases where access is difficult, it is imperative that caution be employed in order to avoid ureteral trauma. Tight ureteral orifices and soft ureteral strictures can be dilated with a balloon or a ureteral catheter. If this is not successful or if it cannot be done safely, a ureteral stent should be placed and repeat ureteroscopy should be attempted after two weeks of passive dilation. Many strictures can be successfully treated with balloon dilation or endoureterotomy followed by ureteral stenting for 8 to 10 weeks (38). Strictures resistant to endoscopic treatment may require open or laparoscopic resection and repair.

SUMMARY

Most major complications can be avoided with careful attention to technique. For each case, safety measures must always be employed. Even so, complications can occur at any time. Fortunately, the majority of complications in modern series are amenable to conservative treatment. As ureteroscope technology evolves, complication rates will continue to decline.

REFERENCES

1. Lyon ES, Kyker JS, Schoenberg HW. Transurethral ureteroscopy in women: a ready addition to the urological armamentarium. J Urol 1978; 119:35–36.
2. Lyon ES, Banno JJ, Schoenberg HW. Transurethral ureteroscopy in men using juvenile cystoscopy equipment. J Urol 1979; 122:152–153.
3. Geavlete P, Georgescu D, Nita G, et al. Complications of 2735 retrograde semirigid ureteroscopy procedures: a single-center experience. J Endourol 2006; 20:179–185.
4. Harmon WJ, Sershon PD, Blute ML, et al. Ureteroscopy: current practice and long-term complications. J Urol 1997; 157:28–32.
5. Schuster TG, Hollenbeck BK, Faerber GJ, Wolf JS Jr. Complications of ureteroscopy: analysis of predictive factors. J Urol 2001; 166:538–540.
6. Chow GK, Patterson DE, Blute ML, et al. Ureteroscopy: effect of technology and technique on clinical practice. J Urol 2003; 170:99–102.
7. Francesca F, Scattoni V, Nava L, et al. Failures and complications of transurethral ureteroscopy in 297 cases: conventional rigid instruments vs. small caliber semirigid ureteroscopes. Eur Urol 1995; 28:112–115.
8. Weinberg JJ, Ansong K, Smith AD. Complications of ureteroscopy in relation to experience: report of survey and author experience. J Urol 1987; 137:384–385.
9. Abdel-Razzak O, Bagley DH. The 6.9 F semirigid ureteroscope in clinical use. 1993; 41:45–48.
10. Butler MR, Power RE, Thornhill JA, et al. An audit of 2273 ureteroscopies—a focus on intraoperative complications to justify proactive management of ureteric calculi. Surg J R Coll Surg Edinb Irel 2004; 2:42–46.
11. Moretti KL, Jose JS. Ureteral intussusception owing to a malignant ureteral polyp. J Urol 1987; 137:493–494.
12. Gabriel JB Jr, Thomas L, Guarin U, et al. Ureteral intussusception by papillary transitional cell carcinoma. Urology 1986; 28:310–312.
13. Duchek M, Hallmans G, Hietala SO, et al. Inverted papilloma with intussusception of the ureter. Case report. Scand J Urol Nephrol 1987; 21:147–149.
14. Bernhard PH, Reddy PK. Retrograde ureteral intussusception: a rare complication. J Endourol 1996; 10:349–351.

15. Chiong E, Consigliere D. Antegrade ureteral intussusception: a rare complication of percutaneous endopyelotomy. Urology 2004; 64:1231, e12–e14.
16. Mazer MJ, Lacy SS, Kao L. "Bell-shaped ureter," a radiographic sign of antegrade intussusception. Urol Radiol 1979; 1:63–65.
17. Hart JB. Avulsion of the distal ureter with Dormia basket. J Urol 1967; 97:62–63.
18. Grasso M, Bagley D. Small diameter, actively deflectable, flexible ureteropyeloscopy. J Urol 1998; 160:1648–1653.
19. de la Rosette J, Skrekas T, Segura JW. Handling and prevention of complications in stone basketing. Eur Urol 2006; 50:991–999.
20. Martin X, Ndoye A, Konan PG, et al. Hazards of lumbar ureteroscopy: apropos of 4 cases of avulsion of the ureter. Prog Urol 1998; 8:358–362.
21. Johnson DB, Pearle MS. Complications of ureteroscopy. Urol Clin North Am 2004; 31:157–171.
22. Honeck P, Wendt-Nordhal G, Hacker A, et al. Risk of collateral damage to endourologic tools by holmium:YAG laser energy. J Endourol 2006; 20:495–497.
23. Alapont JM, Broseta E, Oliver F, et al. Ureteral avulsion as a complication of ureteroscopy. Int Braz J Urol 2003; 29:18–23.
24. Bonfig R, Gerharz EW, Riedmiller H. Ileal ureteric replacement in complex reconstruction of the urinary tract. BJU Int 2004; 93:575–580.
25. Bluebond-Langner R, Rha KH, Pinto PA, et al. Laparoscopic-assisted renal autotransplantation. Urology 2004; 63:853–856.
26. Grasso M. Complications of ureteropyeloscopy. In: Taneja SS, Smith RB, Ehrlich RM, eds. Complications of Urologic Surgery, 3rd ed. Philadelphia, PA: Saunders, 2001:268–276.
27. Kramolowsky EV. Ureteral perforation during ureterorenoscopy: treatment and management. J Urol 1987; 138:36–38.
28. Stoller ML, Wolf JS Jr, Hofmann R, Marc B. Ureteroscopy without routine balloon dilation: an outcome assessment. J Urol 1992; 147:1238–1242.
29. Abdel-Razzak OM, Bagley DH. Clinical experience with flexible ureteropyeloscopy. J Urol 1992; 148:1788–1792.
30. Green DF, Lytton B. Early experience with direct vision electrohydraulic lithotripsy of ureteral calculi. J Urol 1985; 133:767–770.
31. Denstedt JD, Clayman RV. Electrohydraulic lithotripsy of renal and ureteral calculi. J Urol 1990; 143:13–17.
32. Sofer M, Watterson JD, Wollin TA, et al. Holmium:YAG laser lithotripsy for upper urinary tract calculi in 598 patients. J Urol 2002; 167:31–34.
33. Bilen CY, Mahalati K, Sahin A, et al. Ureteroscopic management of lower ureteral stones: two years' experience. Int Urol Nephrol 1997; 29:301–306.
34. Sun Y, Wang L, Liao G, et al. Pneumatic lithotripsy versus laser lithotripsy in the endoscopic treatment of ureteral calculi. J Endourol 2001; 15:587–590.
35. Sozen S, Kupeli B, Tunc L, et al. Management of ureteral stones with pneumatic lithotripsy: report of 500 patients. J Endourol 2003; 17:721–724.
36. Aghamir SK, Mohseni MG, Ardestani A. Treatment of ureteral calculi with ballistic lithotripsy. J Endourol 2003; 17:887–890.
37. Hofbauer J, Hobarth K, Marberger M. Electrohydraulic versus pneumatic disintegration in the treatment of ureteral stones: a randomized, prospective trial. J Urol 1995; 153:623–625.
38. Chen GL, Bagley DH. Ureteroscopic surgery for upper tract transitional-cell carcinoma: complications and management. J Endourol 2001; 15:399–404.
39. Al-Awadi K, Kehinde EO, Al-Hunayan A, Al-Khayat. Iatrogenic ureteric injuries: incidence, aetiological factors and the effect of early management on subsequent outcome. Int Urol Nephrol 2005; 37:235–241.
40. Lytton B, Weiss RM, Green DF. Complications of ureteral endoscopy. J Urol 1987; 137:649–653.
41. Evans CP, Stoller ML. The fate of the iatrogenic retroperitoneal stone. J Urol 1993; 150:827–829.
42. Lopez-Alcina E, Broseta E, Oliver F, et al. Paraureteral extrusion of calculi after endoscopic pulsed-dye laser lithotripsy. J Endourol 1998; 12:517–521.
43. Grasso M, Liu JB, Goldberg B, Bagley DH. Submucosal calculi: endoscopic and intraluminal sonographic diagnosis and treatment options. J Urol 1995; 153:1384–1389.
44. Lam JS, Gupta M. Ureteroscopic management of upper tract transitional cell carcinoma. Urol Clin North Am 2004; 31:115–128.
45. Lim DJ, Shattuck MC, Cook WA. Pyelovenous lymphatic migration of transitional cell carcinoma following flexible ureteroscopy. J Urol 1993; 149:109–111.
46. Hendin BN, Streem SB, Levin HS, et al. Impact of diagnostic ureteroscopy on long-term survival in patients with upper tract transitional cell carcinoma. J Urol 1999; 161:783–785.
47. Raney AM. Electrohydraulic ureterolithotripsy. Urology 1978; 12:84–85.
48. Santa-Cruz RW, Leveillee RJ, Krongrad A. Ex vivo comparison of four lithotriptors commonly used in the ureter: what does it take to perforate? J Endourol 1998; 12:417–422.

49. Razvi HA, Denstedt JD, Chun SS, Sales JL. Intracorporeal lithotripsy with the holmium:YAG laser. J Urol 1996; 156:912–944.
50. Grasso M. Experience with the holmium laser as an endoscopic lithotrite. Urology 1996; 48:199.
51. Kim FJ, Herrell SD, Jahoda AE, Albala DM. Complications of acucise endopyelotomy. J Endourol 1998; 12:433–436.
52. Giddens JL, Grasso M. Retrograde ureteroscopic endopyelotomy using the holmium:YAG laser. J Urol 2000; 164:509–512.
53. Bagley DH, Liu JB, Goldberg B. Endoluminal sonographic imaging of the ureteropelvic junction. J Endourol 1996; 10:105–110.
54. Hudson RG, Conlin MJ, Bagley DH. Ureteric access with flexible ureteroscopes: effect of the size of the ureteroscope. BJU Int 2005; 95:1043–1054.
55. Carey RI, Gomez CS, Maurici G, et al. Frequency of ureteroscope damage seen at a tertiary care center. J Urol 2006; 176:607–610.
56. Cheung MC, Lee F, Leung YL, et al. Outpatient ureteroscopy: predictive factors for postoperative events. Urology 2001; 58:914–918.
57. Pearle MS, Pierce HL, Miller GL, et al. Optimal method of urgent decompression of the collecting system for obstruction and infection due to ureteral calculi. J Urol 1998; 160:1260–1264.
58. Knopf HJ, Graff, HJ, Schulze H. Perioperative antibiotic prophylaxis in ureteroscopic stone removal. Eur Urol 2003; 44:115–118.
59. Denstedt JD, Wollin TA, Sofer M, et al. A prospective randomized controlled trial comparing non-stented versus stented ureteroscopic lithotripsy. J Urol 2001; 165:1419–1422.
60. Cheung MC, Lee F, Leung YL, et al. A prospective randomized trial on ureteral stenting after ureteroscopic holmium laser lithotripsy. J Urol 2003; 169:1257–1260.
61. Ford TF, Parkinson MC, Wickham JE. Clinical and experimental evaluation of ureteric dilatation. Br J Urol 1984; 56:460–463.
62. Lam JS, Gupta M. Tips and tricks for the management of retained ureteral stents. J Endourol 2002; 16:733–741.
63. Weizer AZ, Auge BK, Silverstein AD, et al. Routine postoperative imaging is important after ureteroscopic stone manipulation. J Urol 2002; 168:46–50.
64. Byrne RR, Auge BK, Kourambas J, et al. Routine ureteral stenting is not necessary after ureteroscopy and ureteropyeloscopy: a randomized trial. J Endourol 2002; 16:9–13.
65. Garvin TJ, Clayman RV. Balloon dilation of the distal ureter to 24F: an effective method for ureteroscopic stone retrieval. J Urol 1991; 146:742–745.
66. Stackl W, Marberger M. Late sequelae of the management of ureteral calculi with the ureterorenoscope. J Urol 1986; 136:386–389.
67. Richter S, Shalev M, Lobik L, et al. Early postureteroscopy vesicoureteral reflux—a temporary and infrequent complication: prospective study. J Endourol 1999; 13:365–366.
68. Puppo P, Ricciotti G, Bozzo W, Introini C. Primary endoscopic treatment of ureteric calculi. A review of 378 cases. Eur Urol 1999; 36:48–52.
69. Krambeck AE, Murat FJ, Gettman MT, et al. The evolution of ureteroscopy: a modern single-institution series. Mayo Clin Proc 2006; 81:468–473.
70. Brito AH, Mitre AI, Srougi M. Ureteroscopic pneumatic lithotripsy of impacted ureteral calculi. Int Braz J Urol 2006; 32:295–309.
71. Dretler SP, Young RH. Stone granuloma: a cause of ureteral stricture. J Urol 1993; 150:1800–1802.
72. Delvecchio FC, Auge BK, Brizuela RM, et al. Assessment of stricture formation with the ureteral access sheath. Urology 2003; 61:518–522.

33 | Complications of Intravesical Therapy

Michael A. O'Donnell and José L. Maymí
Department of Urology, University of Iowa, Iowa City, Iowa, U.S.A.

INTRODUCTION

With an overall recurrence rate approaching 70% after surgical treatment alone, non-muscle-invasive (superficial) bladder cancer is among the most difficult to eradicate and most costly of all human cancers (1,2). To reduce recurrence and repetitive surgery, adjuvant topical therapy in the form of instillation of either cytotoxic chemotherapeutic or immunotherapeutic agents directly into the bladder (intravesical administration) has become a major part in the treatment algorithm. But while even progression to invasive disease can be prevented in some cases, no therapy to date has been shown to actually improve the survival of patients with superficial bladder cancer (3). Since topical treatment can lead to a variety of local and/or systemic complications, it is incumbent on the administering physician to fully understand the potential toxicity of this therapy to make the best decision on its appropriate use.

INTRAVESICAL CHEMOTHERAPY—GENERAL PRINCIPLES RELATED TO EFFICACY AND TOXICITY

The scientific rationale behind the use of intravesical chemotherapy is to introduce a cytotoxic drug at relatively high concentration directly to the tumor cells while minimizing systemic exposure. Two general formats have been widely used. A single dose of perioperative chemotherapy has been advocated on the basis of Class A medical evidence demonstrating a 39% relative reduction in the odds of tumor recurrence (4). The reputed basis of efficacy is prevention of tumor cell re-implantation shortly following transurethral resection of the bladder (TURB) tumor. The more commonly used format is repetitive, usually weekly, chemotherapy over four to eight weeks occasionally followed by further (usually monthly) maintenance treatments, of which, the utility of the latter is still under debate (5,6). Urothelial tumor–drug contact is very important in the whole process. For this reason, best results are nearly always obtained with as complete a prior tumor resection as possible. For any remaining residual disease, whether microscopic or not, the administered drug must penetrate into the full depth of the tumor to be effective. The variables affecting tumor eradication include the nature of the drug (mechanism of action), concentration at the tumor site, ability to penetrate, contact time with the tumor, and stability in the urine (7). Since dwell time in the bladder is limited by bladder capacity (typically 2 hours) and ongoing urine production (with progressive drug dilution), the drug usually has to be administered several times over a certain period of time to produce an efficient anti-cancer response.

Unfortunately, local toxicity (usually in the form of cystitis) is also directly related to effective drug exposure (time and concentration) as well as the drug's intrinsic irritability on normal urothelium or exposed resected stroma. Systemic toxicity depends on drug absorption and the unique properties of the agent. Factors affecting drug absorption include not only effective drug exposure but also its molecular weight and integrity of the bladder wall. A large deep tumor resection will expose a larger thin surface area facilitating absorption while an inflamed bladder from a co-existent urinary tract infection can do the same. Worse yet, an unrecognized bladder perforation or traumatic catheterization can allow direct extravasation of most of the administered dose.

TABLE 1 Classification of Cytotoxic Chemotherapeutic Drugs

Biologic class	Subtype	Drugs	Molecular weight (Da)	Systemic toxicity
Topoisomerase inhibitors	Anthracyclines	Doxorubicin (adriamycin)	580	Cardiomyopathy, myelosuppression, mucositis, local
		Epirubicin	580	Less cardiotoxic
		Valrubicin	724	Even less cardiotoxic
	Anthracendioines	Mitoxantrone	444	Myelosuppression, N/V, Mucositis
Alkylating agents	Ethylenimine	Thiotepa	189	Myelosuppression, N/V, Mucositis
	Bioreductive alkylator	Mitomycin-C	334	Myelosuppression, N/V, mucositis, dermatitis, asthenia, fibrosis, CHF, hemolytic uremic syndrome, hypersensitivity
	Platinum analogs	Cisplatin	300	Renal, neuropathy, N/V, myelosuppression, electrolyte disturbances, anaphylactoid rxns
Antimetabolites	Anti-folate	Methotrexate	454	Myeolosuppression, mucositis, renal, pneumonitis, hepatic fibrosis
	Pyrimidine analogues	Gemcitabine	300	Myelosuppression, N/V, flu-like symptoms
Mitotic spindle inhibitors	Taxanes	Docetaxel	862	Myelosuppression, cardiac arrhythmia, alopecia, neuropathy, capillary leak, hypersensitivity

Abbreviations: CHF, congestive heart failure; N/V, nausea/vomiting.

Cytotoxic drugs that have been used for intravesical chemotherapy are listed in Table 1 and can be catalogued by the mechanistic class of agent to which they belong. Systemically, all have the potential for inducing myelosuppression as well as a variety of other side effects. Until recently, class-specific drugs were limited to topoisomerase inhibitors, primarily anthracyclines, and alkylating agents, primarily thiotepa and mitomycin-C. Although gemcitabine and taxanes have been used extensively against metastatic bladder cancer, intravesical clinical experience with gemcitabine in Phase I/II trials was first reported in 2002 and with docetaxel in 2006. There are a few drugs, such as cisplatin, mitoxantrone, and methotrexate that have been used intravesically but have lost favor due to reduced efficacy and/or toxicity.

Another important feature of chemotherapeutic drugs is their tendency for venous irritation and tissue damage after inadvertent extravasation during intravenous drug administration. This property of intrinsic local tissue reactivity has been well studied and has allowed drugs to be catalogued according to the level of contact toxicity (8). Vesicant agents are those that are destructive to local tissues and can cause extensive tissue necrosis, sometimes requiring skin grafting and resulting in permanent disability. For this reason they are usually delivered via central access lines. Non-vesicant agents can still be highly irritating but are seldom destructive. The relative categorization of some of the major chemotherapeutic drugs according to their vesicant/irritant status is provided in Table 2. It is noteworthy that the two most commonly used chemotherapeutic drugs for intravesical therapy, the anthracyclines and mitomycin-C, belong to the vesicant subclass. At the same time, the most common dose-limiting side effect of these intravesical agents is local in origin manifested as irritable cystitis with urgency, frequency, dysuria, bladder pain, and/or hematuria.

TABLE 2 Classification of Chemotherapeutics by Vesicant/Irritant Status

Vesicant	Irritant	Minimal	None
All anthracyclines	Cisplatin	Methotrexate	Bleomycin
All vinca alkaloids	Carboplatin	Mitoxantrone	Gemcitabine
Mitomycin-C	Etoposide	Pemetrexed	Cytarabine
Cisplatin (high-dose)	Ifosphamide	Thiotepa	5-Fluorouracil
Paclitaxel	Docetaxel		
	Busulfan		

INTRAVESICAL CHEMOTHERAPEUTIC AGENTS
Thiotepa

Thiotepa is a polyfunctional alkylating agent related chemically and pharmacologically to nitrogen mustard. It results in DNA cross-linkage thereby interfering with protein synthesis to exert its cytotoxic effect. This mechanism is non-cell cycle-specific but more prominent in rapidly dividing cells. On the basis of tissue concentration studies, it is reported that thiotepa has only modest differential affinity for neoplasms (9).

Thiotepa is the smallest of all other intravesical chemotherapeutic agents, with a molecular weight of 189 Da increasing its potential for systemic absorption (10). Ultrastructural studies have also revealed that thiotepa directly induces disruption of microvilli and tight junctions, possibly further enhancing mucosal permeability (11). Typically, thiotepa is used at a dose of 30 to 60 mg dissolved in 30 to 60 cc of water or saline and delivered once per week for six weeks. Approximately 20% of the drug at a concentration of one mg/mL is absorbed within one hour of instillation from the normal bladder but this increases markedly in the presence of inflammation, tumor diathesis, and after transurethral resection (TUR) in which cases 50% to 100% of the drug can be absorbed (12). A cumulative drug effect has also been reported in elderly and debilitated patients as well as those treated with prior pelvic radiation (13).

Thiotepa has been used intravesically for the treatment of bladder cancer since the early 1960s and much information on its local and systemic toxicity has been accumulated (14). During its first two decades of use, the incidence of leukopenia [white blood cells (WBC) <3000] was reported in 17% (range 8–54%) of 401 patients from nine series reviewed (15). Thrombocytopenia (platelets <100,000) was found in 9% (range 3–31%). Higher doses, biweekly administration, and one to two years of maintenance therapy were generally associated with an increased incidence of these side effects. Six treatment-related deaths due to acute nonlymphocytic leukemia-myelodysplastic syndrome have been reported, almost all of which were the result of long-term therapy (mean 42 months) (16). On this basis, it has been advised to limit thiotepa dosing to 30 mg in 30 cc and discontinue its use after one year. Weekly monitoring of WBC counts with dose interruption to maintain WBC >4000 and platelets >100,000 while on active therapy is also recommended. An updated 1999 compilation by the American Urological Association (AUA) Bladder Cancer Guidelines Panel estimated the incidence of thiotepa-induced myelosuppression at 13% (range 8–19%) (Table 3) (17). Rarely, fever, nausea/vomiting, dermatitis, and stomatitis have been reported. The use of thiotepa has been diminished due to all these serious systemic side effects and with the arrival of safer drugs.

Local side effects of thiotepa are generally restricted to irritative symptoms ranging from 12% to 69% in earlier studies, with dose and duration dependence (15). A more recent compilation reported frequency to be 11%, hematuria 13%, dysuria 30%, and contracted bladder 3% (17). These side effects only rarely result in interruption of therapy. Other rare complications from case reports include infertility, eosinophilic cystitis, hemorrhagic cystitis, and vesicoureteral reflux (18–21). Single-dose perioperative therapy using thiotepa (recommended dose 30 mg in 30 cc for 30 minutes delivered within 6 hours of resection) has been of variable effectiveness in preventing tumor recurrence, with the largest study using a more dilute formulation (30 mg in 60 cc) given 24 hours after TUR showing no benefit (22–26). A very low incidence of cystitis (<1%) and transient leukopenia (0–10%) have been reported with this regimen.

Mitomycin C

Mitomycin C (MMC) is a bioreductive alkylating agent isolated from *Streptomyces caespitosus* that requires intracellular enzymatic reduction by quinone reductase to become activated (27). While not cell cycle-specific, increased susceptibility is seen during late G1 and early S phases of DNA synthesis (28). Its major mechanism of action is through DNA cross-linking but generation of reactive oxygen species also contributes to its activity (29,30).

Mitomycin C has a molecular weight of 334 Da and is typically used in doses of 20 to 40 mg in 20 to 40 cc of water or saline. MMC's larger size is assumed to contribute to its limited systemic absorption. Indeed, numerous pharmocodynamic studies of absorption of MMC in animal and human bladders under various conditions have consistently demonstrated little systemic absorption, typically <1% of the administered dose (corresponding to plasma levels of

TABLE 3 Summary of Toxicity Reported for Common Intravesical Agents

Toxicity	Thiotepa	MMC	Doxorubicin	BCG
Local				
Frequency/nocturia	11 (1–42)	42 (26–59)	27 (23–32)	63 (48–76)
Dysuria	30 (10–57)	35 (30–41)	20 (8–39)	75 (64–84)
Irritative symptoms	13 (7–21)	18 (12–26)	21 (13–30)	Too varied to calculate
Pain/cramps	NR	10 (6–14)	12 (4–25)	12 (7–18)
Hematuria	13 (4–23)	16 (7–28)	19 (12–29)	29 (22–36)
Incontinence	NR	1 (0.4–4)	9 (3–18)	4 (3–6)
Bladder contracture[a]	3 (0.3–13)	5 (2–11)	3 (0.8–6)	3 (2–5)
Systemic				
Flu-like	11 (4–23)	20 (4–48)	7 (3–13)	24 (18–31)
Fever/chills	4 (1–10)	3 (1–7)	4 (2–9)	27 (22–32)
Arthalgias	NR	9 (0.1–47)	1 (0.1–5)	5 (1–13)
Myelosuppression	13 (8–19)	2 (0.3–7)	0.8 (0.2–2)	1 (0.1–4)
Nausea/vomiting[a]	9 (0.8–31)	9 (1–26)	8 (4–13)	9 (6–14)
Skin rash	2 (0.4–4)	13 (8–19)	2 (0.5–6)	6 (3–10)
Other	0.2 (0–2)	3 (0.5–8)	0.2 (0–2)	23 (19–27)
Infectious				
Bacterial cystitis[a]	7 (2–16)	20 (17–23)	6 (2–12)	20 (13–28)
Epid/prost/urethral	0.4 (0–4)	4 (2–9)	2 (0.1–7)	5 (4–8)
Pneumonia	NR	0.2 (0–2)	NR	1 (0.2–3)
Systemic	0.3 (0–3)	NR	NR	4 (2–5)
Treatment continuation				
Incomplete	5 (2–11)	9 (2–14)	7 (2–16)	8 (5–10)
Interruption	6 (3–11)	11 (8–16)	2 (0.1–8)	7 (5–11)

Note: Values given are percentages.
[a]Corresponding rates for TUR alone (without chemotherapy) are 0.8 for bladder contracture, 0.9 for nausea/vomiting and 20 for bacterial cystitis.
Abbreviations: BCG, bacillus Calmette-Guerin; MMC, mitomycin C; NR, not reported.
Source: Adapted from the AUA Bladder Cancer Guidelines Panel Report on the Management of Non-Muscle-Invasive Bladder Cancer, 1999.

under 40 ng/mL) (31–33). Under conditions of extensive resection, active inflammation or infection, or prior radiation levels of three to five times higher have been reported (34,35). Methods to increase the depth of penetration of MMC by using higher concentrations (e.g., 40 mg in 20 cc), or coincident microwave hyperthermia, or electromotive therapy have also resulted in two to five times higher serum levels (36–38). However, because the level of MMC required for myelosuppression is estimated to be >400 ng/mL (10 times the typical levels), bone marrow toxicity is only very rarely observed (average 2% incidence) (39). Serious systemic side effects, including severe bone marrow suppression and death after intravesical mitomycin have occurred but have almost uniformly been reported in cases of suspected bladder perforation (40,41). Necrosis of the glans penis and urethral sloughing following MMC administration were also found after traumatic catheterization and are consistent with the known strong vesicant properties of MMC (42,43).

Local toxicity in the form of chemical cystitis is the most frequent side effect of MMC therapy and occurs in about 18% of patients (range 12–26%) (17). Importantly, chemical cystitis must be distinguished from bacterial cystitis that also occurs with a similar frequency in these patients. Milder manifestations of frequency or dysuria are even more common in 42% and 35% of the patients, respectively. Hematuria is found in 16% and pain in 10% while actual incontinence is rare in 1% (Table 3). Treatment interruption or discontinuation occurs in about 10% of patients largely due to these local effects. As with other agents there is some suggestion that these side effects are dose exposure-related. The more serious side effect of bladder contracture, the end result of severe chemical cystitis, appears highest with mitomycin than any other agent at approximately 5% with rates as high as 23% reported for patients treated for two years (44). This may be a function of MMC's strong vesicant nature, allergic/hypersensitivity, and/or fibrosis potential. Eosinophilic infiltrates and even inflammatory mass lesions have been reported to be a result of MMC therapy (45). It is thus important to withhold therapy at the first sign of severe cystitis (i.e., moderate to severe symptoms persisting beyond one week).

Moderate relief of chemical cystitis can be achieved with an oral prednisone taper or even intravesical steroids (46).

Another significant side effect associated primarily with MMC is a desquamatous, eczematous rash most commonly appearing on the palms, soles, chest, face, and genitals in approximately 13% of treated patients (17). This rash is often associated with coincident chemical cystitis. The origin of this rash is not completely clear but is suspected to be the result of a delayed hypersensitivity reaction, possibly exacerbated by contact sensitivity in certain areas (palms and genitals) (47). Evidence for the hypersensitivity phenomenon includes its occurrence only after prior MMC exposure, association with eosinophils, skin patch recall, and occurrence with systemic MMC therapy (hand–foot syndrome) (48,49). These rashes usually respond to cessation of further therapy and institution of either topical or a systemic steroid taper (50). Minor rashes responding to treatment do not necessarily require cessation of further treatment. Avoiding inadvertent extended patient skin contact with the drug is recommended during instillation and after voiding.

Other rare complications have been described in case reports with the use of intravesical MMC. Sonneveld et al. described in a case report the development of a secondary non-Hodgkin lymphoma behind the bladder approximately 5 years after 26 intravesical instillations of MMC to treat recurrent papillary tumors (51). Slowly healing eschars with bladder calcifications at tumor resection sites have also been described with intravesical mitomycin, especially with perioperative instillation (Fig. 1). Usually they cause no symptoms and respond to conservative management (52). Occasionally, transmural muscle necrosis can also result (53).

Single-dose postoperative mitomycin (40 mg in 40 cc for 30–60 minutes) has emerged as a viable means to reduce tumor recurrence post-TURB (54). In a large study by the Medical Research Council in England in which 300 patients received postoperative MMC, the incidence of side effects was "extremely low," although delayed healing at the resection site was seen in some cases. In another study, chemical cystitis and a slight allergic skin reaction were noted in only two of 57 patients (3.5%) (55). Local side effects, however, are increased if additional weekly therapy continues after the initial post-TUR dose and resulted in 3% discontinuation rate for cystitis in the early versus 0% in the late initiation group (56). Single-dose perioperative mitomycin is contraindicated in the setting of a suspected bladder perforation as documented by extensive pelvic tissue damage and even death (40,41).

The Anthracyclines (Doxorubicin, Epirubicin, and Valrubicin)

The anthracycline family includes doxorubicin as well as all its derivatives including epirubicin, pirarubicin, and valrubicin (among others). All of these have been tested as intravesical agents with doxorubicin tested the most, followed by epirubicin and valrubicin. All the members of the anthracycline family are relatively large molecules with molecular weights exceeding 500 Da. Doxorubicin and epirubicin are both 580 Da, while pirarubicin (853 Da) and valrubicin (724 Da) are even larger due to side-chain modifications that affect solubility and biodistribution. Less cardiotoxicity is seen with these derivatives.

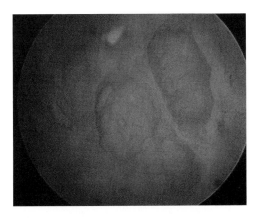

FIGURE 1 Calcification after intravesical mitomycin instillation.

Doxorubicin hydrochloride (Adriamycin®, Pharmacia Inc., Kalamazoo, Michigan, U.S.A.) was originally isolated from *Streptomyces caesius.* Its mechanism of action primarily involves inhibition of topoisomerase II but intercalation of the drug between adjacent base pairs of the DNA double helix and free radical formation also contribute to its efficacy (57). There is also evidence of direct cytotoxicity through interaction with the cell membrane (58). Doxorubicin is relatively non-cell cycle-specific but most active in the S phase of DNA replication (59). The common dose for most of the anthracyclines is 50 mg in 50 cc of water or saline but higher concentrations of 80 to 90 mg in 50 cc have also been described.

Because of their larger molecular weights, systemic absorption of the anthracycline drugs is very low and systemic side effects very rare (60,61). Indeed, myelosuppression occurs in <1% of patients (17). Allergic reactions, primarily skin rash, have been reported in 2% of patients treated with Adriamycin® but have also been documented with epirubicin and valrubicin (62–64). These allergic reactions are usually treated according to their symptoms, mainly by using antihistaminic drugs and supportive measures. Fever (4%) and nausea/vomiting (1–2%) have also been reported (17). As with all intravesical drugs, integrity of the bladder wall is important in limiting absorption with lower levels of absorption found during later instillations. One severe local reaction with adriamycin and three with epirubicin (and one death) from bladder perforations have been reported (65,66). Yoshimura et al. described chemical pericystitis in a patient who underwent transurethral resection of the bladder tumor, with a subsequent instillation of Adriamycin (65). The patient had fever lasting more than 2 weeks, lower abdominal pain, and mild hydronephrosis of the left kidney. A computed tomography (CT) showed an irregular thickening of his left bladder wall. Due to symptom persistence, an exploratory laparotomy was performed. The left perivesical space was found replaced by a scar and edematous tissue. Yoshimura et al. presumed that extravasation of doxorubicin was responsible. Because classic signs of peritonitis may not always be present, a CT scan (preferably CT cystogram) should be performed in all suspected perforations after TURB and perioperative drug instillation. In one documented case of valrubicin leakage, no accompanying local untoward effects were observed (64). Valrubicin has also been used for intraperitoneal chemotherapy of ovarian disease (67).

Not unexpectedly, given their vesicant profile, local side effects are more commonly seen with all anthracyclines administered intravesically. Chemical cystitis (urgency, frequency, and dysuria) has been reported in about a quarter of the patients (range 8–39%) treated with Adriamycin, with hematuria in 19% (17). The cystitis rate with epirubicin may be lower (Table 4). Although a direct comparative study by Eto et al. (74) with low doses of epirubicin and Adriamycin yielded similar results, Ali-El-Dein (72) demonstrated a more favorable local and systemic toxicity profile with more conventional higher doses of epirubicin versus Adriamycin.

Valrubicin is a semi-synthetic derivative of doxorubicin with a higher molecular weight of 724 Da. The modifications increase the hydrophobicity of the drug requiring a lipid expedient, Cremophor® (BASF, Mount Olive, New Jersey, U.S.A.), for dissolution. It more rapidly traverses the cell membrane and accumulates in the cell cytoplasm while showing minimal absorption across the bladder wall and very little (<1%) systemic absorption (64). For this reason, much higher doses of the drug can be given intravesically, up to 800 mg in its Food and Drug Administration (FDA)-approved format. Valrubicin was approved in the United States for intravesical use in patients who failed bacillus Calmette-Guerin (BCG) treatment [Valstar package insert (Medeva—US), Rev 10/98, Rec 1/99, Celltech Pharmaceuticals, Rochester, New York, U.S.A.]. This drug, in its intravesical route, has been studied in several clinical trials, with a total of 184 patients (Table 5).

Valrubicin intravesical therapy is most commonly associated with localized adverse events exceeding that of the other anthracyclines. Chemical cystitis and hematuria are found in the majority of patients. More serious systemic effects were found with postoperative therapy (76). One patient with a perforated bladder developed neutropenia 2 weeks after the treatment. He also presented with moderate anemia and mild thrombocytopenia that were probably related to the treatment. Another patient experienced mild post-infusion contact dermatitis, having a rash in the groin area. The third patient had a new diagnosis of cancer unrelated to valrubicin and the fourth patient had an exacerbation of his chronic obstructive pulmonary disease unrelated to the therapy.

TABLE 4 Toxicity Reported from Intravesical Epirubicin Trials

Study	No. patients	Induction dose (mg)	Dose frequency	Chemical cystitis	Systemic effects
Matsumura et al. (68)	35	50–80	q d × 3/wk × 2 wk	26% (both doses similar)	None
Burk et al. (69)	911	30–50–80	q wk × 8	15% (all doses)	None
Cumming et al. (70)	37	50	q wk × 8	38% (chemical) 43% (bacterial)	NR
Oosterlinck et al. (63)	204	80	Post-TURB	6.8%	0.9% allergic
Kurth et al. (71)	34	30–80	q wk × 8	2.9%	0.6% nausea, hypotension
Ali-El-Dein et al. (72)	55	50	Post-TURB	22% (6% major)	None
	59	50	q wk × 8	25% (8% major)	None
Ali-El-Dein et al. (73)	57	50	q wk × 8 then q mo × 4	16% (8% major)	None
	56	80		24% (9% major)	None
	56	50 ADR		42% (13% major)	5% allergic, fever, decreased platelet counts
Eto et al. (74)	75	30	2×/wk × 4 then q mo × 11	10% pain; 15% freq, 5% hemat	NR
	75	30 ADR		15% pain; 15% freq, 0% hemat	

Abbreviations: ADR, Adriamycin®; freq, frequency; hemat, hematuria; NR, none recorded, Post-TURB, post-transurethral resection of the bladder.

Gemcitabine

Gemcitabine is a pyrimidine antimetabolite, analogous to cytosine arabinoside, with a molecular weight of 300 Da. Its mechanism of action involves incorporation of the pyrimidine base analog into DNA by one of the metabolites [2′, 2′-difluorodeoxycytidine (dFdCTP)], resulting in chain termination (79). In addition, gemcitabine inhibits ribonucleotide reductase, an enzyme necessary for DNA synthesis (80). It was first approved in the United States to treat pancreatic cancer (81) but has since been found to be effective in other tumors such as non-small-cell lung cancer, leiomyosarcoma, and ovarian cancer (82). Phase III clinical trial revealed similar survival rates in patients but reduced toxicity with metastatic urothelial cancer treated with gemcitabine plus cisplatin versus the conventional treatment with methotrexate, vinblastine, doxorubicin, and cisplatin (83).

The dose of gemcitabine most commonly being used for intravesical therapy is 1000, 1500, or 2000 mg dissolved in 50 to 100 cc of water or saline. Buffering has been used by some investigators to raise its pH from 2.5 to a more physiologic range by adding 50 to 100 mEq. of bicarbonate (84). However, there is no evidence that this affects efficacy and/or toxicity.

Studies of the intravesical pharmacodynamics of gemcitabine in the non-post-surgical state have revealed the low serum absorption (0.5–5.5%) expected based on its 300-Da molecular

TABLE 5 Toxicity Reported from Valrubicin Trials

Study	No. patients	Induction dose (mg)	Dose frequency	Chemical cystitis (%)	Hematuria (%)	UTI (%)	Other adverse effects
Greenberg et al. (75)	32	200–900	q wk × 6 wk	90	22	13	Minor and transient
Patterson et al. (76)	22	400–800	Post-TURB × 1	100	59	NR	Myelo-suppression (1 patient) Nausea—27% Vomiting—14%
Steinberg et al. (77)	90	800	q wk × 6 wk	90	17	18	Asthenia—7% Urinary retention—6%
Newling et al. (78)	40	800	q wk × 6 wk	77.5	27.5	NR	NR

Abbreviations: NR, none recorded; TURB, transurethral resection of the bladder, UTI, urinary tract infection.

weight (85). This corresponds to an absorption of between 10 and 110 mg from the bladder, well below the dose typically used systemically, >1500 mg. Furthermore, plasma levels of the active metabolite 2′, 2′-difluorodeoxyuridine (dFdU) have also been recorded in the low micromolar range (86). In a study by Palou et al. in which gemcitabine was given immediately after TURB and six random bladder biopsies, maximum levels of 4.5 and 6.1 µg/mL were recorded in two patients and attributed to bladder perforations, even though the bladder perforation remained clinically unrecognized without apparent increase in local or systemic toxicity (87). This would still correspond to a dose 10–15% of that typically given for systemic therapy.

Table 6 summarizes the clinical trials using gemcitabine as the intravesical agent with a total of 92 patients. It should be noted that in these studies rather strict criteria for assessing toxicity were used based on National Cancer Institute and World Health Organization grading scales. Toxicities are graded from 1 to 5: 1, mild side effects; 2, moderate side effects; 3, severe side effects; 4, life-threatening or disabling side effects; 5, fatal.

No interruption of the treatment was reported in these six cohorts of patients during the treatment and all toxicities were short-term, nonlimiting, and reversible. Most were grade I (minimal) or grade II (moderate). Most authors concluded that gemcitabine was well tolerated with regard to local cystitis. This may be related to the non-vesicant activity of the drug. This has also been this author's personal experience excepting worse local toxicity in patients with baseline bladder irritability, where pH buffering of the acidic solution may be helpful. Transient nausea and occasional vomiting occurring usually 24 hours after instillation is the most common other side effect that responds well to anti-emetic drugs such as ondansetron (Zofran®, GlaxoSmithKline, Philadelphia, Pennsylvania, U.S.A.).

Docetaxel

Docetaxel is a relatively high-molecular-weight (862 Da) semi-synthetic compound derived from the needles of the pacific yew tree, *Taxus baccata*. Its mechanism of action is primarily through microtubular stabilization and prevention of the depolymerization necessary for proper spindle activity during mitosis (91). Docetaxel is active against a wide range of solid cancers and has shown substantial activity even as a single agent against metastatic bladder cancer (92,93). It has been particularly active in combinations with other chemotherapeutic agents such as cisplatin or gemcitabine (94,95). It is conventionally formulated at a dose of 37.5 mg in 50 cc of normal saline for intravenous use.

TABLE 6 Toxicity from Intravesical Gemcitabine

Study	No. patients	Induction dose (mg)	Dose frequency	Chemical cystitis	Hematuria (%)	Other adverse events
Dalbagni et al. (84)	18	500–2000	2×/wk × 6 wk (repeat cycle with 1 wk break)	39%	29	[a]UTI (1), Myelo-suppression (1), Hand-foot syndrome (2), Asthenia (4), Nausea (4), Vomiting (1)
Laufer et al. (85)	15	500–2000	q wk × 6 wk	67%	67	[b]
Witjes et al. (88)	10	1000–2000	q wk × 6 wk	40%	NR	Headaches, fatigue, and heavy legs (30%)
De Berardinis et al. (89)	12	500–2000	q wk × 6 wk	One patient	NR	[c]
Serretta et al. (90)	27	500–2000	q wk × 6 wk	11.1%	NR	Nausea (11.1%) Fatigue (3.7%)
Palou et al. (87)	10	1500–2000	Post-TURB × 1	One patient	NR	Liver toxicity (2)

[a]Toxicities were seen ≥1000 mg. Most toxicities were grade 1 or 2. Four were grade 3.
[b]Majority of toxicities were grade 1. Three patients had grade 2 urinary frequency or dysuria. Two patients experienced grade 3 toxicity, one with an epididimitis and other with urinary retention. Other adverse events included: leucopenia, anemia, thrombocytopenia, incontinence, bladder spasms, proteinuria, elevated blood urea nitrogen, fatigue, headache, chills, pruritus, hyperglycemia, rhinitis, dizziness, pelvic pain, diarrhea, myalgia, arthralgia, hyperkalemia, cough, nausea, and hypertension.
[c]No hematological (leukopenia, neutropenia, thrombocytopenia, and anemia) toxicities more than grade 1 were reported.
Abbreviations: NR, not reported; UTI, urinary tract infection.

There has been only one Phase I clinical trial of intravesical docetaxel reported, but its novelty, activity, and tolerability deserve mention (96). In this dose-escalating trial, docetaxel was administered beginning at 5 mg in 40 cc saline, increasing to 75 mg in 100 cc over a total of six dose ranges once a week for 6 weeks. All patients were pretreated with oral dexamethasone to decrease the probability of a hypersensitivity reaction, estimated to occur with a frequency of 6.5% with systemic therapy (97). There was no systemic absorption noted in any patient. Three patients reported urinary frequency (grade I), four patients experienced dysuria (grade I), five had hematuria (2 grade I, 3 grade II), and three had transient facial flushing (grade I). These mild toxicities occurred at all dose levels without a clear indication of dose effect. All resolved without any clinical intervention. No dose-limiting toxic levels was reached. Five of these all pretreated BCG-failure patients are disease-free at 14 months of follow-up (98).

This author has also had direct experience with treating eight patients with the 37.5 mg in 50 cc dose of docetaxel alone or in combination with other agents (gemcitabine or mitomycin) without dexamethasone pretreatment, and has also found minimal local or systemic toxicity. The non-vesicant (irritant) nature of docetaxel may be responsible for its lack of association with significant chemical cystitis. While allergic or hypersensitivity reactions have not yet been reported with intravesical use, pretreatment with steroids or anti-histamines or availability of an anaphylactic kit should be considered.

Other Intravesical Chemotherapeutic Drugs

Largely now of historical interest, ethoglucid is a 262-Da molecular weight compound that functions as an alkylating agent. Its use was greatest in the 1970s through early 1990s when it was used as an alternative to the smaller, more absorptive thiotepa (15). Given usually as a 100-mL 1% solution, it was associated with moderate frequency, urgency, and dysuria (59% in one study) as well as bladder contractures in 20% (99). Bone marrow suppression was found in 4% although other authors did not report significant myelosuppression (100). It largely fell out of favor when a comparative trial against adriamycin demonstrated no advantage.

Mitoxantrone (molecular weight 444 Da), like the anthracyclines, functions as a topoisomerase II inhibitor but is a non-vesicant. It continues to be studied as a potential adjunctive agent but has less popularity in most of Europe and North America. Comparative trials with mitomycin have shown mitoxantrone to be and trials with adriamycin or interferon have shown it to be inferior near-equivalent in efficacy (101–103). A trial against TURB alone revealed it to be marginally better in efficacy (104). Systemic toxicity is rare and reported only in cases of bladder perforation (105,106). Chemical cystitis is variable and appears to depend significantly on the dose, commonly used at 5, 10, or 20 mg in 50 cc (101,102,105–107). The incidence of chemical cystitis varies from 21% to 63%.

Cisplatin (molecular weight 300 Da) is a very active alkylating agent used for the systemic treatment of advanced bladder cancer. However, its intravesical use in bladder cancer has been squelched by a combination of low efficacy versus thiotepa and adriamycin as well as significant unheralded systemic toxicity (108,109). Seven of 68 patients in one clinical trial suffered an anaphylactic reaction with hypotension, all occurring sometime after their eighth instillation. Anaphylaxis has been previously reported by other investigators and is a known potentially lethal side effect of all platinum-containing compounds (110).

Methotrexate (molecular weight 454 Da) is a well-known anti-folate chemotherapeutic that is part of many advanced bladder cancer multidrug regimens, most notably methotrexate, vinblastine, doxorubicin, cisplatin (MVAC) (111). A phase I/II trial of intravesical methotrexate was well tolerated to the highest dose tested of 500 mg/m^2 (roughly 800 mg) weekly for six weeks with negligible serum absorption and no systemic toxicity. However, no clinical response was observed.

COMBINATION INTRAVESICAL CHEMOTHERAPY

While multi-agent chemotherapy has become the norm in the systemic treatment of most human malignancies, this strategy has not found a place in topical intravesical use against bladder cancer. However, small limited trials provide some early insight into this possibility.

Attempts at using mitomycin (20 mg on day 1) in close sequence with adriamycin (40 mg on day 2) have shown significant activity [e.g., 81% complete response to carcinoma in situ (CIS)] but at the expense of moderate to severe chemical cystitis in over one-half of the treated patients, one-third of whom had to terminate therapy prematurely (112,113). More tolerable results have been obtained with the combination of the non-vesicant agent cytarabine of mitomycin (114,115). Cytarabine (molecular weight 243 Da) shares a similar mechanism of action as gemcitabine. Local irritation without systemic toxicity was reported in 10% to 40% of patients (116). Similar tolerable results have been reported for sequential intravesical gemcitabine (1000 mg in 50 cc saline × 1.5 hours) followed immediately by mitomycin (40 mg in 20 cc water × 2 hours), with local cystitis and transient nausea/vomiting attributed to MMC and gemcitabine, respectively (117). This same author had successfully tested other sequential combinations including gemcitabine (1000 mg in 50 cc saline)/docetaxel (37.5 mg in 50 cc saline), adriamycin (50 mg in 50 cc water)/gemcitabine (1000 mg in 50 cc saline), and docetaxel (37.5 mg in 50 cc saline)/mitomycin (40 mg in 20 cc water) with best local tolerability in the first and moderate but tolerable chemical cystitis in the next two regimens. On the basis of these observations, it can be hypothesized that non-vesicant combinations have the least local toxicity, followed by single-vesicant/non-vesicant combinations, followed by dual-vesicant combinations. Further studies need to be done to validate this theory.

INTRAVESICAL IMMUNOTHERAPY—PRINCIPLES AND TREATMENT ISSUES

There are two major immunotherapeutic drugs in use for superficial bladder cancer, the live attenuated cow tuberculosis (*Mycobacterium bovis*) vaccine, BCG, and the (usually recombinant) human immunostimulant protein, interferon-alpha (IFN-α). Unlike cytotoxic chemotherapeutic drugs that act as direct inhibitors of cell proliferation or inducers of cell death, immunotherapeutic drugs work in a more indirect manner, requiring subsequent mobilization of immune effector cells. As such, neither BCG nor IFN-α has any place in the immediate postoperative setting. In the case of IFN-α, it is essentially ineffective (118). In the case of BCG, it is contraindicated because of the higher chance of systemic intravesation, leading to potential sepsis (119,120). Immunotherapeutics also display nonlinear pharmacological properties including parabolic dose–response curves and memory along with significant individual variation. As the exact mechanistic basis for the anti-cancer properties of both BCG and IFN-α is not completely known, much of clinical practice with these biological response modifiers is based on empiric studies.

In North America, intravesical BCG is used twice as often as intravesical cytotoxic chemotherapy while the opposite is true in Europe. The reason for this discrepancy is not altogether clear but may relate to historical use patterns as well as a different appreciation for the toxicity associated with BCG use. This may also relate to a stronger immune reaction in those with prior tuberculosis (TB) exposure or BCG immunization common in Europe but rare in North America. BCG is still the agent of choice in most of the world for the treatment of the high-grade surface-spreading form of bladder cancer known as CIS and the only agent known to reduce the risk of progression to muscle-invasive disease (120). IFN-α is among the least used intravesical agents, especially as a single agent but has some use in combination with BCG.

The format of administration of BCG and/or IFN-α resembles that of cytotoxic chemotherapeutics in that once weekly administration for six to eight weeks is the norm with variable maintenance (rebooster) treatments. The drugs are commonly mixed with 50 cc of saline for a 2-hour retention time. As with chemotherapy, toxicity can be both local and/or systemic.

Local Toxicity Associated with BCG

For patients previously naïve to BCG or TB it is very unusual to have much in the way of local toxicity or bladder irritability during the first few weekly doses of BCG. Thereafter, patients commonly begin to experience frequency, urgency, and dysuria beginning shortly after the first 2-hour void that escalates over the ensuing 6 to 12 hours. These symptoms usually resolve by 24 hours initially but with increasing re-treatment tend to become more intense sooner with a longer time (3–7 days) to completely dissipate. The local toxicity situation with BCG/TB-exposed patients is more accelerated. Using a validated questionnaire, Bohle et al. addressed the symptoms during the course of 6-week instillations of BCG (121). Even after the first instillation, 50% of the patients complained of dysuric episodes. During subsequent instillations there was an increase up to 80% of patients with dysuric complaints. In a study by Saint et al., cystitis of 2 to 48 hours duration was noted in 46%, 48 hour to 7 days in 38% and >7 days duration in 12% (122). Increased duration was seen after the fourth induction treatment. Along with this increased intensity of irritable symptoms, the likelihood of gross hematuria also increases such that roughly one-third of patients suffer from this side effect (17). The recorded incidence of these varied symptoms is listed in Table 3 and is notably greater for BCG than for any of the cytotoxic chemotherapeutics. Indeed, in a meta-analysis of BCG versus mitomycin comparative clinical trials, there was a statistically increased higher incidence of cystitis (54% vs. 39%) for BCG-treated patients (123). Interestingly, the total discontinuation or treatment interruption rate is similar between MMC and BCG, each at roughly 10%.

Whether maintenance therapy is associated with a higher frequency and/or degree of cystitis is still a matter of debate. There was no significant increased association of increased cystitis incidence with BCG maintenance or non-maintenance therapy in chemotherapy versus BCG meta-analysis; however, no direct maintenance versus non-maintenance comparison studies were included and most of the studies were of European origin (124). Three separate comparison trials for toxicity have suggested some worsened cystitis in the maintenance group. Hudson et al. reported dysuria in 67% of patients with a single 6-week induction cycle of BCG, while this increased to 81% in the monthly maintenance arm (125). However, this was not statistically significant. Lamm et al. reported that only 16% of patients randomized to a miniseries of 3-weekly maintenance treatments actually received all their scheduled doses, presumably due to toxicity (126). Saint et al. reported a similar (19%) completion rate for all maintenance doses in a smaller trial of similar design (122). Furthermore, 57% had dose reduction for toxicity and 39% had treatment discontinued. Even if maintenance therapy is associated with higher local toxicity, the clinical significance of this is uncertain as most side effects are reversible.

The histological changes found in the bladder after BCG therapy imply a generalized inflammatory process with pronounced mononuclear inflammatory infiltrate and epithelial sloughing (127). Granulomas are present in roughly a quarter of the cases. Visual abatement of most bladder inflammation occurs after 6 weeks but full resolution of granulomatous changes may take 6 months or longer (128). Figure 2 demonstrates a case of severe BCG inflammation with granuloma formation.

Most cystitis symptoms can be controlled with the appropriate use of acetaminophen, non-steroidal anti-inflammatory drugs (NSAIDs), urinary analgesics, and antispasmodics. Importantly, despite most patients experiencing some temporary toxicity from BCG therapy, two studies have shown that this does not adversely affect their overall long-term quality of life (121,129). Furthermore, local toxicity does not correlate with clinical response to BCG (130).

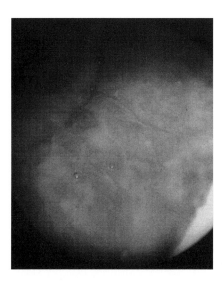

FIGURE 2 Severe bacillus Calmette-Guerin inflammation with granuloma formation.

Asymptomatic prostatitis, estimated as occurring in up to 40% of patients and often associated with an abnormal digital rectal examination, does not require specific therapy (131). However, it may be difficult to distinguish from the nodularity associated with prostate cancer (132). Prolonged symptomatic BCG cystitis and/or prostatitis (estimated incidence <5%) can be troublesome during therapy and in the post-BCG observation period (17). This is particularly more likely to occur during re-treatment or prolonged maintenance therapy. This situation is best avoided by withholding BCG treatment until all significant symptoms from the prior instillation have subsided. A one to two week delay has not been shown to reduce BCG efficacy in such a setting (133,134). Reinstitution of BCG at a lower dose or premature termination of further treatment for this cycle may also be appropriate. If localized severe cystitis does occur and conservative symptomatic treatment measures fail, this condition can be treated with oral fluoroquinolones (3–12 weeks) or oral isoniazid. A short, two to three week, oral steroid taper sandwiched between antibiotic coverage has also been shown to be helpful in refractory cases (135). The incidence of permanent bladder contracture after BCG is estimated as 2–3% (17,136,137).

Systemic Side Effects of BCG

Systemic side effects of BCG occur in one of two major forms, infectious and non-infectious. Fever/chills and a flu-like illness is reported in roughly a quarter of patients receiving BCG (Table 3) and has actually been associated with an improved cancer prognosis (138). In roughly 3% of patients body temperature exceeds 39.5°C (139). Not all fevers are a sign of BCG infection but rather may be the result of spillover of BCG-induced pyrogenic inflammatory cytokines from the bladder into the bloodstream (137). Unfortunately, in the acute setting it may be impossible to distinguish an infectious event from a non-infectious event. Such patients are best seen, evaluated, and sometimes hospitalized for observation. At a minimum, a flouroquinolone antibiotic should be considered since it will treat the majority of non-BCG bacterial urinary tract infections (UTIs) and has reasonable anti-mycobacterial activity until the patient declares him/herself symptom-free. Patients with self-limiting fevers <48 hours may be re-treated with NSAID prophylaxis (e.g., ibuprofen 600 mg q 6 hours × 3 beginning two hours prior to therapy) and at a reduced dose of BCG (140).

Clinical signs of a more serious process, such as BCG intravesation into the bloodstream (BCGosis), include exaggerated manifestations of the above-mentioned systemic effects particularly if they occur early during the initial course of induction therapy, within 2 hours after BCG instillation, or in the setting of traumatic catheterization (or too early instillation post-TURB). In the extreme case, a picture resembling gram-negative bacterial sepsis may emerge with the rapid and sequential appearance of skin mottling, chills, rigors, high temperatures (often over 39.5°C), and hypotension likely as a result of high levels of cytokines released directly into the bloodstream (the so-called cytokine storm) (141,142). The estimated incidence of this life-threatening event may be as high as 0.4% and several deaths have been reported (137,143,144). Prompt fluid resuscitation measures should be instituted as well as anti-pyretics, anti-tuberculosis antibiotics, and systemic steroids that have been shown to be life-saving in such instances (142,145,146).

Fevers without associated hypotension that begin after 24 hours, persist more than 48 hours, or relapse in a diurnal pattern (usually in the early evenings) following the cortisol cycle are more indicative of an established BCG infection (BCGitis). Organ-specific manifestations may be present, suggesting epididymal-orchitis, pneumonitis, or hepatitis that occur with a cumulative incidence of 2% to 4% (17,147). CT scans may show a pattern typical of miliary spread in the liver or lung (148). Other rare documented sites of BCG dissemination include infection of aneurysms/prosthetic material; renal, vertebral, and pelvic abscesses; and granulomatous penile ulceration (149–153). These patients often require hospitalization and the administration of double or triple drug therapy such as isoniazid (INH) (300 mg/day), rifampin (600 mg/day) ± ethambutol (1200 mg/day). A second or third generation fluoroquinolone may be added or substituted since it covers most gram-negative bacterial infections and has moderate activity against BCG. BCG is resistant to both pyrizidimide and cycloserine. It is reasonably sensitive to amikacin but less to gentamicin or tobramycin (154). Resolution of fever and associated symptoms is typically slow given the slow 24 to 48 hour replication time for BCG. Failure to improve on such therapy within a week or significant clinical deterioration should lead to the addition of systemic steroids (e.g., prednisone 40 mg/day tapered over two to six weeks but occasionally longer) (155). Antituberculosis drugs should be continued for 3, 6, or 12 months, depending on the severity of the presenting illness. Liver enzyme monitoring is required for INH and rifampin.

Other non-infectious systemic side effects of BCG may be related to an immune hypersensitivity state. Minor examples include arthralgias and skin rashes occurring in 5% to 6% of patients (17). However, more severe cases involve polyarthritis, Reiter's syndrome (urethritis, arthritis, conjunctivitis), and frank anaphylactic reactions (139,156,157). Most require immediate and permanent cessation of further therapy along with steroid therapy.

Methods to Prevent or Minimize BCG Complications

The more serious infectious side effects of BCGosis and BCGitis are best prevented by careful atraumatic catheter placement and withholding treatment in the event of any gross blood or severe pain. At least one and preferably two to three weeks should elapse after TURB before initiation of BCG. In general, manipulation such as urethral dilation, should not be performed immediately prior to BCG instillation. BCG should never be administered under high pressure but ideally dripped into the bladder under gravity. Caution should be exercised in treating immunosuppressed patients with BCG. Patients on low-dose oral or inhaled steroids have been successfully treated as have a few transplant patients on stronger anti-rejection medications (158,159). However, there have been documented cases of re-activation TB or BCG sepsis in immunocompromised patients (160,161).

All patients with symptoms of bladder irritability should be investigated with urinalysis and/or culture. BCG should be delayed if bacteriuria is indicated or if symptoms are moderate or greater to reduce the risk of inducing a sustained BCG cystitis (162). Routine use of peri-catherization antibiotics is not recommended, but if clinically indicated penicillins, cephlosporins, trimethoprim/sulfonamides, and nitrofurantoin are preferred since they are not cidal to BCG (154).

Several further adjustments to the BCG regimen may help reduce its local and systemic toxicity. Dose reduction of BCG (to one-half, one-third, or one-fourth standard dose) has been actively explored and in such studies a 50% to 75% reduction in BCG dose results in a 30% to 50% drop in serious morbidity without a significant impact on anti-cancer efficacy (163–164). This may be a problem during initial therapy in BCG-naïve populations in North America for high-grade papillary disease or CIS (165,166). However, this approach may be useful during re-induction and/or maintenance therapy when dropout from toxicity are higher. While controlled studies have not yet been performed to validate their utility, other regimen modifications include reducing the dwell time to 30 minutes or applying treatments on an every other week schedule (167,168). Pretreating patients with INH has not been shown to diminish either the associated symptomatology or the incidence of serious BCG infection (169). Administering 200 mg of ofloxacin 6 and 18 hours after each BCG treatment, however, significantly decreased by 18.5% the incidence of moderate and severe adverse events resulting in better compliance with full BCG treatment (170). Importantly, no obvious detriment to BCG efficacy was apparent in either study.

Side Effects of IFN-α Therapy

As a large protein with a molecular weight close to 20,000 Da there is minimal absorption of IFN-α after intravesical instillation. Typically, doses in the range of 50 to 100 million units (MU) are administered weekly. No dose-limiting toxicity was seen even with doses as high as 1000 MU (171). IFN-α is one of the best tolerated agents, causing minimal cystitis in 0% to 11% of patients (172,173). Systemic side effects include fever and a flu-like syndrome associated with fatigue and malaise occurring in under 15% of all but the highest dose trial. There was a 3% discontinuation in one trial and 4% in another (171,178). Table 7 lists the frequency of these side effects amongst multiple trials (171,174–181). Rare cases of confusion and suicidal ideation were also reported (178).

TABLE 7 Toxicity Reported from Intravesical Interferon Trials

Study	No. patients	Interferon dose (MU)	Cystitis (%)	Flu-like (%)
Torti et al. (171)	35	50–1000	0	27
Glashan et al. (174)	38	10	0	8
	47	100	0	14
Kostakopoulos et al. (175)	30	10	0	3
Portillo et al. (176)	45	60	0	0
Bartoletti et al. (177)	20	54	0	0
Malmstrom et al. (178)	27	30	0	11
	27	50	0	11
	27	80	11	11
Papatsoris et al. (179)	53	100	9	NR
DaSilva et al. (180)	64	60	0	0
	63	100	0	0
Giannakopoulos et al. (181)	22	40	0	0
	24	60	0	0
	23	80	0	0

Abbreviation: NR, not reported.

Combined BCG plus IFN-α Therapy

The theoretical advantage of combined BCG plus IFN-α therapy is reported to be the favorable immune synergy in eliciting a more productive cell-mediated T-helper type I immune response (182). Tolerability and toxicity data were reported from an interim analysis of 490 patients, approximately half of whom were BCG-naïve and received standard-dose BCG plus IFN-α (50 MU) while prior BCG-failure patients received one-third dose BCG plus IFN-α (50 MU) (183). While some degree of cystitis was present in over 80% of patients in both groups, need for medication was approximately 15%, delay or further BCG dose decrease in only 4% and dropout rate during induction in 2% to 3%. Furthermore, using only three 3-week maintenance cycles with further automatic BCG dose reduction to one-tenth, over 90% of eligible patients completed all three maintenance cycles. Systemic side effects were moderate or greater in <15% of patients. Serious adverse events occurred in 5.3% of patients and were primarily inflammatory or infectious in origin. Furthermore, they were approximately 50% lower in the low-dose BCG treated groups.

SUMMARY

Intravesical therapy with cytotoxic chemotherapy or immunotherapeutics share several common features of inducing local toxicity in the form of chemical or inflammatory cystitis. In the chemotherapy group this is more prevalent with known vesicant agents and during long-term therapy with high drug concentrations. The incidence of cystitis is highest overall with BCG and least with IFN-α. Despite these side effects, less than 10% of patients actually have to discontinue intravesical therapy and most of these patients recover well. Systemic side effects to chemotherapeutics depend greatly on absorption of drug and the toxicities inherent to each drug as well as occasional serious allergic reactions. Unrecognized bladder perforation can exaggerate these toxicities, leading to deadly consequences. In the case of BCG, attention must be given to avoiding serious infections associated with improper catheter placement and patient selection. Prompt recognition and specific therapy are required to avoid potentially lethal septic complications. Additional vigilance is required to recognize hypersensitivity immune reactions and in preventing local toxicity from escalating to serious levels. Knowledge and appreciation of the properties of these powerful drugs will help maximize their therapeutic utility.

REFERENCES

1. Haukaas S, Daehlin L, Maartmann-Moe H, et al. The long-term outcome in patients with superficial transitional cell carcinoma of the bladder: a single-institutional experience. BJU Int 1999; 83: 957–963.

2. Avritscher EB, Cooksley CD, Grossman HB, et al. Clinical model of lifetime cost of treating bladder cancer and associated complications. Urology 2006; 68:549–553.

3. Sylvester RJ, van der Meijden AP, Witjes JA, et al. Bacillus calmette-guerin versus chemotherapy for the intravesical treatment of patients with carcinoma in situ of the bladder: a meta-analysis of the published results of randomized clinical trials. J Urol 2005; 174:86–91.

4. Sylvester RJ, Oosterlinck W, van der Meijden AP. A single immediate postoperative instillation of chemotherapy decreases the risk of recurrence in patients with stage Ta T1 bladder cancer: a meta-analysis of published results of randomized clinical trials. J Urol 2004; 171:2186–2190.

5. Baselli EC, Greenberg RE. Maintenance therapy for superficial bladder cancer. Oncology (Williston Park) 2001; 15:85–88.

6. Huncharek M, Geschwind JF, Witherspoon B, et al. Intravesical chemotherapy prophylaxis in primary superficial bladder cancer: a meta-analysis of 3703 patients from 11 randomized trials. J Clin Epidemiol 2000; 53:676–880.

7. Highley MS, van Oosterom AT, Maes RA, et al. Intravesical drug delivery. Pharmacokinetic and clinical considerations. Clin Pharmacokinet 1999; 37:59–73.

8. Ener RA, Meglathery SB, Styler M. Extravasation of systemic hemato-oncological therapies. Ann Oncol 2004; 15:858–862.

9. Bibby MC, McDermott BJ, Double JA, et al. Influence of the tissue distribution of ThioTEPA and its metabolite, TEPA, on the response of murine colon tumours. Cancer Chemother Pharmacol 1987; 20:203–206.

10. Masters JR, McDermott BJ, Harland S, et al. ThioTEPA pharmacokinetics during intravesical chemotherapy: the influence of dose and volume of instillate on systemic uptake and dose rate to the tumour. Cancer Chemother Pharmacol 1996; 38:59–64.

11. Weaver D, Khare N, Haigh J, et al. The effect of chemotherapeutic agents on the ultrastructure of transitional cell carcinoma in tissue culture. Invest Urol 1980; 17:288–292.

12. Lunglmayr G, Czech K. Absorption studies on intraluminal thio-tepa for topical cytostatic treatment of low-stage bladder tumors. J Urol 1971; 106:72–74.

13. Veenema RJ, Dean AL Jr, Uson AC, Roberts M, Longo F. Thiotepa bladder instillations: therapy and prophylaxis for superficial bladder tumors. J Urol 1969; 101:711–715.

14. Jones HC, Swinney J. Thiotepa in the treatment of tumours of the bladder. Lancet 1961; 2:615–618.

15. Thrasher JB, Crawford ED. Complications of intravesical chemotherapy. Urol Clin N Am 1992; 19:529–539.

16. Silberberg JM, Zarrabi MH. Acute nonlymphocytic leukemia after thiotepa instillation into the bladder: report of 2 cases and review of the literature. J Urol 1987; 138:402–403.

17. Smith JA Jr, Labasky RF, Cockett AT, et al. Bladder cancer clinical guidelines panel summary report on the management of nonmuscle invasive bladder cancer (stages Ta, T1 and TIS). The American Urological Association. J Urol 1999; 162:1697–1701.

18. Homonnai TZ, Paz G, Servadio C. Sterilisation following instillation of thiotepa into the urinary bladder. Br J Urol 1982; 54:60.

19. Choe JM, Kirkemo AK, Sirls LT. Intravesical thiotepa-induced eosinophilic cystitis. Urology 1995; 46:729–731.

20. Treible DP, Skinner D, Kasimain D, et al. Intractable bladder hemorrhage requiring cystectomy after use of intravesical thiotepa. Urology 1987; 30:568–570.

21. Mukamel E, Glanz I, Nissenkorn I, Cytron S, Servadio C. Unanticipated vesicoureteral reflux: a possible sequela of long-term thio-tepa instillations to the bladder. J Urol 1982; 127:245–246.

22. Medical Research Council. The effect of intravesical thiotepa on the recurrence rate of newly diagnosed superficial bladder cancer. An MRC Study. MRC Working Party on Urological Cancer. Br J Urol 1985; 57:680–685.

23. Zincke H, Utz DC, Taylor WF, et al. Influence of thiotepa and doxorubicin instillation at time of transurethral surgical treatment of bladder cancer on tumor recurrence: a prospective, randomized, double-blind, controlled trial. J Urol 1983; 129:505–509.

24. Zincke H, Benson RC Jr, Hilton JF, et al. Intravesical thiotepa and mitomycin C treatment immediately after transurethral resection and later for superficial (stages Ta and Tis) bladder cancer: a prospective, randomized, stratified study with crossover design. J Urol 1985; 134:1110–1114.

25. Burnand KG, Boyd PJ, Mayo ME, et al. Single dose intravesical thiotepa as an adjuvant to cystodiathermy in the treatment of transitional cell bladder carcinoma. Br J Urol 1976; 48:55–59.

26. Gavrell GJ, Lewis RW, Meehan WL, Leblanc GA. Intravesical thio-tepa in the immediate postoperative period in patients with recurrent transitional cell carcinoma of the bladder. J Urol 1978; 120:410–411.

27. Xu BH, Gupta V, Singh SV. Mechanism of differential sensitivity of human bladder cancer cells to mitomycin C and its analogue. Br J Cancer 1994; 69:242–246.

28. Badalament RA, Farah RN. Treatment of superficial bladder cancer with intravesical chemotherapy. Semin Surg Oncol 1997; 13:335–341.

29. Iyer VN, Szybalski W. A molecular mechanism of mitomycin action: linking of complementary DNA strands. Proc Natl Acad Sci U S A 1963; 50:355–362.

30. Lown JW. The molecular mechanism of antitumor action of the mitomycins. In: Carter SK, Crooke ST, eds. Mitomycin C: Current Status and New Developments. Orlando, FL: Academic Press, 1979:5.

31. Dalton JT, Wientjes MG, Badalament RA, et al. Pharmacokinetics of intravesical mitomycin C in superficial bladder cancer patients. Cancer Res 1991; 51:5144–5152.

32. De Bruijn EA, Sleeboom HP, van Helsdingen PJ, et al. Pharmacodynamics and pharmacokinetics of intravesical mitomycin C upon different dwelling times. Int J Cancer 1992; 51:359–364.

33. van Helsdingen PJ, Rikken CH, Sleeboom HP, et al. Mitomycin C resorption following repeated intravesical instillations using different instillation times. Urol Int 1988; 43:42–46.

34. Wajsman Z, Dhafir RA, Pfeffer M, et al. Studies of mitomycin C absorption after intravesical treatment of superficial bladder tumors. J Urol 1984; 132:30–33.

35. Schmidbauer CP, Porpaczy P, Georgopoulos A, et al. Absorption of doxorubicin-hydrochloride and mitomycin-C after instillation into noninfected and infected bladders of dogs. J Urol 1984; 131: 818–821.

36. Au JL, Badalament RA, Wientjes MG, et al; International Mitomycin C Consortium. Methods to improve efficacy of intravesical mitomycin C: results of a randomized phase III trial. J Natl Cancer Inst 2001; 93:597–604.

37. Paroni R, Salonia A, Lev A, et al. Effect of local hyperthermia of the bladder on mitomycin C pharmacokinetics during intravesical chemotherapy for the treatment of superficial transitional cell carcinoma. Br J Clin Pharmacol 2001; 52:273–278.

38. Di Stasi SM, Giannantoni A, Stephen RL, et al. Intravesical electromotive mitomycin C versus passive transport mitomycin C for high risk superficial bladder cancer: a prospective randomized study. J Urol 2003; 170:777–782.

39. Crooke ST, Henderson M, Samson M, et al. Phase I study of oral mitomycin C. Cancer Treat Rep 1976; 60:1633–1636.

40. Zein TA, Friedberg N, Kim H. Bone marrow suppression after intravesical mitomycin C treatment. J Urol 1986; 136:459–460.

41. Racioppi M, Porreca A, Foschi N, et al. Bladder perforation: a potential risk of early endovesical chemotherapy with mitomycin C. Urol Int 2005; 75:373–375.

42. Brady JD, Assimos DG, Jordan GH. Urethral slough: a rare and previously unreported complication of intravesical mitomycin. J Urol 2000; 164:1305.

43. Neulander EZ, Lismer L, Kaneti J. Necrosis of the glans penis: a rare complication of intravesical therapy with mitomycin c. J Urol 2000; 164:1306.

44. Eijsten A, Knonagel H, Hotz E, et al. Reduced bladder capacity in patients receiving intravesical chemoprophylaxis with mitomycin C. Br J Urol 1990; 66:386–388.

45. Clark T, Chang SS, Cookson MS. Eosinophilic cystitis presenting as a recurrent symptomatic bladder mass following intravesical mitomycin C therapy. J Urol 2002; 167:1795.

46. Jauhiainen K, Sotarauta M, Permi J, et al. Effect of mitomycin C and doxorubicin instillation on carcinoma in situ of the urinary bladder. A Finnish multicenter study. Eur Urol 1986; 12:32–37.

47. de Groot AC, Conemans JM. Systemic allergic contact dermatitis from intravesical instillation of the antitumor antibiotic mitomycin C. Contact Dermatitis 1991; 24:201–209.

48. Colver GB, Inglis JA, McVittie E, et al. Dermatitis due to intravesical mitomycin C: a delayed-type hypersensitivity reaction? Br J Dermatol 1990; 122:217–224.

49. Rao S, Cunningham D, Price T, et al. Phase II study of capecitabine and mitomycin C as first-line treatment in patients with advanced colorectal cancer. Br J Cancer 2004; 91:839–843.

50. DeFuria MD, Bracken RB, Johnson DE, et al. Phase I-II study of mitomycin C topical therapy for low-grade, low stage transitional cell carcinoma of the bladder: an interim report. Cancer Treat Rep 1980; 64:225–230.

51. Sonneveld P, Kurth KH, Hagemeyer A, et al. Secondary hematologic neoplasm after intravesical chemotherapy for superficial bladder carcinoma. Cancer 1990; 65:23–25.

52. Llopis M, Moreno J, Botella R, et al. Incrusted cystitis after intravesical mitomycin C treatment. Acta Urol Belg 1993; 61:21–23.

53. Nieuwenhuijzen JA, Bex A, Horenblas S. Unusual complication after immediate postoperative intravesical mitomycin C instillation. Eur Urol 2003; 43:711–712.

54. Tolley DA, Parmar MK, Grigor KM, et al. The effect of intravesical mitomycin C on recurrence of newly diagnosed superficial bladder cancer: a further report with 7 years of follow up. J Urol 1996; 155:1233–1238.

55. Solsona E, Iborra I, Ricos JV, et al. Effectiveness of a single immediate mitomycin C instillation in patients with low risk superficial bladder cancer: short and long-term followup. J Urol 1999; 161: 1120–1123.

56. Bouffioux C, Kurth KH, Bono A, et al. Intravesical adjuvant chemotherapy for superficial transitional cell bladder carcinoma: results of 2 European Organization for Research and Treatment of Cancer randomized trials with mitomycin C and doxorubicin comparing early versus delayed instillations and short-term versus long-term treatment. European Organization for Research and Treatment of Cancer Genitourinary Group. J Urol 1995; 153:934–941.

57. Carter SK. Adriamycin-a review. J Natl Cancer Inst 1975; 55:1265–1274.

58. Triton TR, Yee G. The anticancer agent adriamycin can be actively cytotoxic without entering cells. Science 1982; 217:248–250.

59. Duque JL, Loughlin KR. An overview of the treatment of superficial bladder cancer. Intravesical chemotherapy. Urol Clin North Am 2000;27:125–135.

60. Wientjes MG, Badalament RA, Au JL. Penetration of intravesical doxorubicin in human bladders. Cancer Chemother Pharmacol 1996; 37:539–546.

61. Nagakura K, Takao M, Odajima K, et al. Serum uptake of doxorubicin intravesically administered soon after transurethral resection of bladder carcinoma. Hinyokika Kiyo 1989; 35:1509–1512.

62. Crawford ED, McKenzie D, Mansson W, et al. Adverse reactions to the intravesical administration of doxorubicin hydrochloride: report of 6 cases. J Urol 1986; 136:668–669.

63. Oosterlinck W, Kurth KH, Schroder F, et al. A prospective European Organization for Research and Treatment of Cancer Genitourinary Group randomized trial comparing transurethral resection followed by a single intravesical instillation of epirubicin or water in single stage Ta, T1 papillary carcinoma of the bladder. J Urol 1993; 149:749–752.

64. Marchetti A, Wang L, Magar R, et al. Management of patients with Bacilli Calmette-Guerin-refractory carcinoma in situ of the urinary bladder: cost implications of a clinical trial for valrubicin. Clin Ther 2000; 22:422–438.

65. Yoshimura A, Ogawa A, Wajiki M, et al. Chemical pericystitis: a rare complication of intravesical doxorubicin. J Urol 1986; 135:1237–1239.

66. Oddens JR, van der Meijden AP, Sylvester R. One immediate postoperative instillation of chemo-therapy in low risk Ta, T1 bladder cancer patients. Is it always safe? Eur Urol 2004; 46: 336–338.

67. Markman M, Homesley H, Norberts DA, et al. Phase 1 trial of intraperitoneal AD-32 in gynecologic malignancies. Gynecol Oncol 1996; 61:90–93.

68. Matsumura Y, Tsushima T, Ozaki Y, et al. Intravesical chemotherapy with 4'-epi-Adriamycin in patients with superficial bladder tumors. Cancer Chemother Pharmacol 1986; 16:176–177.

69. Burk K, Kurth KH, Newling D. Epirubicin in treatment and recurrence prophylaxis of patients with superficial bladder cancer. Prog Clin Biol Res 1989; 303:423–434.

70. Cumming JA, Kirk D, Newling DW, et al. A multi-centre phase two study of intravesical epirubicin in the treatment of superficial bladder tumour. Eur Urol 1990; 17:20–22.

71. Kurth K, Vijgh WJ, ten Kate F, et al. Phase I/II study of intravesical epirubicin in patients with carci-noma in situ of the bladder. J Urol 1991; 146:1508–1512.

72. Ali-el-Dein B, Nabeeh A, el-Baz M, et al. Single-dose versus multiple instillations of epirubicin as prophylaxis for recurrence after transurethral resection of pTa and pT1 transitional-cell bladder tumours: a prospective, randomized controlled study. Br J Urol 1997; 79:731–735.

73. Ali-el-Dein B, el-Baz M, Aly AN, et al. Intravesical epirubicin versus doxorubicin for superficial bladder tumors (stages pTa and pT1): a randomized prospective study. J Urol 1997; 158:68–73.

74. Eto H, Oka Y, Ueno K, et al. Comparison of the prophylactic usefulness of epirubicin and doxo-rubicin in the treatment of superficial bladder cancer by intravesical instillation: a multicenter randomized trial. Kobe University Urological Oncology Group. Cancer Chemother Pharmacol 1994; 35(Suppl):S46–S51.

75. Greenberg RE, Bahnson RR, Wood D, et al. Initial report on intravesical administration of N-trifluo-roacetyladriamycin-14-valerate (AD 32) to patients with refractory superficial transitional cell carci-noma of the urinary bladder. Urology 1997; 49:471–475.

76. Patterson AL, Greenberg RE, Weems L, et al. Pilot study of the tolerability and toxicity of intravesical valrubicin immediately after transurethral resection of superficial bladder cancer. Urology 2000; 56:232–235.

77. Steinberg G, Bahnson R, Brosman S, et al. Efficacy and safety of valrubicin for the treatment of Bacillus Calmette-Guerin refractory carcinoma in situ of the bladder. The Valrubicin Study Group. J Urol 2000; 163:761–767.

78. Newling DW, Hetherington J, Sundaram SK, et al. The use of valrubicin for the chemoresection of superficial bladder cancer–a marker lesion study. Eur Urol 2001; 39:643–647.

79. Hendricksen K, Witjes JA. Intravesical gemcitabine: an update of clinical results. Curr Opin Urol 2006; 16:361–366.

80. Hertel LW, Boder GB, Kroin JS, et al. Evaluation of the antitumor activity of gemcitabine (2',2'-difluoro-2'-deoxycytidine). Cancer Res 1990; 50:4417–4422.

81. Burris HA III, Moore MJ, Andersen J, et al. Improvements in survival and clinical benefit with gem-citabine as first-line therapy for patients with advanced pancreas cancer: a randomized trial. J Clin Oncol 1997; 15:2403–2413.

82. Schiller JH, Harrington D, Belani CP, et al; Eastern Cooperative Oncology Group. Comparison of four chemotherapy regimens for advanced non-small-cell lung cancer. N Engl J Med 2002; 346: 92–98.

83. von der Maase H, Hansen SW, Roberts JT, et al. Gemcitabine and cisplatin versus methotrexate, vinblastine, doxorubicin, and cisplatin in advanced or metastatic bladder cancer: results of a large, randomized, multinational, multicenter, phase III study. J Clin Oncol 2000; 18:3068–3077.

84. Dalbagni G, Russo P, Bochner B, et al. Phase II trial of intravesical gemcitabine in bacille Calmette-Guerin-refractory transitional cell carcinoma of the bladder. J Clin Oncol 2006; 24:2729–2734.

85. Laufer M, Ramalingam S, Schoenberg MP, et al. Intravesical gemcitabine therapy for superficial transitional cell carcinoma of the bladder: a phase I and pharmacokinetic study. J Clin Oncol 2003; 21:697–703.

86. De Berardinis E, Antonini G, Peters GJ, et al. Intravesical administration of gemcitabine in superficial bladder cancer: a phase I study with pharmacodynamic evaluation. BJU Int 2004; 93:491–494.

87. Palou J, Carcas A, Segarra J, et al. Phase I pharmacokinetic study of a single intravesical instillation of gemcitabine administered immediately after transurethral resection plus multiple random biopsies in patients with superficial bladder cancer. J Urol 2004; 172:485–488.

88. Witjes JA, van der Heijden AG, Vriesema JL, et al. Intravesical gemcitabine: a phase 1 and pharmacokinetic study. Eur Urol 2004; 45:182–186.

89. De Berardinis E, Antonini G, Peters GJ, et al. Intravesical administration of gemcitabine in superficial bladder cancer: a phase I study with pharmacodynamic evaluation. BJU Int 2004; 93:491–494.

90. Serretta V, Galuffo A, Pavone C, et al. Gemcitabine in intravesical treatment of Ta-T1 transitional cell carcinoma of bladder: Phase I-II study on marker lesions. Urology 2005; 65:65–69.

91. Ringel I, Horwitz SB. Studies with RP 56976 (taxotere): a semisynthetic analogue of taxol. J Natl Cancer Inst 1991; 83:288–291.

92. de Wit R, Kruit WH, Stoter G, et al. Docetaxel (Taxotere): an active agent in metastatic urothelial cancer; results of a phase II study in non-chemotherapy-pretreated patients. Br J Cancer 1998; 78:1342–1345.

93. Dimopoulos MA, Bakoyannis C, Georgoulias V, et al. Docetaxel and cisplatin combination chemotherapy in advanced carcinoma of the urothelium: a multicenter phase II study of the Hellenic Cooperative Oncology Group. Ann Oncol 1999; 10:1385–1388.

94. Garcia del Muro X, Marcuello E, Guma J, et al. Phase II multicentre study of docetaxel plus cisplatin in patients with advanced urothelial cancer. Br J Cancer 2002; 86:326–330.

95. Pectasides D, Visvikis A, Aspropotamitis A, et al. Chemotherapy with cisplatin, epirubicin and docetaxel in transitional cell urothelial cancer. Phase II trial. Eur J Cancer 2000; 36:74–79.

96. McKiernan JM, Masson P, Murphy AM, et al. Phase I trial of intravesical docetaxel in the management of superficial bladder cancer refractory to standard intravesical therapy. J Clin Oncol 2006; 24:3075–3080.

97. Stanford BL, Shah SR, Ballard EE, et al. A randomized trial assessing the utility of a test-dose program with taxanes. Curr Med Res Opin 2005; 21:1611–1616.

98. Masson P, Murphy AM, Goetzl MA, et al. Long-term follow up of intravesical docetaxel for the treatment of superficial bladder cancer resistant to standard intravesical therapy. J Urol 2006; 175(Suppl. 4):273, abstract no. 846.

99. Robinson MR, Shetty MB, Richards B, et al. Intravesical epodyl in the management of bladder tumors: combined experience of the Yorkshire Urological Cancer Research Group. J Urol 1977; 118:972–973.

100. Kurth KH, Schroder FH, Tunn U, et al. Adjuvant chemotherapy of superficial transitional cell bladder carcinoma: preliminary results of a European organization for research on treatment of cancer. Randomized trial comparing doxorubicin hydrochloride, ethoglucid and transurethral resection alone. J Urol 1984; 132:258–262.

101. Ricos Torrent JV, Monros Lliso JL, Iborra Juan I, et al. Mitoxantrone (MTX) versus mitomycin C (MMC) in the ablative treatment of Ta, T1 superficial bladder tumors. Phase III, randomized prospective study. Arch Esp Urol 1992; 45:647–652.

102. Huang JS, Chen WH, Lin CC, et al. A randomized trial comparing intravesical instillations of mitoxantrone and doxorubicin in patients with superficial bladder cancer. Chang Gung Med J 2003; 26:91–97.

103. Papatsoris AG, Deliveliotis C, Giannopoulos A, et al. Adjuvant intravesical mitoxantrone versus recombinant interferon-alpha after transurethral resection of superficial bladder cancer: a randomized prospective study. Urol Int 2004; 72:284–291.

104. Flamm J, Donner G, Oberleitner S, et al. Adjuvant intravesical mitoxantrone after transurethral resection of primary superficial transitional cell carcinoma of the bladder. A prospective randomised study. Eur J Cancer 1995; 31A:143–146.

105. Yaman LS, Yurdakul T, Zissis NP, et al. Intravesical mitoxantrone for superficial bladder tumors. Anticancer Drugs 1994; 5:95–98.

106. Stewart DJ, Green R, Futter N, et al. Phase I and pharmacology study of intravesical mitoxantrone for recurrent superficial bladder tumors. J Urol 1990; 143:714–716.

107. Serretta V, Corselli G, Pavone C, et al. Intravesical mitoxantrone in superficial bladder tumours (Ta-T1). Eur J Cancer 1993; 29A:1899–1900.

108. Blumenreich MS, Needles B, Yagoda A, et al. Intravesical cisplatin for superficial bladder tumors. Cancer 1982; 50:863–865.

109. Bouffioux C, Denis L, Oosterlinck W, et al. Adjuvant chemotherapy of recurrent superficial transitional cell carcinoma: results of a European organization for research on treatment of cancer randomized trial comparing intravesical instillation of thiotepa, doxorubicin and cisplatin.

The European Organization for Research on Treatment of Cancer Genitourinary Group. J Urol 1992; 148:297–301.

110. Zanotti KM, Markman M. Prevention and management of antineoplastic-induced hypersensitivity reactions. Drug Saf 2001; 24:767–779.

111. Sternberg CN, Yagoda A, Bander NH, et al. Phase I/II trial of intravesical methotrexate for superficial bladder tumors. Cancer Chemother Pharmacol 1986; 18:265–269.

112. Sekine H, Ohya K, Kojima SI, et al. Equivalent efficacy of mitomycin C plus doxorubicin instillation to bacillus Calmette-Guerin therapy for carcinoma in situ of the bladder. Int J Urol 2001; 8:483–486.

113. Fukui I, Sekine H, Kihara K, et al. Sequential instillation therapy with mitomycin C and adriamycin for superficial bladder tumors. Cancer Chemother Pharmacol 1987; 20(Suppl):S52–S55.

114. Yoshida O, Miyakawa M, Watanabe H, et al. Study of combination chemotherapy with cytosine arabinoside in the intravesical treatment of superficial bladder tumors. Hinyokika Kiyo 1983; 29: 357–364.

115. Kinoshita N, Tochigi H, Yanagawa M, et al. Clinical study of intravesical instillation therapy of superficial bladder tumor–combination therapy of mitomycin C, adriamycin, peplomycin and cytosine arabinoside. Hinyokika Kiyo 1990; 36:257–263.

116. Sakamoto N, Naito S, Kumazawa J, et al.; Kyushu University Urological Oncology Group. Prophylactic intravesical instillation of mitomycin C and cytosine arabinoside for prevention of recurrent bladder tumors following surgery for upper urinary tract tumors: a prospective randomized study. Int J Urol 2001; 8:212–216.

117. Maymi JL, Saltsgaver N, O'Donnell MA. Intravsical sequential gemcitabine-mitomycin chemotherapy as salvage treatment for patients with refractory superficial bladder cancer. J Urol 2006; 175(Suppl. 4):271, abstract no. 840.

118. Rajala P, Liukkonen T, Raitanen M, et al. Transurethral resection with perioperative instilation on interferon-alpha or epirubicin for the prophylaxis of recurrent primary superficial bladder cancer: a prospective randomized multicenter study—Finnbladder III. J Urol 1999; 161:1133–1135.

119. Lamm DL. Complications of bacillus Calmette-Guerin immunotherapy. Urol Clin North Am 1992; 19:565–572.

120. Sylvester RJ, van der Meijden AP, Lamm DL. Intravesical bacillus Calmette-Guerin reduces the risk of progression in patients with superficial bladder cancer: a meta-analysis of the published results of randomized clinical trials. J Urol 2002; 168:1964–1970.

121. Bohle A, Balck F, von Weitersheim J, et al. The quality of life during intravesical bacillus Calmette-Guerin therapy. J Urol 1996; 155:1221–1226.

122. Saint F, Irani J, Patard JJ, et al. Tolerability of bacille Calmette-Guerin maintenance therapy for superficial bladder cancer. Urology 2001; 57:883–888.

123. Bohle A, Jocham D, Bock PR. Intravesical bacillus Calmette-Guerin versus mitomycin C for superficial bladder cancer: a formal meta-analysis of comparative studies on recurrence and toxicity. J Urol 2003; 169:90–95.

124. van der Meijden AP, Sylvester RJ, Oosterlinck W, et al. EORTC Genito-Urinary Tract Cancer Group. Maintenance Bacillus Calmette-Guerin for Ta T1 bladder tumors is not associated with increased toxicity: results from a European Organisation for Research and Treatment of Cancer Genito-Urinary Group Phase III Trial. Eur Urol 2003; 44:429–434.

125. Hudson MA, Ratliff TL, Gillen DP, et al. Single course versus maintenance bacillus Calmette-Guerin therapy for superficial bladder tumors: a prospective, randomized trial. J Urol 1987; 138: 295–298.

126. Lamm DL, Blumenstein BA, Crissman JD, et al. Maintenance bacillus Calmette-Guerin immunotherapy for recurrent TA, T1 and carcinoma in situ transitional cell carcinoma of the bladder: a randomized Southwest Oncology Group Study. J Urol 2000; 163:1124–1129.

127. Pagano F, Bassi P, Milani C, et al. Pathologic and structural changes in the bladder after BCG intravesical therapy in men. Prog Clin Biol Res 1989; 310:81–91.

128. Prescott S, James K, Hargreave TB, et al. Immunopathological effects of intravesical BCG therapy. Prog Clin Biol Res 1989; 310:93–105.

129. Mack D, Frick J. Quality of life in patients undergoing bacille Calmette-Guerin therapy for superficial bladder cancer. Br J Urol 1996; 78:369–371.

130. Sylvester RJ, van der Meijden AP, Oosterlinck W, et al. EORTC Genito-Urinary Tract Cancer Group. The side effects of Bacillus Calmette-Guerin in the treatment of Ta T1 bladder cancer do not predict its efficacy: results from a European Organisation for Research and Treatment of Cancer Genito-Urinary Group Phase III Trial. Eur Urol 2003; 44:423–428.

131. Oates RD, Stilmant MM, Freedlund MC, et al. Granulomatous prostatitis following bacillus Calmette-Guerin immunotherapy of bladder cancer. J Urol 1988; 140:751–754.

132. Oppenheimer JR, Kahane H, Epstein JI. Granulomatous prostatitis on needle biopsy. Arch Pathol Lab Med 1997; 121:724–729.

133. Lamm DL. Bacillus Calmette-Guerin immunotherapy for bladder cancer. J Urol 1985; 134:40–47.

134. Brosman SA. Experience with bacillus Calmette-Guerin in patients with superficial bladder carcinoma. J Urol 1982; 128:27–30.

135. Wittes R, Klotz L, Kosecka U. Severe bacillus Calmette-Guerin cystitis responds to systemic steroids when antituberculous drugs and local steroids fail. J Urol 1999; 161:1568–1569.

136. Orihuela E, Herr HW, Pinsky CM, et al. Toxicity of intravesical BCG and its management in patients with superficial bladder tumors. Cancer 1987; 60:326–333.

137. Lamm DL, Steg A, Boccon-Gibod L, et al. Complications of bacillus Calmette-Guerin immunotherapy: review of 2602 patients and comparison of chemotherapy complications. Prog Clin Biol Res 1989; 310:335–355.

138. Luftenegger W, Ackermann DK, Futterlieb A, et al. Intravesical versus intravesical plus intradermal bacillus Calmette-Guerin: a prospective randomized study in patients with recurrent superficial bladder tumors. J Urol 1996; 155:483–487.

139. Lamm DL, Stogdill VD, Stogdill BJ, et al. Complications of bacillus Calmette-Guerin immunotherapy in 1,278 patients with bladder cancer. J Urol 1986; 135:272–274.

140. O'Donnell MA, Burns JA. Intravesical bacille Calmette-Guerin in the treatment and prophylaxis of urothelial bladder cancer. In: Droller MJ, ed. Atlas of Clinical Oncology: Urothelial Tumors. London: BC Decker, 2004:229–231.

141. Aikawa N. Cytokine storm in the pathogenesis of multiple organ dysfunction syndrome associated with surgical insults. Nippon Geka Gakkai Zasshi 1996; 97:771–777.

142. Rival G, Garot D, Mercier E, et al. Acute respiratory failure and septic shock induced by Mycobacterium bovis. A rare side effect of intravesical BCG therapy. Presse Med 2006; 35:980–982.

143. Rawls WH, Lamm DL, Lowe BA, et al. Fatal sepsis following intravesical bacillus Calmette-Guerin administration for bladder cancer. J Urol 1990; 144:1328–1330.

144. Deresiewicz RL, Stone RM, Aster JC. Fatal disseminated mycobacterial infection following intravesical bacillus Calmette-Guerin. J Urol 1990; 144:1331–1333.

145. Steg A, Leleu C, Debre B, et al. Systemic bacillus Calmette-Guerin infection in patients treated by intravesical BCG therapy for superficial bladder cancer. Prog Clin Biol Res 1989; 310:325–334.

146. DeHaven JI, Traynellis C, Riggs DR, et al. Antibiotic and steroid therapy of massive systemic bacillus Calmette- Guerin toxicity. J Urol 1992; 147:738–742.

147. Lamm DL, van der Meijden PM, Morales A, et al. Incidence and treatment of complications of bacillus Calmette-Guerin intravesical therapy in superficial bladder cancer. J Urol 1992; 147:596–600.

148. Elkabani M, Greene JN, Vincent AL, et al. Disseminated Mycobacterium bovis after intravesicular bacillus Calmette-Guerin treatments for bladder cancer. Cancer Control 2000; 7:476–481.

149. Kamphuis JT, Buiting AG, Misere JF, et al. BCG immunotherapy: be cautious of granulomas. Disseminated BCG infection and mycotic aneurysm as late complications of intravesical BCG instillations. Neth J Med 2001; 58:71–75.

150. Guerra CE, Betts RF, O'Keefe RJ, et al. Mycobacterium bovis osteomyelitis involving a hip arthroplasty after intravesicular bacille Calmette-Guerin for bladder cancer. Clin Infect Dis 1998; 27:639–640.

151. Hakim S, Heaney JA, Heinz T, et al. Psoas abscess following intravesical bacillus Calmette-Guerin for bladder cancer: a case report. J Urol 1993; 150:188–189.

152. Siskron FT, IV, Venable DD, Gonzalez E, et al. Granulomatous mass in a nonrefluxing renal unit after bacillus Calmette-Guerin therapy for bladder cancer. J Urol 1997; 158:882–883.

153. French CG, Hickey L, Bell DG. Caseating granulomas on the glans penis as a complication of bacille calmette-guerin intravesical therapy. Rev Urol 2001; 3:36–38.

154. Durek C, Rusch-Gerdes S, Jocham D, et al. Sensitivity of BCG to modern antibiotics. Eur Urol 2000; 37(Suppl 1):21–25.

155. Anonymous. Case records of the Massachusetts General Hospital. Weekly clinicopathological exercises. Case 29–1998. A 57-year-old man with fever and jaundice after intravesical instillation of bacille Calmette-Guerin for bladder cancer [(clinical conference)]. N Engl J Med 1998; 339:831–837.

156. Tinazzi E, Ficarra V, Simeoni S, et al. Reactive arthritis following BCG immunotherapy for urinary bladder carcinoma: a systematic review. Rheumatol Int 2006; 26:481–488.

157. Hodish I, Ezra D, Gur H, et al. Reiter's syndrome after intravesical bacillus Calmette-Guerin therapy for bladder cancer. Isr Med Assoc J 2000; 2:240–241.

158. Yossepowitch O, Eggener SE, Bochner BH, et al. Safety and efficacy of intravesical bacillus Calmette-Guerin instillations in steroid treated and immunocompromised patients. J Urol 2006; 176:482–485.

159. Palou J, Angerri O, Segarra J, et al. Intravesical bacillus Calmette-Guerin for the treatment of superficial bladder cancer in renal transplant patients. Transplantation 2003; 76:1514–1516.

160. Izes JK, Bihrle W III, Thomas CB. Corticosteroid-associated fatal mycobacterial sepsis occurring 3 years after instillation of intravesical bacillus Calmette-Guerin. J Urol 1993; 150:1498–1500.

161. Gonzalez OY, Musher DM, Brar I, et al. Spectrum of bacille Calmette-Guerin (BCG) infection after intravesical BCG immunotherapy. Clin Infect Dis 2003; 36:140–148.

162. van der Meijden AP. Practical approaches to the prevention and treatment of adverse reactions to BCG. Eur Urol 1995; 27(Suppl 1):23–28.

163. Takashi M, Wakai K, Ohno Y, et al. Evaluation of a low-dose intravesical bacillus Calmette-Guerin (Tokyo strain) therapy for superficial bladder cancer. Int Urol Nephrol 1995; 27:723–733.

164. Martinez-Pineiro JA, Solsona E, Flores N, et al. Improving the safety of BCG immunotherapy by dose reduction. Cooperative Group CUETO, Eur Urol 1995; 27(Suppl 1):13–18.

165. Pagano F, Bassi P, Piazza N, et al. Improving the efficacy of BCG immunotherapy by dose reduction. Eur Urol 1995; 27(Suppl 1):19–22.

166. Morales A, Nickel JC, Wilson JW. Dose-response of bacillus Calmette-Guerin in the treatment of superficial bladder cancer. J Urol 1992; 147:1256–1258.

167. Andius P, Fehrling M, Holmang S. Intravesical bacillus Calmette-Guerin therapy: experience with a reduced dwell-time in patients with pronounced side-effects. BJU Int 2005; 96:1290–1293.

168. Bassi P, Spinadin R, Carando R, et al. Modified induction course: a solution to side-effects? Eur Urol 2000; 37(Suppl 1):31–32.

169. van der Meijden AP, Brausi M, Zambon V, et al; Members of the EORTC Genito-Urinary Group. Intravesical instillation of epirubicin, bacillus Calmette-Guerin and bacillus Calmette-Guerin plus isoniazid for intermediate and high risk Ta, T1 papillary carcinoma of the bladder: a European Organization for Research and Treatment of Cancer genito-urinary group randomized phase III trial. J Urol 2001; 166:476–481.

170. Colombel M, Saint F, Chopin D, et al. The effect of ofloxacin on bacillus calmette-guerin induced toxicity in patients with superficial bladder cancer: results of a randomized, prospective, double-blind, placebo controlled, multicenter study. J Urol 2006; 176:935–939.

171. Torti FM, Shortliffe LD, Williams RD, et al. Alpha-interferon in superficial bladder cancer: a Northern California Oncology Group Study. J Clin Oncol 1988; 6:476–483.

172. Brown DH, Wagner TT, Bahnson RR. Interferons and bladder cancer. Urol Clin North Am 2000; 27:171–178.

173. Belldegrun AS, Franklin JR, O'Donnell MA, et al. Superficial bladder cancer: the role of interferon-alpha. J Urol 1998; 159:1793–1801.

174. Glashan RW. A randomized controlled study of intravesical alpha-2b-interferon in carcinoma in situ of the bladder. J Urol 1990; 144:658–661.

175. Kostakopoulos A, Deliveliotis C, Mavromanolakis E, et al. Intravesical interferon alfa-2b administration in the treatment of superficial bladder tumors. Eur Urol 1990; 18:201–203.

176. Portillo J, Martin B, Hernandez R, et al. Results at 43 months' follow-up of a double-blind, randomized, prospective clinical trial using intravesical interferon alpha-2b in the prophylaxis of stage pT1 transitional cell carcinoma of the bladder. Urology 1997; 49:187–190.

177. Bartoletti R, Massimini G, Criscuolo D, et al. Interferon alfa 2a in superficial bladder cancer prophylaxis: toleration and long-term follow-up. A phase I-II study. Anticancer Res 1991; 11:2167–2170.

178. Malmstrom PU. A randomized comparative dose-ranging study of interferon-alpha and mitomycin-C as an internal control in primary or recurrent superficial transitional cell carcinoma of the bladder. BJU Int 2002; 89:681–686.

179. Papatsoris AG, Deliveliotis C, Giannopoulos A, et al. Adjuvant intravesical mitoxantrone versus recombinant interferon-alpha after transurethral resection of superficial bladder cancer: a randomized prospective study. Urol Int 2004; 72:284–291.

180. da Silva FC, Furtado L, Reis M, et al. Comparison of two doses of interferon-alpha-2b in intravesical prophylaxis of superficial bladder tumors. Portuguese Genito-Urinary Group. Eur Urol 1995; 28:291–296.

181. Giannakopoulos S, Gekas A, Alivizatos G, et al. Efficacy of escalating doses of intravesical interferon alpha-2b in reducing recurrence rate and progression in superficial transitional cell carcinoma. Br J Urol 1998; 82:829–834.

182. Luo Y, Chen X, Downs TM, et al. IFN-alpha 2B enhances Th1 cytokine responses in bladder cancer patients receiving Mycobacterium bovis bacillus Calmette-Guerin immunotherapy. Immunology 1999; 162:2399–2405.

183. O'Donnell MA, Lilli K, Leopold C. National Bacillus Calmette-Guerin/Interferon Phase 2 Investigator Group. Interim results from a national multicenter phase II trial of combination bacillus Calmette-Guerin plus interferon alfa-2b for superficial bladder cancer. J Urol 2004; 172:888–893.

34 | Complications of External-Beam Radiation Therapy

Clair Beard
Department of Radiation Oncology, Dana-Farber/Brigham and Women's Cancer Center, Boston, Massachusetts, U.S.A.

INTRODUCTION

External-beam radiation therapy (EBRT) has been used to treat patients with prostate cancer for at least five decades and has always been associated with a risk of normal tissue complications. However, radiation therapy equipment has changed radically over time, as have the risks of morbidity. The first teletherapy units were of low energy. Treatment planning was performed based on bony landmarks and low doses of radiotherapy were delivered with generally poor results. With the development of linear accelerators in the early 1970s and fluoroscopic simulation, it became possible to target the prostate more accurately and to deliver radiation in the range of 6500 rad (or cGy). Most of the patients treated in the era before the use of prostate-specific antigen (PSA) assays, had advanced disease so cancer control was modest and complications were recognized, but generally accepted, as a necessary part of treatment. A major step forward in the realm of EBRT came with the advent of computed tomogrpahy (CT)-based planning and shaped or conformal blocks. A randomized trial performed in England, comparing relatively low-dose radiation given by means of either standard treatment or conformal radiotherapy (CRT), demonstrated lower complication rates with conformal treatment (1). Radiation oncologists were now able to deliver doses as high as 70 to 75 Gy, but with complications that will be discussed later in this chapter. More recently, intensity-modulated radiotherapy (IMRT), a more sophisticated type of three-dimensional CRT (3DCRT), has become the standard therapy at many institutions in the United States and abroad. IMRT is costly and difficult to deliver, but exciting in that it allows protection of normal tissue in a way that was not previously possible. An example of 3DCRT and IMRT in the same patient is shown in Figure 1. The conformality of the IMRT around the prostate can be seen on inspection of the isodose curves, which are closer to the prostate and yield a smaller dose to the normal tissues, such as rectum and bladder.

INFORMING PATIENTS ABOUT THE POSSIBILITY OF NORMAL-TISSUE COMPLICATIONS

Any patient who chooses to receive EBRT is potentially at risk for complications, either temporary or permanent. Whether men assume an active or a collaborative role in making the choice to receive radiation, their understanding of potential complications is important in order to prevent decisional conflict and regret after treatment (2–4). A study by Clark et al. at the Boston University School of Public Health (5) revealed that, while treatment-related side effects do not necessarily change measures of overall health status or health-related quality of life, there can be other effects. Patients who experience difficulty with urinary control also report significantly lower sexual intimacy and sexual confidence, as well as awkwardness and anxiety about sexual interaction. In that study, patients who reported frequent diarrhea, urgency, or pain with bowel movements also reported lower scores on sexual intimacy, marital affection, masculine self-esteem, and greater health worry. On a more positive note, when patients feel confident that their prostate cancer is controlled and that the decision was well informed, their degree of satisfaction is higher. Thus it behooves the treating clinician to carefully and methodically inform patients about complication risks.

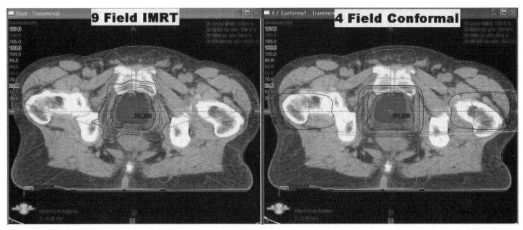

FIGURE 1 Comparison of IMRT and 3DCRT plans on the same patient. The prostate is the gray structure in the center. The lines represent isodose lines. Inspection shows better conformation to the prostate and better avoidance of the rectum with 9-field IMRT. *Abbreviations*: 3DCRT, three-dimensional CRT; IMRT, intensity-modulated radiotherapy.

Selection for EBRT

Not all prostate-cancer patients are equally likely to receive EBRT. Patients with advanced prostate cancer receive EBRT if they do not have the option for brachytherapy or surgery. Other patients choose EBRT because of fear of surgery, economic concerns with loss of work, or fear of surgical risks of incontinence (3). However, the Prostate Cancer Outcomes Study, a study of pre-diagnosis urinary, bowel, and sexual function, revealed that *baseline* incontinence, erectile

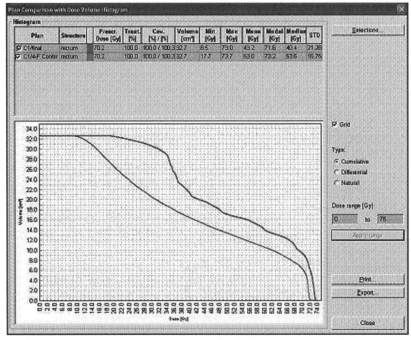

FIGURE 2 Comparison of dose-volume histograms using IMRT and 3DCRT. Dose-volume histograms demonstrate the difference in rectal dose between the two plans. The area below the top line is the rectal dose delivered by the 3DCRT plan. The area below the bottom line is the rectal dose delivered by IMRT. The difference is significant. *Abbreviations*: 3DCRT, three-dimensional CRT; IMRT, intensity-modulated radiotherapy.

dysfunction, and significant comorbidity are more prevalent in patients receiving radiotherapy. This is consistent with the fact that older patients are more likely to receive radiation (6). The authors of these studies (3,5,6) end by stating that better information on baseline function and the risks and benefits of prostate cancer treatment should be provided to patients.

With regard to baseline function, there are some general guidelines for patient selection. Patients with a history of inflammatory bowel disease, such as ulcerative colitis or Crohn's disease, are considered to be at risk for radiation-induced complications (7). Most radiation oncologists approach them gingerly. Diabetes, a common comorbid condition in patients who receive EBRT, was shown in one report to be associated with more late grade 2 gastrointestinal (GI) tract toxicity (28% vs. 17%; $p = 0.011$), late grade 2 genitourinary (GU) toxicity (14% vs. 6%; $P = 0.001$), and increased late grades 3 and 4 GI complications (8). These results were confirmed by other studies as well (9–11). Morbid obesity is not in and of itself a contraindication for EBRT, but data from the University of California at San Francisco (UCSF) demonstrated a high prevalence of technical treatment errors related to difficulty with patient positioning in this population and had specific recommendations for their treatment (12).

Having established the importance of patient health status, education, and concern about potential complications, this chapter will discuss common radiation-induced complications, using patient-reported outcomes whenever possible, with an understanding that observational studies provide useful information as well (4). Most of the available data are based on CRT and the reader must understand that over time we will need to re-evaluate our health-related quality-of-life expectations as radiotherapy delivery becomes more refined.

RECTAL COMPLICATIONS
General Information

Portions of the anterior rectal wall, by virtue of their relationship to the posterior edge of the prostate, receive full-dose radiotherapy in patients treated for prostate cancer (13). Prior to conformal radiation, radiation proctopathy and proctitis were considered an unfortunate and unavoidable consequence of treatment (14,15). With the advent of CRT, the incidence of bowel complications decreased, but there were still patients who experienced permanent distressing alteration in rectal function. With the advent of IMRT and image-guided radiotherapy (IGRT), which will be discussed later in this chapter, radiation oncologists are seeing fewer and fewer of the problematic rectal function changes that we had become accustomed to. While IMRT and IGRT are too new to have long-term complication data, the early data on improved rectal function are very exciting and a great relief to radiation oncologists.

Pathological Changes in the Rectum after EBRT

As shown in Figure 1, the portion of rectum included in the radiation fields is quite different for conventional treatment, conformal radiation, and IMRT. There is no way, however, that any treatment technique can completely avoid some radiation dose to the rectum. Whenever prostate radiation is given, it may be possible to exceed the tolerance of an individual's normal rectal mucosa, resulting in short-term complications, such as proctopathy and, for some patients, radiation proctitis (13). Microscopic changes in the rectal mucosa may be seen shortly after initiation of radiation and include damage to the epithelial cells of the mucosa and distortion of the vascular endothelial cells, as shown in Figure 3A (14,15). The pathophysiology of early-radiation bowel reaction may be caused by inflammatory mediators (16). Studies have shown that levels of leukotriene B4, thromboxane B2, and prostaglandin E2 all rise markedly in the rectum as a response to radiation therapy (17). If the patient fails to heal, these injuries can progress to thinning and loss of the mucosal epithelial layer, loss of the lamina propria lymphocytes, eosinophilic crypt abscess formation, and swelling of the arteriolar endothelium (13,18–20). In some patients, persistent and progressive mucosal ulcers occur with associated submucosal edema as shown in Figure 3B. More commonly, neovascularization and dilation of small vessels develop (20). Late effects of radiation injury to the intestine include telangiectasia formation and mucosal atrophy (21). In extreme cases, progressive ischemia and fibrosis can lead to stricture formation, fistulization, and perforation.

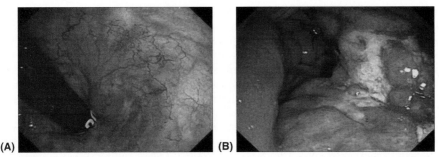

FIGURE 3 (**A**) Mild case of radiation proctopathy. (**B**) Severe case of radiation proctitis. Both images Courtesy of Dr. David Carr-Locke, Brigham and Women's Hospital.

Symptoms of Radiation Proctopathy and Proctitis

Acute radiation proctopathy, by definition, occurs during and up to six weeks after completion of radiation therapy. Patients may experience urgency, tenesmus, increased frequency of bowel movements, occasional diarrhea, or hemorrhoidal bleeding (22). Chronic radiation proctitis is defined when clinical symptoms persist or appear 6 to 12 months after the conclusion of radiation therapy. Symptoms of chronic radiation proctitis are the result of the pathophysiologic changes occurring in the rectum. Hematochezia or rectal bleeding is the most common symptom and occurs as a result of rupture of the fragile radiation-induced telangiectasias, as well as oozing from friable ischemic mucosa, as shown in Figure 3B. This can be particularly serious for patients on warfarin or other anticoagulants, and rectal bleeding can be severe enough to result in significant anemia and the necessity of transfusions. In a recent study, only patients on anticoagulants developed chronic rectal bleeding, (Anthony V. D'Amico, personal communication) as shown in Figure 4.

There can be other symptoms of radiation proctitis. Patients can experience difficulty with elimination or, more commonly, frequent elimination, particularly in the morning. Rarely, they can have urgency with occasional fecal incontinence, with the latter attributed to changes in

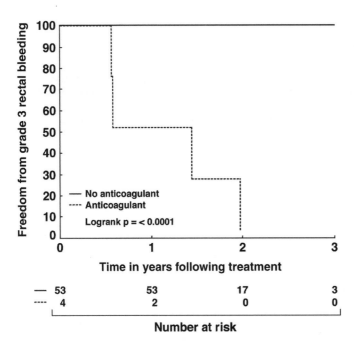

FIGURE 4 Freedom from grade 3 rectal bleeding between patients taking anticoagulants and those who were not. These unpublished data were collected as part of a prospective phase II dose escalation trial performed at Dana-Farber Cancer Institute and Brigham and Women's Hospital. *Source*: From Ref. 22.

anal–rectal function. Yeoh et al. performed a retrospective study of anal–rectal monometry before and after radiation therapy in 35 patients (23). Although no alteration in sphincter morphology occurred, upon completion of radiation therapy most patients experienced a lower threshold volume per perception of rectal distention, which correlated with symptoms of urgency and fecal incontinence. Decreased rectal compliance, potentially related to fibrosis, may be responsible for this particular symptom. In a study from the Royal Marsden Hospital in London, Andreyev et al. (24) retrospectively recorded consecutive series of patients with lower GI symptoms that started after radiotherapy, who were referred during a 32-month period to their gastroenterology clinic. In that series, more than one half the patients had at least two diagnoses, ranging from bacterial overgrowth to colitis or a new primary gastrointestinal cancer. They make the excellent point that any patient developing rectal symptoms after radiotherapy should be carefully evaluated, and it is our clinical practice at the Brigham and Women's Hospital to refer all such patients for a full colonoscopy, or a sigmoidoscopy if a colonoscopy has been recently done.

Measurement of Rectal Symptoms

Measuring the incidence of rectal complications with radiotherapy is considerably more difficult than defining them descriptively. Early on, most of the available information came from chart reviews of the patients' on-treatment notes during radiotherapy and follow-up appointments. This was extremely misleading since it is well established that physicians discover and report far fewer complications than patients do. The most commonly used tool for measuring acute and long-term bladder and bowel toxicity consists of the radiation therapy oncology g'roup (RTOG) Acute Radiation Morbidity Scoring Criteria (25). This is a physician-based scoring system that assigns a toxicity grade based on symptoms reported by the patient. A portion of this tool is shown in Table 1. The disadvantages of this tool are that it is not self-administered nor was it ever validated. Another tool that is gaining popularity is the expanded prostate

TABLE 1 Radiation Therapy Oncology Group Acute Radiation Morbidity Scoring Criteria for Lower Gastrointestinal and Genitourinary Toxicities

Organ/tissue	[0]	[1]	[2]	[3]	[4]
Lower gastrointestinal including pelvis	No change	Increased frequency or change in quality of bowel habits not requiring medication/rectal discomfort not requiring analgesics	Diarrhea requiring parasympatholytic drugs (e.g., Lomotil)/mucus discharge not necessitating sanitary pads/rectal or abdominal pain requiring analgesics	Diarrhea requiring parenteral support/severe mucus or blood discharge necessitating sanitary pads/abdominal distention (flat plate radiograph demonstrates distended bowel loops)	Acute or subacute obstruction, fistula or perforation; gastrointestinal bleeding requiring transfusion; abdominal pain or tenesmus requiring tube decompression or bowel diversion
Genitourinary	No change	Frequency of urination or nocturia twice pretreatment habit/dysuria, urgency not requiring medication	Frequency of urination or nocturia that is less frequent than every hour. Dysuria urgency, bladder spasm requiring local anesthetic (e.g., Pyridium)	Frequency with urgency and nocturia hourly or more frequently/dysuria, pelvis pain, or bladder spasm requiring regular, frequent narcotic/gross hematuria with/without clot passage	Hematuria requiring transfusion/acute bladder obstruction not secondary to clot passage, ulceration or necrosis

Source: Reprinted with permission from Elsevier Publishing.

cancer index composite (EPIC) (26). This instrument was developed based on advice of an expert panel and of prostate cancer patients. It is both reliable and valid and tests a broad spectrum of urinary, bowel, sexual, and hormonal symptoms. It is short, easy to fill out, and compliance with the tool is high. Unlike other tools, it has a small section on bother associated with symptoms which characterizes symptoms on a scale of one through five as being "no problem," "a very small problem," "a small problem," "a moderate problem," or "a big problem." EPIC can be used to measure long-term complications and has been recently studied and validated in short-term acute bowel toxicity (27).

Technical Factors Associated with Rectal Function Changes after Radiation

Most radiation oncologists believe that the dose to and volume of rectum treated are the most important factors in the development of radiation proctitis. Early experience with 3DCRT at Fox Chase Cancer Center (28), the University of Chicago (29), and UCSF (30) suggested that rectal toxicity was reduced compared with conventional therapy. The new 3DCRT technology allowed more accurate measurement of the dose to the rectum. Initial studies recognized the very close relationship between chronic rectal toxicity and the volume of the rectal wall irradiated to doses greater than 50 Gy (9,31–36). One particularly important and demonstrative study was a randomized trial performed at MD Anderson Cancer Center in Houston (37). In that trial, patients were randomized to either 70 or 78 Gy. The first 100 patients with two-year follow up were evaluated for rectal side effects. The 70-Gy group actually had more changes in bowel function than the high-dose group (34% vs. 10%), more frequent bowel movements (47% vs. 27%), and more urgent bowel movements (37% vs. 18%) ($p < 0.040$ for all three comparisons). However, when the entire group of 305 patients was evaluated four years later, a very different picture evolved (38). Rectal side effects were significantly greater in the 78-Gy group. Grade 2 or higher toxicity rates at six years were 12% for the patients who received 70 Gy and 26% for the patients who received 78 Gy ($p = 0.001$). For the patients in 78-Gy arm, grade 2 or higher rectal toxicity correlated highly with the proportion of rectum treated to greater than 70 Gy. If 25% or less of the rectum received 70 Gy, the risk of rectal bleeding was on the order of 10%. If the volume of rectum receiving 70 Gy was greater than 25%, the risk of rectal reaction was almost 40%. Confirmatory data came from other groups as well. In a series of 171 patients treated with CRT at Memorial Sloan-Kettering Cancer Center, grade 2 or higher rectal bleeding correlated with the percentage of volume of rectal wall exposed to 46 Gy (34). Similar data were reported by researchers at Massachusetts General Hospital (see Table 2) (39,40).

Treatment and Prevention of Proctitis

Given the association between inflammatory changes and subsequent rectal bleeding or proctopathy, a number of groups have looked at pharmacologic mechanisms to prevent radiation symptoms. Misoprostol, a prostaglandin E1 analog, was used for many years in the treatment of gastric and duodenal ulcers. A small randomized trial with only 16 patients suggested misoprostol to be beneficial in patients receiving pelvic radiotherapy (49). However, in a large prospective randomized trial with 100 patients, misoprostol not only failed to decrease the incidence and severity of radiation-induced acute proctopathy but also actually increased the risk of rectal bleeding in the treatment arm ($p = 0.03$) (50). Similar results were seen with sucralfate, an aluminum sucrose octasulphate designed to "coat" the rectum and prevent inflammation in a trial of 44 patients (51). That prospective randomized trial was actually stopped early when patients of the treatment arm developed significantly more diarrhea than the controls.

Recently, a new class of functional drugs that metabolize to 5-aminosalicylic acid (5-ASA) has been developed and used in inflammatory bowel disease. Balsalazide belongs to this class and appears to be a potent inhibitor of the synthesis and release of a number of intestinal pro-inflammatory mediators as well as an inhibitor of natural killer cells, mast cells, neutrophils, mucosal lymphocytes, and macrophages (52). In a small randomized trial of 27 patients, proctitis ($p = 0.04$), urethritis, fatigue, and diarrhea were all decreased in the treatment arm. To date, this represents the most promising pharmacologic approach to preventing radiation-induced proctitis.

TABLE 2 Risk of Rectal Complications after External-Beam Radiation Therapy

Institution	Number of patients	Technique	Dose (Gy)	Scoring system	Grade 2 and 3 early	Grade 2 and 3 late
Peeters et al. Netherlands Cancer Institute (41)	669	3DCRT	68 78	RTOG		23.2% (68 Gy) 26.5% (78 Gy) P = NS
Dearnaley et al. Institute of Cancer Research (42)	126 (patients received AA)	3DCRT	64 74	RTOG LENT/SOMA	30% 38%	16% 26% >74 Gy, P = 0.02
Schultheiss et al. Fox Chase Cancer Center (43)	616	3DCRT	65	RTOG/EORTC	NS	3.4% G3 Rectal bleeding
Michalski et al. Washington University (44)	225 (100 at 78 Gy)	3DCRT	78	RTOG	NS	3% at 78 Gy
Michalski et al. Mallinkrodt Institute of Radiology (45)	288	3DCRT	68.4 73.8 79.2	RTOG	0–20% 8%	
Boersma et al. Netherlands Cancer Institute (31)	130	3DCRT	70–78	RTOG LENT/SOMA	NS	14% RTOG 20% LENT/SOMA
Chou et al. University of California Davis (46)	198	3DCRT	66–79 (median 73.8)	RTOG	66% Grade 1 and 2 No dose effect	
Vargas et al. William Beaumont Hospital (47)	331	IMRT	75.6 median	NCI Common Toxicity Criteria	Acute rectal toxicity predicted long-term rectal toxicity, P = 0.001	9%, 18%, 25% Depending upon volume of rectum treated
Storey et al. M.D. Anderson Cancer Center (48)	189	3DCRT	70 78	RTOG Late Effects Normal Tissue Task Force Criteria	2 years	70 Gy 14% 78 Gy 21%
Dearnaley et al. Royal Marsden NHS Trust and the Institute of Cancer Research (1)	225	Conv. 3DCRT	64	RTOG	M 3.6 years	Con G≥1 56% 3DCRT G≥1 37% P = 0.0004 Con G2 15% 3DCRT G2 5%, P = 0.01

Abbreviations: 3DCRT, three-dimensional conformal radiotherapy; AA, adrogen ablation; IMRT, intensity-modulated radiotherapy; EORTC, European Organization for Research and Treatment of Cancer; LENT/SOMA, late effects normal tissues/subjective, objective, management, analytic; NCI, National Cancer Institute; NS, not significant; RTOG, radiation therapy oncology group.

Technical Factors Designed to Prevent Proctitis

We have discussed the benefits of IMRT and shown the increased conformality of the high-dose region with respect to the prostate. However, even with IMRT, a margin of normal tissue beyond the imaged prostate must be treated. This is done for several reasons. First, the prostate moves from day to day as a result of bladder and rectal emptying and filling. This is referred to as inter-fraction motion. There are also the issues of set-up error and small patient movements during therapy. Daily imaging of the prostate before each treatment allows the treating clinician to decrease the margin of normal tissue by correcting for small changes in prostate location from day to day. This is referred to as IGRT. IGRT can be accomplished with placement of radio-opaque gold seed markers within the prostate and special imaging hardware that localizes the prostate each day before treatment. Ultrasound imaging of the prostate done in the linear accelerator treatment room can also be performed each day before treatment but may be less accurate than the implanted seeds. Some linear accelerators are fashioned with an imaging CT scan either attached to or, more commonly, in the room with the treatment unit. A high-quality CT scan is performed each day to localize the prostate and the radiation fields are adjusted as needed.

While IGRT is a very important component of IMRT, there is more to consider. IMRT can take up to 25 minutes to administer. Even when the patient lies quietly and is immobilized with an external device, cine-magnetic resonance imaging demonstrates that, although infrequent, prostate motion of up to 5 mm may occur in patients with an empty rectum, and up to 10 mm in those with a full rectum (53). This sort of motion effectively removes the prostate from the high-dose radiation beam. One way to overcome this intrafraction motion is with an internal immobilization device. Placement of an endorectal balloon allows immobilization and localization (Fig. 5). It has the additional benefit of pushing the lateral and posterior rectal wall away from the prostate and thus promoting rectal sparing (54,55). Decreased rectal toxicity with this approach has been demonstrated by the group at Baylor College of Medicine in Houston, Texas (56), and by the Dana-Farber/Brigham and Women's Cancer Center (22). In the latter study, patient tolerance of balloon placement was studied and found to be high. No patients discontinued use of the balloon in that 100-patient study (22). Similar data were presented by Ronson et al. from Loma Linda. In that study, 3474 or 97.6% of their balloon-immobilized patients tolerated the balloon placement for their entire course of radiation therapy (57).

Treatment of Radiation Proctitis

For many years, bloody radiation proctitis was best treated with formalin instillation. Either the rectum was irrigated (generally for patients with transfusion-dependent proctitis) or, for less dramatic cases, formalin was applied directly with a cotton swab to the blood vessels that seemed to be bleeding. The results were imperfect and complications of the formalin instillation could be severe, such as pain, incontinence, and formalin-induced colitis (58,59). Two newer therapies have almost completely replaced formalin instillation: hyperbaric oxygen treatment and argon plasma coagulation (APC). Hyperbaric oxygen is defined as the therapeutic administration of 100% oxygen at environmental pressures greater than 1 atm absolute (60). Typically, treatment is given in an airtight vessel (multi-patient chambers are now available) pressurized to 2 to 2.5 atm absolute for 60 to 120 minutes daily for a total of 30 to 60 sessions. Hyperbaric

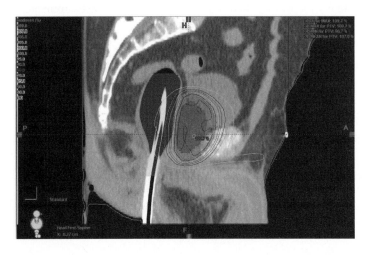

FIGURE 5 Endorectal balloon immobilization device used at Brigham and Women's Hospital. The endorectal balloon effectively wedges the prostate between the balloon and pubic symphysis, minimizing intrafraction prostate motion to a mean value of 1.3 mm. Usually between 80 and 100 mL of air is inserted into the balloon. *Source*: From Ref. 152.

oxygen appears to stimulate angiogenesis and reduces tissue edema. It is believed that this leads to normalized tissue metabolism and tissue regeneration (61,62). Jones et al. from Princess Margaret Hospital reported their results in 10 treated patients. Of the 10, only two did not experience significant improvement from hyperbaric oxygen therapy (63).

APC is a more convenient method of managing chronic rectal bleeding from radiation. There have been several case studies reporting experience with APC for radiation proctitis and the convenience of this procedure makes it an attractive alternative to hyperbaric oxygen for patients with rectal bleeding. In one study, a single treatment prevented further rectal bleeding in 21 patients (81%) (64). However, as noted by Kwon and Carr-Locke in their recent editorial on the subject, most patients will need two if not three treatments for lasting results (65).

BLADDER DYSFUNCTION
General Information

Bladder dysfunction, while more common than rectal dysfunction, is clearly less bothersome to patients and less well studied. However, this does not mean that it is less important. We know from Clark et al. that severe incontinence or obstructive or irritative symptoms are associated with substantially diminished ability to live without vigilance or frustration regarding urinary control (5). Sexual intimacy, marital affection, and masculine self-esteem can also be affected. Incontinence, while uncommon after radiation therapy, in that study was associated with preoccupation with both avoiding leakage and the location of bathrooms, and with feeling dirty, helpless, and embarrassed when control was lost. In a study looking at the information required by patients with early-stage prostate cancer in choosing a course of treatment (66), respondents were asked to designate each item on a checklist of 59 items as "necessary" or "not necessary" to the decision-making process. The sixth largest percentage of respondents felt that information about treatment effect on bladder function was necessary for making their decision. Only concerns about cancer control were rated "necessary" by a greater number of respondents.

Histological Changes in the Bladder after Radiation

The pathophysiology of radiation effect on the bladder and urethra is not well studied. Presumably, the same types of changes that one sees with rectal biopsy would also be seen in the bladder during or after radiation in patients with symptoms (67). These would be changes such as fibrosis, progressive endarteritis, thinning of the bladder mucosa and muscular tissues, and inflammation of telangiectasia. The cellular effect of radiation on the normal bladder epithelium is not known, except for some evidence from the Academy of Medical Sciences of Ukraine in Kiev (68). Two hundred and four patients with chronic cystitis after the Chernobyl accident underwent bladder biopsies with immunohistochemical studies. Chemical evidence of oxidative stress generated by the ionizing radiation was present as evidenced by elevated levels of 8-hydroxy-2-deoxyguanosine, 8-oxoguanine-DNA-glycosylase, apurinic/apyrimidinic endonuclease, and xerodermapigmentosum A endonuclease. While these findings are not strictly applicable to patients undergoing therapeutic radiation, there are likely to be similarities. One major difference is, of course, that the Ukrainian patients had chronic exposure over years, which probably overwhelmed their DNA-damage repair.

Risk Factors for Bladder Function Change after Radiation

Given that bladder symptoms are common, although generally not severe, there is great interest in attempting to establish which patients are most at risk for bladder symptoms. When clinicians switched from standard radiotherapy to conformal radiation, they were able to shape their blocks around the prostate and treat less of the bladder, although the amount of the urethra exposed to radiation did not change. Perez et al. (69) reported a statistically significant decrease in moderate dysuria and difficulty urinating in patients treated with 3DCRT in contrast to those treated with standard radiotherapy. Most of the groups that have looked at prior transurethral resection of the prostate (TURP) demonstrated a worsening of bladder function among patients so treated for almost any bladder symptom studied (70–73).

Since it is established that many of the patients who receive radiotherapy are older, sicker, or have advanced disease, it is interesting to evaluate their baseline bladder function and any effect that it might have on subsequent bladder complications. In a prospective Phase 2 dose-escalation trial at Brigham and Women's Hospital (22), baseline bladder function was ascertained on all patients. Eighteen of 46 (39%) reported baseline nocturia, 32 (70%) reported daytime frequency, and 23 (50%) reported mild to moderate urgency. In that study, three categories actually improved during radiotherapy, presumably due to the pharmacokinetic intervention. Similar data are reported by Hanlon et al. (74) at Fox Chase Cancer Center. These data are important because only a small number of investigators have examined if the presence of urinary dysfunction at presentation correlates with late GU toxicity. Liu et al. (73) at the British Columbia Cancer Agency specifically identified associations between late grade 2 or 3 toxicity and prior TURP, coexisting GU disease, and acute GU toxicity.

Pretreatment with hormones was also found to be a statistically significant predictor of poor GU function ($p < 0.001$), defined as grade 2 or worse acute GU toxicity, in a study reported by Peeters et al. from the Netherlands Cancer Institute (75). In that study, treating a larger volume was not directly related to acute grade 2 or 3 toxicity, whereas neoadjuvant hormone therapy was related. Nearly one half of the patients not treated with hormone therapy had grade 2 toxicity or worse during treatment as compared with 73% of those who received neoadjuvant hormone therapy. The authors found this interesting, but were unable to provide an explanation for the phenomenon.

Incidence and Types of Bladder Function Changes after Radiation

Only limited data are available on the urodynamic change after radiotherapy. Seventeen unselected patients were accrued into a single-arm prospective study by Choo et al. (76). None reported changes in self-assessed urologic symptoms at 18 months post-radiation compared to pre-radiation baseline using three separate quality-of-life tools. All underwent formal urodynamic testing. There was a statistically significant reduction in their bladder capacity at 18 months post-radiation compared to that at pre-radiation baseline, in both the supine and upright positions (reductions of 100 and 54 mL, respectively). Other parameters that showed statistically significant changes were reduction in bladder volume at first sensation in both the supine and upright positions and decrease in bladder volume at desired void in the supine position. However, no changes were noted with regard to pressure at capacity, pressures at first sensation, and at desire to void, maximum flow rate, voiding pressure, voided volume, or post-void residual volume. The authors concluded that while there were changes, as evidenced by the urodynamics, the changes were well tolerated and patients were satisfied with their bladder function.

Patients who receive radiotherapy are at risk for daytime increased frequency, increased nocturia, slow flow of urine, dysuria, urgency, and incontinence. The most important long-term effect is hematuria, which can be mild to severe. On review of the literature, many of the investigators focus on incontinence as a comparison to the incontinence rates seen with radical prostatectomy. Some of these data come from the Prostate Cancer Outcomes Study (77), which was designed to assess bodily function in men with clinically localized prostate cancer treated either with radical prostatectomy or EBRT. At five years, 41% of radiotherapy patients were incontinent compared to 15.3% of radical prostatectomy patients. Cross-sectional analysis revealed that initially more men in the EBRT group than in the radical prostatectomy group reported baseline incontinence. In keeping with other reports, the cohort had a high level of distress due to urinary dysfunction and patients were bothered either a lot or somewhat by incontinence, urinary frequency, and nocturia.

Some of the best long-term data come from Massachusetts General Hospital, where 167 men were treated between 1976 and 1992 in a proton-combination protocol (70). The median follow up in that group was 13.1 years. Genitourinary toxicity accumulated progressively during the entire follow-up period, with an actuarial incidence rate of 59% at five years, when considering all possible types of bladder dysfunction. Of note is that the actuarial risk of grade 2 or greater hematuria was 21% at five years and 47% at 15 years, although the risk for grade 3 hematuria was much lower. Some of this is probably secondary to the perineural proton boost technique, which is no longer used, but does provide an important point about long-term follow up for prostate cancer patients.

A questionnaire given to patients at Eastern Virginia Medical School (78) one year after treatment indicated that 70.6% of patients who had received radiotherapy indicated that they had either never experienced urine leakage, or had experienced it less than one time per month. Ten percent of irradiated patients had incontinence more than two times per day. Ninety-one percent of irradiated patients never used a pad. However, single-institutional data reported by Zelefsky et al. (79) reported no incontinence in their patient population, although they did have other bladder symptoms which will be reported later. The differences in the incidences quoted may certainly be due to differences in patient population and treatment technique. They may also be due to failure to use common validated quality-of-life tools. Miller et al. (80) from the University of Michigan contacted early-stage prostate cancer patients six years after treatment and asked them to complete a health-related quality-of-life assessment tool which included physical and mental component scores as well as prostate cancer-specific quality-of-life items, including those for urinary irritative and obstructive symptoms, urinary incontinence, and bowel, sexual, and hormonal domains. One interesting and previously unreported fact that the University of Michigan study brought to light was that urinary incontinence worsened among 3DCRT patients over time starting around five years after treatment, although the risk was low. Despite this, their health-related quality of life remained largely favorable up to eight years after radiation treatment.

Most of the gold-standard publications reported by radiation oncologists evaluating symptoms after radiotherapy use the RTOG Acute Radiation Morbidity Scoring Criteria shown in Table 1 (25). These scales are designed specifically to look at severity of dysfunctions rather than individual types of dysfunction per se. Patients needing more serious intervention have higher scores on the RTOG scale. The methodology varies from report to report, but most are physician-based assessments of toxicity taken from the patient record and recorded during direct patient interviews. Most of the available data are taken from reports on CRT. The RTOG has recently reported on the results of RTOG 9406 (45). This is a dose-escalation trial with dose levels of 68.4, 73.8, and 79.2 Gy. Data are multi-institutional. Acute tolerance to 3DCRT was very good to all three dose levels; half of the patients had either no or grade 1 toxicity, 0% to 3% experienced grade 3 bladder toxicity and there were no grade 4 or 5 toxicities. The late toxicity results of the highest doses have recently been reported (44). Again, late toxicity was excellent, with 62% to 64% of patients having either no or mild grade 1 late toxicity. A small number of patients had grade 2 toxicity, but of the 225 patients, only four experienced grade 3 toxicity, with no grade 4 or 5 toxicity seen. The most common grade 3 late effect was hematuria, and one patient developed a rectal–urethral fistula requiring surgery. Although there was a trend toward increased toxicity with 79.2 Gy compared to 78 Gy, the difference was not statistically significant.

Using a modified RTOG toxicity scale, Beckendorf et al. (81) reported the results of 306 patients who were randomized to receive 70 or 80 Gy at 17 institutions. Acute toxicity was acceptable, but the percentages were higher in the groups that used slightly larger fields. During radiation, 80% of patients complained of bladder side effects, including treatment interruption for five patients, one of whom required hospitalization for urinary catheterization. There was no difference however between the two arms. A multivariate analysis was undertaken looking at the age of patients, comorbidity, T-stage, arm of treatment, and relative volume of bladder wall or rectum receiving more than 65-, 70- or 72-Gy. The only independent variable that was significant was the size of the target volume. Recovery was rapid for patients in the study, and by two months only 15% (at 70 Gy) and 25% (at 80 Gy) were reporting urinary toxicity.

In Dr. Zelefsky's report on 743 patients treated with high-dose 3DCRT (82), the 5-year actuarial incidences of the development of grade 2 and grade 3 late GU toxicities were 10% and 3%, respectively. Doses greater than 75.6 Gy ($p = 0.008$) and acute GU symptoms ($p = 0.001$) were the independent predictors of grade >2 late GU toxicity.

These studies serve to emphasize an important point: within reason, bladder side effects are less dose-dependent than rectal side effects. We believe that this is due to the fact that many of the urinary side effects experienced by patients are attributed to the urethra, which passes directly through the prostate and which cannot be spared at any dose level. This has implications for IMRT planning which will be discussed later in the chapter.

Treatment of Bladder Function Changes after Radiation

Given that patients either have GU dysfunction at baseline, particularly lower urinary tract symptoms, or will develop it at least temporarily during treatment, it seems reasonable to offer treatment. At Memorial Sloan-Kettering, patients were given either terazosin hydrochloride (THC) or nonsteroidal anti-inflammatory drugs (NSAIDs) (83). Treatment with THC resulted in significant resolution of urinary symptoms in 67% of patients. Only 16% of patients responded to NSAIDs. A similar pilot study was undertaken at the Harvard Joint Center for Radiation Therapy (84). Twenty-six consecutive patients were given tamsulosin hydrochloride, a superselective alpha1A-adrenergic antagonist. Sixty-two percent (16/26) responded to 0.4 mg, but half subsequently progressed. Three quarters of the patients who progressed, however, achieved a durable response with a 0.8-mg dose. Symptoms were controlled in 77% (20/26) of these patients.

Hemorrhagic Cystitis: A Special Consideration

Hemorrhagic cystitis can be seen anywhere from two months to >10 years after pelvic radiation. Treatment varies from institution to institution. Some start with bladder irrigation with continuous saline, followed by cystoscopy infalgration (85). Alum silver nitrate bladder irrigation can be done as well as formalin instillation. In the most severe cases, selective embolization of the hypogastric arteries, urinary diversion, and cystectomy may be ultimately necessary, although this is extremely rare.

While radiation-induced hemorrhagic cystitis has a characteristic appearance on magnetic resonance imaging (MRI) (86), it is essential that any irradiated patient presenting with hematuria, microscopic or gross, be thoroughly evaluated for a second malignancy. Our practice at the Brigham and Women's Hospital and Dana-Farber Cancer Institute is to do urine cytology, cystoscopy, and CT-based imaging of the kidneys, urethra, and bladder in all patients who develop hematuria after radiation therapy. MRI follow up is needed.

When simple local therapies fail, patients are commonly referred for hyperbaric oxygen therapy. Hyperbaric oxygen therapy improves regional tissue oxygenation in previously irradiated tissue and results in neovascularization and capillary growth into hypoxic and scarred submucosal tissues (67). Hyperbaric oxygen treatment is not simple to deliver. Patients must remain in the hyperbaric chamber with 100% oxygen for 90 minutes, breathing at 2.36 atmospheres absolute pressure per session. There are 5-minute air breaks after every 30 to 45 minute session. Generally, 40 sessions are planned, but patients may receive up to 60 sessions if their symptoms persist. Previously, single-person horizontal units were the only form of hyperbaric oxygen chamber available. Now multi-person chambers are becoming increasingly available, where patients may sit, read, and socialize during treatment.

Almost all patients benefit to some degree from hyperbaric oxygen treatment (87–90), but recent data from the Section of Urology and Renal Transplantation and Center for Hyperbaric Medicine at Virginia Mason Medical Center (67) indicate that among 60 patients, 48 (80%) had either total or partial resolution of hematuria. However, for those treated within six months of hematuria onset, 96% (27/28) had complete or excellent partial symptomatic resolution ($p = 0.003$). Prior intravesicular chemical installation did not affect the clinical outcome.

SEXUAL FUNCTION AFTER EBRT
General Information

Sexual dysfunction is probably the most common consequence of prostate cancer treatment. While most clinicians are aware that young sexually active men with prostate cancer will have concerns about the potential for sexual dysfunction, they should also be aware that a cross-sectional study of sexuality and aging in male veterans revealed that many men remain interested in sex and eroticism well into old age (91). In another study of 212 patients from British Columbia, most patients (84%) reported that they had received or had access to some type of information on erectile dysfunction, usually from their urologist (92). In that study, 81% of patients would have preferred written information both before and after treatment. Providing patients with this information is not simple. First, there has not been a clear definition of potency or impotence. The National Institutes of Health Consensus on Erectile Dysfunction defined impotence as the consistent inability to obtain and maintain a penile erection sufficient to permit satisfactory sexual intercourse (93). This somewhat conventional definition implies the presence of a willing and healthy partner. Some authors (94,95) believe that this definition is inappropriate, and would prefer a broader definition of potency to include masturbation. These authors would also be interested in studying other aspects of sexual health, such as rigidity of erections, presence of spontaneous daytime erections or morning or night erections, presence of a willing partner, and psychological factors that might contribute to erectile dysfunction. For example, should a patient who is able to achieve a soft, short-lived erection be considered potent? Most of the data on radiation-induced sexual function changes lack this sort of detail.

Historically, the most practical way to learn about sexual health in prostate cancer patients has been by using a questionnaire. There was no consensus on which questionnaire was best, or on how the questions should be asked, so much of the information available to patients and clinicians was difficult to interpret. Recently, the international index of erectile function (IIEF) has been introduced, translated into many languages, and validated (96). Though not specifically designed for prostate cancer patients, the hope is that it will allow intra-study comparison.

Etiology of Sexual Function Changes after EBRT

Post-irradiation erectile dysfunction is thought to be due to vascular damage. The pioneer in this area is Dr. Goldstein from the Boston University Medical Center who performed a detailed study of 23 patients (97). The 23 patients underwent nocturnal penile tumescence testing, bulbo-cavernous reflex latency, penile Doppler ultrasonography, endocrine screening, and perineal electromyography. Two underwent selective pudendal arteriography. The neurological examinations were normal, but the penile Doppler evaluations were abnormal in all patients. The authors concluded that post-radiation erectile dysfunction was due to vascular damage at the base of the penis. Dr. Zelefsky and colleagues from Memorial Sloan-Kettering evaluated 98 patients after EBRT or prostatectomy approximately a year after treatment (98). Duplex ultrasonography of the penis was performed before and after an intracavernosal injection of prostaglandin. The EBRT patients either had arteriogenic dysfunction with poor penile blood-flow rates, or cavernosal dysfunction with poor cavernosal distensability. Arteriogenic dysfunction was rare.

Incidence of Erectile Dysfunction after EBRT

Most of the data presently available come from the era of conformal radiation. Representative data are included in Table 3 from both retrospective and prospective studies. The range of erectile dysfunction listed by the authors is extremely broad and most studies lacked baseline data. Cormorbid disease was not rigorously recorded in most of the studies, but did correlate with a higher incidence of erectile dysfunction in one study (107). Although two studies showed no influence of the volume of tissue irradiated on erectile dysfunction (37,108), a third prospective study saw less erectile dysfunction in patients treated with CRT compared to those who received whole-pelvis irradiation (99).

Other Forms of Sexual Dysfunction

There are other forms of sexual dysfunction after EBRT. Patients report loss of libido (104), as there can be a decrease in serum testosterone levels due to scatter radiation to the testicles during therapy. Even without androgen suppression therapy, some patients do not recover their pretreatment testosterone levels (109). Ejaculatory disorders occur as well. Ejaculatory disturbance can include reduction or absence of ejaculate volume, discomfort during ejaculation, and hemospermia. A complete lack of ejaculation can occur and has been reported in 2% to 56% of patients (104,110–112). Occasionally, patients have concerns about their fertility. These patients should bank sperm prior to any radiotherapy treatment.

TABLE 3 Risk of Erectile Dysfunction after External-Beam Radiation Therapy

Author	Number of patients	Median age of patients	Tool used to ascertain potency	Percentage of patients potent prior to treatment	Percentage of patients potent after treatment (mean follow-up)
Beard et al. (99)	121	69	Talcott adaptation of Fowler Instrument (prospective)	WP 94 SF 82 CRT 85	WP-56 SF-68 CRT-80 P = 0.31 (12 months)
Crook et al. (100)	192	70	Fowler tool sent one 1 year after RT	82	35 (33 months)
Fossa et al. (101)	114	69	I-PSS	19	39
Fransson and Widmark (102)	199	71	Self-assessment questionnaire sent after XRT	n.a.	44 (48 months)
Hamilton et al. (103)	457	n.a.	Self-administered tool 12–24 months after diagnosis	55	42 at 12 months 32 at 24 months
Helgason et al. (104)	53	70	Radiumhelmut scale of sexual functioning sent two 2 years after EBRT	66	50
Pilepich et al. (105)	230	71	MD assessment (prospective)	44	28
Turner et al. (106)	290	69	Three 3-tier scale recorded at each visit by MD (prospective)	63	68 at 12 months 41 at 24 months

Abbreviations: CRT, conformal radiotherapy; I-PSS, international prostate symptom score; MD, medical doctor; n.a., not available; SF, small field; WP, whole pelvis; EBRT, external-beam radiation therapy.

Prevention of Erectile Dysfunction after EBRT

While it may not be possible to prevent ejaculatory dysfunction, there is great interest in reducing the component of erectile dysfunction that occurs when the penile bulb and crura are irradiated. An association between the dose of radiation to the bulb of the penis and subsequent erectile dysfunction was first demonstrated by Fisch et al. at UCSF (113). In that study, patients receiving a dose of less than 40 Gy to 70% of the bulb of the penis had a much greater likelihood of maintaining potency ($p = 0.03$). Patients who received 70 Gy or more to 70% of the bulb of the penis developed erectile dysfunction. These data are similar to that of Merrick et al. (114) in their brachytherapy patient population. However, a letter written by Dr. Mulhall to the editor of the *Journal of Urology* shortly after Dr. Fisch published his work is worth mentioning (115). Dr. Mulhall pointed out that the bulb of the penis, commonly recognized by urologists as the urethral bulb, but more correctly called the corpus spongiosum, plays no significant role in the genesis or maintenance of erection. On the other hand, radiation of the immediately adjacent corpora cavernosa is implicated in post-radiation erectile dysfunction. Subsequent publications report the dose to both areas. Both are quite difficult to avoid using CRT. However, the proximal penile tissues can be contoured and subdivided into the corpora cavernosa and the corpus spongiosum and entered into the computer as critical structures to be avoided using IMRT plans. Sethi et al. from Loyola University Medical Center reported a 50% reduction in dose to the critical penile structures with IMRT (116). Similar data were reported in a planning study by Kao et al. (117). IMRT reduced the mean penile bulb dose compared with 3DCRT from 48.9 to 33.2 Gy ($p < 0.001$), the percentage of the penile bulb receiving greater than 40 Gy from 67.2% to 37.7% ($p < 0.001$), and the dose received by greater than 95% of the penile bulb from 11.7 to 5.3 Gy ($p = 0.003$). Because the erectile tissue is close to the prostatic apex, a structure that is notoriously difficult to see at CT simulation, there is real interest in using MR-CT fusion to better identify these critical structures. That MRI is superior to CT for the imaging of the erectile tissue is established (118). Although these data have to be confirmed by larger studies, it seems warranted to limit the dose to the corpus spongiosum and corpora cavernosa, with IMRT whenever possible.

Treatment of Erectile Dysfunction after EBRT

Until such time as erectile dysfunction can be avoided entirely, men will wish to be sexually active despite their erectile dysfunction. Data from the Surveillance, Epidemiology and End-Results Prostate Cancer Outcome Study of 1977 men with localized prostate cancer who received either EBRT or radical prostatectomy revealed that overall 58.5% of the men used some form of treatment for erectile dysfunction during the 60 months following the prostate cancer diagnosis (119). Sildenafil was the preferred initial treatment for erectile dysfunction in that study, but is not generally effective in men with complete loss of erectile function (120), and appears to be associated with decreasing efficacy with time (121,122). While the Prostate Cancer Outcome Study showed that sildenafil and other newer related agents were definitely the most widely used form of treatment for erectile dysfunction, they were not considered as helpful by users as penile prosthesis, vacuum erection devices, or penile injection therapy (107).

Sildenafil was tested in open-label studies and reported to be effective in 90% of patients. Zelefsky et al. reported on 50 patients a median of 19 months after EBRT (123). In that population, treatment with sildenafil resulted in an improvement in firmness of erections in 54% of patients. Similar data were reported by Kedia et al. (124) and Weber et al. (125). Incrocci et al. performed a randomized, double-blinded placebo-controlled cross-over trial with 60 patients who complained of erectile dysfunction 39 months after EBRT (126). In that trial, 55% of patients had successful intercourse using sildenafil at a 100-mg dose with mild or moderate side effects. However, a follow-up study showed that at two years, only 24% were still using the drug because of lack of efficacy (60%), cost (24%), or side effects (16%) (127).

FATIGUE
Incidence and Etiology of Fatigue

Fatigue is considered one of the most common symptoms reported by cancer patients, including those with prostate cancer. It is difficult to define because it is a non-specific, multidimensional concept, and one that is highly subjective. Possible causes of fatigue are listed in Table 4 (128). The most common definition is that cancer-related fatigue (CRF) is the persistent feeling of overwhelming tiredness related to cancer or cancer treatment that interferes with the usual functioning in daily life (129). In fact, 91% of patients in one study done at the National Cancer Institute reported that CRF "prevented a normal life" (130). CRF is often unrelated to physical activity and may not be relieved by sleep or rest (131).CRF also has a number of correlates, including pain, depression, and sleep disturbance, which may result from either cancer treatment or the cancer itself, as shown in Table 4 (132). There are a number of modern instruments designed to measure fatigue. The Piper Fatigue Scale, the Schwartz Center Fatigue Scale, and the Fatigue Assessment Questionnaire are specifically designed to investigate radiation-related fatigue (133). Whatever tool is used, it is generally accepted that fatigue scores increase gradually during the course of radiotherapy and decrease shortly after completion (132,134). Because fatigue is difficult to study, it is underestimated by both physicians and nurses (133). The reported range of fatigue is broad, from 4% to 91% (135). There are some data specific to prostate cancer patients. In one prospective study of 337 patients (99), the Profile of Mood State (POMS) indicated that vigor decreased and fatigue increased for all patients who received radiotherapy, more so for those treated with whole-pelvis radiation. Poor vigor and fatigue were still present at the 3- and 12-month time points of the study. Similar associations between increasing field size and fatigue have been reported in other patient populations (136–138). In two other studies looking at only prostate-cancer patients (101,139), the incidence of fatigue was not given, but it was described as the most common long-term complication of radiotherapy, particularly for patients who had androgen-suppression treatment with their radiotherapy. Prevalence and prevalence odds ratio of fatigue were estimated by Forlenza et al. (140) using the very large Swedish Twin Registry as controls and linked with the Swedish National Registry-based data for cancer patients. Prostate cancer patients were included in the study. Men with prostate cancer were twice as likely to report chronic fatigue not affecting activity, and almost three times more likely to report chronic fatigue affecting their activity, than were age-matched controls. The authors specifically stated that they lacked the data to speculate as to why the fatigue might

TABLE 4 Potential Causes of Radiotherapy-
Related Fatigue in Cancer Patients

Biochemical factors
   Serum interleukins
   Reverse triiodothyronine
   Decline in neuromuscular efficiency

Physical factors
   Pulse change with orthostatic stress

Psychological disturbances
   Stress
   Sleep disturbances
   Depression
   Anxiety

Radiotherapy complications
   Myelosupression
   Diarrhea
   Malnutrition
   Dehydration
   Electrolyte disorders
   Dyspnea
   Nausea/vomiting
   Hormonal or immune insufficiency
   Change in weight

Concomitant or previous therapies
   Chemotherapy
   Hormonotherapy
   Biologic response modifiers (e.g., interferon)
   Surgery
   Pharmacological therapy (e.g., analgesics)

Co-existing morbidities
   Pain
   Myelosupression
   Anemia
   Infection
   Malnutrition
   Dehydration
   Electrolyte disorders
   Concomitant diseases (e.g., heart or renal insufficiency)
   Immobilization (functional disability)

Source: Reprinted with permission from Elsevier publishing.

be occurring in prostate-cancer patients. However Dr. Vordermark and colleagues (141) investigated 103 prostate cancer patients and looked at urinary function, rectal function, and fatigue. In that study, long-term severe fatigue was both more frequent than in the sample of the general population and was significantly correlated with severe urinary and/or rectal symptoms.

Treatment of Fatigue

Having established that fatigue is more of a problem than previously recognized in a radiotherapy population, we must consider management of fatigue and its associated symptoms. Fatigue associated with electrolyte abnormalities, low blood counts, or medication reactions can be medically managed. In our clinic, sleepless patients are offered short-term sleeping medicines, as good rest is considered a critical part of our treatment protocol. We recommend a highly nutritious diet and mild exercise. For many years it was common practice to encourage patients receiving radiotherapy to rest and to avoid physical effort. Windsor et al. (142), from the Ninewells Hospital and Medical School in Dundee, Scotland performed a prospective, randomized trial on 66 men with localized prostate cancer in order to determine whether aerobic exercise would reduce the incidence of fatigue and prevent deterioration of physical functioning during radiotherapy. There were no significant differences between the two groups at baseline or midway through radiotherapy treatment. However by the end of treatment, men in the control group had significantly increased fatigue scores from baseline ($p = 0.013$) with no significant increases observed in the exercise group. Although the exercise intervention was home-based, moderate-intensity continuous walking for 30 minutes on at least three days of each week, the exercise group actually experienced improvement in exercise tolerance by the end of radiotherapy. While more studies of this sort are needed to confirm these results, it may be that good health habits are as or more important during or after a course of radiotherapy than before.

SECOND MALIGNANCIES

It is well known that radiation is carcinogenic. Most of the information on radiation-induced carcinogenesis comes from A-bomb survivors in Japan, from radiation accidents, from individuals medically exposed, and from second cancers in patients who received radiotherapy (143). The risk of second malignancies after exposure to radiotherapy is a complex topic (144). Single-institutional studies lack the statistical power to detect a relatively small increased incidence of radiation-induced malignancies. In addition, it is not clear if patients who undergo radiotherapy also have a higher than normal risk of a second cancer because of their lifestyle or because of a genetic predisposition. In calculating the risk of developing a fatal second malignancy, the most commonly-used risk coefficients were compiled in 1993, by the National Council on Radiation Protection and Measurements (NCRPM) (145). The risk of second malignancies from radiation treatment is likely not a serious concern until at least five years after treatment because of the latency period of tumors (145). For patients who must receive radiation therapy, the issue is somewhat academic, but for others who have other choices of treatment (e.g., low-risk prostate cancer patients who might choose radical prostatectomy), quantifying the risks for radiation-induced second malignancy might be helpful and informative as the patient attempts to make his treatment choice.

One method of attempting to estimate the risk of second malignancy after radiation is to follow up a group of patients treated at a single institution, as was done at the Mayo Clinic Cancer Registry for patients who received EBRT for prostate cancer (146). With more than 12,353, man-years of follow up, no statistically significant increase in the risk of bladder cancer was demonstrated. If patients did develop bladder cancer after their radiotherapy, the incidence was no higher than that seen in the Surveillance, Epidemiology and End-Results study. This retrospective review implied that the risk of bladder cancer was not increased after EBRT. A separate explanation is that even a large study such as this would have limited power to detect and quantify realistic increases in rates of second malignancies.

A more common approach to this issue involves retrospective studies based on data collected from large tumor registries. Brenner et al. from the Center for Radiological Research at Columbia University (147) used data from the National Cancer Institute Surveillance, Epidemiology and End-Results (SEER) program (148). There were 122,123 men in the database who had prostate cancer as their first primary tumor and who survived for more than two months after their initial diagnosis. Of the 51,584 men with prostate cancer who received radiotherapy, 3549 (6.9%) developed second malignancies. Of the 70,539 men who underwent surgery, 5055 (7.2%) developed second malignancies. Overall, 8604 developed secondary malignancies, which was significantly less than the 9905 expected. The effect was found in both the radiotherapy group and the surgical-treatment group. However, when the analysis was restricted to subjects less than 60 years of age at diagnosis, the standardized incidence ratio (observed/expected) for all malignancies at all times in the radiotherapy group was 1.05 compared with 0.89 when there was no age restriction.

The data indicated that there was little evidence of difference in the risk of leukemia or lymphatic or hematopoietic malignancy for patients treated with radiotherapy versus surgery (147). There was a risk of developing second solid tumors and it was significantly greater after radiotherapy than after surgery (by 6%). The risk increased as a function of time. Risks were highest for bladder, lung, and rectal cancer, as well as for sarcoma. While the risks sound high when presented as percentages, among the 17,327 men who underwent radiotherapy and survived more than five years, there were an estimated 139 extra solid tumors, corresponding to one of 125 men or one of 465 person-years of risk. A follow-up study published by Dr. Baxter et al. (149) revealed that the relative risk of rectal cancer was 1.7 for the radiation group compared with the surgery-only group. Interestingly, the incidence of colonic tumors did not increase in the irradiated patients. An interesting debate expressed in a correspondence published in the journal *Gastroenterology* between Dr. Brenner and Dr. Baxter followed (150). Dr. Brenner believed that sites at highest risk for prostate cancer patients were bladder and lung, with the lung cancers due to scattered radiation. Dr. Baxter's opinion was that most studies demonstrate that the major carcinogenic effect from radiation is within the high-dose region. Although the absolute risk of a radiation-induced malignancy in the prostate-cancer population is small, it is a source of interest and concern for radiation oncologists. Hall and Wuu (143) and Kry et al. (151) from the University of Texas MD Anderson Cancer Center have written at length about the relationship between radiation technique and second cancers. Machine energy, field size, dose, and IMRT versus 3DCRT are all relevant. As our patients live longer after treatment for their prostate cancer, without doubt there will be more information on this risk of a second cancer and the ways to prevent it.

REFERENCES

1. Dearnaley DP, Khoo VS, Norman AR, et al. Comparison of radiation side-effects of conformal and conventional radiotherapy in prostate cancer: a randomised trial. Lancet 1999; 353(9149):267–272.
2. Davison BJ, Goldenberg SL. Decisional regret and quality of life after participating in medical decision-making for early-stage prostate cancer. BJU Int 2003; 91(1):14–17.
3. Holmboe ES, Concato J. Treatment decisions for localized prostate cancer: asking men what's important. J Gen Intern Med 2000; 15(10):694–701.
4. Wei JT, Dunn RL, Sandler HM, et al. Comprehensive comparison of health-related quality of life after contemporary therapies for localized prostate cancer. J Clin Oncol 2002; 20(2):557–566.
5. Clark JA, Inui TS, Silliman RA, et al. Patients' perceptions of quality of life after treatment for early prostate cancer. J Clin Oncol 2003; 21(20):3777–3784.
6. Harlan LC, Potosky A, Gilliland FD, et al. Factors associated with initial therapy for clinically localized prostate cancer: prostate cancer outcomes study. J Natl Cancer Inst 2001; 93(24):1864–1871.
7. Willett CG, Ooi CJ, Zietman AL, et al. Acute and late toxicity of patients with inflammatory bowel disease undergoing irradiation for abdominal and pelvic neoplasms. Int J Radiat Oncol Biol Phys 2000; 46(4):995–998.
8. Herold DM, Hanlon AL, Hanks GE. Diabetes mellitus: a predictor for late radiation morbidity. Int J Radiat Oncol Biol Phys 1999; 43(3):475–479.
9. Skwarchuk MW, Jackson A, Zelefsky MJ, et al. Late rectal toxicity after conformal radiotherapy of prostate cancer (I): multivariate analysis and dose-response. Int J Radiat Oncol Biol Phys 2000; 47(1):103–413.
10. Schultheiss TE, Lee WR, Hunt MA, et al. Late GI and GU complications in the treatment of prostate cancer. Int J Radiat Oncol Biol Phys 1997; 37(1):3–11.
11. Akimoto T, Muramatsu H, Takahashi M, et al. Rectal bleeding after hypofractionated radiotherapy for prostate cancer: correlation between clinical and dosimetric parameters and the incidence of grade 2 or worse rectal bleeding. Int J Radiat Oncol Biol Phys 2004; 60(4):1033–1039.
12. Millender LE, Aubin M, Pouliot J, et al. Daily electronic portal imaging for morbidly obese men undergoing radiotherapy for localized prostate cancer. Int J Radiat Oncol Biol Phys 2004; 59(1):6–10.
13. Hong JJ, Park W, Ehrenpreis ED. Review article: current therapeutic options for radiation proctopathy. Aliment Pharmacol Ther 2001; 15(9):1253–1262.
14. Berthrong M, Fajardo LF. Radiation injury in surgical pathology. Part II. Alimentary tract. Am J Surg Pathol 1981; 5(2):153–178.
15. Tarpila S. Morphological and functional response of human small intestine to ionizing irradiation. Scand J Gastroenterol Suppl 1971; 12:1–52.
16. Jahraus CD, Bettenhausen D, Malik U, et al. Prevention of acute radiation-induced proctosigmoiditis by balsalazide: a randomized, double-blind, placebo controlled trial in prostate cancer patients. Int J Radiat Oncol Biol Phys 2005; 63(5):1483–1487.
17. Cole AT, Slater K, Sokal M, et al. In vivo rectal inflammatory mediator changes with radiotherapy to the pelvis. Gut 1993; 34(9):1210–1214.
18. Hasleton PS, Carr N, Schofield PF. Vascular changes in radiation bowel disease. Histopathology 1985; 9(5):517–534.
19. Sher ME, Bauer J. Radiation-induced enteropathy. Am J Gastroenterol 1990; 85(2):121–128.

20. Swaroop VS, Gostout CJ. Endoscopic treatment of chronic radiation proctopathy. J Clin Gastroenterol 1998; 27(1):36–40.
21. Denham JW, O'Brien PC, Dunstan RH, et al. Is there more than one late radiation proctitis syndrome? Radiother Oncol 1999; 51(1):43–53.
22. Woel R, Beard C, Chen MH, et al. Acute gastrointestinal, genitourinary, and dermatological toxicity during dose-escalated 3D-conformal radiation therapy (3DCRT) using an intrarectal balloon for prostate gland localization and immobilization. Int J Radiat Oncol Biol Phys 2005; 62(2):392–396.
23. Yeoh EK, Russo A, Botten R, et al. Acute effects of therapeutic irradiation for prostatic carcinoma on anorectal function. Gut 1998; 43(1):123–127.
24. Andreyev HJ, Vlavianos P, Blake P, et al. Gastrointestinal symptoms after pelvic radiotherapy: role for the gastroenterologist? Int J Radiat Oncol Biol Phys 2005; 62(5):1464–1471.
25. Cox JD, Stetz J, Pajak TF. Toxicity criteria of the Radiation Therapy Oncology Group (RTOG) and the European Organization for Research and Treatment of Cancer (EORTC). Int J Radiat Oncol Biol Phys 1995; 31(5):1341–1346.
26. Wei JT, Dunn RL, Litwin MS, et al. Development and validation of the expanded prostate cancer index composite (EPIC) for comprehensive assessment of health-related quality of life in men with prostate cancer. Urology 2000; 56(6):899–905.
27. Muanza TM, Albert PS, Smith S, et al. Comparing measures of acute bowel toxicity in patients with prostate cancer treated with external beam radiation therapy. Int J Radiat Oncol Biol Phys 2005; 62(5):1316–1321.
28. Yan D, Lockman D, Brabbins D, et al. An off-line strategy for constructing a patient-specific planning target volume in adaptive treatment process for prostate cancer. Int J Radiat Oncol Biol Phys 2000; 48(1):289–302.
29. Martinez AA, Yan D, Lockman D, et al. Improvement in dose escalation using the process of adaptive radiotherapy combined with three-dimensional conformal or intensity-modulated beams for prostate cancer. Int J Radiat Oncol Biol Phys 2001; 50(5):1226–1234.
30. Fleming I, Cooper J, Henson D, et al., eds. AJCC Cancer Staging Handbook. 5th ed. Philadelphia, PA: Lippincott Williams and Wilkins, 1998.
31. Boersma LJ, van den Brink M, Bruce AM, et al. Estimation of the incidence of late bladder and rectum complications after high-dose (70–78 Gy) conformal radiotherapy for prostate cancer, using dose-volume histograms. Int J Radiat Oncol Biol Phys 1998; 41(1):83–92.
32. Fiorino C, Cozzarini C, Vavassori V, et al. Relationships between DVHs and late rectal bleeding after radiotherapy for prostate cancer: analysis of a large group of patients pooled from three institutions. Radiother Oncol 2002; 64(1):1–12.
33. Huang EH, Pollack A, Levy L, et al. Late rectal toxicity: dose-volume effects of conformal radiotherapy for prostate cancer. Int J Radiat Oncol Biol Phys 2002; 54(5):1314–1321.
34. Jackson A, Skwarchuk MW, Zelefsky MJ, et al. Late rectal bleeding after conformal radiotherapy of prostate cancer. II. Volume effects and dose-volume histograms. Int J Radiat Oncol Biol Phys 2001; 49(3):685–698.
35. Kupelian PA, Reddy CA, Carlson TP, et al. Dose/volume relationship of late rectal bleeding after external beam radiotherapy for localized prostate cancer: absolute or relative rectal volume? Cancer J 2002; 8(1):62–66.
36. Wachter S, Gerstner N, Goldner G, et al. Rectal sequelae after conformal radiotherapy of prostate cancer: dose-volume histograms as predictive factors. Radiother Oncol 2001; 59(1):65–70.
37. Nguyen LN, Pollack A, Zagars GK. Late effects after radiotherapy for prostate cancer in a randomized dose-response study: results of a self-assessment questionnaire. Urology 1998; 51(6):991–997.
38. Pollack A, Zagars GK, Starkschall G, et al. Prostate cancer radiation dose response: results of the M. D. Anderson phase III randomized trial. Int J Radiat Oncol Biol Phys 2002; 53(5):1097–1105.
39. Benk VA, Adams JA, Shipley WU, et al. Late rectal bleeding following combined X-ray and proton high dose irradiation for patients with stages T3-T4 prostate carcinoma. Int J Radiat Oncol Biol Phys 1993; 26(3):551–557.
40. Hartford AC, Niemierko A, Adams JA, et al. Conformal irradiation of the prostate: estimating long-term rectal bleeding risk using dose-volume histograms. Int J Radiat Oncol Biol Phys 1996; 36(3):721–730.
41. Peeters ST, Heemsbergen WD, van Putten WL, et al. Acute and late complications after radiotherapy for prostate cancer: results of a multicenter randomized trial comparing 68 Gy to 78 Gy. Int J Radiat Oncol Biol Phys 2005; 61(4):1019–1034.
42. Dearnaley DP, Hall E, Lawrence D, et al. Phase III pilot study of dose escalation using conformal radiotherapy in prostate cancer: PSA control and side effects. Br J Cancer 2005; 92(3):488–498.
43. Schultheiss TE, Hanks GE, Hunt MA, et al. Incidence of and factors related to late complications in conformal and conventional radiation treatment of cancer of the prostate. Int J Radiat Oncol Biol Phys 1995; 32(3):643–649.
44. Michalski JM, Winter K, Purdy JA, et al. Toxicity after three-dimensional radiotherapy for prostate cancer on RTOG 9406 dose level V. Int J Radiat Oncol Biol Phys 2005; 62(3):706–713.

45. Michalski JM, Purdy JA, Winter K, et al. Preliminary report of toxicity following 3D radiation therapy for prostate cancer on 3DOG/RTOG 9406. Int J Radiat Oncol Biol Phys 2000; 46(2):391–402.

46. Chou RH, Wilder RB, Ji M, et al. Acute toxicity of three-dimensional conformal radiotherapy in prostate cancer patients eligible for implant monotherapy. Int J Radiat Oncol Biol Phys 2000; 47(1):115–119.

47. Vargas C, Martinez A, Kestin LL, et al. Dose-volume analysis of predictors for chronic rectal toxicity after treatment of prostate cancer with adaptive image-guided radiotherapy. Int J Radiat Oncol Biol Phys 2005; 62(5):1297–1308.

48. Storey MR, Pollack A, Zagars G, et al. Complications from radiotherapy dose escalation in prostate cancer: preliminary results of a randomized trial. Int J Radiat Oncol Biol Phys 2000; 48(3):635–642.

49. Khan AM, Birk JW, Anderson JC, et al. A prospective randomized placebo-controlled double-blinded pilot study of misoprostol rectal suppositories in the prevention of acute and chronic radiation proctitis symptoms in prostate cancer patients. Am J Gastroenterol 2000; 95(8):1961–1966.

50. Hille A, Christiansen H, Pradier O, et al. Effect of pentoxifylline and tocopherol on radiation proctitis/enteritis. Strahlenther Onkol 2005; 181(9):606–614.

51. Hovdenak N, Sorbye H, Dahl O. Sucralfate does not ameliorate acute radiation proctitis: randomised study and meta-analysis. Clin Oncol (R Coll Radiol) 2005; 17(6):485–491.

52. Prakash A, Spencer CM. Balsalazide. Drugs 1998; 56(1):83–89; discussion 90.

53. Ghilezan MJ, Jaffray DA, Siewerdsen JH, et al. Prostate gland motion assessed with cine-magnetic resonance imaging (cine-MRI). Int J Radiat Oncol Biol Phys 2005; 62(2):406–417.

54. Sanghani MV, Ching J, Schultz D, et al. Impact on rectal dose from the use of a prostate immobilization and rectal localization device for patients receiving dose escalated 3D conformal radiation therapy. Urol Oncol 2004; 22(3):165–168.

55. Teh BS, Dong L, McGary JE, et al. Rectal wall sparing by dosimetric effect of rectal balloon used during intensity-modulated radiation therapy (IMRT) for prostate cancer. Med Dosim 2005; 30(1):25–30.

56. Teh BS, McGary JE, Dong L, et al. The use of rectal balloon during the delivery of intensity modulated radiotherapy (IMRT) for prostate cancer: more than just a prostate gland immobilization device? Cancer J 2002; 8(6):476–483.

57. Ronson BB, Yonemoto LT, Rossi CJ, et al. Patient tolerance of rectal balloons in conformal radiation treatment of prostate cancer. Int J Radiat Oncol Biol Phys 2006; 64(5):1367–1370.

58. Pikarsky AJ, Belin B, Efron J, et al. Complications following formalin installation in the treatment of radiation induced proctitis. Int J Colorectal Dis 2000; 15(2):96–99.

59. Konishi T, Watanabe T, Kitayama J, et al. Endoscopic and histopathologic findings after formalin application for hemorrhage caused by chronic radiation-induced proctitis. Gastrointest Endosc 2005; 61(1):161–164.

60. Bennett M, Feldmeier J, Hampson N, et al. Hyperbaric oxygen therapy for late radiation tissue injury. Cochrane Database Syst Rev 2005; (3):CD005005.

61. O'Sullivan B, Levin W. Late radiation-related fibrosis: pathogenesis, manifestations, and current management. Semin Radiat Oncol 2003; 13(3):274–289.

62. Zel G. Hyperbaric oxygen therapy in urology. AUA Update Ser 1990; 9:114.

63. Jones K, Evans AW, Bristow RG, et al. Treatment of radiation proctitis with hyperbaric oxygen. Radiother Oncol 2006; 78(1):91–94.

64. Sebastian S, O'Connor H, O'Morain C, et al. Argon plasma coagulation as first-line treatment for chronic radiation proctopathy. J Gastroenterol Hepatol 2004; 19(10):1169–1173.

65. Kwon RS, Carr-Locke DL. Are we making progress with argon plasma coagulation in chronic radiation proctopathy? J Gastroenterol Hepatol 2005; 20(2):171–172.

66. Feldman-Stewart D, Brundage MD, Nickel JC, et al. The information required by patients with early-stage prostate cancer in choosing their treatment. BJU Int 2001; 87(3):218–223.

67. Chong KT, Hampson NB, Corman JM. Early hyperbaric oxygen therapy improves outcome for radiation-induced hemorrhagic cystitis. Urology 2005; 65(4):649–653.

68. Romanenko A, Morimura K, Wei M, et al. DNA damage repair in bladder urothelium after the Chernobyl accident in Ukraine. J Urol 2002; 168(3):973–977.

69. Perez CA, Michalski JM, Purdy JA, et al. Three-dimensional conformal therapy or standard irradiation in localized carcinoma of prostate: preliminary results of a nonrandomized comparison. Int J Radiat Oncol Biol Phys 2000; 47(3):629–637.

70. Gardner BG, Zietman AL, Shipley WU, et al. Late normal tissue sequelae in the second decade after high dose radiation therapy with combined photons and conformal protons for locally advanced prostate cancer. J Urol 2002; 167(1):123–126.

71. Maartense S, Hermans J, Leer JW. Radiation therapy in localized prostate cancer: long-term results and late toxicity. Clin Oncol (R Coll Radiol) 2000; 12(4):222–228.

72. Zelefsky MJ, Fuks Z, Hunt M, et al. High dose radiation delivered by intensity modulated conformal radiotherapy improves the outcome of localized prostate cancer. J Urol 2001; 166(3):876–881.

73. Liu M, Pickles T, Agranovich A, et al. Impact of neoadjuvant androgen ablation and other factors on late toxicity after external beam prostate radiotherapy. Int J Radiat Oncol Biol Phys 2004; 58(1):59–67.

74. Hanlon AL, Watkins Bruner D, Peter R, et al. Quality of life study in prostate cancer patients treated with three-dimensional conformal radiation therapy: comparing late bowel and bladder quality of life symptoms to that of the normal population. Int J Radiat Oncol Biol Phys 2001; 49(1):51–59.

75. Peeters ST, Hoogeman MS, Heemsbergen WD, et al. Volume and hormonal effects for acute side effects of rectum and bladder during conformal radiotherapy for prostate cancer. Int J Radiat Oncol Biol Phys 2005; 63(4)1142–1152.

76. Choo R, Do V, Herschorn S, et al. Urodynamic changes at 18 months post-therapy in patients treated with external beam radiotherapy for prostate carcinoma. Int J Radiat Oncol Biol Phys 2002; 53(2):290–296.

77. Potosky AL, Davis WW, Hoffman RM, et al. Five-year outcomes after prostatectomy or radiotherapy for prostate cancer: the prostate cancer outcomes study. J Natl Cancer Inst 2004; 96(18):1358–1367.

78. McCammon KA, Kolm P, Main B, et al. Comparative quality-of-life analysis after radical prostatectomy or external beam radiation for localized prostate cancer. Urology 1999; 54(3):509–516.

79. Zelefsky MJ, Fuks Z, Wolfe T, et al. Locally advanced prostatic cancer: long-term toxicity outcome after three-dimensional conformal radiation therapy—a dose-escalation study. Radiology 1998; 209(1):169–174.

80. Miller DC, Sanda MG, Dunn RL, et al. Long-term outcomes among localized prostate cancer survivors: health-related quality-of-life changes after radical prostatectomy, external radiation, and brachytherapy. J Clin Oncol 2005; 23(12):2772–2780.

81. Beckendorf V, Guerif S, Le Prise E, et al. The GETUG 70 Gy vs. 80 Gy randomized trial for localized prostate cancer: feasibility and acute toxicity. Int J Radiat Oncol Biol Phys 2004; 60(4):1056–1065.

82. Zelefsky MJ, Leibel SA, Gaudin PB, et al. Dose escalation with three-dimensional conformal radiation therapy affects the outcome in prostate cancer. Int J Radiat Oncol Biol Phys 1998; 41(3): 491–500.

83. Zelefsky MJ, Ginor RX, Fuks Z, et al. Efficacy of selective alpha-1 blocker therapy in the treatment of acute urinary symptoms during radiotherapy for localized prostate cancer. Int J Radiat Oncol Biol Phys 1999; 45(3):567–570.

84. Prosnitz RG, Schneider L, Manola J, et al. Tamsulosin palliates radiation-induced urethritis in patients with prostate cancer: results of a pilot study. Int J Radiat Oncol Biol Phys 1999; 45(3): 563–566.

85. Neheman A, Nativ O, Moskovitz B, et al. Hyperbaric oxygen therapy for radiation-induced haemorrhagic cystitis. BJU Int 2005; 96(1):107–109.

86. Worawattanakul S, Semelka RC, Kelekis NL. Post radiation hemorrhagic cystitis: MR findings. Magn Reson Imaging 1997; 15(9):1103–1106.

87. Corman JM, McClure D, Pritchett R, et al. Treatment of radiation induced hemorrhagic cystitis with hyperbaric oxygen. J Urol 2003; 169(6):2200–2202.

88. Bevers RF, Bakker DJ, Kurth KH. Hyperbaric oxygen treatment for haemorrhagic radiation cystitis. Lancet 1995; 346(8978):803–805.

89. Bui QC, Lieber M, Withers HR, et al. The efficacy of hyperbaric oxygen therapy in the treatment of radiation-induced late side effects. Int J Radiat Oncol Biol Phys 2004; 60(3):871–878.

90. Peusch-Dreyer D, Dreyer KH, Muller CD, et al. Management of postoperative radiation injury of the urinary bladder by hyperbaric oxygen (HBO). Strahlenther Onkol 1998; 174 Suppl 3:99–100.

91. Mulligan T, Moss CR. Sexuality and aging in male veterans: a cross-sectional study of interest, ability, and activity. Arch Sex Behav 1991; 20(1):17–25.

92. Davison BJ, Keyes M, Elliott S, et al. Preferences for sexual information resources in patients treated for early-stage prostate cancer with either radical prostatectomy or brachytherapy. BJU Int 2004; 93(7):965–969.

93. NIH Consensus Conference. Impotence. NIH Consensus Development Panel on Impotence. JAMA 1993; 270(1):83–90.

94. Incrocci L. Sexual function after external-beam radiotherapy for prostate cancer: What do we know? Crit Rev Oncol Hematol 2006; 57(2):165–173.

95. Schover LR, Fouladi RT, Warneke CL, et al. Defining sexual outcomes after treatment for localized prostate carcinoma. Cancer 2002; 95(8):1773–1785.

96. Rosen RC, Riley A, Wagner G, et al. The international index of erectile function (IIEF): a multidimensional scale for assessment of erectile dysfunction. Urology 1997; 49(6):822–830.

97. Goldstein I, Feldman MI, Deckers PJ, et al. Radiation-associated impotence. A clinical study of its mechanism. JAMA 1984; 251(7):903–910.

98. Zelefsky MJ, Eid JF. Elucidating the etiology of erectile dysfunction after definitive therapy for prostatic cancer. Int J Radiat Oncol Biol Phys 1998; 40(1):129–133.

99. Beard CJ, Propert KJ, Rieker PP, et al. Complications after treatment with external-beam irradiation in early-stage prostate cancer patients: a prospective multiinstitutional outcomes study. J Clin Oncol 1997; 15(1):223–229.

100. Crook J, Esche B, Futter N. Effect of pelvic radiotherapy for prostate cancer on bowel, bladder, and sexual function: the patient's perspective. Urology 1996; 47(3):387–394.

101. Fossa SD, Woehre H, Kurth KH, et al. Influence of urological morbidity on quality of life in patients with prostate cancer. Eur Urol 1997; 31(Suppl. 3):3–8.

102. Fransson P, Widmark A. Self-assessed sexual function after pelvic irradiation for prostate carcinoma. Comparison with an age-matched control group. Cancer 1996; 78(5):1066–1078.

103. Hamilton AS, Stanford JL, Gilliland FD, et al. Health outcomes after external-beam radiation therapy for clinically localized prostate cancer: results from the Prostate Cancer Outcomes Study. J Clin Oncol 2001; 19(9):2517–2526.

104. Helgason AR, Fredrikson M, Adolfsson J, et al. Decreased sexual capacity after external radiation therapy for prostate cancer impairs quality of life. Int J Radiat Oncol Biol Phys 1995; 32(1):33–39.

105. Pilepich MV, Krall JM, al-Sarraf M, et al. Androgen deprivation with radiation therapy compared with radiation therapy alone for locally advanced prostatic carcinoma: a randomized comparative trial of the Radiation Therapy Oncology Group. Urology 1995; 45(4):616–623.

106. Turner SL, Adams K, Bull CA, et al. Sexual dysfunction after radical radiation therapy for prostate cancer: a prospective evaluation. Urology 1999; 54(1):124–129.

107. Mantz CA, Song P, Farhangi E, et al. Potency probability following conformal megavoltage radiotherapy using conventional doses for localized prostate cancer. Int J Radiat Oncol Biol Phys 1997; 37(3):551–557.

108. Fransson P, Bergstrom P, Lofroth PO, et al. Prospective evaluation of urinary and intestinal side effects after BeamCath stereotactic dose-escalated radiotherapy of prostate cancer. Radiother Oncol 2002; 63(3):239–248.

109. Pickles T, Graham P. What happens to testosterone after prostate radiation monotherapy and does it matter? J Urol 2002; 167(6):2448–2452.

110. McGowan DG. Radiation therapy in the management of localized carcinoma of the prostate: a preliminary report. Cancer 1977; 39(1):98–103.

111. Borghede G, Sullivan M. Measurement of quality of life in localized prostatic cancer patients treated with radiotherapy. Development of a prostate cancer-specific module supplementing the EORTC QLQ-C30. Qual Life Res 1996; 5(2):212–222.

112. van Heeringen C, De Schryver A, Verbeek E. Sexual function disorders after local radiotherapy for carcinoma of the prostate. Radiother Oncol 1988; 13(1):47–52.

113. Fisch BM, Pickett B, Weinberg V, et al. Dose of radiation received by the bulb of the penis correlates with risk of impotence after three-dimensional conformal radiotherapy for prostate cancer. Urology 2001; 57(5):955–959.

114. Merrick GS, Wallner K, Butler WM, et al. A comparison of radiation dose to the bulb of the penis in men with and without prostate brachytherapy-induced erectile dysfunction. Int J Radiat Oncol Biol Phys 2001; 50(3):597–604.

115. Mulhall JP, Yonover PM. Correlation of radiation dose and impotence risk after three-dimensional conformal radiotherapy for prostate cancer. Urology 2001; 58(5):828.

116. Sethi A, Mohideen N, Leybovich L, et al. Role of IMRT in reducing penile doses in dose escalation for prostate cancer. Int J Radiat Oncol Biol Phys 2003; 55(4):970–978.

117. Kao J, Turian J, Meyers A, et al. Sparing of the penile bulb and proximal penile structures with intensity-modulated radiation therapy for prostate cancer. Br J Radiol 2004; 77(914):129–136.

118. Buyyounouski MK, Horwitz EM, Uzzo RG, et al. The radiation doses to erectile tissues defined with magnetic resonance imaging after intensity-modulated radiation therapy or iodine-125 brachytherapy. Int J Radiat Oncol Biol Phys 2004; 59(5):1383–1391.

119. Stephenson RA, Mori M, Hsieh YC, et al. Treatment of erectile dysfunction following therapy for clinically localized prostate cancer: patient reported use and outcomes from the Surveillance, Epidemiology, and End Results Prostate Cancer Outcomes Study. J Urol 2005; 174(2):646–650; discussion 650.

120. McMahon CG. High dose sildenafil citrate as a salvage therapy for severe erectile dysfunction. Int J Impot Res 2002; 14(6):533–538.

121. El-Galley R, Rutland H, Talic R, et al. Long-term efficacy of sildenafil and tachyphylaxis effect. J Urol 2001; 166(3):927–931.

122. Ohebshalom M, Parker M, Guhring P, et al. The efficacy of sildenafil citrate following radiation therapy for prostate cancer: temporal considerations. J Urol 2005; 174(1):258–262; discussion 262.

123. Zelefsky MJ, McKee AB, Lee H, et al. Efficacy of oral sildenafil in patients with erectile dysfunction after radiotherapy for carcinoma of the prostate. Urology 1999; 53(4):775–778.

124. Kedia S, Zippe CD, Agarwal A, et al. Treatment of erectile dysfunction with sildenafil citrate (Viagra) after radiation therapy for prostate cancer. Urology 1999; 54(2):308–312.

125. Weber DC, Bieri S, Kurtz JM, et al. Prospective pilot study of sildenafil for treatment of postradiotherapy erectile dysfunction in patients with prostate cancer. J Clin Oncol 1999; 17(11):3444–3449.

126. Incrocci L, Koper PC, Hop WC, et al. Sildenafil citrate (Viagra) and erectile dysfunction following external beam radiotherapy for prostate cancer: a randomized, double-blind, placebo-controlled, cross-over study. Int J Radiat Oncol Biol Phys 2001; 51(5):1190–1195.

127. Incrocci L, Hop WC, Slob AK. Efficacy of sildenafil in an open-label study as a continuation of a double-blind study in the treatment of erectile dysfunction after radiotherapy for prostate cancer. Urology 2003; 62(1):116–120.

128. Jereczek-Fossa BA, Marsiglia HR, Orecchia R. Radiotherapy-related fatigue. Crit Rev Oncol Hematol 2002; 41(3):317–325.

129. Mock V, Atkinson A, Barsevick A, et al. NCCN Practice Guidelines for Cancer-Related Fatigue. Oncology (Williston Park) 2000; 14(11A):151–161.

130. Curt GA, Breitbart W, Cella D, et al. Impact of cancer-related fatigue on the lives of patients: new findings from the Fatigue Coalition. Oncologist 2000; 5(5):353–360.

131. Morrow GR, Andrews PL, Hickok JT, et al. Fatigue associated with cancer and its treatment. Support Care Cancer 2002; 10(5):389–398.

132. Smets EM, Visser MR, Willems-Groot AF, et al. Fatigue and radiotherapy: (A) experience in patients undergoing treatment. Br J Cancer 1998; 78(7):899–906.

133. Jereczek-Fossa BA, Marsiglia HR, Orecchia R. Radiotherapy-related fatigue: how to assess and how to treat the symptom. A commentary. Tumori 2001; 87(3):147–151.

134. Smets EM, Visser MR, Willems-Groot AF, et al. Fatigue and radiotherapy: (B) experience in patients 9 months following treatment. Br J Cancer 1998; 78(7):907–912.

135. Patrick DL, Ferketich SL, Frame PS, et al. National Institutes of Health State-of-the-Science Conference Statement: Symptom Management in Cancer: Pain, Depression, and Fatigue, July 15–17, 2002. J Natl Cancer Inst 2003; 95(15):1110–1117.

136. Okuyama T, Akechi T, Kugaya A, et al. Factors correlated with fatigue in disease-free breast cancer patients: application of the Cancer Fatigue Scale. Support Care Cancer 2000; 8(3):215–222.

137. Kiebert GM, Curran D, Aaronson NK, et al. Quality of life after radiation therapy of cerebral low-grade gliomas of the adult: results of a randomised phase III trial on dose response (EORTC trial 22844). EORTC Radiotherapy Co-operative Group. Eur J Cancer 1998; 34(12):1902–1909.

138. Schwartz AL, Nail LM, Chen S, et al. Fatigue patterns observed in patients receiving chemotherapy and radiotherapy. Cancer Invest 2000; 18(1):11–19.

139. Walker BL, Nail LM, Larsen L, et al. Concerns, affect, and cognitive disruption following completion of radiation treatment for localized breast or prostate cancer. Oncol Nurs Forum 1996; 23(8): 1181–1187.

140. Forlenza MJ, Hall P, Lichtenstein P, et al. Epidemiology of cancer-related fatigue in the Swedish twin registry. Cancer 2005; 104(9):2022–2031.

141. Vordermark D, Schwab M, Flentje M, et al. Chronic fatigue after radiotherapy for carcinoma of the prostate: correlation with anorectal and genitourinary function. Radiother Oncol 2002; 62(3):293–297.

142. Windsor PM, Nicol KF, Potter J. A randomized, controlled trial of aerobic exercise for treatment-related fatigue in men receiving radical external beam radiotherapy for localized prostate carcinoma. Cancer 2004; 101(3):550–557.

143. Hall EJ, Wuu CS. Radiation-induced second cancers: the impact of 3D-CRT and IMRT. Int J Radiat Oncol Biol Phys 2003; 56(1):83–88.

144. Hall EJ, Martin SG, Amols H, et al. Photoneutrons from medical linear accelerators--radiobiological measurements and risk estimates. Int J Radiat Oncol Biol Phys 1995; 33(1):225–230.

145. National Council on Radiation Protection and Measurements. Risk estimates for radiation protection. Report no. 115. Bethesda, MD, 1993.

146. Chrouser K, Leibovich B, Bergstralh E, et al. Bladder cancer risk following primary and adjuvant external beam radiation for prostate cancer. J Urol 2005; 174(1):107–110; discussion 110–101.

147. Brenner DJ, Curtis RE, Hall EJ, et al. Second malignancies in prostate carcinoma patients after radiotherapy compared with surgery. Cancer 2000; 88(2):398–406.

148. Ries L, Kosary C, Hankey B, et al., eds. SEER Cancer Statistics Review 1973–1994. Bethesda, MD: National Institutes of Health, National Cancer Institute; 1997 DHHS Pub No. (NIH)97–2789.

149. Baxter NN, Tepper JE, Durham SB, et al. Increased risk of rectal cancer after prostate radiation: a population-based study. Gastroenterology 2005; 128(4):819–824.

150. Brenner DJ, Hall EJ, Curtis RE, et al. Prostate radiotherapy is associated with second cancers in many organs, not just the colorectum. Gastroenterology 2005; 129(2):773–774; author reply 774–775.

151. Kry SF, Salehpour M, Followill DS, et al. The calculated risk of fatal secondary malignancies from intensity-modulated radiation therapy. Int J Radiat Oncol Biol Phys 2005; 62(4):1195–1203.

152. D'Amico AV, Manola J, Loffredo M, et al. A practical method to achieve prostate gland immobilization and target verification for daily treatment. Int J Radiat Oncol Biol Phys 2001; 51(5):1431–1436.

35 | Complications of Prostate Brachytherapy: Cause, Prevention, and Treatment

Larissa J. Lee and Anthony L. Zietman
Department of Radiation Oncology, Massachusetts General Hospital and
Harvard Medical School, Boston, Massachusetts, U.S.A.

INTRODUCTION

Brachytherapy is a technique for the treatment of prostate cancer that has a long history. Early in the twentieth century, Hugh Hampton Young was implanting prostates with radium needles and later radon seeds, and was witness to remarkable tumor regression. The technique, though initially popular, fell from grace due to the considerable dangers inherent in handling sources which emitted tissue-destructive alpha particles and high-energy penetrating photons. Alternative radioactive sources such as iodine-125 were ultimately developed which emit less penetrating forms of radiation and the technique once again achieved popularity in the 1970s only to fall from favor due to the difficulties inherent in freehand source placement during an open procedure and the new enthusiasm for linear accelerator-based external radiation. Brachytherapy is now in its third incarnation this time returning in parallel with the development of transrectal ultrasound (TRUS). Radioactive sources can now be placed using 18 gauge needles and a transperineal approach. The use of ultrasound guidance and a perineal template allows for precise source placement, and the entire procedure can be performed in less than an hour, with the patient able to go home the same day. Excellent cancer control rates are now being reported. It is interesting to note that the wave of enthusiasm for this new iteration of the technique preceded the publication of any evidence of efficacy. It was to a large extent driven by public interest, the Internet, and a perception that the morbidity associated with brachytherapy was substantially less than that with radical prostatectomy and conventional external beam radiation. It has, however, subsequently become clear that, while quick and convenient, it is not without its own unique set of associated morbidity. In retrospect this is not surprising as brachytherapy delivers high and ablative doses of radiation to the prostate as shown by the extremely low prostate specific antigen (PSA) values subsequently achieved in those cured of their cancer. These same radiation doses are also delivered to the bladder neck, prostatic urethra, external sphincter, and neurovascular bundles. In this chapter we discuss the consequences of high-dose radiation to these structures. Though most published data refer to the "classic" implantation of the prostate with permanent sources such as iodine and palladium, the same patterns are also likely to be seen with the newer forms of temporary high dose-rate (HDR) brachytherapy using iridium.

TECHNICAL ASPECTS

Two broad approaches can be taken to the implantation of sources within the prostate. The first, or preplanned technique, begins with a "volume study" prior to the day of the implant. TRUS is used to make a three-dimensional map of the prostate which is downloaded onto a planning computer. The appropriate number of seeds, their strength (activity), and their arrangement can be calculated. The seeds are then ordered and are implanted in a rapid procedure under anesthesia in the operating room (OR). The second approach is to plan, load seeds into needles, and a single-step implantation in the OR. This has the advantage of guaranteeing that the prostate has the same shape and orientation at the time of planning and implantation because they are almost simultaneous events. It also allows for the real-time compensation of any "cold spots" in the implant with additional seeds. The disadvantage is that more time is actually spent in the OR. While the use of preplanning or real-time dosimetry may affect the speed and convenience of the implant, it is not clear whether either affects the morbidity associated with the procedure.

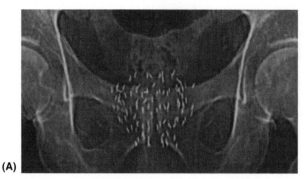
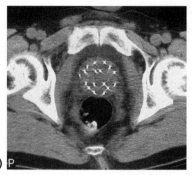

(A)   **(B)** P

FIGURE 1 Plain radiograph (**A**) and CT scan (**B**) showing contemporary prostate brachytherapy using 125-iodine seeds. Note the relative central sparing seen on the transverse CT cut (**B**).

Both approaches aim to place seeds in an arrangement that is a compromise between homogeneous loading in which seeds are evenly scattered across the prostate and peripheral loading in which they are placed just within the capsule. The first arrangement delivers radiation doses that are extremely high centrally, whereas the latter concentrates the dose peripherally. It is known as modified peripheral loading in which a few sources are placed centrally though away from the urethra in order to reduce the amount of activity required peripherally (Fig. 1). This means that the rectum is exposed to more tolerable doses of radiation.

URINARY MORBIDITY
Acute Urinary Morbidity

Urinary symptoms are among the most commonly reported side effects following brachytherapy. Most patients develop some degree of urinary irritative or obstructive symptoms, including urinary frequency, urgency, dysuria, incomplete voiding, weak stream, or less commonly, acute urinary retention. Numerous quality-of-life studies have been performed to assess urinary morbidity following brachytherapy by using the International Prostate Symptom Score (IPSS) or Radiation Therapy Oncology Group (RTOG) criteria. The IPSS was developed by the American Urological Association (AUA) as a measure of symptom relief following prostatectomy for benign prostatic hyperplasia (BPH), and has been validated as a useful tool in assessing urinary morbidity after prostate brachytherapy. Mild to moderate urinary symptoms in the first month following brachytherapy are very common, reported by the majority of patients. In a large prospective study from Memoral Sloan-Kettering Cancer Center (MSKCC), 37% of patients reported grade 1 urinary toxicity, 41% grade 2 toxicity, and 2.2% grade 3 urinary toxicity (1). Several series have shown that urinary symptoms peak at one to two months after implantation and return to preimplantation baseline levels within one year (2,3). Thus, although most men may be expected to experience some degree of urinary symptoms following brachytherapy, symptoms are generally short-lived and improve rapidly within several months.

Several studies have shown that the prostate may swell substantially in the first week after implantation and with this comes a risk of acute urinary retention. Prolonged urinary retention can significantly affect the quality of life, increase the risk of catheter-related urinary tract infections, and lead to potentially morbid surgical efforts to relieve it them. Following the procedure, there are two risk periods for acute retention. The first is within 24 hours and is seen in men who had precarious flow preprocedure, the second occurs in the second week when the cumulative effect of the radiation triggers an inflammatory prostatitis. Earlier studies in which unselected patients were implanted report an overall incidence of acute urinary retention of between 5% and 25%. Men with larger prostate volumes and substantial preimplant urinary symptoms, reflected by a higher AUA score, appear to be at greatest risk for this complication. In patients with large prostates with volumes exceeding 90 cm^3, the risk of acute urinary retention may exceed 40% (4). The incidence drops sharply to 3% and 6% in glands measuring less than 45 or 45 to 60 cm^3, respectively, but is as high as 28% in glands measuring 60 to 90 cm^3.

The American Brachytherapy Society considers a prostate volume of greater than 60 cm³ a relative contraindication for brachytherapy (5). In addition, patients with significant urinary symptoms prior to brachytherapy are more likely to suffer acute urinary retention. Terk et al. (6) demonstrated that patients with an IPSS score of more than 20 had a 29% risk of urinary retention, as compared to patients with less severe urinary symptoms. Patients with moderate urinary symptoms and an IPSS score of 10 to 19 had an 11% risk, while patients with minimal symptoms (IPSS < 10) had a risk of only 2% of developing urinary retention. Urodynamic studies, post-void residual urine volume, and maximum flow rate are not reliable predictors for acute urinary retention. However, patients with evidence of urinary obstruction are considered poor candidates for brachytherapy.

Given the relatively short time course to the development of urinary retention, acute prostate swelling is most likely related both to needle trauma and the early effects of radiation. Post-implantation prostatic ultrasound and computed tomography (CT) studies have shown that the prostate may increase in size by approximately 20% to 40%. Several studies have shown that the number of needle incursions is also related to the risk of urinary retention (7). Furthermore, a learning curve exists in brachytherapy technique, as the incidence of urinary retention has been shown to decrease in single-institution studies when efforts were made to reduce the number of needles per case and reduce OR time (8).

Gross hematuria is common in patients immediately following seed implantation and is generally of little clinical significance. Occasionally, patients will develop urinary retention, requiring catheter placement and bladder irrigation. A minority of patients report intermittent gross hematuria that generally resolves within three months (9). The cause of hematuria is most often attributed to procedural trauma, radiation urethritis, prostatitis, or cystitis. It is reasonable to consider a hematuria work-up for genitourinary malignancy if the clinical situation merits.

Patient Selection

To minimize urinary morbidity, careful patient selection is employed by the urologist and radiation oncologist. Relative contraindications to brachytherapy include large prostate size and significant urinary symptoms as measured by the AUA score. In practice, patients with significant voiding symptoms or a post-void residual greater than 100 cc are considered poor brachytherapy candidates (10). Patients with prostate volumes greater than 50 to 60 cm³ are expected to suffer more substantial, although temporary, urinary symptoms. In a large retrospective analysis by Gelblum et al. (1), pretreatment AUA scores of greater than 7 were associated with greater grade 2 urinary morbidity and a longer time to resolution of symptoms. Median lobe hyperplasia is also considered a relative contraindication to seed implantation secondary to anatomic considerations, although an increased risk of post-implant morbidity has not yet been substantiated (11). The median lobe may swell during the acute phase causing ball-valve obstruction of the bladder neck (Fig. 2). Patients with a history of

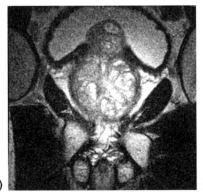 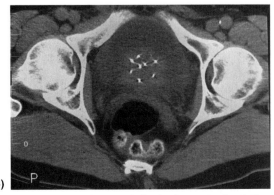

(A) **(B)**

FIGURE 2 **(A)** Coronal MRI showing large intravesical median lobe, a relative contraindication for prostate brachytherapy; **(B)** subsequent acute urinary retention due to aggressive median lobe implantation and edema. *Abbreviation*: MRI, magnetic resonance imaging.

poorly controlled diabetes and wound-healing problems should be carefully considered as potential brachytherapy candidates, as they are at increased risk of developing postoperative complications.

Prevention

Alpha-blockers are considered the most effective treatment for acute urinary morbidity following brachytherapy. They are widely prescribed for relief of the common irritative and obstructive symptoms that many patients experience. The rationale for the prophylactic use of alpha-blockers is to reduce urinary symptoms and shorten their time course. In two recent randomized trials, prophylactic use of alpha-blockers hastened the resolution of urinary symptoms, but did not affect the peak severity of symptoms or significantly decrease the incidence of acute urinary retention (12,13). Nonetheless, alpha-blockers are commonly prescribed at the time of brachytherapy to patients with mild preimplant urinary symptoms or large prostatic volumes who are at risk for more post-procedure voiding complications.

The role of androgen deprivation in the prevention of urinary morbidity is not firmly established. Androgen deprivation has been shown to consistently reduce prostatic volume by approximately 30% to 40%. The rationale for the use of androgen deprivation is to reduce the size of the prostate to make an implant technically easier and to reduce the risk of acute urinary retention. Several reports have found that androgen deprivation is associated with increased acute urinary morbidity. In a retrospective study by Sacco et al. (14), the risk of urinary retention in patients who received androgen suppression was greater than that in volume-matched controls, and the prostate volume at the time of diagnosis was found to be more predictive of urinary retention than the volume at the time of implant.

Anti-inflammatory medications such as steroids may be effective in reducing urinary morbidity by preventing prostatic edema. Post-implant volume may increase by 20% on postoperative day 1 compared with the preplanning volume (15). Peri-operative steroid administration is commonly used to prevent acute edema when radiation implants are performed in other sites in the body such as the base of tongue where swelling can lead to airway obstruction. Some investigators have shown that they can reduce prostate volume within 4 weeks (16). In a retrospective study, the incidence of acute urinary retention was reduced from 18.8% to 8.2% by the routine use of a two-week course of dexamethasone (14).

Technique

Brachytherapy technique also has a significant impact on urinary morbidity. Central sparing of the urethra is now routinely performed through the adoption of peripheral loading patterns that limit radiation dose to the urethra. During the procedure itself, the urethra is marked with a catheter and care is taken not to pass the needles through nor leave seeds in the proximity of the urethra. Attention should also be paid to the doses delivered to the bladder neck and external sphincter and, although there are no data yet to document a reduction in morbidity, this is indeed likely.

Treatment

Alpha-blockers are considered the first-line treatment for urinary symptoms after brachytherapy. Alpha-blockers are effective at relieving obstructive symptoms such as incomplete voiding, weak stream, and acute urinary retention by relaxing the prostatic smooth muscle. Patients with irritative symptoms also benefit with the use of alpha-blockers by promoting complete bladder emptying. Local bladder anesthetics such as pyridium are frequently used for patients with significant dysuria. Non-steroidal anti-inflammatory drugs (NSAIDs) may also provide relief of irritative symptoms in select patients. In patients with urinary urgency, anticholinergics such as Tolterodine (Detrol, Pfizer) and antispasmodics such as oxybutynin (Ditropan, Alta) relieve smooth muscle contractions of the bladder. However, these medications should be used with caution as they may precipitate acute urinary retention.

Late Urinary Toxicity

Late urinary complications of brachytherapy include persistent urinary frequency, chronic urinary retention, incontinence, and urethral stricture. Though these late complications of brachytherapy are uncommon they can profoundly affect the quality of life of patients in whom they occur. The acute irritative and obstructive symptoms measured by the AUA score have been found to return to baseline within 12 months following implantation. One recent study found that there was no difference in long-term urinary quality of life between patients treated with brachytherapy and age-matched controls with newly diagnosed prostate cancer (17).

When prolonged urinary retention occurs it is best managed conservatively. Our policy is to leave the catheter in situ for two weeks and then attempt a voiding trial. If the patient fails, the catheter is reinserted and a trial occurs a week later. If he fails again then he is taught clean intermittent self-catheterization. For almost all patients, spontaneous voiding will ultimately occur although it may take several months. A small proportion of patients require a post-implant transurethral prostatic resection (TURP) to relieve prolonged urinary obstruction refractory to medical management. Post-implantation TURP is associated with a significant rate of urinary incontinence, with a reported incidence 18% to 50% (18–20). In addition, patients with a large or poorly healed TURP defect may be at greater risk for urethral necrosis and stricture (Fig. 3). It is better to wait at least six months before attempting any surgical relief and probably better to begin with a transurethral incision of the prostate or a very cautious and limited TURP.

The incidence of brachytherapy-related urethral stricture is reported to be between 0% and 12%, and has been correlated with the dose to the bulbo-membranous urethra (21). Patients with urethral stricture may present with obstructive symptoms such as weak stream or straining while voiding. The first step in management of a urethral stricture is urethral dilation or internal urethrotomy. Rarely, conversion to a suprapubic catheter or self-catheterization is required for recurrent strictures. The median time to development of a urethral stricture is approximately 24 months, but can occur many years after brachytherapy.

Superficial urethral necrosis is a more devastating complication of brachytherapy that is associated with severe dysuria and incontinence. The risk of urethral necrosis is minimized with peripheral seed loading to avoid excess dose to the urethra. It is strongly associated with prior or subsequent prostatic surgical procedures.

GASTROINTESTINAL MORBIDITY
Acute Gastrointestinal Morbidity

Rectal symptoms are far less common than urinary symptoms following prostate brachytherapy. Side effects that are commonly reported include diarrhea, mucus discharge, rectal bleeding, and urgency. Most studies have used the RTOG criteria to score rectal symptoms. The RTOG toxicity score reflects the degree of proctitis, with grade 1 considered as mild symptoms of proctitis requiring no treatment and grade 2 as rectal symptoms managed by medical therapy. Gelblum and Potters (22) reported the incidence of grade 1 and 2 rectal toxicity to be 9.4% and

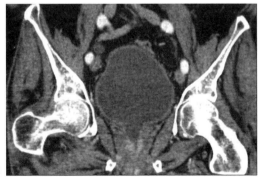
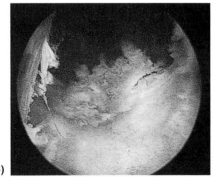

(A) (B)

FIGURE 3 (**A**) Coronal CT scan showing a deep TURP defect prior to brachytherapy; (**B**) subsequent superficial urethral necrosis following brachytherapy. *Abbreviations*: CT, computed tomography; TURP, transurethral resection of the prostate.

6.6%, respectively, with a peak incidence at eight months. Only 0.5% of patients experienced grade 3 rectal toxicity, and were documented to have rectal ulceration by colonoscopy. A recent prospective study used the National Cancer Institute (NCI) Common Toxicity Criteria system as a more comprehensive tool to examine acute rectal toxicity after brachytherapy. Adverse events such as diarrhea, incontinence, urgency, proctitis, pain, spasm and hemorrhage were individually scored from grade 1–5. Overall, the highest rate of grade 1–2 toxicity was observed for diarrhea, with an incidence of 17.5%. All the individually reported events were observed in at least 5% of patients with grade 1–2 toxicity with the exception of rectal spasms. There were no reported toxicities greater than grade 2 (23).

Treatment

For patients that experience acute rectal toxicity, symptom management with dietary changes or medication can be of great benefit. A high-fiber diet or the addition of a bulking agent such as Metamucil [(Psyllium) Procter & Gamble] can reduce the number of daily bowel movements and lessen rectal irritation. Diarrhea can also be effectively controlled with antidiarrheal agents such as Imodium (leperamide) (Janssen Pharmaceutica) or Lomotil, Pfizer (diphenoxylate lactopine). For patients with rectal bleeding, tenesmus or pain, suppositories containing a steroid can provide a local anti-inflammatory effect.

Late Gastrointestinal Morbidity

Manifestations of late radiation toxicity include rectal bleeding, pain, diarrhea, urgency and fecal incontinence that develop 6 to 18 months after treatment. Sigmoidoscopy or colonoscopy can confirm the diagnosis in the presence of characteristic mucosal changes (Fig. 4). The rectal mucosa often appears pale and friable with multiple telangectasias. Multiple studies have found that the incidence of radiation proctitis is related to the length or volume of rectum exposed to radiation as well as the maximum dose. If the rectal surface area receiving 100 Gy, 150 Gy, or 200 Gy is below 30%, 20%, or 10%, respectively, the risk of late morbidity can be reduced to less than 5% (24). Brachytherapy technique again plays a critical role in determining the risk of complications. The placement of perirectal seeds within 2 mm of the anterior rectal wall has been found to be related to late rectal bleeding (25).

One of the more devastating and rare complications of prostate brachytherapy is the development of a rectal fistula. Patients who develop rectourethral or rectovesical fistulas may present with pain, hematuria, rectal bleeding, intractable urinary tract infections, fecaluria, or urine via the rectum. The incidence of rectal fistula has been reported to be less than 1%, and is likely related to the radiation dose to the anterior rectal wall. It may be increased in men who have combined external beam radiation and brachytherapy. Patient factors such as underlying vascular disease, poorly controlled diabetes, and smoking history may also contribute. Rectal biopsy has also been correlated as a significant risk factor for the development of fistula (26).

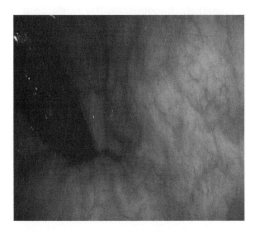

FIGURE 4 Anterior rectal erythema and angio-ectasia commonly seen after brachytherapy and the cause of late, post-implant bleeding.

Prevention

Because the incidence of radiation proctitis is related both to the volume and maximum radiation dose to the anterior rectal wall, technical and planning considerations are paramount. In addition, preventative medical strategies have also been explored. Amifostine is a radioprotectant that has been shown to reduce normal tissue toxicity in head and neck cancer. Intravenous administration is unfortunately associated with hypotension and nausea, limiting its widespread use. More recently, intrarectal administration has shown promising results in the prevention of rectal toxicity. Several studies have demonstrated a reduction in grades 1–2 rectal morbidity with intrarectal amifostine that was well tolerated without systemic side effects (27–29). The role of amifostine in limiting rectal morbidity is currently under investigation for patients undergoing external beam radiation therapy, and has yet to be established for brachytherapy patients.

Salicylates such as sulfasalazine and balasalazide are well-established anti-inflammatory medications for the treatment of inflammatory bowel disease and idiopathic colitis. These agents may have a role in preventing acute gastrointestinal toxicity, but longer follow up is needed to evaluate their role in preventing late radiation injury (30,31). In addition, sucralfate has been proposed to reduce radiation-induced mucosal injury by forming a protective barrier over the anterior rectal wall. Unfortunately, multiple randomized studies have not shown a benefit for preventing acute radiation proctitis (32,33).

There are three ways of preventing fistula formation. The first is meticulous technique in placing the posterior seeds with careful observation during implantation using TRUS in both the transverse and sagittal planes. The second is to advise the gastroenterologist to avoid the temptation to treat asymptomatic angioectasia seen on routine colonoscopy. The third is to avoid treating men with inflammatory bowel disease. A clear correlation exists between inflammatory bowel disease (IBD) and severe radiation injury after external beam radiation, and may represent a relative contraindication for brachytherapy.

Treatment

For patients that develop signs of late radiation toxicity, including rectal bleeding, tenesmus and pain, steroid suppositories or rectal foam are both safe and effective. If bleeding from rectal angioectasias is significant and refractory to conservative medical therapy, argon plasma coagulation (APC) may be used to arrest the bleeding. APC uses high-frequency energy that is transmitted to friable tissue by ionized gas. The efficacy of APC for persistent rectal bleeding has been demonstrated in multiple studies (34). Rectal pain and cramping may occur in some patients after treatment, but no major complications have been reported. Conservative management of rectal fistula is often ineffective, although small fistulae may heal after endoscopic clamping and sealing with fibrin plugs (Fig. 5). Surgical intervention is often required to alleviate symptoms by diversion of the fecal stream by colostomy or ileostomy. Definitive resection of the fistula is performed prior to ostomy closure.

SEXUAL MORBIDITY

Brachytherapy carries an inherent risk of long-term sexual dysfunction, similar to the other curative modalities for early-stage disease. The putative mechanism of radiation-induced erectile dysfunction is arterial damage to the neurovascular bundles that travel along the posterolateral aspect of the prostate or possibly demyelination. Structural alterations in corporal smooth muscle, venous insufficiency, and endothelial dysfunction may also play an important role. The risk of erectile dysfunction following brachytherapy has been widely reported from 6% to 61%, confounded by the method of data collection (physician- vs patient-reported), differences in followup, and the use of invalidated reporting tools. The effect of treatment is often obscured by the natural loss of erections with age and the relatively high incidence of erectile dysfunction prior to treatment. Nevertheless, a prospective study by Merrick et al. (35) found the potency preservation rate after brachytherapy to be 50% at three years using a validated quality-of-life instrument, the International Index of Erectile Function (IEFF). Potters et al. reported the rate of potency preservation to be as high as 76% at five years for brachytherapy alone. Potency preservation was, however, significantly lower at 56% when brachytherapy was combined with external beam radiation therapy and fell to 29% with the addition of

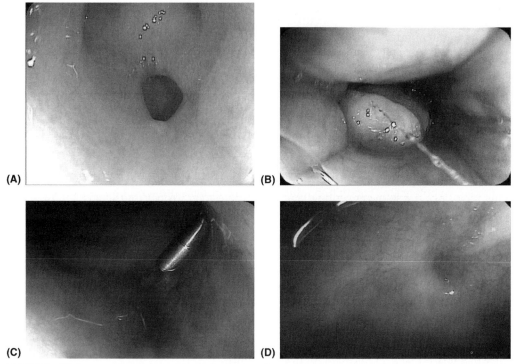

FIGURE 5 (**A**) Deep rectal ulcer present developing 2 years after combined prostate brachytherapy and external radiation; (**B**) application of fibrin plug, repeated on three occasions; (**C**) clip closure of ulcer containing plug; (**D**) complete ulcer healing 3 months later.

neoadjuvant hormones (36). The median time to the development of brachytherapy-induced erectile dysfunction is reported as 6 to 17 months, mostly occurring within two years. Preimplant potency, age, and the presence of vascular disease or diabetes are also important predictors of post-implant erectile dysfunction.

The sum total of sexual morbidity is wider than the loss of erectile function and includes hematospermia and orgasmalgia. Hematospermia is common in the first several weeks after seed implantation, but is generally short-lived. Patients may also experience burning with orgasm, or orgasmalgia, for a limited period of time (37). Decreased ejaculate volume is common and relates to the ultimate ablation of the glandular tissue in the prostate.

Technique

Careful attention to brachytherapy technique likely has a significant impact on the preservation of potency. Extra-prostatic and particularly peri-apical seed placement should be performed judiciously, and color Doppler may be used to assess the location of the neurovascular bundle. Erectile dysfunction has been correlated with surgical trauma following radical prostatectomy, and needle trauma to the neurovascular bundles or venous bodies during an implant is a likely factor in immediate post-implant impotence. Initial studies have not correlated the risk of erectile dysfunction with radiation dose to the neurovascular bundle, although followup has been limited (38) and knowledge of the exact location of the NVBs in any individual patient poor. Laboratory evidence and clinical studies have suggested that dose to the penile bulb after external radiation was also strongly associated with potency. The same group has demonstrated that the radiation dose to the penile bulb was highly correlated with the risk of erectile dysfunction after brachytherapy. On day 0 CT-based dosimetry scans, a radiation dose of less than 50 Gy delivered to 50% of the penile bulb was highly correlated with post-treatment potency (39). However, another prospective study failed to confirm this finding (40). It is not yet clear if the true dose-limiting structure is the penile bulb itself, or a surrogate for the adjacent neurovascular structures.

Treatment

Radiation-induced erectile dysfunction has a significant response rate of up to 85% with phosphodiesterase (PDE-5) inhibitors. PDE-5 inhibitors increase cyclic GMP levels within the corpora cavernosae to promote nitric oxide-induced vasodilation required to maintain an erection. These medications, which include sildenafil (Viagra®, Pfizer), vardenafil (Levitra®, Bayer), and tadalafil (Cialis®, Lilly ICOS) are well tolerated with minimal side effects, which may include headache, lightheadedness, or flushing. A small proportion of men experience blue-tinted vision while taking sildenafil. Because these medications are potent vasodilators, they are absolutely contraindicated with the concurrent use of nitrates, given the risk of life-threatening hypotension. The PDE-5 inhibitors vary in their duration of effectiveness, with sildenafil being the shortest acting drug lasting four hours, and tadalafil the longest lasting up to 36 hours. There is, as yet, no evidence that prophylactic use of these drugs can prevent the development of impotence though several studies are currently testing the hypothesis.

Men who do not respond to medical treatment may consider slightly more invasive approaches to induce an erection. Self-injection of the corpora cavernosae with a prostaglandin such as Caverject® (Pfizer) can reproducibly produce an erection in greater than 85% of men, although it is frequently discontinued due to penile pain and prolonged erection. Intraurethral installation of prostaglandin is a second less invasive method. Vacuum-assisted devices and penile prostheses are reserved for men who do not respond to the first- and second-line therapies. These devices are not in any way contraindicated by the prior use of brachytherapy although insertion of penile prostheses may be more difficult if there is deep perineal fibrosis.

REPRODUCTIVE CAPACITY

When localized prostate cancer is treated by radiation, infertility can occur in several ways: direct damage to the sperm themselves while in the seminal vesicles; damage to the testicular germinal centers and hormonal supporting cells from scattered radiation; fibrotic obstruction of ducts for sperm transportation; and from the development of erectile impotence. As treatment commonly induces at least one of these problems and because patients tend to be older, with older partners, fertility is an issue rarely considered. Indeed, it is usually assumed that brachytherapy will inevitably cause infertility.

A small series reported by Grocela et al. (41) shows that viable sperm may be seen in the ejaculate of some men up to 22 months after prostate brachytherapy and that pregnancy may be possible, while none of the couples consented to genetic testing to prove paternity. Morphology of the sperm in this small series was within normal limits though sperm counts were normal and semen volume low.

It has long been recognized that external radiation to the testes can induce azoospermia. In adults, Leydig cell dysfunction requires doses in excess of 20 Gy but spermatogonia are far more sensitive. Single direct doses of just 4 to 6 Gy may produce azoospermia lasting five years or more (42). Scattered doses have been calculated for the remaining testis of men being treated for seminoma. Two-thirds develop oligospermia or even azoospermia after doses between 0.2 and 1.3 Gy. Recovery, however, occurs in the majority of these men. There are little data on teratogenesis among the progeny of children born to men who have received prior testicular irradiation.

There is a great deal of uncertainty about the testicular radiation doses that brachytherapy patients receive due to variability in testicular position but they can be estimated to be in the range of 0.03 to 2.5 Gy delivered at a very low dose rate over months (Fig. 6). These are doses that might be expected to induce oligospermia but not necessarily permanent azoospermia. There is likely a lower biologic effect on the testis from low-dose brachytherapy than there is from the pulsed external beam radiation effects that have been reported in the literature.

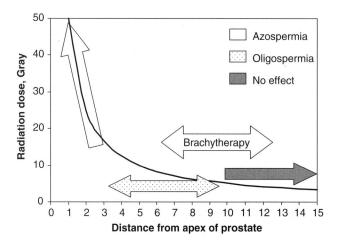

FIGURE 6 Radiation dose received by the testis as a function of testicular distance from the apex of the prostate. *Source*: From Ref. 41.

The cases reported by Grocela et al. (41) advocate caution and suggest that men being treated with prostate brachytherapy should be counseled regarding the possibility of continued fertility.

CONCLUSIONS

Morbidity following prostate brachytherapy comes in two waves. The first or acute wave is the consequence of needle trauma coupled with a radiation prostatitis or urethritis. This is usually temporary and can be managed medically. The second wave arises months or years later and is the result of late changes in the vasculature of the irradiated epithelial and mesenchymal tissues. These changes may be irreversible. Management of these late complications should always begin conservatively as heavily irradiated tissues are notoriously slow to heal and overly aggressively treatment may worsen the situation.

REFERENCES

1. Gelblum DY, Potters L, Ashley R, Waldbaum R, Wang XH, Leibel S. Urinary morbidity following ultrasound-guided transperineal prostate seed implantation. Int J Radiat Oncol Biol Phys 1999; 45(1):59–67.
2. Cesaretti JA, Stone NN, Stock RG. Urinary symptom flare following I-125 prostate brachytherapy. Int J Radiat Oncol Biol Phys 2003; 56(4):1085–1092.
3. Lee WR, McQuellon RP, Harris-Henderson K, Case LD, McCullough DL. A preliminary analysis of health-related quality of life in the first year after permanent source interstitial brachytherapy (PIB) for clinically localized prostate cancer. Int J Radiat Oncol Biol Phys 2000; 46(1):77–81.
4. Landis DM, Schultz D, Cormack R, et al. Acute urinary retention after magnetic resonance image-guided prostate brachytherapy with and without neoadjuvant external beam radiotherapy. Urology 2005; 65(4):750–754.
5. Nag S, Beyer D, Friedland J, Grimm P, Nath R. American Brachytherapy Society (ABS) recommendations for transperineal permanent brachytherapy of prostate cancer. Int J Radiat Oncol Biol Phys 1999; 44(4):789–799.
6. Terk MD, Stock RG, Stone NN. Identification of patients at increased risk for prolonged urinary retention following radioactive seed implantation of the prostate. J Urol 1998; 160(4):1379–1382.
7. Buskirk SJ, Pinkstaff DM, Petrou SP, etal. Acute urinary retention after transperineal template-guided prostate biopsy. Int J Radiat Oncol Biol Phys 2004; 59(5):1360–1366.
8. Keyes M, Schellenberg D, Moravan V, et al. Decline in urinary retention incidence in 805 patients after prostate brachytherapy: the effect of learning curve? Int J Radiat Oncol Biol Phys 2006; 64(3):825–834.
9. Barker J Jr, Wallner K, Merrick G. Gross hematuria after prostate brachytherapy. Urology 2003; 61(2):408–411.
10. Beekman M, Merrick GS, Buller WM, Wallner KE, Allen ZA, Galbreath RW. Selecting patients with pretreatment postvoid residual urine volume less than 100 mL may favorably influence brachytherapy-related urinary morbidity. Urology 2005; 66(6):1266–1270.

11. Nguyen J, Wallner K, Han B, Sutlief S. Urinary morbidity in brachytherapy patients with median lobe hyperplasia. Brachytherapy 2002; 1(1):42–47.

12. Elshaikh MA, Ulchaker JC, Reddy CA, et al. Prophylactic tamsulosin (Flomax) in patients undergoing prostate 125I brachytherapy for prostate carcinoma: final report of a double-blind placebo-controlled randomized study. Int J Radiat Oncol Biol Phys 2005; 62(1):164–169.

13. Merrick GS, Butler WM, Wallner KE, Lief JH, Galbreath RW. Prophylactic versus therapeutic alpha-blockers after permanent prostate brachytherapy. Urology 2002; 60(4):650–655.

14. Sacco DE, Daller M, Grocela JA, Babayan RK, Zietman AL. Corticosteroid use after prostate brachytherapy reduces the risk of acute urinary retention. BJU Int 2003; 91(4):345–349.

15. Prestidge BR, Bice WS, Kiefer EJ, Prete JJ. Timing of computed tomography-based postimplant assessment following permanent transperineal prostate brachytherapy. Int J Radiat Oncol Biol Phys 1998; 40(5):1111–1115.

16. Speight JL, Shinohara K, Pickett B, Weinberg VK, Hsu IC, Roach M, 3rd. Prostate volume change after radioactive seed implantation: possible benefit of improved dose volume histogram with perioperative steroid. Int J Radiat Oncol Biol Phys 2000; 48(5):1461–1467.

17. Merrick GS, Butler WM, Wallner KE, Galbreath RW, Lief JH. Long-term urinary quality of life after permanent prostate brachytherapy. Int J Radiat Oncol Biol Phys 2003; 56(2):454–461.

18. Hu K, Wallner K. Urinary incontinence in patients who have a TURP/TUIP following prostate brachytherapy. Int J Radiat Oncol Biol Phys 1998; 40(4):783–786.

19. Merrick GS, Butler WM, Wallner KE, Galbreath RW. Effect of transurethral resection on urinary quality of life after permanent prostate brachytherapy. Int J Radiat Oncol Biol Phys 2004; 58(1):81–88.

20. Kollmeier MA, Stock RG, Cesaretti J, Stone NN. Urinary morbidity and incontinence following transurethral resection of the prostate after brachytherapy. J Urol 2005; 173(3):808–812.

21. Merrick GS, Butler WM, Wallner KE, et al. Risk factors for the development of prostate brachytherapy related urethral strictures. J Urol 2006; 175(4):1376–1380; discussion 1381.

22. Gelblum DY, Potters L. Rectal complications associated with transperineal interstitial brachytherapy for prostate cancer. Int J Radiat Oncol Biol Phys 2000; 48(1):119–124.

23. Shah JN, Ennis RD. Rectal toxicity profile after transperineal interstitial permanent prostate brachytherapy: use of a comprehensive toxicity scoring system and identification of rectal dosimetric toxicity predictors. Int J Radiat Oncol Biol Phys 2006; 64(3):817–824.

24. Waterman FM, Dicker AP. Probability of late rectal morbidity in 125I prostate brachytherapy. Int J Radiat Oncol Biol Phys 2003; 55(2):342–353.

25. Mueller A, Wallner K, Merrick G, et al. Perirectal seeds as a risk factor for prostate brachytherapy-related rectal bleeding. Int J Radiat Oncol Biol Phys 2004; 59(4):1047–1052.

26. Theodorescu D, Gillenwater JY, Koutrouvelis PG. Prostatourethral-rectal fistula after prostate brachytherapy. Cancer 2000; 89(10):2085–2091.

27. Ben-Josef E, Han S, Tobi M, et al. A pilot study of topical intrarectal application of amifostine for prevention of late radiation rectal injury. Int J Radiat Oncol Biol Phys 2002; 53(5):1160–1164.

28. Kouloulias VE, Kouvaris JR, Pissakas G, et al. Phase II multicenter randomized study of amifostine for prevention of acute radiation rectal toxicity: topical intrarectal versus subcutaneous application. Int J Radiat Oncol Biol Phys 2005; 62(2):486–493.

29. Singh AK, Menard C, Guion P, et al. Intrarectal amifostine suspension may protect against acute proctitis during radiation therapy for prostate cancer: a pilot study. Int J Radiat Oncol Biol Phys 2006; 65(4):1008–1013.

30. Kilic D, Egehan I, Ozenirler S, Dursun A. Double-blinded, randomized, placebo-controlled study to evaluate the effectiveness of sulphasalazine in preventing acute gastrointestinal complications due to radiotherapy. Radiother Oncol 2000; 57(2):125–129.

31. Jahraus CD, Bettenhausen D, Malik U, Sellitti M, St Clair WH. Prevention of acute radiation-induced proctosigmoiditis by balsalazide: a randomized, double-blind, placebo controlled trial in prostate cancer patients. Int J Radiat Oncol Biol Phys 2005; 63(5):1483–1487.

32. O'Brien PC, Franklin CI, Dear KB, et al. A phase III double-blind randomised study of rectal sucralfate suspension in the prevention of acute radiation proctitis. Radiother Oncol 1997; 45(2):117–123.

33. Kneebone A, Mameghan H, Bolin T, et al. The effect of oral sucralfate on the acute proctitis associated with prostate radiotherapy: a double-blind, randomized, trial. Int J Radiat Oncol Biol Phys 2001; 51(3):628–635.

34. Silva RA, Correia AJ, Dias LM, Viana HL, Viana RL. Argon plasma coagulation therapy for hemorrhagic radiation proctosigmoiditis. Gastrointest Endosc 1999; 50(2):221–224.

35. Merrick GS, Butler WM, Wallner KE, et al. Erectile function after prostate brachytherapy. Int J Radiat Oncol Biol Phys 2005; 62(2):437–447.

36. Potters L, Torre T, Fearn PA, Leibel SA, Kattan MW. Potency after permanent prostate brachytherapy for localized prostate cancer. Int J Radiat Oncol Biol Phys 2001; 50(5):1235–1242.

37. Merrick GS, Wallner K, Butler WM, Galbreath RW, Lief JH, Benson ML. A comparison of radiation dose to the bulb of the penis in men with and without prostate brachytherapy-induced erectile dysfunction. Int J Radiat Oncol Biol Phys 2001; 50(3):597–604.

38. Merrick GS, Butler WM, Dorsey AT, Lief JH, Donzella JG. A comparison of radiation dose to the neurovascular bundles in men with and without prostate brachytherapy-induced erectile dysfunction. Int J Radiat Oncol Biol Phys 2000; 48(4):1069–1074.
39. Merrick GS, Wallner K, Butler WM, Lief JH, Sutlief S. Short-term sexual function after prostate brachytherapy. Int J Cancer 2001; 96(5):313–319.
40. Macdonald AG, Keyes M, Kruk A, Duncan G, Moravan V, Morris WJ. Predictive factors for erectile dysfunction in men with prostate cancer after brachytherapy: is dose to the penile bulb important? Int J Radiat Oncol Biol Phys 2005; 63(1):155–163.
41. Grocela JA, Mauceri T, Zietman AL. New life after prostate brachytherapy. Br J Urol 2005; 96:781–782.
42. Clifton D, Bremner W. The effect of testicular X-irradiation on spermatogenesis in man: a comparison with the mouse. J Androl 1983; 4:387–392.

36 | Complications of Chemotherapy for Urologic Cancer

Elisabeth M. Battinelli and Marc B. Garnick
Division of Hematology and Oncology, Department of Medicine, Beth Israel Deaconess Medical Center, Harvard Medical School, Boston, Massachusetts, U.S.A.

The field of urological malignancies represents the combination of many medical specialties including oncology (both radiation and medical), urology, and other specialized surgeries in an attempt to provide a multidisciplinary approach to treatment. Medical treatment of these diseases includes not only chemotherapy but also many biologic treatments as well as targeted drugs. For a list of the chemotherapeutic agents discussed in Table 1. Here with review the basic treatment modalities of the urological malignancies and elaborate on the risks and complications associated with these specific treatments that are of special interest to the practicing urologist and uro-oncologist.

CHEMOTHERAPY FOR TESTICULAR CANCER
Treatment Regimens

Testicular germ-cell tumors are remarkable in that they are uniquely sensitive to chemotherapeutic agents. The most frequently used regimen is the bleomycin, etoposide (BEP) and cisplatin. Bleomycin is a cytotoxic agent as it generates activated free radicals, which cause breaks in single- and double-stranded DNA leading to cell death. Its main side effects include skin reactions, pulmonary toxicity, and rarely myelosuppression. Etoposide is a topoisomerase II inhibitor that is derived from a plant alkaloid. Its main side effects include myelosuppression, gastrointestinal upset, anorexia, alopecia, and an increased risk of secondary malignancies including acute myelogenous leukemia. Cisplatin is a platinum analog, which covalently binds to DNA resulting in the formation of DNA adducts, leading to the inhibition of DNA synthesis and function. Its main side effects include nephrotoxicity, gastrointestinal upset, myelosuppression, neurotoxicity, ototoxicity, hypersensitivity reactions, and transient elevation in liver function tests, hair loss, secretion of antidiuretic hormone (SIADH), vascular events, and a metallic taste sensation, leading to loss of appetite.

Using the BEP regimen in the adjuvant setting in early-stage disease has resulted in a long-term disease-free survival of 96%. In arranging a treatment plan for patients with chemotherapy, the number of cycles and the specific treatment regimen are decided based on the stage and the histology of the testicular cancer. In addition to the standard use of paraortic subdiaphragmatic low-dose radiation therapy, stage I seminoma can also be treated with the single agent carboplatin (1,2). Carboplatin has a mechanism of action and side-effect profile similar to that of cisplatin but is associated with less neurotoxicity and less myelosuppression. Reiter et al. (2) showed that patients receiving postoperative courses of carboplatin had a disease-free survival of >74 months. If stage I disease is consistent with non-seminoma, then two cycles of BEP may be recommended (3). However, the specific treatment choice is often debated and includes active surveillance or retroperitoneal lymph node dissection. For stage II disease, chemotherapy is used in the adjuvant setting after retroperitoneal lymph node dissection and may consist of two cycles of BEP (4). Again this treatment was associated with a decreased rate of relapse and disease-free survival of greater than 85 months, which was the median follow-up time for the study. For patients with more advanced-stage testicular cancer, the usual regimen involves three or four cycles of BEP. If the patient has a contraindication to bleomycin, an alternative approach is the use of etoposide, ifosfamide, and cisplatin (VIP) which has been shown in two randomized trials to have equal efficacy (5). The progression-free survival rates were 64% and 58% and the overall survival rates were 69% and 67% in the VIP and BEP arms,

TABLE 1   Major Chemotherapy Drugs used in the treatment of Urologic Cancers

Antimetabolites
   Methotrexate
Anthracyclines
   Doxorubicin
Alkylating agents
   Cyclophosphamide
   Ifosfamide
Antitumor antibiotics
   Bleomycin
   Mitoxantrone
Platinum analogs
   Carboplatin
   Cisplatin
Taxanes
   Paclitaxel
Topoisomerase inhibitors
   Etoposide
Vinca alkaloids
   Vinblastine
   Vincristine
   Vinorelbine

respectively, in the study by Hinton et al. (5). They further classified their patient population into good-, intermediate-, and poor-risk patients and found that for patients in the intermediate- or poor-risk group the standard BEP treatment remained the treatment of choice. For those however, who were not able to receive bleomycin due to concomitant pulmonary disease, the VIP regimen is a viable option.

Toxicities

There are many toxicities associated with these regimens. Since however this disease is considered curable in the right clinical setting, a higher level of toxicity is often tolerated in anticipation of a potential cure. The associated toxicities include myelosuppression, pulmonary toxicity, nephrotoxicity, infertility, cardiac toxicity, neurotoxicity, and the risk of a second malignancy.

Nephrotoxicity

Nephrotoxicity is related to the use of cisplatin. Attempts have been made to reduce the nephrotoxic effects mainly by hydrating the patient during drug administration. The consequences of receiving cisplatin include a decline in glomerular filtration rate, increase in serum creatinine levels, hypomagnesemia, and salt wasting.

Raynaud's Phenomenon and Hypomagnesemia

Other associated toxicities include vascular abnormalities including Raynaud's phenomenon and the risk of thromboembolic events. As with other cancers, the risk of thromboembolic events is also increased in the setting of testicular cancer. In a study by Weijl et al. in which patients with testicular cancer were followed up for 6 weeks after the initial treatment with a chemotherapeutic regimen, the thrombosis rate in this group was 8.4%, with 16.7% of these events being arterial and 83.3% being venous thromboembolic events (6). Raynaud's phenomenon has been shown to occur in 7% of patients who receive BEP (7). In this study by Berger et al. (7), the development of Raynaud's phenomenon was associated with increased cumulative dose of bleomycin and also receiving bleomycin with vinblastine instead of etoposide. As a result of hypomagnesemia that can result when using cisplatin, the patients could also develop other electrolyte-related abnormalities including hypophosphatemia and hypokalemia. For this reason, electrolytes should be monitored closely in patients receiving this regimen.

Neuropathy

Neuropathy also frequently results from the use of cisplatin-based regimens. Typically, patients with testicular cancer who receive the cisplatin-based regimens may experience neuropathy concurrent with the therapy and as late as three months after the completion of therapy (8). In a study by von Schlippe et al. (8), 29 patients with metastatic germ-cell tumors undergoing combination cisplatin-based chemotherapy were followed up for development of neurological toxicity. At the end of the chemotherapy, only 11% of patients had parasthesias; however, by three months after the completion of chemotherapy, 65% reported neurological complaints. These symptoms did abate within the first year of treatment with only 17% of patients having persistent symptoms.

Infertility and Reproductive Disorders

Cisplatin also appears to be responsible for the infertility associated with the BEP regimen. This is thought to be due to a decrease in spermatogenesis and is usually associated with three or more cycles of BEP (9). However, it has been shown that in approximately 70% of men who receive BEP sperm recovery will take place within three years of receiving the regimen (10). In a study by Lampe et al., the time to recovery of spermatogenesis was nearly complete within five years of receiving chemotherapy (11). Sixty-four percent of 178 patients however, had recovery of their sperm counts within one year.

Cardiovascular Complication, Myocardial Ischemia, Lipid Abnormalities, and Hypertension

Cardiac toxicity is also associated with the BEP regimen. The main cardiac-associated toxicities include hypertension, atherosclerosis, coronary artery disease, and dyslipidemia. Hypertension has been observed to develop in patients who had previously received cisplatin-based chemotherapy regimens as part of their treatment of testicular cancer (12). Patients have also been shown to have a higher rate of cardiovascular disease. The rate of myocardial infarction was found to be 6% in patients who had received a cisplatin-based regimen for treatment of their testicular cancer (12). Interestingly, the patients also had an elevated rate of hypercholesterolemia and hypertension, which would potentially put them at risk of having a cardiovascular event. Another study conducted in Britain by Huddart et al. showed a two-fold increased risk of myocardial infarction in patients who received chemotherapy as part of their treatment for testicular cancer, which was not associated with increased baseline cardiac risk factors (13).

Pulmonary Toxicity

Pulmonary toxicity is usually due to bleomycin and is characterized as pneumonitis and pulmonary fibrosis. The chance of developing pulmonary toxicity appears to be dose-related and is greatly increased in patients who receive greater than 360 units of bleomycin. This is the major cause of chemotherapy-associated mortality in testicular cancer, accounting for 50% of treatment-related deaths. The patient should therefore be monitored carefully and bleomycin be discontinued at the earliest sign of pulmonary toxicity. It is hence recommended that the patient have pulmonary function tests prior to each cycle with specific attention to the diffusing capacity of carbon monoxide (DLCO) since a decrease in DLCO is associated with bleomycin-induced pulmonary toxicity (14). It is generally recommended that bleomycin be stopped when DLCO falls by 40% or <60% of the patient's baseline.

Acute Respiratory Distress Syndrome in Bleomycin-Treated Patients Who Undergo Surgery

Perhaps one of the most devastating consequences of chemotherapy for germ-cell tumors of the testis is the development of pulmonary problems in the postoperative patient who has undergone bleomycin therapy. If this complication develops, it is usually fatal. Development of acute respiratory distress syndrome has occurred in patients who received anesthesia who had previously been treated with bleomycin (15). It is recommended that patients who were exposed to bleomycin in the preoperative setting receive low concentrations of inspired oxygen during the perioperative period, with careful monitoring of fluid replacement and restriction of crystalloids instead of colloids for resuscitation. The toxicity is postulated to be due to high concentrations of oxygen leading to increased free radicals in the lungs (15).

Development of Second Cancers Secondary to Chemotherapy

There is also concern regarding the development of second malignancies in those patients who have received chemotherapy for testicular cancer (16). It has been estimated that treatment with three to four cycles of BEP results in an increase of leukemia in 3.2% of those who received a cumulative cisplatin dose of 650 mg and six-fold higher in those who received higher doses (17). However, prolonged use of etoposide for autologous transplantation has been associated with higher rates of leukemia and has been estimated at 2.6% for those who receive an etoposide dose more than 2000 mg/m^2 (18).

CHEMOTHERAPY REGIMENS FOR ADVANCED UROTHELIAL CANCER

Bladder cancer can be considered as a continuum of disorders including superficial, invasive, and metastatic disease. Chemotherapy is mainly employed in the metastatic setting although recent evidence has suggested that it may also have a role in the neoadjuvant and adjuvant settings for invasive cancers.

Superficial Bladder Cancer

Superficial bladder cancer includes the early stages of disease, tumors confined to the urothelium above the basement membrane (Ta), and tumors that extend into the lamina propria but remain superficial to the muscularis propria (T1). Although carcinoma in situ is considered here, this lesion is often associated with both clinical and genetic features of invasion early in its course and represents a very different biology than superficial disease of low malignant potential. The usual management of these early-stage bladder cancers involves cytoscopic resection with or without intravesical therapy. The decision to utilize intravesical therapy in addition to surgery is based on several prognostic factors. These include the number and size of the tumors, histology, and whether this is a primary or a recurrent lesion. Based on these risk factors, patients are placed into two categories: low risk and high risk. Low-risk disease is unifocal, has no associated carcinoma in situ, and is located in an accessible part of the bladder; residual disease is less than T1 on restaging. High-risk disease is multifocal, is associated with carcinoma in situ, the tumors are located in the dome and anterior wall of the bladder, and the residual disease is T1 on restaging (19). Intravesical therapy is usually used in the adjuvant setting as prophylaxis against disease recurrence. The standard intravesical therapies include bacillus Calmette-Guerin (BCG) and mitomycin C. All intravesical therapies do have some common side effects, which include bladder irritation, resulting in dysuria and polyuria. However, other intravesical treatments have specific side effects, which will be discussed below.

Bacillus Calmette-Guerin

This is the live attenuated form of *Mycobacterium bovis*, thought to be the most useful agent for superficial bladder cancer. Usual side effects include hematuria, pneumonitis, arthralgias, rash, granulomatous prostatitis, and epididymitis (20).

Mitomycin C

This is an alkylating agent also used for intravesical installation. The main side effects of this medication include bladder cystitis and myelosuppression, both of which occur infrequently. The response rate was associated with a five-year disease-free survival of 25% versus 41% in those who did not receive mitomycin C (21). Other treatment options include anthracyclines such as doxorubicin, epirubicin, valrubicin, interferon, thiotepa, and gemcitabine.

Thiotepa

Thiotepa is an ethylenimine analog chemically related to nitrogen mustard and therefore functions as an alkylating agent. Its ability to be absorbed when used for intravesicular therapy is variable. It has been associated with myelosuppression even when used in the intravesicular manner. In a study by Hollister et al., thrombocytopenia was the most common hematologic toxicity, although leucopenia and anemia were also seen (Hollister reference).

Acute suppression occurred usually within the three months of therapy and was related to the dose of thiotepa used. Based on these findings, the dosage used and the length of therapy are regulated.

Advanced Bladder Cancer

In the setting of metastatic bladder cancer, chemotherapy has been shown to improve outcomes. The median survival for patients who receive supportive care alone is only four to six months whereas those who receive treatment with cisplatin-based chemotherapy regimens have survival ranging from 12 to 14 months (22). There have been a number of prognostic factors that have been correlated with survival and response to chemotherapy. These include non-transitional cell histology, poor performance status (23), sites of metastasis being lymph nodes, lung, and soft tissue as opposed to bone and liver, elevated serum alkaline phosphatase and lactic dehydrogenase, expression of the multidrug resistance transporter (MDR) *P*-glycoprotein (24), and p53 overexpression (25). The expression of p53 was shown to be particularly important in T2 and T3a tumors and was associated with a decreased survival rate of 41% as compared to 77% in those without the mutation.

Single-Agent Chemotherapy
Cisplatin

The most effective single agents for TCCs are cisplatin and methotrexate. Cisplatin is a platinum analog, which covalently binds to DNA resulting in formation of DNA adducts, leading to the inhibition of DNA synthesis and function. Its main side effects include nephrotoxicity, gastrointestinal upset, myelosuppresion, neurotoxicity, ototoxicity, hypersensitivity reactions, and transient elevation in liver function tests, hair loss, SIADH, vascular events, and a metallic taste sensation leading to loss of appetite.

Methotrexate

Methotrexate is an antimetabolite, which inhibits dihydrofolate reductase (DHFR), resulting in reduced folate levels and ultimately inhibition of DNA synthesis. Its main side effects include myelosuppression, mucositis, renal failure, pneumonitis, skin rash, and neurotoxicity. The response rate however, to single-agent therapy has been low with most studies showing only a 3% to 9% response to cisplatin as a single agent (22). Use of single-agent therapy for bladder cancer has fallen out of favor as a result of the better overall response rates with multi-agent regimens.

Combination Agent Chemotherapy

The most common combination regimens include methotrexate, vinblastine, doxorubicin, and cisplatin (MVAC); cyclophosphamide, doxorubicin, and cisplatin (CISCA); methotrexate and vinblastine with or without cisplatin (CMV/MV); and most recently gemcitabine plus cisplatin. The MVAC regimen has long been considered the first-line treatment for metastatic bladder cancer. Response rates have been shown to be as high as 50% to 60% when compared to CISCA and CMV regimens with a median survival of 7 to 13 months (26,27). The regimen however is very toxic and is particularly difficult for elderly patients or those with multiple comorbidities.

MVAC-Associated Toxicities

The main toxicity includes bone marrow suppression leading to febrile neutropenia, mucositis, hearing loss, nephrotoxicity, and peripheral neuropathy. The majority of these side effects are due to cisplatin. It has been shown that treatment-related deaths can be as high as 3% to 4% (28,29). The majority of deaths appear to occur when this regimen is used in the metastatic setting since its use in the neoadjuvant setting is not associated with any treatment-related deaths (30). This is most likely due to the fact that only three cycles of MVAC are given in the neoadjuvant setting as opposed to six cycles in the metastatic setting. The main reason for death appears to be the result of neutropenic sepsis and infection (31,32). The overall cause of these deaths is usually neutropenic sepsis. It appears to be lower when granulocyte colony-stimulating factor (G-CSF) is used. Due to this concern high-grade myelosuppressive episodes are the main dose-limiting events. High-grade neutropenia occurs in 62% to 85% of patients with 14% to 26% experiencing febrile episodes during times of neutropenia, of these approximately 10% have neutropenic sepsis. High-grade anemia and thrombocytopenia occur in 20% of patients. This may be problematic in patients with bladder lesions due to increased risk of bleeding. Another major toxicity associated with this regimen is mucositis, which can occur in 20% of patients. Interestingly, although the above-mentioned toxicities can be associated with morbidity and mortality, patients receiving this drug in a recent trial comparing the MVAC regimen to gemcitabine and cisplatin reported a good quality of life with improved mentation and pain (32).

Gemcitabine/Cisplatin-Associated Toxicities

More recently, the combination of gemcitabine and cisplatin has been shown to have efficacy in advanced bladder cancer. In phase II studies, the response rate was 52% and the median survival was 13 months (33,34). Although there are associated toxicities due to cisplatin, they are less frequent, since the dose is less than that used in the MVAC regimen. In comparative studies gemcitabine plus cisplatin was associated with similar response rates and survival times but less toxicity (32). In this study, the treatment-related death rate for gemcitabine plus cisplatin in comparison to MVAC was 1% versus 3%. There was also less neutropenic fever (1% vs. 12%) and less mucositis (1% vs. 22%). With this regimen, myelosuppression as well as renal toxicity are the main dose-limiting toxicities. Neutropenia can occur in 71% of patients, thrombocytopenia in 57%, anemia in 27%, and gastrointestinal disturbance in 22% (32). However, in the von der Maase trial (32) in which gemcitabine and cisplatin were compared to MVAC, the rate of febrile neutropenia was lower (2% vs. 14%) and neutropenic sepsis occurred in only 1% as opposed to 12%. More patients in the gemcitabine and cisplatin arm had weight gain and many also had an improvement from baseline of 10 points or more in performance status over a four-week period.

Because of these associated toxicities and the fact that carboplatin is better tolerated, it has been considered as a substitute for cisplatin, especially in those patients with comorbidities that would preclude the use of cisplatin. There have been two randomized trials that show that carboplatin is less effective than cisplatin in treating bladder cancer (35,36). In the Bellmunt trial, survival in the cisplatin arm was 16 months versus only nine months in the carboplatin arm (35). In the Petrioli study (36), cisplatin was also shown to be superior with a response rate of 71% as opposed to 41% in the carboplatin-treated patient. No carboplatin regimen has therefore ever been shown to prolong survival in patients or provide a benefit in terms of quality of life. It is therefore recommended that the use of carboplatin only be considered in patients who have a major contraindication to receiving cisplatin such as renal insufficiency or known neurologic compromise.

CHEMOTHERAPY REGIMENS FOR RCC

Renal cell carcinoma (RCC) is well known to be a very chemotherapy-resistant cancer. When surgery is not an option, as occurs in locally advanced or metastatic RCC, the main treatment approach has been chemotherapy and immune-based therapies. The rate of response of RCC has been estimated to be as low as 4% to 6% (37). In a review by Yagoda et al., of 3635 patients with RCC who had been treated with either single-agent or combination chemotherapy regimens, only 5.6% achieved a complete or a partial response (38). In another study by Amato in which 50 trials of chemotherapy were reviewed, the response rate was estimated at 6% (39).

One possible explanation for this is the presence of MDR (P-glycoprotein/P-170) in the proximal tubule cells. It has been shown that the MDR gene is over-expressed in patients with RCC (40). The protein that is encoded by this gene results in the drug being extracted from the cells. There have been studies to try to block the MDR pathway concomitantly with chemotherapy treatment but they have had limited success (41,42).

Single-Agent Regimens
Vinblastine
Some of the single-agent regimens that have been used in the past include vinblastine which has been associated with a 16% response (43). Vinblastine is a plant alkaloid that inhibits tubulin polymerization, thereby inhibiting mitosis and leading to cell cycle arrest. Its main side effects

include myelosuppression, mucositis, alopecia, hypertension, neurotoxicity, skin irritation with infusion, inappropriate SIADH, and vascular events including stroke, Raynaud's phenomenon, ileus, and constipation, and myocardial infarctions. Follow-up studies showed that the response rate was more in the range of 2.5% to 5% (44,45). As discussed below, the main treatment of RCC is immunotherapy.

Infusional Floxuridine

Another single agent used is infusional floxuridine which was initially thought to have a response rate of 20% but then was shown to only have a response in 0% to 14% of patients when given in a non-circadian infusional regimen (46). Floxuridine is a fluoropyrimidine deoxynucleoside analog, which incorporates the metabolite floxuridine triphosphate into RNA resulting in inhibition of DNA synthesis and function. Its main side effects include hepatotoxicity, gastrointestinal upset, hand–foot syndrome, myelosuppresion, neurotoxicity, and blepharitis.

Combined Chemotherapy Regimens
Gemcitabine and 5-FU

One chemotherapy regimen that has been shown to have limited success in RCC is the combination of gemcitabine and continuous infusion of 5-fluorouracil (5-FU) (47,48). Gemcitabine is an antimetabolite that results in chain termination and inhibition of DNA synthesis, the main side effects of which include myelosuppression, gastrointestinal upset, hepatotoxicity, pulmonary toxicity, infusion reaction, and a flu-like syndrome. 5-FU is a fluoropyrimidine analog with mechanism of action and side effects similar to those of floxuridine. In a phase II study by Rini et al. (48), 39 patients who received gemcitabine and infusional 5-FU with metastatic RCC had a response rate of 17% with a median progression-free survival of 29 weeks. Similar rates were also seen when gemcitabine was combined with capecitabine, an orally active form of 5-FU (49). Of note, this regimen may be especially useful in patients with papillary histology, which is particularly resistant even to immune-based therapy.

Immune-based Therapies for RCC

Immune-based therapy is the main systemic therapy used to treat RCC. Both interferon alfa (IFN-α) and interleukin-2 (IL-2) have been shown to have some success in treating RCC (50). In an attempt to determine who would be the best candidate for immune-based therapies, Motzer et al. established five prognostic factors associated with a lower likelihood of responding to immune-based therapy (51). These factors included low hemoglobin, high lactate dehydrogenase, and high serum calcium levels, no history of prior nephrectomy, and a low Karnofsky performance status. If three or more of these factors were present, the patient was less likely to benefit from immune-based therapy.

Interferon

Interferon treatment is associated with a response rate of 14% (52). IL-2 which is the only FDA-approved regimen for RCC has response rates as high as 21% in some patients. Although it was initially thought that treatment with IFN-α resulted in a survival benefit, multivariate analysis of the three trials using interferon therapy showed that the duration of response was only 12.2 months and five-year survival rate was 3%. IFN-α is approved in Europe for the treatment of RCC. The main side effects are similar to those seen with IL-2 and include flu-like symptoms, mental status changes, and depression. Patients are often started preemptively on antidepressant medications when it is thought that this may become an issue with treatment.

Interleukin-2

The response to low-dose IL-2 is 13%. Many patients however cannot tolerate IL-2 due to comorbidities and also because of the associated capillary leak syndrome which is its main toxicity (53). The duration of the response is on average 54 months (54). The high-dose intravenous dosing schedule is often associated with significant morbidity and mortality and requires hospitalization in wards equipped to manage the toxicity. The main side effects include capillary leak syndrome as mentioned above, hypotension, systemic symptoms including flu-like symptoms, weight loss, abnormal liver function tests, and depression.

Targeted Therapies for RCC

New advances in our understanding of cancer genetics have led to the development of targeted therapy for metastatic RCC. Both the sporadic and the hereditary forms of RCC (especially clear cell histology) are associated with mutations in the von Hippel-Lindau (VHL) gene. This gene appears to be involved via Knudson's "two hit" model which states that one copy of a defective gene is inherited and the second copy occurs as a sporadic event leading to oncologic transformation. It has been shown by Latif et al. that the initial event in the development of RCC is loss of function mutations in the VHL gene (55). The usual role of VHL gene is in the hypoxin inducible factor (HIF) pathway. VHL binds to hydroxylated HIF-1α and polyubiquinates leading to proteosome-mediated degradation of HIF. During hypoxia, HIF-1α is not hydroxylated and therefore cannot bind to the VHL and instead accumulated and complexes with HIF-1β which then translocates into the nucleus of the cell and binds to the hypoxia-responsive element (HRE), leading to expression of HIF genes. In a similar manner, when the VHL gene is mutated, the VHL protein is not able to form a complex with HIF-1α and therefore it is not degraded, making it available to complex with HIF-1β leading to upregulation of HIF genes. Some of the downstream targets of the HRE include vascular endothelial growth factor (VEGF), platelet derived growth factor (PDGF), and erythropoietin. Many of these genes are involved in angiogenesis and may function to feed tumor development.

Multi-Kinase Inhibitors

Based on a better understanding of the molecular aspects of RCC development, it has been possible to design therapeutic targets of these pathways. Two such drugs that have recently been approved for the treatment of RCC are sunitinib and sorafenib. Sunitinib is a orally bioavailable small molecule that inhibits multiple split kinase domain receptor tyrosine kinases (RTKs) including VEGF and PDGF (56). This drug has been shown in clinical trials to have a partial response rate of 40% and 27% of patients had stable disease for at least three months. This was associated with a median time to progression of 8.7 months (57). The medication itself was well tolerated with only fatigue as the dose-limiting side effect. Other side effects include diarrhea, nausea, stomatitis, and erythema of the soles of the feet and palms of the hands.

The other FDA-approved drug is sorafenib, which is also a small bioavailable molecule, acting as a Raf-kinase inhibitor and subsequently leading to inhibition of several RTKs including VEGF, FLT3 receptor, and PDGF. The response rate has been dramatic with 78% of patients in a phase III trial having stable disease compared to 55% in the placebo arm of the study. Similar side effects were seen with this medication including hand–foot syndrome, diarrhea, hair loss, fatigue, nausea, and hypertension (57).

Another molecule that also works by interacting with the VEGF pathway is bevacizumab, a recombinant monoclonal antibody that binds VEGF, blocking its ability to interact with its receptor. In a phase II trial this medication was associated with a 10% partial response rate and a median time to progression of 4.8 months as compared to 2.5 months (58). This drug although given in the intravenous form, is very well tolerated, with only hypertension and rash as the main toxicities.

One possible means by which to gain improved results may be the use of these new agents in combination to block many pathways simultaneously. It is yet to be determined, however, if the toxicity of the combination would be tolerated as many of these agents have overlapping side effects. It is also not known, if these medications may enhance the effects of immunotherapy, thereby leading to higher response rates.

CHEMOTHERAPY FOR PROSTATE CANCER

Previously, prostate cancer was also thought to be a chemoresistant cancer. Prior treatment options centered around the use of mitoxantrone plus a corticosteroid for palliative treatment, whereas newer regimens involve the use of docetaxel. This regimen however was not associated with a survival endpoint. In the landmark TAX-327 trial, 1006 men with metastatic hormonally refractory prostate cancer (HRPC) who had receive docetaxel at two different schedule or mitoxantrone. Patients receiving docetaxel had a longer median survival of 18.9 months versus 16.5 months, with overall decrease of prostate specific antigen (PSA) with 48%, 45%, and 32% respectively, for the two doses if docetaxel or mitoxantrone, and an improvement in overall pain levels. In a second study using docetaxel, a survival benefit was also seen (60). In this SWOG 9916 study, docetaxel plus estramustine phosphate was compared to mitoxantrone plus prednisone and showed a survival benefit with a median survival of 17.5 months for the docetaxel arm versus 15.6 months for the mitoxantrone arm. The median time to progression was 6.3 months in those patients who received docetaxel and estramustine and 3.2 months in the group given mitoxantrone and prednisone. The PSA also decreased 50% and 27% and an objective tumor response was seen in 17% and 11% of patients, respectively, who had measureable disease. Based on these results, the FDA-approved docetaxel as a first-line treatment for HRPC. The approved regimen however, recommends the use of prednisone instead of estramustine due to the inherent risk of thromboembolic events when using estramustine. The reported rate of thromboembolic events, particularly when estramustine is combined with taxanes has been estimated to be 10% (61). The overall risk appears to be greater for venous than arterial events which was estimated at 5% in comparison to 1% in a meta-analysis (61).

These chemotherapeutic agents however, are also associated with numerous toxicities. Docetaxel is derived from the needles of the European yew tree. Its mechanism of action is ignition of microtubules by enhanced tubulin polymerization leading to inhibition of microtubules. It is metabolized by the P450 system in the liver. Docetaxel is associated with a number of toxicities including gastrointestinal disturbance (40%), myelosuppression, alopecia (80%), fluid retention (50%), mucositis, and peripheral neuropathy. Treatment-related deaths have been estimated at 0.3% to 2.4% (59,60). The main risk appears to be due to the vascular complications that were elucidated above. Studies have been carried out to try to decrease the overall risk of thromboembolic events, thereby decreasing the risk of potential death of the patient by anticoagulation. Use of aspirin or low-dose anticoagulation has been suggested for prophylaxis while on an estramustine regimen, however, this has not been tested in a randomized clinical trial to date (60).

Mitoxantrone is also associated with toxicity. This is an anthracenedione analog, which intercalates into DNA resulting in inhibition of DNA synthesis and also inhibits topoisomerase II. It is also metabolized by the P450 system. Major toxicities include myelosuppression, gastrointestinal upset (70%), mucositis, diarrhea, and cardiotoxicity which can result in atrial arrhythmias and usually occurs within the first 24 to 48 hours; however, there is also a risk of dilated cardiomyopathy with congestive heart failure if the cumulative dose exceeds 140 mg/m^2, hair loss (40%), and a blue coloration of the fingernails and urine. The risk of cardiac toxicity can be substantial. In a study comparing mitoxantrone to docetaxel the risk was estimated to be as high as 7% (60). It has been estimated that patients receiving a cumulative mitoxantrone dose of greater than100 mg/m^2 have a 15% risk of cardiac toxicity (62). The estimated decrease in left ventricular ejection fraction (LVEF) that is seen with this drug is 10% (59). It is advised that patients receiving this medication have their LVEF monitored every four cycles as was done in the study by Petrylak et al. (60). The dose-limiting toxicity however associated with this drug is myelosuppression. The rate of high-grade neutropenia has been estimated to be anywhere between 35% and 63%, depending on the starting dose (60). The rate of thrombocytopenia has been estimated at 6% (62). Because of the associated bone marrow suppression it has been suggested that patients should initially be treated with a dose of 12 mg/m^2 and then transitioned to 14 mg/m^2 based on their degree of myelosuppression (59,60).

HORMONAL THERAPY FOR PROSTATE CANCER

Initial management of prostate cancer usually involves androgen deprivation, which is used mainly in conjunction with radiation therapy. Androgen deprivation is achieved through the use of luteinizing hormone-releasing hormone agonists (LHRH®, Astra Zineca), which results in inhibition of follicle stimulating hormone (FSH) and LH release. The main agonists used are goserelin (Zoladex) and leuprolide (Lupron®, TAP Pharmaceutica) and buserelin. This provides an alternative to surgical castration for the treatment of metastatic prostate cancer. The main side effects of androgen deprivation are mainly loss of body hair, weight gain, gynecomastia, loss of libido, impotence, breast enlargement, and hot flashes. Less common side effects include nausea, vomiting, polyuria and polydipsia, and peripheral edema. Moreover, patients on androgen deprivation also experience a 10% decline in hemoglobin level, which is responsive to erythropoietin injections. A long-term side effect that is under-appreciated is the development of osteoporosis. The fracture rate for men on androgen deprivation is usually 9% to 40%. The reduction in bone mineral density can be seen as early as six to nine months after initiation of therapy. Bisphosphonates have been shown to reverse bone loss in men undergoing androgen deprivation. The fracture rate unfortunately remains the same in these patients (63). Due to ease of administration, zoledronic acid is the preferred treatment. Zoledronic acid is given as a 4-mg intravenous infusion over 15 minutes every three months to prevent osteopenia secondary to androgen deprivation. There are many side effects of this medication the most notable of which is osteonecrosis of the jaw which is a real concern in patients with poor dentition.

During the initial treatment with LHRH agonists there can be an initial rise in testosterone due to increased LH and FSH levels. This is referred to as the "flare" and can usually occur anytime within the first few weeks of initiating treatment. This can result in worsening of symptoms related to prostate cancer including worsening bone pain or worsened uretheral obstruction (64). Because of this, concurrent anti-androgen therapy is usually undertaken in the early weeks of treatment. Due to these concerns, these agents are contraindicated in any patient with impending spinal cord compression or urinary obstruction. An LHRH antagonist, abarelix, has recently been approved and is not associated with the initial surge in testosterone. It is indicated in patients with neurologic compromise, urinary obstruction and severe pain from metastatic prostate cancer (65).

There are also non-steroidal anti-androgens such as bicalutamide and flutamide available, which block activation of the androgen receptor itself and therefore are not associated with reduced testosterone levels. This mainly leads to fewer side effects related to hypogonadism. Namely, the patients report less hot flashes (13% vs. 50%) and increased libido (66). These drugs however are associated with higher rates of gynecomastia (47% vs. 3.8%). The rates of osteoporosis are also lower with the non-steroidal anti-androgens when compared to castration (67). Patients taking the non-steroidal anti-androgen, bicalutamide, have an increased risk of developing liver function test abnormalities requiring frequent blood tests to monitor transaminases.

Other drugs that are used to block the production of androgen by the adrenal is the antifungal agent ketoconazole, which directly inhibits adrenal androgen synthesis, and corticosteroids, which reduce pituitary production of adrenocorticotrophic hormone, thereby leading to decreased synthesis of androgens. The usual side effects of this treatment include those associated with prolonged steroid use as well as gastrointestinal upset and neurotoxicity which can occur with the use of ketoconazole (68).

REFERENCES

1. Schmoll HJ, Souchon R, Krege S, et al. European consensus on diagnosis and treatment of germ cell cancer: a report of the European Germ Cell Cancer Consensus Group (EGCCCG). Ann Oncol 2004; 15(9):1377–1399.
2. Reiter WJ, Brodowicz T, Alavi S, et al. Twelve-year experience with two courses of adjuvant single-agent carboplatin therapy for clinical stage I seminoma. J Clin Oncol 2001; 19(1):101–104.
3. Amato RJ, Ro JY, Ayala AG, Swanson DA. Risk-adapted treatment for patients with clinical stage I nonseminomatous germ cell tumor of the testis. Urology 2004; 63(1):144–148; discussion 8–9.
4. Behnia M, Foster R, Einhorn LH, Donohue J, Nichols CR. Adjuvant bleomycin, etoposide and cisplatin in pathological stage II non-seminomatous testicular cancer. The Indiana University experience. Eur J Cancer 2000; 36(4):472–475.
5. Hinton S, Catalano PJ, Einhorn LH, et al. Cisplatin, etoposide and either bleomycin or ifosfamide in the treatment of disseminated germ cell tumors: final analysis of an intergroup trial. Cancer 2003; 97(8):1869–1875.
6. Weijl NI, Rutten MF, Zwinderman AH, et al. Thromboembolic events during chemotherapy for germ cell cancer: a cohort study and review of the literature. J Clin Oncol 2000; 18(10):2169–2178.

7. Berger CC, Bokemeyer C, Schneider M, Kuczyk MA, Schmoll HJ. Secondary Raynaud's phenomenon and other late vascular complications following chemotherapy for testicular cancer. Eur J Cancer 1995; 31A:2229–2238.

8. von Schlippe M, Fowler CJ, Harland SJ. Cisplatin neurotoxicity in the treatment of metastatic germ cell tumour: time course and prognosis. Br J Cancer 2001; 85(6):823–826.

9. Fossa SD, Kravdal O. Fertility in Norwegian testicular cancer patients. Br J Cancer 2000; 82(3):737–741.

10. Petersen PM, Hansen SW, Giwercman A, Rorth M, Skakkebaek NE. Dose-dependent impairment of testicular function in patients treated with cisplatin-based chemotherapy for germ cell cancer. Ann Oncol 1994; 5(4):355–358.

11. Lampe H, Horwich A, Norman A, Nicholls J, Dearnaley DP. Fertility after chemotherapy for testicular germ cell cancers. J Clin Oncol 1997; 15(1):239–245.

12. Meinardi MT, Gietema JA, van der Graaf WT, et al. Cardiovascular morbidity in long-term survivors of metastatic testicular cancer. J Clin Oncol 2000; 18(8):1725–1732.

13. Huddart RA, Norman A, Shahidi M, et al. Cardiovascular disease as a long-term complication of treatment for testicular cancer. J Clin Oncol 2003; 21(8):1513–1523.

14. McKeage MJ, Evans BD, Atkinson C, Perez D, Forgeson GV, Dady PJ. Carbon monoxide diffusing capacity is a poor predictor of clinically significant bleomycin lung. New Zealand Clinical Oncology Group. J Clin Oncol 1990; 8(5):779–783.

15. Goldiner PL, Carlon GC, Cvitkovic E, Schweizer O, Howland WS. Factors influencing postoperative morbidity and mortality in patients treated with bleomycin. Br Med J 1978; 1(6128):1664–1667.

16. Travis LB, Curtis RE, Storm H, et al. Risk of second malignant neoplasms among long-term survivors of testicular cancer. J Natl Cancer Inst 1997; 89(19):1429–1439.

17. Travis LB, Andersson M, Gospodarowicz M, et al. Treatment-associated leukemia following testicular cancer. J Natl Cancer Inst 2000; 92(14):1165–1171.

18. Houck W, Abonour R, Vance G, Einhorn LH. Secondary leukemias in refractory germ cell tumor patients undergoing autologous stem-cell transplantation using high-dose etoposide. J Clin Oncol 2004; 22(11):2155–2158.

19. Nieder AM, Brausi M, Lamm D, et al. Management of stage T1 tumors of the bladder: International Consensus Panel. Urology 2005; 66(6 suppl 1):108–125.

20. Lamm DL, Stogdill VD, Stogdill BJ, Crispen RG. Complications of bacillus Calmette-Guerin immunotherapy in 1,278 patients with bladder cancer. J Urol 1986; 135(2):272–274.

21. Au JL, Badalament RA, Wientjes MG, et al. Methods to improve efficacy of intravesical mitomycin C: results of a randomized phase III trial. J Natl Cancer Inst 2001; 93(8):597–604.

22. Loehrer PJ, Sr., Einhorn LH, Elson PJ, et al. A randomized comparison of cisplatin alone or in combination with methotrexate, vinblastine, and doxorubicin in patients with metastatic urothelial carcinoma: a cooperative group study. J Clin Oncol 1992; 10(7):1066–1073.

23. Raghavan D, Shipley WU, Garnick MB, Russell PJ, Richie JP. Biology and management of bladder cancer. N Engl J Med 1990; 322(16):1129–1138.

24. Kim WJ, Kakehi Y, Yoshida O. Multifactorial involvement of multidrug resistance-associated [correction of resistance] protein, DNA topoisomerase II and glutathione/glutathione-S-transferase in nonP-glycoprotein-mediated multidrug resistance in human bladder cancer cells. Int J Urol 1997; 4(6):583–590.

25. Sarkis AS, Bajorin DF, Reuter VE, et al. Prognostic value of p53 nuclear overexpression in patients with invasive bladder cancer treated with neoadjuvant MVAC. J Clin Oncol 1995; 13(6):1384–1390.

26. Boccardo F, Pace M, Guarneri D, Canobbio L, Curotto A, Martorana G. Carboplatin, methotrexate, and vinblastine in the treatment of patients with advanced urothelial cancer. A phase II trial. Cancer 1994; 73(7):1932–1936.

27. Logothetis CJ, Dexeus FH, Chong C, et al. Cisplatin, cyclophosphamide and doxorubicin chemotherapy for unresectable urothelial tumors: the M.D. Anderson experience. J Urol 1989; 141(1):33–37.

28. Witjes JA, Wullink M, Oosterhof GO, de Mulder P. Toxicity and results of MVAC (methotrexate, vinblastine, adriamycin and cisplatin) chemotherapy in advanced urothelial carcinoma. Eur Urol 1997; 31(4):414–419.

29. Bamias A, Aravantinos G, Deliveliotis C, et al. Docetaxel and cisplatin with granulocyte colony-stimulating factor (G-CSF) versus MVAC with G-CSF in advanced urothelial carcinoma: a multicenter, randomized, phase III study from the Hellenic Cooperative Oncology Group. J Clin Oncol 2004; 22(2):220–228.

30. Grossman HB, Natale RB, Tangen CM, et al. Neoadjuvant chemotherapy plus cystectomy compared with cystectomy alone for locally advanced bladder cancer. N Engl J Med 2003; 349(9):859–866.

31. Sternberg CN, de Mulder PH, Schornagel JH, et al. Randomized phase III trial of high-dose-intensity methotrexate, vinblastine, doxorubicin, and cisplatin (MVAC) chemotherapy and recombinant human granulocyte colony-stimulating factor versus classic MVAC in advanced urothelial tract tumors: European Organization for Research and Treatment of Cancer Protocol no. 30924. J Clin Oncol 2001; 19(10):2638–2646.

32. von der Maase H, Hansen SW, Roberts JT, et al. Gemcitabine and cisplatin versus methotrexate, vinblastine, doxorubicin, and cisplatin in advanced or metastatic bladder cancer: results of a large, randomized, multinational, multicenter, phase III study. J Clin Oncol 2000; 18(17):3068–3077.

33. Kaufman D, Raghavan D, Carducci M, et al. Phase II trial of gemcitabine plus cisplatin in patients with metastatic urothelial cancer. J Clin Oncol 2000; 18(9):1921–1927.

34. Moore MJ, Winquist EW, Murray N, et al. Gemcitabine plus cisplatin, an active regimen in advanced urothelial cancer: a phase II trial of the National Cancer Institute of Canada Clinical Trials Group. J Clin Oncol 1999; 17(9):2876–2881.

35. Bellmunt J, Ribas A, Eres N, et al. Carboplatin-based versus cisplatin-based chemotherapy in the treatment of surgically incurable advanced bladder carcinoma. Cancer 1997; 80(10):1966–1972.

36. Petrioli R, Frediani B, Manganelli A, et al. Comparison between a cisplatin-containing regimen and a carboplatin-containing regimen for recurrent or metastatic bladder cancer patients. A randomized phase II study. Cancer 1996; 77(2):344–351.

37. Yagoda A, Abi-Rached B, Petrylak D. Chemotherapy for advanced renal-cell carcinoma: 1983–1993. Semin Oncol 1995; 22(1):42–60.

38. Yagoda A, Petrylak D, Thompson S. Cytotoxic chemotherapy for advanced renal cell carcinoma. Urol Clin North Am 1993; 20(2):303–321.

39. Amato RJ. Chemotherapy for renal cell carcinoma. Semin Oncol 2000; 27(2):177–186.

40. Fojo AT, Shen DW, Mickley LA, Pastan I, Gottesman MM. Intrinsic drug resistance in human kidney cancer is associated with expression of a human multidrug-resistance gene. J Clin Oncol 1987; 5(12):1922–1927.

41. Hao D, Huan SD, Stewart DJ, Segal RJ, Yau JC. A pilot study of low dose hydroxyurea as a novel resistance modulator in metastatic renal cell cancer. J Chemother 2000; 12:360–366.

42. Bates S, Kang M, Meadows B, et al. A Phase I study of infusional vinblastine in combination with the P-glycoprotein antagonist PSC 833 (valspodar). Cancer 2001; 92(6):1577–1590.

43. Kuebler JP, Hogan TF, Trump DL, Bryan GT. Phase II study of continuous 5-day vinblastine infusion in renal adenocarcinoma. Cancer Treat Rep 1984; 68(6):925–926.

44. Pyrhonen S, Salminen E, Ruutu M, et al. Prospective randomized trial of interferon alfa-2a plus vinblastine versus vinblastine alone in patients with advanced renal cell cancer. J Clin Oncol 1999; 17(9):2859–2867.

45. Fossa SD, Droz JP, Pavone-Macaluso MM, Debruyne FJ, Vermeylen K, Sylvester R. Vinblastine in metastatic renal cell carcinoma: EORTC phase II trial 30882. The EORTC Genitourinary Group. Eur J Cancer 1992; 28A:878–880.

46. Milowsky MI, Nanus DM. Chemotherapeutic strategies for renal cell carcinoma. Urol Clin North Am 2003; 30(3):601–609.

47. Mani S, Vogelzang NJ, Bertucci D, Stadler WM, Schilsky RL, Ratain MJ. Phase I study to evaluate multiple regimens of intravenous 5-fluorouracil administered in combination with weekly gemcitabine in patients with advanced solid tumors: a potential broadly active regimen for advanced solid tumor malignancies. Cancer 2001; 92(6):1567–1576.

48. Rini BI, Vogelzang NJ, Dumas MC, Wade JL III, Taber DA, Stadler WM. Phase II trial of weekly intravenous gemcitabine with continuous infusion fluorouracil in patients with metastatic renal cell cancer. J Clin Oncol 2000; 18(12):2419–2426.

49. Waters JS, Moss C, Pyle L, et al. Phase II clinical trial of capecitabine and gemcitabine chemotherapy in patients with metastatic renal carcinoma. Br J Cancer 2004; 91(10):1763–1768.

50. Cohen HT, McGovern FJ. Renal-cell carcinoma. N Engl J Med 2005; 353(23):2477–2490.

51. Motzer RJ, Mazumdar M, Bacik J, Russo P, Berg WJ, Metz EM. Effect of cytokine therapy on survival for patients with advanced renal cell carcinoma. J Clin Oncol 2000; 18(9):1928–1935.

52. Wirth MP. Immunotherapy for metastatic renal cell carcinoma. Urol Clin North Am 1993; 20(2):283–295.

53. Yang JC, Sherry RM, Steinberg SM, et al. Randomized study of high-dose and low-dose interleukin-2 in patients with metastatic renal cancer. J Clin Oncol 2003; 21(16):3127–3132.

54. Fisher RI, Rosenberg SA, Fyfe G. Long-term survival update for high-dose recombinant interleukin-2 in patients with renal cell carcinoma. Cancer J Sci Am 2000; 6(suppl 1):S55–S57.

55. Latif F, Tory K, Gnarra J, et al. Identification of the von Hippel-Lindau disease tumor suppressor gene. Science 1993; 260(5112):1317–1320.

56. Fabian MA, Biggs WH III, Treiber DK, et al. A small molecule-kinase interaction map for clinical kinase inhibitors. Nat Biotechnol 2005; 23(3):329–236.

57. Patel PH, Chaganti RS, Motzer RJ. Targeted therapy for metastatic renal cell carcinoma. Br J Cancer 2006; 94(5):614–619.

58. Yang JC, Haworth L, Sherry RM, et al. A randomized trial of bevacizumab, an anti-vascular endothelial growth factor antibody, for metastatic renal cancer. N Engl J Med 2003; 349(5):427–434.

59. Tannock IF, de Wit R, Berry WR, et al. Docetaxel plus prednisone or mitoxantrone plus prednisone for advanced prostate cancer. N Engl J Med 2004; 351(15):1502–1512.

60. Petrylak DP, Tangen CM, Hussain MH, et al. Docetaxel and estramustine compared with mitoxantrone and prednisone for advanced refractory prostate cancer. N Engl J Med 2004; 351(15):1513–1520.

61. Lubiniecki GM, Berlin JA, Weinstein RB, Vaughn DJ. Thromboembolic events with estramustine phosphate-based chemotherapy in patients with hormone-refractory prostate carcinoma: results of a meta-analysis. Cancer 2004; 101(12):2755–2759.
62. Kantoff PW, Halabi S, Conaway M, et al. Hydrocortisone with or without mitoxantrone in men with hormone-refractory prostate cancer: results of the cancer and leukemia group B 9182 study. J Clin Oncol 1999; 17(8):2506–2513.
63. Smith MR, Eastham J, Gleason DM, Shasha D, Tchekmedyian S, Zinner N. Randomized controlled trial of zoledronic acid to prevent bone loss in men receiving androgen deprivation therapy for non-metastatic prostate cancer. J Urol 2003; 169(6):2008–2012.
64. Loblaw DA, Mendelson DS, Talcott JA, et al. American Society of Clinical Oncology recommendations for the initial hormonal management of androgen-sensitive metastatic, recurrent, or progressive prostate cancer. J Clin Oncol 2004; 22(14):2927–2941.
65. Koch M, Steidle C, Brosman S, et al. An open-label study of abarelix in men with symptomatic prostate cancer at risk of treatment with LHRH agonists. Urology 2003; 62(5):877–882.
66. Iversen P, Tyrrell CJ, Kaisary AV, et al. Casodex (bicalutamide) 150-mg monotherapy compared with castration in patients with previously untreated nonmetastatic prostate cancer: results from two multicenter randomized trials at a median follow-up of 4 years. Urology 1998; 51(3):389–396.
67. Sieber PR, Keiller DL, Kahnoski RJ, Gallo J, McFadden S. Bicalutamide 150 mg maintains bone mineral density during monotherapy for localized or locally advanced prostate cancer. J Urol 2004; 171(6 pt 1):2272-6, quiz 435.
68. Small EJ, Halabi S, Dawson NA, et al. Antiandrogen withdrawal alone or in combination with ketoconazole in androgen-independent prostate cancer patients: a phase III trial (CALGB 9583). J Clin Oncol 2004; 22(6):1025–1033.

37 | Vascular Complications of Urologic Surgery

Jonathan D. Gates
Division of Vascular and Endovascular Surgery, Harvard Medical School and Division of Trauma, Burns, and Surgical Critical Care, Trauma Center, Brigham and Women's Hospital, Boston, Massachusetts, U.S.A.

INTRODUCTION

Vascular complications may occur in any clinical scenario and obtaining a satisfactory outcome sometimes taxes even the most experienced surgeons. The impact of intra-operative vascular complications may be mitigated through thoughtful preoperative preparation and knowledge of vascular reconstructive techniques. Unexpected intra-operative bleeding is best managed using the time-tested approach of the trauma surgeon, which is access, exposure, control, and repair. Even in the postoperative state, vascular issues may arise.

PREOPERATIVE PREPARATION

Given the fact that preoperative imaging is so prevalent with magnetic resonance imaging, computed tomography (CT) angiography and formal arteriograms, concomitant vascular problems are often identified before surgery. Issues such as incidental aortic aneurysms, arterial occlusive disease, renal artery stenosis, or renal artery aneurysms may be identified and discussed before the incision is made.

Wide preparation of the skin allows access to various body cavities for both proximal and distal control as well as access to "spare" parts for vascular reconstruction. The most extensive preparation may require a chin to knees exposure in the event that the intra-caval renal tumor extends into the right atrium. A midline abdominal incision allows access to the entire length of the inferior venal cava and an extension as a median sternotomy allows for potential cardiopulmonary bypass. If the saphenous vein is needed for a vascular conduit or a vein patch then the limb should be circumferentially prepared to provide easy access to the thigh for harvest of the vein.

If one anticipates the potential for large blood loss then the temperature in the room should be elevated and the Bair Hugger applied to those areas not in the surgical field. A level 1 infuser or similar rapid transfusion devices are helpful to deliver warm fluids and blood products rapidly. Avoidance of hypothermia is critical to prevent coagulopathy in a patient with extensive blood loss. The cell saver has limited utility in urologic surgery given the preponderance of interventions for various tumors.

It is wise to have immediate access to a laparotomy kit with vascular instrumentation even when performing a laparoscopic procedure should a vascular injury arise. Should conversion to open exploration be required, further assistance in the form of additional nursing personnel and a vascular surgeon would be desirable. A call to the blood bank should be made immediately to alert them to the potential need for additional blood products in the form of packed red blood cells, fresh frozen plasma, and even cryoprecipitate.

Instrumentation

An array of vascular instruments should include soft-jawed clamps with rubber inserts and the fine-toothed vascular clamps of the DeBakey variety. The renal arteries are best controlled with the smaller bulldog clamps.

Temporary indwelling vascular shunts are useful for hemorrhage control with concomitant distal perfusion technique. The Argyle straight shunts (15cm long) are packaged in a group of four ranging in diameter from 8 to 14 Fr to approximate the size of the recipient vessels.

These are secured in place with either commercially available Rumel tourniquets or an easily fashioned homemade variety (1). The Pruitt-Inahara shunt is longer and is used to bridge larger defects and has the advantage of intra-luminal balloons for blood loss control and for secure placement.

Fogarty balloon catheters were originally designed as embolectomy catheters for removal of intravascular debris, yet they also serve as a method for intravascular control. These catheters are manufactured in a variety of sizes; however, the catheters in the 4 to 6 Fr range reflect the size of the inflated balloon and are most useful for small-to-medium-sized vessels. An aortic occluding balloon catheter is available for intravascular control of the larger vessels. A three-way stopcock allows positioning and inflation of the balloon without further stabilization.

Monofilament vascular sutures of Prolene ranging in size from 50 to 2-0 should be available. The finer sutures are good for delicate work as in lateral repairs of limited vascular defects. The 3-0 Prolene suture comes with a larger radius needle making it easier to "find" the other end of the needle as it is passed through the tissue to facilitate repair of an actively bleeding vessel. The finer needles become lost to view in that scenario.

Vascular Grafts

The final component of preoperative preparation for the potential vascular complication is vascular graft availability. The autogenous greater saphenous vein has always been the preferable conduit for vascular reconstruction. It is usually readily available, is relatively resistant to infection, and given the normal intima is relatively resistant to occlusion in low flow situations. The major downside is that about 20% of the time it is either unavailable through previous harvest or of inadequate caliber (2). The saphenous vein is often a useful conduit for renal artery repair. Renal artery replacement with the autogenous hypogastric artery is acceptable. It is probably prudent to be sure that both hypogastric vessels are widely patent and free of disease prior to sacrificing one as a conduit.

Large vessel reconstructions with autogenous vein may include segments of the superficial femoral vein or the internal jugular vein. The former is hampered by tedious dissection deep in the thigh and the latter often requires a separate operative field distant from the original site.

Synthetic vascular grafts for reconstruction include polytetrafluoroethylene (PTFE) and Dacron and the biologic grafts of human cadaveric aorta and heterografts that include bovine carotid arteries (3).

Polytetrafluoroethylene is a chemically inert polymer composed of carbon and fluorine extruded in a manufacturing process that creates microscopic porosities within the graft. These porosities or nodes allow tissue ingrowth for graft incorporation into the local tissues. These grafts are available in sizes ranging from 3 to 20 mm (4).

Dacron is a multifilament yarn tightly woven into a mesh that no longer requires preclotting. These large-caliber grafts are most successful for reconstruction of the abdominal aorta and iliac arteries. Long-term patency of these grafts in large blood flow areas is excellent. Short segment synthetic grafts (6 mm) have also been used for proximal renal artery repair and bypass with good success (4).

The cadaveric aortic graft has prove relatively resistant to degenerative change and infection and may be used in infected fields (5). The bovine carotid artery graft usually measures about 7mm in size and is suitable for arterial replacement in infected fields as well.

LAPAROSCOPIC SURGERY

Laparoscopic surgery is quite safe but there is always the possibility of vascular injury related to Veress needle or trocar placement. The confluence of the iliac veins at the inferior vena cava, the distal aorta, and the proximal iliac arteries are at highest risk (6). In addition, the epigastric vessels in the anterior abdominal wall are at risk of trocar injury.

The risk of vascular injury from the Veress needle during laparoscopy is relatively uncommon. Hurd et al. (7) concluded from a review of CT scans that the umbilicus is at or just cephalad to the aortic bifurcation and consistently located cephalad to the point where the left common iliac vein crosses the midline. The incidence of major vascular injury associated with laparoscopy is difficult to determine. Mintz's survey of 100,000 laparoscopic procedures in France in the 1970s suggested that three major vascular injuries occurred for each 10,000 procedures (8). Parsons et al. (9) reported on 894 urologic laparoscopies at a single institution in 2004. The most common intra-operative complication was vascular injury with an incidence of 2.5%. In general the reported rate of major vascular injury from laparoscopy is thought to be between 0.5% and 2.5% (9–12).

A hard sign of vascular injury is obvious bleeding within the operative field. The more subtle retroperitoneal injury may present with hemodynamic instability alone as the blood loss is contained and hidden in the retroperitoneum. Active bleeding, hypotension, and retroperitoneal collections of blood identified in proximity to major vascular structures during laparoscopy would all mandate conversion to open exploration.

ARTERIAL COMPLICATIONS
Overall Approach

Arteries most at risk of injury during urologic surgery include the renal, juxtarenal and infrarenal aorta, and the iliac arteries. I have found that the majority of the retroperitoneal urologic tumors approximate but do not infiltrate these arterial structures.

Several generalizations are important when dealing with vascular injuries. The basic tenet of safe surgery is to first obtain proximal and distal control before entering into any retroperitoneal hematomas or bleeding vascular structures. If the central hematoma is located at the juxtarenal level then that may dictate supraceliac control. Supraceliac control in the abdomen is best obtained with a nasogastric tube first placed in the stomach. This will serve not only to decompress the stomach but also serve as a landmark to identify the esophagus and bluntly reflect it to the patient's left. Deeper dissection into the retroperitoneum brings the surgeon's hand on top of the anterior aorta and the right and left crus are reflected away from the aorta to allow placement of a clamp on either side. There is no need to dissect behind the aorta for there is a risk of disrupting the posterior origins of the lumbar vessels. Should the suspected injury be even higher on the aorta, then intrathoracic control may be prudent.

Once that is obtained, the hematoma may be opened and the vascular clamps replaced closer to the site of the injury to minimize the blood loss through collaterals entering the controlled segment. Only at this point, should systemic heparinization be considered. In the event of torrential blood loss before vascular control, therapeutic heparinization may be avoided due to the natural tendency toward coagulopathy from dilution of the coagulation factors, acidosis, and hypothermia.

A thorough visualization of the injury is critical to an assessment of how it should be repaired. It is critical to note and almost superfluous to point out that you cannot fix what you cannot see. Debridement of the vascular wall to create a smooth nonthrombogenic intimal surface is an important step. Any irregularity left on the flow surface could serve as a nidus for platelet deposition and subsequent occlusion.

In the process of repairing an intraoperative arterial injury, debridement of the damaged segment is required. If this is incomplete, then there will be a flap of intima that may serve as a leading edge for intimal dissection from prograde blood flow resulting in thrombosis of the vascular repair. If the dissection of the wall of the artery is deep into the media, then it may appear as a subadvential hematoma when observed from outside of the vessel. If there were a suspicion of poor distal flow from intimal dissection, then re-exploration, proper debridement, and possible interposition grafting would be needed.

Following repair of the injured vessels, flushing of the operative site with heparinized saline solution removes any fibrinous debris and platelet clumps. This is followed by transient removal of the proximal clamp first for additional prograde flushing followed by transient removal of the distal clamp for retrograde flushing. The suture line is completed and prograde blood flow restored to the distal vasculature. Occasionally there is troublesome bleeding from the suture line, which may be dealt with through placement of additional fine sutures, or if the needle holes were bleeding then thrombin-soaked gelfoam applied to the suture line would be appropriate. Heparin reversal with Protamine is used on occasion in the event of troublesome needle hole bleeding following repair of large high-flow vessels.

Arterial Reconstruction

Several options are available for control and repair of the bleeding site. Branch avulsions off the infrarenal aorta may often be controlled with digital compression followed by direct compression with a vascular forceps (13). A full-thickness figure-of-eight suture placed beneath the occluding forceps may be all that is required. If the defect is larger, then direct digital compression is used until appropriate instrumentation is available and these small defects may be controlled with a side-biting Satinsky clamp. The lateral repair is then performed either directly onto the vessel or more commonly is bolstered with a pledget of Teflon or bovine pericardium to prevent tearing of the vessel. If the lateral defect in the arterial wall is larger, the Satinsky clamp may be inadequate for control and formal proximal and distal control is needed. It is always surprising how much dissection is needed to apply the Satinsky clamp to provide adequate occlusion yet at the same time allow sufficient exposure of the arterial wall for repair.

If primary closure of the defect results in significant narrowing of the vessel wall, then it would be appropriate to patch the vessel. We have moved away from PTFE patch material because of the tendency for needle hole bleeding. Better hemostatic substitutes may be found in Dacron, saphenous vein, or bovine pericardial patches. The bovine pericardium is available in many different sizes and lends itself to repair of larger defects, whereas the saphenous vein is suitable only for small defects.

Larger defects in the artery may require debridement followed by end-to-end repair. These often require mobilization of the artery in order to reapproximate a 1- to 2-cm defect. In an effort to achieve a tension-free anastomosis, selective ligation of branch vessels will allow the ends to come together. Often, complete transaction of an artery is accompanied by a wide displacement due to the intrinsic elastance of the vascular wall resulting in the need for interposition grafting and the selection of a synthetic graft for replacement.

Some of the retroperitoneal renal and testicular tumors tend to have areas of sterile necrosis and are not infected. In the event of an infected field, the autogenous tissues are superior, secondary alternatives would be the bovine carotid artery for medium-sized vessels and the cadaveric aorta for larger vessels. The gold standard vascular reconstruction of the infrarenal aorta in an infected field remains the extra-anatomic axillobifemoral bypass; however, it would be unlikely to be needed in the urologic patient population.

It is appropriate to consider additional pharmacologic agents following operative arterial repair. Usually, the anti-platelet agents, aspirin or plavix are more than sufficient to reduce platelet adhesion at the site of the repair.

VENOUS COMPLICATIONS
Overall Approach

The inferior vena cava (IVC) originates through the confluence of the iliac veins at the fifth lumbar vertebra and serves as a valveless conduit measuring 1.5 cm in width. There are four to five pairs of lumbar veins that drain into the posterior portion of the infrarenal IVC. In addition, the right gonadal, right adrenal, renal veins, the phrenic veins, and the hepatic veins all drain into the IVC before it enters the pericardium. Venous injuries may occur from the laparoscopic or open approach. The venous structures, perhaps through their thinner walls leave a less distinct dissection plane and appear to be more closely invested with tumor than the arterial structures. Most venous repairs or reconstructions should also be treated with pharmacologic agents to avoid stagnation of blood and maintain patency. There is a small amount of literature support for the use of intermittent pneumatic calf compression and low molecular weight dextran-40 for at least 24 hours in improving patency of venous repairs (14). There have been some reports of pulmonary embolism (PE) following IVC repair (15). Available options are to maintain the patient on a brief course of Dextran-40 followed by three months of anticoagulation with either coumadin or plavix.

Renal, adrenal, and metastatic testicular tumors often encroach on the iliac vessels and the IVC. The renal tumors are notorious for their propensity to enter into the IVC through the renal vein (Fig. 1). Careful dissection around the tumor in order to gain proximal and distal control of the venous structures should be performed if it appears that they may be involved. The large

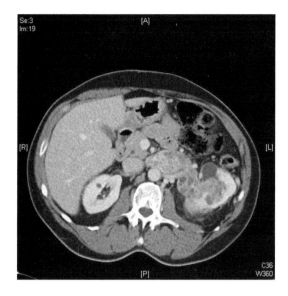

FIGURE 1 Renal cell carcinoma of the left kidney infiltrating the left renal vein. *Source*: Abdominal CT scan (Brigham and Women's Hospital).

renal tumors usually allow easy exposure of the infrarenal IVC; however, suprarenal exposure may be difficult as the mass approaches the undersurface of the liver. Often the intracaval portion of the tumor is not fixed to the wall of the IVC and the mobile tumor can be milked out of the suprarenal IVC prior to clamping. Caval thrombectomy has been shown to have an acceptable operative morbidity and mortality but as expected, advanced stage renal carcinoma dictates a shortened survival (16).

If the intracaval tumor extends into the retrohepatic, supradiaphragmatic IVC or the right atrium, then cardiopulmonary bypass may be warranted. This would allow full visualization of the tumor and ensure adequate resection. If an extensive reconstruction of the retrohepatic IVC or hepatic veins were required, then deep hypothermia with cardiac standstill would allow a bloodless field for optimal reconstruction.

Inadvertent injury to the IVC during the dissection should initially be controlled with direct pressure with a rolled up gauze pad until further exposure is obtained. Aortic control or compression is the ultimate proximal control for intraabdominal bleeding. Venous bleeding differs from arterial bleeding in that the venous blood loss wells up into the wound under low pressure making it difficult to identify the source of the injury. Clamp control of the IVC is critical with particular attention to the lumbar vessels, which may continue to bleed into the field after what appears to be adequate control. This should prompt a posterior search for the culprit vessels. The lumbar vessels are short and thin-walled as well as tethered by the local periadventitial tissues. Careful dissection is imperative to avoid avulsion of these veins (17). Control of these vessels sometimes requires vessel loops or ligation and division for additional mobility. They are short and tenuous requiring careful silk ties for control. Avulsion of these vessels may be problematic and are best dealt with through suture ligation on the side of the IVC and often the distal end retracts into the psoas muscle requiring a figure-of-eight suture for control. If it appears that the injury is at the confluence of the iliac veins, then temporary division of the right common iliac artery may facilitate exposure (18).

Venous Reconstruction

Vena caval repair techniques are similar to those of arterial repair. The two differ in that ligation of the infrarenal IVC is usually well tolerated as opposed to arterial ligation, which is often accompanied by distal ischemia. In general, the concept for venous reconstruction is to keep it simple to reduce the amount of raw intimal surface exposed to blood flow. Hopefully, this will reduce the exposure of the platelets to the thrombogenic subintimal tissues. It is important to point out that one must be vigilant about releasing the distal clamp before the suture line is complete to flush any residual air out of the vessel to prevent air embolism.

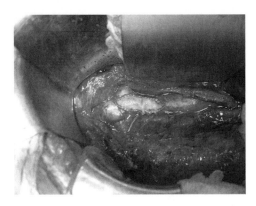

FIGURE 2 Patch angioplasty of the anterior pararenal inferior vena cava with bovine pericardium.

Lateral repair is the most common technique (17). Through-and-through IVC injuries are more commonly seen with penetrating rather than operative trauma. The posterior injury may be treated through an extension of the anterior injury or through careful rotation of the IVC. If the repair narrows the vessel by 50% or greater, consideration should be given to patch angioplasty with saphenous vein or bovine pericardium (Fig. 2).

The more complicated panel grafts or even externally supported PTFE are less than desirable for long-term patency may be compromised.

Deep Venous Thrombosis

The recumbent position, inactivity and perioperative bleeding and thrombosis place any of the general surgical and urologic patients at risk for venous thromboembolic events including deep venous thrombosis (DVT) and PE (19,20). A particular group at high risk of DVT includes those undergoing pelvic surgery for malignancy (20).

The incidence of DVT in the hospitalized patient population has increased as sicker patients recover from otherwise previously fatal disease. In the trauma patient population alone, the incidence of thromboembolic events has been reported to be as high as 58% of patients (21). Unfortunately, the majority of patients with a DVT are asymptomatic. The classic finding of a positive Homans' sign is present in less than 10% of patients with DVT. Our ability to detect DVT with readily available DVT ultrasound and detect PE with the ubiquitous chest CT scan with intravenous contrast (PE protocol) has led to heightened awareness of thromboembolic venous events in hospitalized patients.

Prophylaxis against DVT was evaluated in a meta-analysis of the 29 available trials for a total of 8000 surgical patients. Low-dose subcutaneous heparin significantly ($P < 0.001$) reduced the incidence of DVT from 25.2% without prophylaxis to 8.7% of those who were appropriately treated (22). In addition, the same studies revealed a reduction in PE from 1.2% in those receiving no heparin to 0.5% in the treated patients. Importantly, major hemorrhage was somewhat greater in those treated with prophylactic heparin than in controls but it never reached significance. Minor hemorrhagic complications of wound hematomas were significantly ($p < 0.001$) elevated in the treated group (6.3%) over the control group (4.1%).

Sequential compression devices (SCDs) for DVT prophylaxis have been shown to increase mean and peak common femoral venous blood flow velocities (23). In addition, SCDs have reportedly had a direct stimulatory effect fibrinolytic activity. Compression devices have been shown to reduce the incidence of venous thromboembolic events (24). It appears that SCDs are comparable to subcutaneous heparin in the ability to reduce DVT in low-risk patients but Velmahos et al. suggested that in the high-risk patient, there may be no benefit of SCD, low-dose heparin, or the combination of the two (25). In those situations additional prophylactic medications are available and may be more useful.

Low molecular weight heparins (LMWHs) are a fragment of the standard unfractionated heparin and are one-third the size with a more uniform molecular weight of 4000 to 6000 (26). The smaller size confers different pharmocokinetics than unfractionated heparin because there is far less binding to endothelium and plasma proteins. They have far better bioavailability at low doses, which may explain improved outcomes in the prevention of venous thromboembolic events. LMWH has been shown to be more effective for DVT prophylaxis than the unfractionated heparin with a similar profile for bleeding risk when compared in trauma patients (26). There are studies in the general surgical literature that support the use of LMWH over unfractionated heparin in the prevention of venous thromboembolic events (27–29).

Oral anticoagulation with coumadin is effective and widely practiced in patients undergoing elective hip joint replacement. Unfortunately, its effectiveness in the urology patient is limited by the risk of intraperitoneal bleeding following extensive retroperitoneal dissection and increased incidence of lymphoceles.

Pulmonary Embolism

Fatal PE is believed to occur in up to 200,000 patients a year in the United States alone. It is thought that as many as 90% of pulmonary emboli may be undetected because of subtle symptoms or misdiagnosis (30). From the above discussion, it is apparent that many urologic patients are at risk of venous thromboembolic events. Subcutaneous unfractionated heparin or LMWH are appropriate for prophylaxis in many of these patients.

In certain clinical scenarios full anticoagulation for DVT or treatment for PE may be contraindicated as in active gastrointestinal hemorrhage, severe thrombocytopenia, or large retroperitoneal dissection.

In addition, 3% to 5% percent of patients treated with intravenous heparin will experience an episode of major bleeding (30). An excessive increase in the activated partial thromboplastin time (APTT) while on heparin or the prothrombin time (PT) while on coumadin may increase that risk. The perioperative state, liver disease, severe thrombocytopenia, and concomitant antiplatelet therapy are strong predictors of a bleed on anticoagulation.

One to five percent of those patients receiving unfractionated heparin have an immune-mediated thrombocytopenia that may result in extension of the previous thrombus or new arterial thrombosis (31). There should be a high suspicion should the platelet count drop below 100,000 or to a value less than 50% of the baseline value. Future studies may show that the synthetic pentasaccharide, fondaparinux may also play a therapeutic role in these scenarios (32).

In those clinical situations where full anticoagulation for acute DVT or PE is contraindicated, one may consider the use of an IVC filter. In 1998, Decousas et al. (33) looked at the short-and long-term effectiveness of the IVC filter. This prospective multicenter study from France demonstrated that the IVC filter reduced the incidence of PE at 12 days compared to the cohort receiving anticoagulation alone ($p = 0.03$). Follow-up at two years demonstrated that this protective advantage of the filter was lost. Interestingly, the IVC filters were noted to be associated with an increased incidence of symptomatic DVT at two years with a 20.8% incidence in the filter group compared to 11.6% in the no-filter group. Other investigators share this concern of long-term increases in DVT secondary to the filter (34). This was the first study to confirm that IVC filters do work in the short term but appear to be superfluous in the long term probably due to collateral development. Over time, it appears that they are now a liability. Hence, the temporary IVC filter seems to be a potential short-term solution for a short-term problem (Fig. 3).

Early temporary filters in the 1980s were designed to remain in place with an external connection to the skin for later recovery. Naturally, the external attachment would predispose the patient to infectious complications and limit the duration of the filter to the order of five days. Unfortunately, the risk period of thromboembolic events often exceeds this time limit.

The approach of the latest generation of IVC filters is a permanent filter design without attachment to the skin, but with the option to be retrieved when no longer clinically needed. These retrievable or better, optional IVC filters have been designed to take advantage of the effectiveness of a permanent filter and yet minimize the complications of a long-term indwelling vascular device approaching the ideal device specifications. These are Food and Drug Administration (FDA)-approved permanent filters that have the potential to be removed. There are no time limits to retrieval imposed by the FDA, but the manufacturer has suggested various time intervals. The optional filters afford the opportunity to protect the patient from PE during

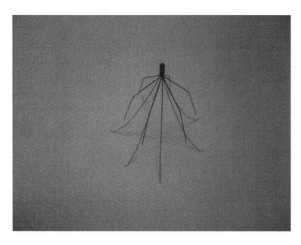

FIGURE 3   Photograph of a retrievable inferior vena cava filter.

a period when they may be at high risk for primary or recurrent PE and may be removed when that high-risk period has passed (Fig. 4).

The three FDA-approved optional filters are the OptEase (Cordis Endovascular®, Miami Lakes, Florida, U.S.A.), Gunther-Tulip (Cook®, Inc., Bloomington, Indiana, U.S.A.), and the Recovery nitinol (C.R. Bard Peripheral Vascular®, Murrey Hill, New Jersey, U.S.A.) filters. They differ in the shape, contact with the wall of the IVC, and the recommended dwell time according to manufacturer. Binkert et al. (35) have reported on retrieval of an optional filter at 317 days without complication on follow-up venogram. The maximal dwell time of optional filters until safe retrieval is possible has not yet been evaluated. Our own experience with retrievals up to 322 days has shown that retrievals after long dwell times are feasible if the filter stays in an untilted position. We expect further design changes, which will allow limitless dwell time and an increasing applicability in the clinical arena.

There have been some sporadic reports of complications of optional filters with respect to migration, deployment, and IVC perforation. In a very few cases there have been reports of fatalities secondary to filter migration. Careful scrutiny is required as we learn more about the indication and behavior of the filters as well as the incidence of PE in various clinical scenarios.

The use and indications for optional filters is appropriately increasing for various indications. Optimal indications and insertion techniques will need to be explored. In an effort to provide useful guidelines for the use of IVC filters, comparative trials examining the role of the optional IVC filters are needed. Future clinical trials must examine the indications for placement and retrieval, optimal dwell time, filter effectiveness and filter-related complications in an effort to provide useful guidelines for the surgical community.

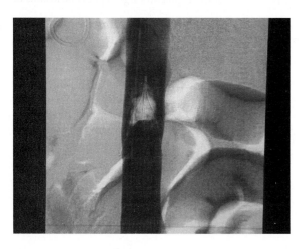

FIGURE 4   A venogram demonstrating a retrievable filter laden with clot from a trapped lower extremity embolus.

SUMMARY

In general, major vascular structures are prominently associated with many urologic procedures. Prevention, preparation, and knowledge management provide the best armamentarium to minimize the effect of vascular complications in the urology patient.

REFERENCES

1. Gates JD, Stieg PE. Carotid artery shunting. Contemp Surg 1996, 49(3):157.
2. Veith FJ, Moss CM, Sprayregen S. Preoperative saphenous venography in arterial reconstructive surgery of the lower extremity. Surgery 1979; 85(3):253–256.
3. Vandecic MO. New graft for the surgical treatment of small vessel diseases. J Cardiovasc Surg 1987; 28(6):711–714.
4. Gates JG, Kent KC. The past, present, and future of small diameter grafts. In: Grooters RK and Nishida H, eds. Alternative Bypass Conduits and Methods for Surgical Coronary Revascularization. Armook, NY: Futura Publishing Company, Inc., 1994:291–315.
5. Gates JD, Warth J, McGowan K. Nocardia associated aortic infection: case report and review of the literature. Vascular Maylitt 2006; 14(3):165–168.
6. Winfield HN, Donovan JF, See WA, et al. Urologic laparoscopic surgery. J Urol 1991; 146:941–948.
7. Hurd WW, Bude RO, DeLancey JL, et al. The relationship of the umbilicus to the aortic bifurcation: Implications for laparoscopic technique. Obstet Gynecol 1992; 80:48–51.
8. Mintz M. Risks and prophylaxis in laparoscopy. A survey of 100,000 cases. J Repro Med 1977; 18:269.
9. Parsons JK, Varkarakis I, Rha KH. Complications of abdominal urologic laparoscopy: longitudinal five-year analysis. Urology 2004; 63(1):27–32.
10. Kleppinger RK. Laparoscopy at a community hospital: An analysis of 4300 cases. J Reprod Med 1977; 19:353.
11. Vallancien G, Cathelineau X, Baumert H. Complications of transperitoneal laparoscopic surgery in urology: review of 1311 procedures at a single center. J Urol 2002; 168(1):23–26.
12. Fahlenkamp D, Rassweiler J, Fornara P. Complications of laparoscopic procedures in urology:experience with 2407 procedures at 4 German centers. J Urol 1999; 162(3 pt 1):765–770.
13. Hertzer NR. Vascular problems in urologic patients. Urol Clin North Am 1985; 12(3):493–506.
14. Hobson RW, Yeager RA, Lynch TG. Femoral venous trauma: techniques for surgical management and early results. Am J Surg 1983; 146(2):220–224.
15. Burch JM, Feliciano DV, Mattox KL, et al. Injuries of the inferior vena cava. Am J Surg 1998; 156:548–552.
16. Li MK, Yip SK, Cheng WS. Inferior vena cava thrombectomy for renal cell carcinoma with thrombus. Ann Acad Med Singapore 1999; 28(4):508–511.
17. Graham JM, Mattox KL, Beall AC Jr. Traumatic injuries of the inferior vena cava. Arch Surg 1978; 113:413–418.
18. Salam A, Stewart MT. New approach to wounds of the aortic bifurcation and inferior vena cava. Surgery 1985; 98:105–108.
19. Upchurch GR Jr, Demling RH, Davies J, et al: Efficacy of subcutaneous heparin in prevention of venous thromboembolic events in trauma patients. Am Sug 1995; 61:749–755.
20. Dalen JE, Alpert JS. Natural history of pulmonary embolism. Prog Cardiovasc Dis 1975; 17:259.
21. Weinmann EE, Salzman EW. Deep vein thrombosis. N Engl J Med 1994; 331:1630–1641.
22. Clagett GP, Reisch JS: Prevention of venous thromboembolism in general surgical patients: Results of a meta-analysis. Ann Surg 1988; 208:227–240.
23. Keith SL, McLaughlin DJ, Anderson FA Jr, et al. Do graduated compression stockings and pneumatic boots have an additive effect on the peak velocity of venous blood flow? Arch Surg 1992; 127:727–730.
24. Dennis JW, Menwat S, Von Thron J, et al. Efficacy of sequential compression devices in multiple trauma patients with severe head injury. J Trauma 1994; 37:205–208.
25. Velmahos GC, Nigro J, Tatevossian R, et al. Inability of an aggressive policy of thromboprophylaxis to prevent deep venous thrombosis (DVT) in critically injured patients: are current methods of DVT prophylaxis sufficient? J Am Coll Surg 1998; 187:529–533.
26. Knudson MM, Morabito D, Paiement GD, et al. Use of low molecular weight heparin in preventing thromboembolism in trauma patients. J Trauma 1996; 41:446–459.
27. Bergqvist D, Burmark US, Frisell J, et al. Thromboprophylactic effect of low molecular weight heparin started in the evening before elective general abdominal surgery: A comparison with low-dose heparin. Semin Thromb Hemost 1990; (16 suppl):19–24.
28. Nurmohamed MT, Rosendaal FR, Buller HR, et al. Low-molecular –weight heparin versus standard heparin in general and orthopedic surgery: A meta-analysis. Lancet 1992; 340:152–156.
29. Hirsh J, Warkentin TE, Raschkle R, et al. Heparin and low molecular weight heparin: Mechanisms of action, pharmacokinetics, dosing considerations, monitoring, efficacy, and safety. Chest 1998; 114:489S–510S.

30. Anderson FA Jr, Wheeler HB, Goldberg RJ, et al. A population-based perspective of the hospital incidence and case-fatality rates of deep venous thrombosis and pulmonary embolism. The Worcester DVT Study. Arch Int Med 1991; 151(5):933–935.
31. Warkentin TE, Levine MN, Hirsh J, et al. Heparin-induced thrombocytopenia in patients treated with low molecular weight heparin or unfractionated heparin. N Engl J Med 1995; 332:1330–1335.
32. Buller HR, Davidson BL, Decousus H, et al. Subcutaneous fondoparinux versus intravenous unfractionated heparin in the initial treatment of pulmonary embolism. N Engl J Med 2003; 349: 1695–1702.
33. Decousas H, Leizorovics A, Parent F, et al. A clinical trial of vena caval filters in the prevention of pulmonary embolism in patients with proximal deep-vein thrombosis. N Engl J Med 1998; 338: 409–415.
34. Rosenthal D, Wellons ED, Levitt AB, et al. Role of prophylactic temporary inferior vena cava filters placed at the ICU bedside under intravascular guidance in patients with multiple trauma. J Vasc Surg 2004; 40:958–964.
35. Binkert CA, Bansal A, Gates JD. IVC filter removal after 317-day implantation. J Vasc Intern Radiol 2005; 16(3):395–398.

It is not the critic who counts: not the man who points out how the strong man stumbles or where the doer of deeds could have done better. The credit belongs to the man who is actually in the arena, whose face is marred by dust and sweat and blood, who strives valiantly, who errs and comes up short again and again, because there is not effort without error or shortcoming, but who knows the great enthusiasms, the great devotions, who spend himself for a worthy cause; who, at the best, knows in the end, the triumph of high achievement, and who, at the worst, if he fails, at least he fails while daring greatly, so that his place shall never be with those cold and timid souls who knew neither victory nor defeat.

—Theodore Roosevelt

Index